Taylor's
**Principles and Practice
of Medical Jurisprudence**

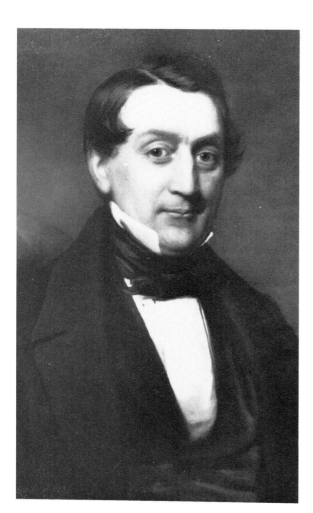

Alfred Swaine Taylor, MD, FRS
1806–1880
For 46 years Lecturer in Medical Jurisprudence
at Guy's Hospital Medical School, London

Taylor's Principles and Practice of Medical Jurisprudence

Edited by

A. Keith Mant
MD(Lond) FRCP FRCPath DMJ

Professor of Forensic Medicine, University of London; Head of the Department of Forensic Medicine, Guy's Hospital, London; Honorary Consultant in Forensic Medicine, King's College Hospital, London; Visiting Lecturer in Medical Jurisprudence and Toxicology, St Mary's Hospital, London

THIRTEENTH EDITION

CHURCHILL LIVINGSTONE
EDINBURGH LONDON MELBOURNE AND NEW YORK 1984

CHURCHILL LIVINGSTONE
Medical Division of Longman Group Limited

Distributed in the United States of America by Churchill
Livingstone Inc., 1560 Broadway, New York, N.Y. 10036, and
by associated companies, branches and representatives
throughout the world.

First edition 1865 (Dr A Swaine Taylor)
Second edition 1873
Third edition 1883 (revised by Dr T Stevenson)
Fourth edition 1894
Fifth edition 1905 (revised by Dr F J Smith)
Sixth edition 1910
Seventh edition 1920
Eighth edition 1928 (revised by Professor Sydney Smith and
Dr W G H Cook)
Ninth edition 1934
Tenth edition 1948
Eleventh edition 1956 (revised by Sir Sydney Smith and Dr
Keith Simpson with collaborators)
Twelfth (Centenary) edition 1965 (revised by Professor Keith
Simpson with collaborators)
Thirteenth edition 1984
Reprinted 1986

ISBN 0 443 01481 7

British Library Cataloguing in Publication Data
Taylor, Alfred Swaine
    Taylor's principles and practice of medical
    jurisprudence.—13th ed.
    1. Medical jurisprudence
    I. Title   II. Mant, A. Keith
    614′.1   RA1051

Library of Congress Cataloging in Publication Data
Taylor, Alfred Swaine, 1806–1880.
    Taylor's Principles and practice of medical
jurisprudence.

    Includes index.
    1. Medical jurisprudence. 2. Medical jurisprudence—
Great Britain. I. Mant, A. Keith. II. Title.
III. Title: Principles and practice of medical
jurisprudence. [DNLM: 1. Jurisprudence. 2. Forensic
medicine. W 700 T238p]
Ra1051.T22   1984   614′.1   83-14287

Produced by Longman Group (FE) Ltd
Printed in Hong Kong

Preface to the Thirteenth Edition

Taylor's first book on medical jurisprudence, *Elements of Medical Jurisprudence*, was published in 1836. This was followed in 1844 by his *Manual of Medical Jurisprudence*, which ran to some 12 editions. The *Principles and Practice of Medical Jurisprudence*, a far more comprehensive book than the manual, first appeared in 1865.

Taylor commented in his earlier editions that science was advancing so rapidly that techniques were out of date within a year of their development and that no book could be kept up to date. Modern science advances even more rapidly and developments in certain fields of forensic science are ever outdated when they first appear in specialist journals.

This 13th edition of 'Taylor' consists of some 17 sections written by 15 contributors—thus losing its old personal touch when one editor revised the previous edition with limited outside assistance. However, it is considered that this edition will fulfil the functions of its predecessors in a more practical manner, as the sections have been written by those with a special interest in the subjects upon which they have written.

Previous editions contained a large amount of historical data—some unchanged since the first edition. There was also an extensive toxicological section dealing with the classical methods for the extraction of metallic and vegetable poisons. It was felt that Taylor had become unbalanced and that, at the expense of historical material which had lost its relevance, it should be rewritten as one volume with its contents orientated more towards the lawyer than the average textbook on medical jurisprudence.

As stated above, advances in certain branches of forensic medicine and especially in forensic science are rapid, and therefore the inclusion of authoritative sections in these fields would serve no useful purpose as there are specialist textbooks on these subjects larger than this entire edition. Toxicology has therefore been limited to the interpretation of blood alcohol and classes of drugs which may be found in drivers of motor vehicles, and serology to the special context of paternity grouping.

It is inevitable when there are a number of authors, the majority of whom are engaged in full time medico-legal work, that some delays will occur in the completion of manuscripts and these delays entail certain revisions in those already completed. I should like to thank all contributors for their forbearance, and especially the publishers.

It is particularly sad that one of our most distinguished contributors, Dr Gavin Thurston, *CBE*, should have died before the publication of this edition.

London, 1984   A.K.M.

Contributors

Philip H. Addison MRCS(Eng) LRCP(Lond)
Formerly Secretary, Medical Defence Union, UK

David A. Ll. Bowen MA MB BChir FRCP FRCP(Edin)
FRCPath DMJ DPath
Professor of Forensic Medicine, University of London at
Charing Cross Hospital Medical School; Lecturer in Forensic
Medicine, University of Oxford, UK

I. D. Bradbrook BSc
Lecturer in Forensic Serology, Guy's Hospital Medical School,
London, UK

John Burton MB(Lond) FFA RCS
Barrister and Honorary Secretary of the Coroners Society of
England and Wales

James Malcolm Cameron MD PhD FRCPath DMJ
Professor of Forensic Medicine, The London Hospital Medical
College; Ver Heyden de Lancey Reader in Forensic Medicine,
The Council of Legal Education, UK

D. J. Gee MB BS FRCPath DMJ
Professor of Forensic Medicine, University of Leeds, UK

T. C. N. Gibbens CBE MD FRCP FRCPsych
Emeritus Professor of Forensic Psychiatry, London University,
UK

Alan Grant MA MD MRCP FRCPath
Honorary Senior Lecturer in Forensic Serology, Guy's
Hospital Medical School, London, UK

B. Hargrove OBE QC LLM PhD
H.M. Recorder of the Crown Court

Colin Hunter-Craig MA MB BChir MRCPath
Consultant Histopathologist, Mid-Downs Health Authority,
West Sussex; Formerly Lecturer in Forensic Medicine, Guy's
Hospital, London, UK

Bernard Knight MD BCh FRCPath DMJ
Barrister and Professor of Forensic Pathology, Welsh National
School of Medicine, University of Wales, Cardiff; Home Office
Pathologist

A. Keith Mant MD(Lond) FRCP FRCPath DMJ
Professor of Forensic Medicine, Guy's Hospital Medical
School, University of London; Senior Lecturer and Consultant
in Forensic Medicine, Kings College Hospital, London; Visit-
ing Lecturer in Medical Jurisprudence and Toxicology, St.
Mary's Hospital, London, UK

David M. Paul MRCS LRCP DRCOG DA DMJ(Clin)
Her Majesty's Coroner to The City of London and to The
Northern District of Greater London; Honorary Lecturer in
Court Practice and Clinical Forensic Medicine, Guy's Hospital
Medical School; Honorary Lecturer in Clinical Forensic
Medicine, St. Bartholomew's Hospital Medical College, Lon-
don, UK.

Peter Pullar MD FRCPath DMJ
Home Office Pathologist; Consultant Pathologist to the Wessex
Department of Forensic Medicine at Winchester; Honorary
Lecturer in Forensic Medicine at Guy's Hospital Medical
School and Southampton University.

B. G. Sims BDS(Lond) LDSRCS(Eng)
Lecturer in Forensic Odontology, The London Hospital
Medical College, London, UK

The Late Gavin Thurston CBE FRCP DMJ
Barrister and H.M. Coroner, Inner West London, UK

P. A. Toseland BSc PhD FRCPath
Consultant Biochemist, Clinical Chemistry, Guy's Hospital,
London, UK

Contents

The development of medico-legal systems

Methods of the official investigation of unnatural deaths can only be fully appreciated in the light of some knowledge of their historical evolution.

Basically, two main systems exist, both of European origin. Most other countries have adopted some modification of one of these two systems, either as a result of a post-colonial inheritance or by direct adoption.

The two main systems have arisen, broadly speaking, from (1) English legal practice, developed from Norman modifications of pre-existing Anglo-Saxon laws or (2) a system developed out of European continental law, originating in the heritage of Roman Law, strongly influenced by the Code Napoleon.

The English system gave rise to the unique office of the 'coroner' which then spread to Wales, Ireland and the numerous British colonies. In modified form, the office still exists in many ex-colonies, including the United States. It should be noted that Scotland is an exception, as the late date of union with England (1707) enabled Scotland to retain its continental-type institutions up to the present day. The coroner system in the United States of America has been progressively modified in many states by conversion to the medical examiner system.

A closer examination of the two major systems will reveal that both have their own faults and advantages.

THE CORONER SYSTEM

The coroner is one of the most ancient offices in English history. An official of this name was in existence in Anglo-Saxon times, during the reign of King Alfred (AD 871–910), long before the Norman Conquest. In AD 925, King Athelstan gave a grant of the coroner's office to John of Beverley.

However, the first official mention of the coroner in the sense that we know it today, comes in the reign of Richard I in the last years of the twelfth century. It seems that the reason for the revival of the coroner at this time was mainly financial stimulus in the face of an acute crisis in the royal treasury. In March of 1194, King Richard was released from captivity in Vienna, where he had been held as hostage by Leopold of Austria: the ransom paid was 1 000 000 marks. In addition to this great burden, England was forced to support Richard's enthusiastic and expensive attendance at the Third Crusade. In the same year, as part of a general increase in fund raising, Richard's very able Justiciar and Chief Minister, Hubert Walter, issued the 'Articles of Eyre', which included provisions for the resuscitation of the office of coroner. Article 20 of the 'Articles of Eyre' provided for the election by every country of three knights and one clerk as 'keepers of the pleas of the Crown'— *custos placitorum coronas*. The coroner had a number of duties, but one of the prime reasons for his re-introduction was to keep a check on the corruption that was rife amongst the sheriffs of the counties, who were the main executives of the law at that time. The coroner was a man of substance, was unpaid and automatically lost his post if he was elected to the office of Sheriff. As 'keeper of the pleas of the Crown' he had to keep a roll of various incidents which were of potential advantage to the King's Treasury, which would act as a check upon the conduct of the sheriff.

These incidents included:

1. Inquests on dead bodies. When a body was found in the open, where the death was sudden or

unexpected or where there were any untoward circumstances, the coroner was obliged to view the body at the earliest possible opportunity. Any person who found a body was obliged to notify the coroner immediately, so that he could attend the scene. Speed was important, as often the local people would hide the body for reasons which will be made obvious. Any failure to summon the coroner or to obstruct him in any way could lead to heavy financial penalties being levied on the local community. Inquests were held with juries but, unlike today, the juries were people who had some personal knowledge or interest in the death and would today be called 'witnesses' rather than jurymen. The jury viewed the body with the coroner and it was their combined observation that sufficed as a post-mortem examination. The presence or absence of wounds was the main criterion.

2. At that time, little more than a century after the Norman Conquest, strife between Saxon and Norman was still commonplace. In an attempt to stamp out clandestine murders of Normans, the law presumed that all persons found dead were Norman victims of assassination, unless the local inhabitants could prove otherwise. Thus, unless there was a 'presentment of Englishry' (or, in Wales, 'Welshry'), the community had a heavy fine called the '*murdrum*' imposed upon them. Long after the necessity for this *lex murdrorum* existed, the practice was continued for purely financial reasons, until it was abolished in 1340.

3. It was also the coroner's duty to arrest anyone indicted for murder at an inquest. The coroner sent a warrant to the sheriff, who made the arrest. This power of committal survived until the end of 1977, when it was abolished as a result of the recommendations of the Inter-departmental Committee on Death Certification and Coroners—the 'Brodrick Report'.[1] Interestingly enough, in the context of medical jurisprudence, the very last case to be sent for trial after almost 800 years usage, was a hospital doctor. She was committed by the Cardiff coroner on 28 December 1971, on a charge of manslaughter by criminal negligence during the intracerebral injection of methotrexate into a child. As with the majority of committals from a coroner's inquest, the subsequent trial at the Crown Court resulted in acquittal.

4. The coroner also had to value any object which was the proximate cause of death, such as a dagger, a sword, any form of transport, etc. This sum was then forfeit to the Crown and the practice continued until the nineteenth century when even objects such as carriages, steam locomotives and ships were valued for forfeiture, after having caused death. The practice of confiscating the value of this '*deodand*' was not abolished until 1846.

5. The coroner was also empowered to confiscate the property of condemned felons and either transfer it to the Crown or sometimes give it to the relatives of the victim by way of compensation. Other similar fiscal duties included taking possession of the lands and chattels belonging to outlaws, those who had abjured the realm after seeking sanctuary in church, suicides or even the *victims* of homicides.

6. Though not a regular function, on the issue of special writ, the coroner was empowered to investigate treasure trove, catches of royal fish (whale and sturgeon), wrecks and other royal interests, all of which had an obvious financial content. The only duties not associated with death that have survived to this day are the treasure trove inquests (Coroner's Act 1887).

The power of the coroner declined rapidly after the fourteenth century, especially with the abolition of the *murdrum* fine and with the rise of the justices of the peace. Though officially the coroner never had any judicial functions, his brief being to 'keep' rather than to 'hold' pleas of the Crown, he did often try criminal pleas, and in 1215 the Magna Carta included a provision (Ch. XXIV) that prohibited coroners (amongst others) from exercising this judicial function, which was from then confined to the County Courts.

With the decline of the medieval inquest, the office of coroner went into limbo for many hundreds of years. By 1500, almost the sole remaining function of the coroner was the holding of inquests into violent deaths, but even these no longer held the same importance as in the thirteenth century. In 1487, Parliament tried to induce the coroner to carry out his duties more diligently by providing a fee for every inquest and a fine if he omitted to do so.

It was not until 1751 that any significant action was taken to improve the status of the coroner. Fees were increased and travelling expenses were granted. But it was the nineteenth century that saw the revival of the office of coroner into what we recognise today. Due to the advent of comprehensive registration of deaths after 1836, the whole administrative system was tightened up and the coroner's function in investigating unusual deaths became strengthened. In the same year of 1836, an Act gave coroners power to order a doctor to perform an autopsy and to attend an inquest: the jury could also demand a second medical opinion. A series of Acts during the latter part of the eighteenth century and further Acts in this century established a salaried, though still mainly part-time, coroner service. The Coroner's Society itself was founded in 1846.

At last proper facilities and incentive for postmortem medical examinations were provided, for until this period the medical aspects of death investigation were virtually nil. The Coroner's Act of 1887 declared that the function of the coroner was no longer that of protecting the financial interests of the Crown, but that of investigating deaths for the benefit of the community. It was with the increased interest in the public health and the collection of statistical data that causes of death became of importance from the medical point of view, rather than the former rough classification into accident, suicide or murder. A Select Committee in 1910 recommended that 'a coroner should have the power to order and pay for a post-mortem in cases of sudden death where the cause is unknown and there is no reason to suspect that death is unnatural or violent'. This led for the first time in 1911 to disposal of coroner's cases without the hitherto inevitable inquest. The Coroner's (Amendment) Act of 1926 gave recognition to the transfer of criminal investigations concerning deaths from the coroner to the police.

In 1935, a Committee of Enquiry under the chairmanship of Lord Wright enquired into the law and practice relating to coroners, though very few of their recommendations have been implemented. In 1971, a further extensive enquiry carried out during the preceding six years was published, the so-called 'Brodrick Report'.[1] Much of the recommendations of this wide-ranging enquiry have now been implemented, mainly those dealing with coroner's practice. Included in the changes brought about between 1977 and 1980 were the abolition of

the coroner's power to commit a person for trial on a charge of criminally causing a death (Criminal Law Act 1977); the abolition of the need for the coroner to view a body before inquest (Coroner's Act 1980); the acceptance of written instead of oral evidence at inquest (Coroner's Rules 1980); the referral of criminally-caused deaths to the Director of Public Prosecution (Coroner's Rules 1977); and the power to dispense with a jury in several types of inquest (Criminal Law Act 1977).

Both the Wright Committee Report and the Brodrick Report re-affirmed confidence in the office of coroner, viewing them favourably in contrast with alternative systems of death investigation.

The main advantages of the coroner system appear to be:

1. The existence of an independent official who can investigate the circumstances without pressures from any other part of the judicial or executive apparatus.

2. The power to summon any evidence or witnesses thought relevant to the case.

3. The high post-mortem rate on reported cases, which in large cities may be of the order of 95–99%.

The system has evolved from almost 800 years of experience in the investigation of unnatural, suspicious or unexpected deaths and in spite of rigorous scrutiny on several occasions during the last century, no better alternative system has been devised.

The coroner's system was introduced progressively into other countries as the English influence spread. It has been mentioned that this came too late in the case of Scotland to displace the well-entrenched legal procedure there, but Anglo-Norman expansion into Wales and Ireland took the legal institutions with it. In the case of Wales, a system of law more highly developed than that of the contemporary Anglo-Saxon laws existed for hundreds of years before the Norman Conquest, codified under Hywel the Good (c. AD 930). This was displaced piecemeal by English incursions, beginning in the south of the country, but the legal system with the coroner did not apply generally until well after the Edwardian Conquest of 1282. With the Act of Union of 1536–37, the law of Wales was completely unified with that of England.

Similarly, English law, carrying the coroner's system with it, was introduced progressively into Ireland following the beginning of the Anglo-Norman Conquest which started in 1169. Today, both the Republic of Ireland and the Province of Ulster both have a coroner's system which is almost identical with that of England, except in minor detail.

The 13 colonies in America were also under English law before Independence and the coroner's system was retained as the United States expanded to its present extent. However, the system has changed considerably, both in the duties and appointment of coroners, where this office is retained, and in the conversion to medical examiner systems in some states. In contrast to England and Wales, where the coroner is a permanent appointee of local government, most American coroners are politically appointed and their tenure of office is dependant upon political power and patronage. Frequently, the American coroner has no qualification either in medicine or law, as is mandatory in England, and there is considerable variation as to his duties and powers in different states. Due to the numerous weaknesses of the system, the introduction of medical examiners has been a feature of parts of the USA during the present century.

MEDICAL EXAMINER SYSTEM

In the English context, there is now a very close relationship between the functions of the coroner and the pathologist, the former being dependent to a considerable extent upon the findings of the latter. In the medical examiner system, this close relationship has been recognised to such an extent that the offices have virtually been fused, the medico-legal expert also having the official executive powers to categorise and dispose of the death. Probably the best known example in the United States is that which exists in New York City, introduced in 1915 after considerable criticism of the previous coroner system. The Chief Medical Examiner must be a medically qualified man and a trained pathologist, his appointment is under the Civil Service, and he is appointed by the Health Department, the office being independent of political vagaries.

The medical examiner has to enquire into deaths which are frankly or suspectedly criminal, suicides, sudden or unexpected, accidents and other similar instances where the medical attendant is unable to certify that death occurred from natural causes. Records must be kept of every enquiry into a death reported to his office and if he discovers or suspects that a death is due to criminal action, he is obliged to notify the District Attorney, who is responsible for initiating prosecutions. The medical examiner's records are made available to the District Attorney and such records are admissable as evidence in American courts. These records are also available to any other interested party, and part of the declared function of the medical examiner's office is to provide a source of expert opinion that is available to either party in a criminal trial. Unlike the coroner, the medical examiner has no power to initiate an enquiry or to hold an inquest.

Cases are referred to the Chief Medical Examiner from a variety of sources: the police, doctors, the city health department and any citizen, have a duty to report any deaths in which there is some cause to think that further investigation is required. The reporting from doctors is sometimes less direct than in the comparable English system: physicians are required to send to the City Health Department a certificate of death and a confidential medical report containing an opinion as to the cause of death, these documents being in a form prescribed under the City Health Code. Where death is not a straightforward natural event occurring during medical treatment, some doctors report directly to the medical examiner, but otherwise the Health Department have a routine check on incoming documents to decide whether or not the case should be referred to the medical examiner's office. This is a more extensive parallel with the screening carried out by the Registrar of Deaths in Britain, who has an obligation to refuse to register certain categories of death and to refer them to the coroner. In New York Health Department, specially trained clerks scrutinize medical reports to ensure that the Chief Medical Examiner is notified of all appropriate deaths within his jurisdiction.

Once reported, the Chief Medical Examiner or one of his expert medical staff examines the body and takes charge of the medico-legal aspects of the investigation. As the majority of such deaths are unnatural, it is the rule for the medical examiner to attend the scene of death. Here he makes a full investigation of the circumstances and is empowered to take charge of any objects which might be relevant in the investigation. He also has the power to decide whether or not an autopsy is required: if not, he can issue a certificate of death.

Where an autopsy is performed, it is done at the Chief Medical Examiner's official premises and if the death is a homicide, the autopsy must be witnessed by at least one other medical examiner. The decision whether to hold an autopsy or not is the responsibility of the Chief Medical Examiner and he may be sued by relatives or other interested persons who dispute his decision.

The advantage of the medical examiner's system is that a large proportion of all deaths are scrutinised by a trained medico-legal expert and undoubtedly any with a criminal, or potentially criminal, element are subjected to a detailed autopsy and full back-up of forensic investigation. However, the system does not investigate the non-criminal death in any depth, as once the attending medical examiner has decided that criminal aspects are absent, the investigation is less thorough than with similar cases under the English coroner's system. The total autopsy rate is much lower under the medical examiner's system, which means that the purely medical and statistical investigation of sudden deaths is less detailed: potentially, there is a greater chance of missing the occult criminal case because of the lack of an autopsy. The 'occupational hazard' of a law suit by relatives against the medical examiner tends to discourage autopsies in cases where it is not deemed particularly necessary from the law enforcement aspect. The advantages of a widespread 'on-scene' scrutiny have to be weighed against the lower autopsy rate when evaluating the relative merits of the two systems.

The position is admirably summarised by the members of the British Inter-departmental Committee on Death Certification and Coroners,[1] which made a detailed survey of other systems for comparison with the coroner's system. They commented: 'But, like the Procurator Fiscal, the enquiry of the medical examiner into deaths from which potentially criminal causes can be rapidly excluded, is thereafter too perfunctory to provide an acceptable model of accurate certification of the medical cause of every death. It has never been possible, even in New York, to produce statistics about causes of death in the form which such records can be produced in England. In many cases, the medical examiner is doing no more than providing evidence of the fact of death of certain individuals which cannot be provided in any other way. Unlike the coroner, his jurisdiction stops well short of adequate enquiry into the circumstances of those deaths which are singled out for special investigation for other than purely medical reasons. Given the predominantly medical bias in the medical examiner's training, it is not surprising that the medical examiner's investigation of the circumstances surrounding a death is sometimes not regarded as sufficiently thorough in removing public doubts and suspicions. When an English coroner accepts jurisdiction over a death, he is obliged to certify the cause of death as well as to provide (in inquest cases) the information required for registration purposes'.

The above description of the New York medical examiner system is paralleled to a great extent by other medical examiner organisations in various states or part of states of the USA. Another well-known model system is that which exists in Virginia. It contrasts with the high density of population in the New York area by having to deal with an area roughly four-fifths of the size of England, with a population of only about 4 000 000. In these circumstances, the Chief Medical Examiner has a number of assistant Chief Medical Examiners to conduct autopsies but also several hundred medical examiners, who are primarily physicians but who attend scenes of death to make the primary decision as to whether further investigation is necessary, especially an autopsy. The autopsy rate in Virginia is around 20%, compared with well over 80% in Great Britain. In the State capital, Richmond, this percentage rises to over 60%, but, again, is comparably much lower than the 97% achieved in some large British cities. For an excellent account of the Virginia medical examiner's system, the reader is referred to the paper by the editor of the present book.[2]

CONTINENTAL (EUROPEAN) SYSTEMS

Though there are considerable national variations between the different nations in Europe, all are much more akin to each other than to the coroner or even the medical examiner system. The common and major difference is that no official comparable to the coroner or medical examiner exists to investigate or supervise the handling of deaths in the community—this interest is retained by the executive and judicial officers of the law enforcement apparatus. Most of the countries have a rigid Criminal Code which defines the procedure for the investigation of criminal or suspicious deaths. Each citizen has a statutory duty to report circumstances relevant to such deaths directly to the police, who are the initiators of all investigations into deaths which are other than innocuous and natural. No enquiry into deaths, comparable with the English inquest, exists on the continent outside the criminal trial.

As an adjunct to this purely law-enforcement-orientated procedure, medico-legal experts (almost always specifically recognised and approved by the legal executive) exist to assist the police in their investigation. They have little or no power to initiate any investigations, but are there to provide expertise upon the request of the police or judiciary. Thus, although the scientific standard of legal medicine may be as high or even higher than anywhere in the world, its application may be frustrated by the absence of any stimulus or even acquiescence from the law enforcement officers.

In practice, this means that in many continental countries, a suspicious death will be referred by the police to a legal medicine institute where an external examination will be conducted. If this examination, taken in conjunction with the circumstances, seems to exclude criminal action, then the matter is dropped. Where criminality is suspected or evident, then the police will probably request an autopsy and report the matter to the Public Prosecutor, in the same manner that the American medical examiner reports to the District Attorney. Depending on the result of the medico-legal investigation, the Public Prosecutor, who often has to be present at the autopsy, may institute criminal proceedings. There are a number of countries where the permission of the Public Prosecutor is

necessary before a request for autopsy from the forensic pathologist is approved.

As with the medical examiner system, this leads to a situation where criminal deaths are thoroughly investigated, but the remainder of unnatural—but apparently innocent—deaths tend to receive much less attention than under the English coroner's system.

As examples of some representative systems, further details are given of the procedure in a few Western European states.

1. Denmark

The organisation of forensic medicine in Denmark is often held up as a model European system and certainly nowhere in the world is the standard of legal medicine so respected as in this relatively small country. From the legal aspect, the system of investigation of deaths is fairly representative of European practice. In Denmark all deceased persons must be examined by a doctor, who has to issue a death certificate. All unnatural deaths (murder, manslaughter and accidents, suicides and where persons are found dead or if there is suspicion of unnatural death) must be notified to the police by a doctor. The police then decide whether an examination in further detail should be performed or not. This examination consists of the drawing-up of a police report and an external medico-legal examination, which is performed by a doctor (preferably the local 'Medical Health Officer') together with a senior police officer. After the examination of the body externally, the police decide whether or not they are satisfied. If they are, the case can be concluded with the issue of a death certificate—if not, an autopsy may be performed.

These medico-legal autopsies are performed by 'State Forensic Pathologists' who are synonymous with the three professors of forensic medicine—the heads of the medico-legal institutes of three of the five Danish universities to which a medical school is attached, i.e., Copenhagen, Aarhus and Odense. These State Forensic Pathologists have assistants and deputies to whom their responsibility may be delegated.

The autopsy reports are always signed by two doctors—the forensic pathologist who performed the autopsy and a medical health officer who has wider ranging responsibilities in Denmark than the comparable title in Britain. One of the State Forensic Pathologists may also be the second signatory to an autopsy. The autopsy reports are passed on to the police, who then decide on subsequent action.

Almost 50 000 deaths occur annually in Denmark and well over 10% are notified to the police. From this latter number, over 20% are subjected to autopsy. The latest official autopsy rate was about 2.5% of the total deaths.

The police must order an autopsy in cases where crime is certain or suspected, where circumstances are so dubious as to require autopsy and where death may be due to recklessness or negligence of a third party, if such action may possibly come to trial.

The State Forensic Pathologists and their co-workers are academic staff of the university service, thus being independent of the prosecution.

If during the preparation of a trial, problems arise from the autopsy findings, the Court may submit written questions to the forensic pathologists or to the Medico-Legal Council, a permanent board of medical experts which gives pre-trial written opinions for the guidance of the courts on any case involving medical or pharmaceutical problems. The Medico-Legal Council belongs to the Ministry of Justice. Thus most medical evidence is agreed before trial and only in quite exceptional cases do forensic pathologists have to appear as expert witnesses in court.

In deaths suspected as homicide, a forensic pathologist from one of the medico-legal institutes or a Medical Health Officer (who are doctors with a broad clinical training who have also attended a special course of four months' duration in forensic medicine) will go to the scene together with the police and carry out the initial forensic investigations on the spot.

The examinations of living persons in criminal cases (victims or offenders) is performed by the medical health officers, in Copenhagen attached to the Medico-Legal Institute. However, any doctor is authorised to make these examinations and give opinions to the police.

Forensic psychiatry is carried out either by medical health officers or by specialists in psychiatry.

In Copenhagen and Aarhus there are specialist clinics in forensic psychiatry.

Thus, the Danish system, exceptionally well organised from the point of view of comprehensiveness and efficiency, is again dependent upon the wishes of the police in investigating cases and the forensic pathologists are somewhat inhibited in their desires to extend the range of cases which should be autopsied.

2. Federal Republic of Germany

In West Germany, a long-established system of handling unnatural deaths is still in use, although it has been the subject of much discussion and criticism by medical and legal authorities. Some modifications have been made in some of the Federal States which comprise West Germany and probably further simplifications and modernisations will be extended in the near future.

At the present time, it is left entirely to the discretion of the doctor certifying the death as to whether he will register a natural or unnatural cause, or suspicion of such cause. If he is not satisfied that the death is natural, his notification to the municipal registrar of deaths will be passed on to the police. These in turn are then bound to inform the Prosecutor's Office (*Staatsanwalt*) to whom it is left to decide whether an autopsy will be requested.

This request has to be referred to a judge in charge of inquests (*Ermittluglungsrichter*) who is empowered to either order an autopsy or reject the Prosecutor's request. In the latter case, the Prosecutor can appeal to a jury of three judges for a final decision.

The autopsy rate on cases reported for medico-legal investigation varies from place to place. In Lubeck it is about 18% but in Heidelberg only about 3%.

Thus, doctors have no power to order an autopsy but only to request the necessity of one through the appropriate channels. If an autopsy is carried out, it must be performed by a 'court doctor' (*Gerichtsarzt*) together with any other doctor except the one who certified the death. A judge and judge's clerk must also be present.

Generally, all staff members of a university department of forensic medicine are entitled and expected to carry out this kind of official medico-legal autopsy, provided that they have been appointed doctors to the court. In some parts of Germany, such as the State of Bavaria and in some large cities such as Stuttgart, Dortmund, Essen, Bremen, there are special medical officers of forensic medicine specifically appointed to perform these autopsies on the judge's request.

Recently a law has come into force in some Federal States obliging the attending doctor to notify the police directly if suspicion of an unnatural death or foul play has arisen. This circumvents the rather clumsy procedure of notification occurring via the registrar of deaths. This is a mandatory rule, though there has never been any bar to a doctor or hospital from notifying the police directly and informally of some suspicious death.

There are no statutory categories of causes of death which are considered to be unnatural and demanding an autopsy. This is left entirely to the certifying doctor's discretion. However, there are three exceptions in which certain causes of death are statutorily reportable. Firstly, death from any of the legally-scheduled occupational diseases must be given to the Professional Accident Insurance Authorities (*Berufsgenossenschaft*) who may or may not order a post-mortem, usually by a specialist pathologist of their choice. Secondly, deaths from infectious diseases must be reported to the Public Health Officer (*Amtsarzt*) who can also order an autopsy. Thirdly, where cremation is desired, permission must be given by the health officer of the district, who—if he has any doubts as to the nature of the death—can also order an autopsy before giving authority for cremation.

The German Penal Code (*Strafgesetzbuch*) and the Penal Proceedings Statutes (*Strafprozessordnung*) make no mention of the topic of unnatural death. The latter statute book contains the rules to be followed at a 'court autopsy' (*Gerichtliche Sektion*) as described above.

The judge in charge may also hold an inquest of his own without invoking the opinion or help of a forensic pathologist or even any doctor at all. He can also inspect the deceased for himself with or without the assistance of a doctor and can give a verdict of his own findings. It should be borne in mind that the German law is only interested in finding out whether a third party is involved and

therefore if a prosecution has to be initiated. Thus, even a law officer is not bound to hand the case over to a judge, but can close the matter at this stage on his own responsibility if he considers that no criminal act was concerned in the death.

It should be added that in some City States (e.g., Hamburg) and in other very large cities, there exist local regulations entitling the municipal authorities to have an autopsy (*Verwaltungsobduktion*) carried out by a qualified pathologist, usually a forensic pathologist, in cases of unattended, uncertified, accidental, or suicidal deaths, or deaths in custody or whilst under medical treatment, etc. These regulations, however, have no legal significance within the wider sphere of German law.

It thus appears that though the professional standard of forensic medicine is exceptionally high in the Federal Republic of Germany and the number of university institutes is proportionately greater than in any other western country, the rather unwieldly system of law, which prevents the medical authorities from initiating forensic autopsies, tends to concentrate forensic efforts only upon criminal cases. Thus, as in other continental countries, the overall autopsy rate on non-natural deaths is unsatisfactorily low.

3. Belgium

The investigation of unnatural deaths in Belgium is very close to that of France, both being direct products of the legal system borne of the Code Napoleon. Again, closely following the continental philosophy, the main legal consideration in the investigation of sudden deaths is to determine whether any criminal element is present and whether any other party needs to be brought to justice. It is not primarily an investigation into the death, from the point of view of classification and investigation of non-criminal factors.

To pursue this function, two officials, both jurists, are involved in the investigation of suspected criminal deaths. The first is the *Procureur du Roi* who is an agent of executive power attached to the court and may be considered to be the Public Prosecutor. The other is the *Juge d'Instruction*, the examining judge who is a member of the judiciary, completely independent of the executive power. A person suspected of having caused or contributed to a death in a criminal manner may be detained by the *Procureur* for up to 24 h, but if this officer believes a longer detention is necessary for the enquiry, he has to entrust the investigation to the *Juge d'Instruction* and request him to issue a warrant. If the judge refuses to do so, the *Procureur* has the right of appeal. Prolonged detention may only be granted by yet another independent magistrate of the judiciary, the President of the Chamber of Council. All investigations and enquiries short of actual trial are conducted in camera, and nothing comparable to the English inquest exists. There is no statutory obligation upon any member of the law enforcement system or the judiciary to employ any particular pathologist and there are no State-recognised pathologists as in, say, Denmark or West Germany. However, from convention and common sense, the excellent institutes of forensic medicine attached to several of the universities such as Gent, Liege, Louvain and Brussels, are widely used.

Unfortunately, a very low autopsy rate exists for all classes of unnatural death which are not frankly or suspectedly criminal. This leads to a curious situation in which exhumations are extremely common, because of the later appearance of cogent reasons why an autopsy is vital, especially in traffic and industrial accidents where large compensation issues become relevant at a later date.

4. The Netherlands

In The Netherlands, the typical continental system was somewhat modified after the Second World War, with centralisation of the forensic pathological facilities at the Medico-Legal Laboratory of the Ministry of Justice, situated at Rijswijk, near The Hague.

In The Netherlands, legal provisions entitle the investigating judge (*Rechter Commissaris*) to take all steps—including an order for an autopsy—at the request of the local Public Prosecutor. The latter official is entitled to request an autopsy in cases of emergency and as most murder investigations constitute such an emergency, a large number of autopsies are initiated by the prosecution in cases where serious crime is apparent or suspected. The police have no authority themselves to order an autopsy.

Statute law has formed legal links between doctors, Registrars of Deaths (*Ambtnaar Burgerlijke Stand*) and the local Public Prosecutors (*Officier van Justitie*). The Law on Disposal of the Dead (*Wet op de Lijkbezorging*) forbids a physician to sign a declaration of death if he is not convinced that his patient has died a natural death. Normally this document has to be produced at the local Registrar's Office where after registration a written consent for burial or cremation will be issued. This is obligatory by law within five days after death.

If death is considered to be unnatural or is suspected to be so, an external examination of the corpse is required by the law to be performed by a Municipal Health Officer (*Gemeentelijk Lijkschouwer*). This medical officer is entitled to issue a death certificate after examination if he considers the death natural: otherwise he is obliged to report to the Public Prosecutor who will then decide if a medico-legal autopsy is necessary. The law requires that a reasonable suspicion of crime has to be present before such an autopsy is requested. Cases in which the cause of death is unknown but in which there is not the slightest suspicion of crime are not covered by the provisions of the statute Law on Disposal of the Dead. Though the ultimate decision rests with the prosecutor, he is usually advised by the police and by the Municipal Health Officer.

The medico-legal external examination of the body (*Lijkschouwing*) is conducted in: (1) all cases in which the attending physician did not feel justified in issuing a certificate of natural death; (2) cases in which death was unattended by any other person; (3) unknown persons found dead; and (4) deaths in prison or in police custody and sometimes deaths in psychiatric hospitals.

The authority of an investigating judge or the public prosecutor to investigate a death is in no way restricted by the previous issue of a certificate of natural death by a physician. They can order a medico-legal autopsy after the attending physician or the Municipal Medical Officer have in good faith certified the death as natural, if police information suggests a suspicion of homicide. Criminal poisoning is proven to be the most frequent cause of death in such cases.

It has become obvious that the system of external examination of the body together with the circumstances is far from being a water-tight procedure.

Serious crimes have escaped attention, as has been proved by exhumations performed later when suspicions of murder emerged. Notwithstanding, this system has proved to be satisfactory in practice: by efficient organisation in collecting medical and police information, the number of cases in which the cause of death is not certain is restricted. With an annual death rate of about 100 000 in a population of about 13 000 000 it is estimated that the frequency of unnatural deaths amounts to 5000–6000.

Due to the selection procedures performed by the Public Prosecutor and the police, the annual number of medico-legal autopsies is constantly about 600. About 40% of these (200–250) are serious crimes including homicide. The remainder are accidents, suicides or natural deaths brought to autopsy because of suspicion of homicide. The total autopsy rate is only between 6 and 10% of all deaths.

The Netherlands Ministry of Justice has established a medico-legal laboratory, which is placed at the disposal of the legal authorities. This laboratory embraces the whole territory of the Kingdom of The Netherlands. District authorities are not obliged to call for assistance by the State Pathologist, but regularly do so. Though the pathologists are directly employed by the Ministry of Justice, they are not in any way bound by the administration in the performance of their scientific work.

Autopsies are performed at any place considered to be suitable, which includes regional hospitals, police headquarters (the larger ones having autopsy facilities) or in the Medico-Legal Laboratory at Rijswijk. Parallel specialist scientific facilities are available from the Forensic Science Laboratory of the Ministry of Justice or from other institutions and transport facilities and technical police assistance have all contributed to build up an efficiently functioning central organisation.

The autopsy report is provided for the benefit of the Court, the prosecution and the defence and by law has to be explained in simple language avoiding technical jargon. The report is accepted in Court as documentary evidence and, if any queries are raised upon it, the expert can be asked to give further information, either during the preliminary examination by the investigating judge or later as an expert witness in the actual trial.

5. Norway

In Norway, the relatives of the deceased person or 'other people present' must present a death certificate to the Court of Probate in order to register the death. This must previously have been certified by any doctor, whether he was the physician of the deceased or not. There are no regulations as in England about the doctor having seen the patient before death during any specified period.

If there is any reason to believe that the death was unnatural and that it may have been the result of a criminal offence, the same persons have a duty to report the death to the police. The law does not impose this duty on the doctor, but it is generally agreed that he has a moral right to report any relevant facts which are within his knowledge. A doctor will, however, hesitate to notify the police except in obvious criminal cases. As only a very small proportion of deaths are obviously criminal, there is sometimes some hesitation on the part of doctors where the circumstances are in doubt.

When the police are notified, they have to investigate the death and to consider whether there is any reason to believe that the death was unnatural and whether it was caused by a criminal offence. If they do so decide, the police must apply to the Court, which has the sole authority to order an autopsy. The Court may order two doctors to perform an autopsy and these experts give a written opinion to the Court.

If the case comes to trial, these experts have to appear in court and give oral testimony. The experts have the right to review in advance all the evidence which will be presented at the trial and during the trial they have the right to examine all the witnesses before they themselves give evidence. The doctors function as medical counsellors to the court and to the parties concerned. Their fee comes from the court and they are therefore completely independent of either the prosecution or defence.

No new legislation has appeared on matters of death certification and investigation of unnatural deaths since 1887 and there is a need for up-to-date revision. As with many other continental systems, the whole machinery is geared solely to the investigation of criminal offences which may have led to death.

For an account of the medico-legal systems in 22

of the European states, the reader is referred to the special issue of the journal Forensic Science[3] in which the present author describes the salient features of each system.

THE DEVELOPMENT OF MEDICAL JURISPRUDENCE AND FORENSIC MEDICINE

Until now, we have examined the origins, development and present state of the death investigation machinery in its official governmental aspects. However, the medical and scientific study of legal problems developed alongside the establishment machinery. Often it responded to the contemporary needs of law enforcement and at other times it was well in advance, even stimulating administrative improvements.

Medical jurisprudence is the older term in English usage, but now *forensic medicine* or *legal medicine* have become more common descriptions, except perhaps in Scotland. The history of legal medicine extends through millennia and probably the best concise account is that of Richard Myers and Robert Britain[4].

The salient points in the history of forensic medicine extend back to the early civilisations of Babylon, Egypt and China, but in the European context, from which virtually all present-day systems have originated, the early sixteenth-century saw the dawn of modern legal medicine, mainly in Italy and Germany.

Various codes and laws which related mainly to the practice of medicine and sometimes to the examination of criminal deaths are extant from Babylon around 2000 BC and from China, India, Egypt, Persia and Greece before the time of Christ. In the Roman period, from which codes of legal practice arose which are the antecedants of continental laws, the famous Twelve Tables of 449 BC set the limits of the duration of pregnancy at 300 days, which was identical with that fixed by the Code Napoleon long afterwards. Medico-legal factors concerning the insane, the unborn child and personal injuries were codified. External post-mortem examination in criminal deaths was obviously carried out, as the body of Julius Caesar was carefully examined by the physician Antistius. The Justinian Code, a vital milestone in the development of law, recognised the status of the doctor as an expert witness and as an impartial assessor. This code, dating from about AD 550, dealt with a considerable number of legal situations in which medical evidence must have been important, especially in connection with sexual and obstetric problems.

Chronologically, the next important event was the publication in China of the book 'Hsi Yuan Lu', a text of medical jurisprudence published about AD 1250, which was reprinted right up to the end of the nineteenth century. However, it was in Europe that legal medicine as we recognise it today began to evolve and as in so many aspects of the Renaissance, it was Italy that took the initiative. Bologna had medico-legal experts as early as the thirteenth century, the emphasis again being upon obstetric, homicidal and toxicological matters. Autopsies were carried out and a number of cities had medico-legal physicians. Pope Innocent III provided for the appointment of doctors to the courts in the thirteenth century and shortly afterwards Pope Gregory IX issued *Decretals* which contained many medico-legal connotations, once more primarily concerned with aspects of reproduction: it was here that the 'Proof of Congress' in alleged impotence was devised. For the next few hundred years in Italy, various Popes ordered further medical assistance to the ecclesiastical courts, mainly in matters of sexology, public health and disposal of the dead.

Though the premier site of the development of forensic medicine in Europe was Italy, it was somewhat haphazard and it was left to the German states to begin the orderly regulation of forensic medicine that still characterises the excellence of their numerous institutes today. The first systematic code of criminal law and procedure in Europe was promulgated by the Bishop of Bamberg in 1507. This *Bamburg Code* required that medical evidence was required in investigation of all deaths from violence and other German states adopted its provisions.

It led within a few decades to the even more comprehensive and famous code of the Emperor Charles V. This *Caroline Code* of 1532 has widespread geographical application over the Empire of Charles and its provisions were more far-reaching than the Bamburg Code. Internal autopsies were made much more frequently under the Code and the range of conditions dealt with included homicide, suicide, abortion, infanticide, serious injuries, complications of pregnancy and a number of other medico-legal matters that look so similar to present day practice. The courts were required to call medical evidence more frequently and the Caroline Code can justly be said to be the charter for modern forensic medicine.

During the rest of the sixteenth century, other codes followed in Germany and their example was reflected in advances in France and Italy.

Publications began to appear in the field of legal medicine, now that a recognised discipline had emerged fortuitously at the time when printing techniques were causing a communication explosion in Europe. The first indiviual names of medico-legists appeared such as Sebidz, Zittmann and Behrens.

The next period was one of consolidation and steady advance in academic legal medicine. Teaching of medical students now included public health and legal medicine, which were closely allied as they still are today in some universities and in the *International Academy of Legal Medicine and Social Medicine.*

In 1575, the famous Ambroise Paré wrote a treatise on the surgery of trauma, including much of medico-legal importance. At the end of the sixteenth century there were a number of other books published, most of which emphasise the sexual and reproductive aspects of medicine, often from a legal point of view. Some of these also included traumatology. In 1598 the famous work of Fidelis of Palermo was published, with four volumes dealing with all manner of medico-legal matters.

In the next century the paramount work was that of Zacchias, one of the physicians to Pope Innocent X. This book, 'Medico-Legal Questions', was published at intervals over 14 years, and dealt with a wide range of forensic subjects, again with considerable importance attached to matters connected with sex and pregnancy.

In this seventeenth century, there were a number of German treatises, including those of Sebitz, Welsch and Johannes Bohn.

In the eighteenth century, France was prominent in legal medicine, with personalities such as Louis,

the first teacher of legal medicine in the country. Three chairs of forensic medicine were created, towards the end of the century, in Paris, Montpellier and Strasbourg. Mahon was the first professor in Paris and published a well known textbook in the first year of the nineteenth century. A subsequent and very famous holder of the Paris chair was Orfila who is well known as the founder of forensic toxicology. His 'Treatise on Poisons' was translated into a number of languages and was the standard textbook for many years.

In Germany at this time, the main figure was that of Casper who taught in Berlin and wrote the classic 'Practical Handbook of Legal Medicine' in 1856.

From this point onward, the era of modern legal medicine in the continental European countries can be said to have commenced. From these energetic beginnings in the sixteenth to the nineteenth centuries, the present extensive network of academic medico-legal institutes was consolidated in Italy, Germany and France and spread to Central and Eastern Europe, which have developed numerous institutes on the German pattern.

The acceptance of the continental institutions in medical jurisprudence was much slower in Great Britain. Although British scientists and men of letters were in constant and close touch with the centres of learning in Europe, the traditional insularity and difference in the legal system have caused the academic acceptance of legal medicine in Britain to be both later and less secure, contrasted with that on the continent. The first Chair in Medical Jurisprudence was established in Edinburgh in 1807, though it was the source of political ridicule at the time. Prior to this, the first publication in legal medicine in English was a translation of Fazelius' 'Elements of Forensic Medicine' of 1767, made by Samuel Farr in 1788.

Scotland took the first real interest in academic forensic medicine, a tradition which it thankfully preserves to this day. Andrew Duncan was the first teacher of legal medicine at Edinburgh, combining his Chair of Physiology with lectures on public health and legal medicine. These lectures were published in 1792 and his personal efforts at arousing interest in legal medicine culminated in the establishment of the Chair in 1807, which was first occupied by Duncan's eldest son, also Andrew. A later incumbent was Sir Robert Christeson, the most well-known of the early nineteenth century British medico-legists. He was primarily a toxicologist and published a treatise on poisons which was very similar to Orfila's book of the same name. The Edinburgh Chair remained pre-eminent for much of the nineteenth century, with famous names such as Traill, Henry Littlejohn and his son of the same name. Much more recent holders of this famous Chair include Sir Sidney Smith and Douglas Kerr, who died in 1960. A Chair was established in the University of Glasgow in 1839 soon after the next Chair in Britain, that at Guy's Hospital in 1834. The latter was held by Alfred Swaine Taylor, probably the most famous name in English legal medicine and originator of the standard work emanating from London, this present book being the direct successor of Taylor's original, well over a century ago.

Legal medicine never became so well established in the universities of England and Wales as it did in Scotland. The established Chairs in London lapsed, even that of Swaine Taylor and the present professorships are but personal Chairs. In fact, there is only one established Chair of Legal Medicine in the whole of England and Wales, at the University of Leeds: even this came near extinction in 1972. Unlike the well-established institutes on the European continent, legal medicine in Britain has had little support from the government and a reluctant partnership with universities, so the quality of British forensic medicine has been due mainly to the quality and enthusiasm of individualists. It was hoped that a turning point might be the Brodrick Report[1] which appeared in 1971 after six years gestation. To date (1982) no implementation has been made of those recommendations which advocate government support for declining academic departments of forensic medicine, which would infuse new life into a small but vital part of the administration of justice in the country.

Like Britain, the development of legal medicine in the United States has been a patchy and individualistic process, rather than the more orderly system on the European continent. The English-styled law was transplanted by the early settlers and the coroner's system and medical examiner's system have developed from that. The medical aspects of law developed slowly until the nineteenth century, again a parallel state of affairs to that in Britain. The first lectures in forensic medicine were given soon after the commencement of those in Edinburgh—J. S. Stringham being the first professor of legal medicine in New York, appointed in 1813. He was in fact an Edinburgh graduate. His contemporary in Philadelphia, Benjamin Rush, was also Edinburgh-trained. Both these early academics wrote the first medico-legal treatises in the New World. Rush was, in fact, one of the signatories to the Declaration of Independence. The first major publication was that of T. R. Beck, Professor of Medical Jurisprudence at Albany, who published 'Elements of Medical Jurisprudence' in 1823. His brother J. B. Beck was professor in the same subject at the College of Physicians and Surgeons in New York and later collaborated with his brother in later editions of the work, which was extremely popular in many countries outside the United States.

Following this, a number of well-known names are recorded in the annals of American legal medicine, including Gross, Amos Dean, Hamilton Godkin and Reese. Later in the century, a major work was that of Whitthaus and Becker. In the early part of this century, practitioners and writers in legal medicine came thick and fast, such as Culbertson, Peterson and Haines and also Herzgog.

In the modern era, the best known textbooks were those of Gonzales, Vance and Helpern in 1937 with a second edition in 1954 adding Umberger as additional author. Alan Moritz contributed the well-known 'Pathology of Trauma' and R. B. H. Gradwohl, a prime mover in the establishment of legal medicine in the United States, edited his 'Legal Medicine' in 1954.

No mention of American legal medicine would be complete without acknowledging the pre-eminence, not only in the USA but world-wide, of the late Professor Milton Helpern, Chief Medical Examiner and Professor of Forensic Medicine in New York. Retiring in 1974, his expertise and leadership in the field of legal medicine has been felt not only in the New World but in many parts of the globe.

In summary, the present state of affairs appears

to be that the scientific and academic face of forensic medicine is often well in advance of the legal and administrative arrangements. In many countries, its full potential cannot be realised, due to frustrations in governmental machinery for applying the technical advances of past years.

ACKNOWLEDGEMENTS

The author is indebted to the following for personal communications concerning continental medico-legal systems: Professor F. Thomas (Belgium); Dr J. Voigt (Denmark); Dr J. Zeldenrust (The Netherlands); Dr J. Giertsen (Norway); Professor F. Schleyer (West Germany).

REFERENCES

1. Report of the Committee on Death Certification and Coroners Command Paper 4810 (1971) London: Her Majesty's Stationery Office.
2. Mant, A. K. (1964) Med.-Legal J., **32**, 86.
3. Knight, B. (1977) For. Sci., **10**, 3.
4. Myers, R. O. & Brittain, R. (1968) In: Gradwohl's 'Legal Medicine' 2nd ed. Bristol.

FURTHER READING

Britain, R. P. (1962) Bibliography of Medico-Legal Works in English. London and New Jersey.
Havard, J. D. J. (1960) The Detection of Secret Homicide. London.
Helpern, M. & Knight, B. (1977) Autopsy—The Memoirs of Milton Helpern. New York: St Martins Press and (1978) London: Harrap.
Knight, B. (1982) Legal Aspects of Medical Practice, 3rd edn. Edinburgh and London: Churchill–Livingstone.
Marhsall, T. K. (1966) Med. Sci. Law, 8, 73.

2

The English legal system

English law, based on the three main sources of custom, case law and statute, owes much of its present superficial form to the historical development of the Courts. Until 1873, when a statutory attempt was made to rationalise the jurisdiction of the main Courts, the growth of the Courts owed more to the competition between different jurisdictions to afford remedies to, and to attract, litigants than to any logical plan to provide nationwide justice. It is vain, therefore, to look for any rational theme in the jurisdictions exercised by the various Courts. Even the well-known division of the law into civil law and criminal laws is only partially observable in the Courts' jurisdictions. For example, the Magistrates' Courts exercise not only a final criminal jurisdiction in relation to the lesser forms of crime but also have jurisdiction to deal with matrimonial matters (where it overlaps with the Family Division of the High Court), adoptions (a jurisdiction it shares with the High Court and the County Court) and also control the issue of various licences, procedures which are in essence administrative rather than judicial.

Another influence on the growth of the legal system was the adversary procedure. The Courts have, until recent years,[1] refused to deal with abstract questions of law so, until a dispute arises between two litigants upon an issue the Courts could not (and still, in the vast majority of cases, do not) give any ruling on the point of law involved. While such a system caused the case law element to be as flexible as was consistent with the doctrine of precedent, it lacked something in certainty and economy. The advantage of the adversary procedure is that the judge is placed in a position where his role is one of assessment of the merits of the two cases before him rather than an investigatory role which

may produce no less just a result but which may antagonise the litigant who believes that he has been unjustly interrogated.

THE SYSTEM OF THE COURTS

Magistrates' Courts

These Courts are the workhorses of the criminal jurisdiction. By far the vast majority of criminal cases are dealt with in the Magistrates' Courts. It is true that many such cases are dealt with by a simple plea of guilty and therefore can be despatched expeditiously but even so it is surprising to find that in some central London Courts case loads of over 80 a day are being despatched with regularity in a single Court.

Magistrates' powers of punishment are generally limited apart from any specific limitation which may be placed by the statute creating the particular offence. In the case of custodial sentences in respect of offences triable either way, a Magistrates' Court on summary conviction may not impose a sentence of imprisonment for more than six months in respect of any one offence and when consecutive sentences are imposed in respect of two or more offences, the maximum length of sentence is 12 months. The maximum fine that may be imposed on conviction of an offence triable either way is £1000. Since the Court will not know the full background of the offender until after he has been found guilty the provision for committal to the Crown Court for sentencing is a necessity.[2a]

The Court's jurisdiction is in two distinct parts. Firstly, it can try summary offences where it has sole jurisdiction and in such cases it reaches a verdict and pronounces the proper sentence. In considering sentence the magistrates may, having heard of an offender's character and previous convictions, commit an offender to the Crown Court for sentence.[2b] This power may only be exercised in respect of summary trial of offences triable either way, unless an offender is committed with a view to a sentence of borstal training being passed, in which case the offence for which he is committed must be punishable with imprisonment.[2b]

In cases where an offence is triable either summarily or by trial on indictment at the Crown Court the offender may elect the mode by which he wishes to be tried. The magistrates may, however, deprive an offender of the opportunity of being tried summarily if they consider that the facts of the offence are so serious that their powers of punishment may be insufficient. Further, some offences are designated by statute as triable only on indictment (e.g., murder, inflicting grievous bodily harm with intent). Where for one reason or another the case is eventually to be tried by judge and jury the magistrates' function is limited to determining whether the prosecution has adduced sufficient evidence to warrant the committal of the accused for trial at the Crown Court.[3]

Since 1967 the need to hear oral evidence from each of the prosecution witnesses has been considerably attenuated and in many cases, where the defence do not claim that upon the statements submitted by the prosecution there is any dispute that a *prima facie* case has been made out, this aspect of the jurisdiction has been reduced almost to the formality of presenting documents to the Court. Upon committal to the Crown Court, the Magistrates' Court has the power to decide whether an accused person shall be admitted to bail or not.

As previously indicated, the Magistrates' Court also has considerable civil jurisdiction and a number of statutes provide that certain matters can be dealt with if information is laid before the Magistrates' Court by a person aggrieved. There is therefore no general jurisdiction and a complainant must be able to point to a statutory power granted to the Court before he can succeed.[4] It follows that there is no power in the Court to initiate proceedings in this respect of its own accord. There must be a complaint made to them first.[5]

In the exercise of its civil jurisdiction the Magistrates' Court supplies a cheap and easily available forum to deal with matrimonial disputes (excluding divorce) and much time is spent in dealing with proceedings under Domestic Proceedings and Magistrates' Courts Act 1978 in relation to the procuring, by spouses, of Orders of separation and maintenance against each other. In the same field, cases concerning the custody of children and their adoption are also within the jurisdiction of this Court.

Magistrates or justices of the peace were originally appointed by the Sovereign granting a commission to particular individuals in an area to keep the King's Peace in a particular area. Today, justices are still appointed on behalf of the Crown by the Lord Chancellor, by the issue of Commissions of the Peace[6], and magistrates so appointed, can be removed by the Lord Chancellor in appropriate cases.

The country is divided into Commission Areas and in each such area the existing Committee of Magistrates will advise the Lord Chancellor's Department as to suitable persons to be appointed. Each magistrate is appointed to one of the Commission Areas in England or Wales and he has jurisdiction (subject to special exceptions) in that area only. A Lay Justice would normally be without legal training and although he undergoes a short period of training prior to sitting in Court, he is obliged to rely heavily upon a clerk (trained in law) to the justices (or his assistant) when dealing with matters of law (as opposed to matters of fact).

In contrast to the Lay Justice, the Stipendiary Magistrate, while he is appointed in the same way, has to be legally qualified in that he must be a barrister or solicitor of not less than seven years standing.[7] The appointments are made on the recommendation of the Lord Chancellor and a similar recommendation is required before the Stipendiary Magistrates can be removed.[8] There are special provisions for the appointment of Metropolitan Stipendiary Magistrates for the London area.[9]

While the Stipendiary Magistrate sits alone, Lay Magistrates will normally sit in a Bench of three or five members. Since 1971, a further duty has been laid upon Lay Magistrates that from time to time when there are appeals from Magistrates' Courts to the Crown Court, one or more Lay Magistrates will sit with a Crown Court Judge in the Crown Court to hear appeals to that Court from the Magistrates' Court. The Magistrates so sitting must not have been concerned with the case under appeal.

Appeals against conviction and sentence are usually to the Crown Court but where either prosecution or defence claim that there is an issue of law involved and that the magistrates are in error, the magistrates may be required to state a case i.e., put their full reasons and findings in writing. If, upon considering such *Case Stated*, either party believes that the magistrates have erred in law, the appeal is then to the Divisional Court of the Queen's Bench Division. From there, by leave, there is a further appeal to the House of Lords.

County Courts

At first sight the County Court appears to be singularly ill-named. It is not the single Court for any particular county. Indeed, in the Metropolitan Area every major district has its own County Court. However, the aim of such Courts has always been to provide *locally* an efficient, uncomplicated and reasonably inexpensive method of resolving civil disputes within certain limitations as to jurisdiction. For this purpose England and Wales are divided into various 'circuits' which are numbered for administrative purposes and appointments are made to such circuits. A circuit may contain a number of County Courts.

The County Court is a creature of statute[10] and its jurisdiction is limited and controlled by the various Acts and Orders which have amended and extended the Courts' original statutory jurisdiction. At present, the Court can hear and determine any action founded on contract or tort or for the payment of money recoverable by statute or any action for the recovery of land or for any of the classes of proceedings in equity, admiralty or probate proceedings mentioned in the County Courts Act 1939 as amended by the Administration of Justice Act 1977, S15. Certain pecuniary limits have been redefined by the County Courts Jurisdiction Order 1981, No.1123. In all actions founded in contract or tort or in actions for money recoverable by statute, or in proceedings relating to solicitors costs under s.69(3) of the Solicitors's Act 1974 and in respect of extortionate credit agreements under the Consumer Credit Act 1974, jurisdiction is limited

to recovery of the sum exclusive of costs of £5000. The equity jurisdiction is limited to £30 000. A plaintiff may proceed in the High Court but he must recover £3000 in order to be entitled to his costs on a High Court scale. In respect of County Court actions there are further limitations imposed in respect of the ordering of costs where the sum recovered falls below certain figures. In addition, certain County Courts have jurisdiction to grant undefended divorces, decrees of nullity and judicial separation and to provide ancillary relief consequent upon such matrimonial decrees. Orders in this sphere of family law are not limited by the financial maxima which apply to ordinary actions and consequently the County Court can now be found dealing with considerable sums by way of property settlements following matrimonial relief. Moreover, the ancillary relief will often be involved with important and controversial questions of the custody of children.

Subject to the limitations described above, County Courts must, in any cause of action for the time being within its jurisdiction, grant such relief as ought to be granted or given in a similar case by the High Court and in as full and ample a manner,[11] but its power to grant injunctions is fettered to cases where a claim for money or other relief is made within the Court's jurisdiction.

The border line between County Court and High Court proceedings can present problems. On the one hand, no action can be commenced in a County Court on any judgment of the High Court or of any other Court in England and Wales[12] but it sometimes occurs that actions are commenced in the High Court (particularly where summary judgment is sought) and, where an application is made to the High Court, an action can be remitted to the County Court and will be remitted in the usual way where the amounts claimed are within the jurisdiction of the County Court.[13]

A number of statutes give the County Court jurisdiction over matters which at first sight would appear to be beyond their normal limits of jurisdiction, for example, the considerable powers under the Rent Acts are in the majority of cases exercisable by the County Court. Further, if a plaintiff who is *prima facie* entitled to a sum which is beyond the limits of the County Court, wishes to utilise the speedier proceedings of the County

Court he can do so by abandoning the excess of his claim above the jurisdiction financial limit. Finally, the jurisdiction can be extended by agreement between the parties to the proceedings that they will agree to the extension of the jurisdiction of the Court either to an unlimited amount or to a specified sum. Such an agreement must be evidenced by a memorandum in writing.[14] The Judge of the County Court will usually sit alone without a jury; he is appointed on the recommendation of the Lord Chancellor as a circuit judge, and once appointed as a circuit judge he can sit in any County Court in England and Wales. However, the Lord Chancellor must assign one or more circuit judges to each district and such appointments can be varied from time to time by the transfer of circuit judges from one district to another.[15] In order to qualify for recommendation by the Lord Chancellor as a Circuit Judge, the candidate must be a barrister of at least 10 years standing or a recorder who has held that office for at least three years.[16] In addition to those who are specifically appointed as circuit judges, every Judge of the Court of Appeal and High Court and every recorder who is a barrister of at least 10 years standing or has held that office for at least five years is by virtue of office capable of sitting as a judge for any County Court district.[17]

Crown Courts

These Courts were established by the Courts Act 1971 following the *Beeching Report* which recommended the removal of the old Courts of Quarter Sessions and the Assize Courts and the amalgamation of those jurisdictions into a single system of Courts administering the criminal law in relation to offences tried on Indictment. The aim was to provide a more extended and rational system of Courts capable of dealing with more serious crime and to deal with it more expeditiously. For this purpose it was necessary to expand appointments to judicial office and to open the post of Circuit Judge to the ranks of solicitors. In its wake the reform brought a vast increase in the number of administrators necessary, or claimed to be necessary, to service the new Crown Courts. There has been some shortening of the period between committal and hearing in the case of indictable offences

but there has also been a substantial increase in the costs of running the Courts.

There are no 'Crown Court Judges' as such, although persons who exercise the jurisdiction of the Court are frequently referred to in common parlance as 'Crown Court Judges'. Any High Court Judge, Circuit Judge or Recorder or Assistant Recorder sitting either alone or with justices of the peace, or any Deputy Circuit Judge can exercise the jurisdiction of the Crown Court but there are limitations as to the types of cases which may be heard by any person apart from a High Court Judge. However, there are dispensing provisions whereby cases of a superior class can be released to a judge (including a recorder or deputy judge) who would not normally be qualified to hear that case. Accordingly a detailed investigation of those categories and limitations on powers of hearing cases is of no real advantage, save that the most serious types of cases such as murder must always be heard by a High Court Judge. The appointment of circuit judges is dealt with in relation to County Court (*supra*). Recorders are appointed from time to time on the recommendation of the Lord Chancellor to the Crown of qualified persons who are barristers or solicitors of at least 10 years standing. Such persons when appointed undertake duties as part time judges of the Crown Court or carry out such other judicial functions as may be required. Unlike the circuit judges, who are appointed until the age of retirement, the recorder is appointed for a limited period, normally three years.[19] He is required to serve a minimum of 20 working days in every year and will not normally be permitted to serve for more than 50 working days in any year.

The Crown Court has jurisdiction to hear all proceedings on indictment,[20] all committals for sentence from Magistrates' Courts[21] and appeals from Magistrates' Courts against both sentence and conviction.[22] In addition, the Court can hear appeals from affiliation orders[23] and appeals against any order requiring a person to enter into recognisances to keep the peace or to be of good behaviour.[24] In addition, to appeal against certain orders made by Magistrates' Courts under various enactments, and under the Licensing Laws, the Crown Court can entertain appeals from decisions of local and other authorities in certain cases.[25] On appeal, the Crown Court can confirm, reverse or vary any decision or may remit or make such order as it thinks just. However, where the Crown Court acts on appeal from a decision by magistrates where the Magistrates have imposed a penalty the Crown Court is normally limited to the extent of the penalty which would be applicable in a Magistrates' Court save where the case has been remitted specifically for sentence.

Where the Crown Court exercises its main jurisdiction by hearing cases on indictment, the judge will sit with a jury of 12 jurors. They will initially be asked to return a unanimous verdict of either guilty or not guilty upon the accused. After 2 h 10 min if no such verdict seems possible, the judge can give a direction that a majority verdict upon which not less than 10 of the jury are agreed will be accepted. On hearing of appeals, save in those cases where he sits with a justice of the peace, the judge will sit alone.

The High Court of Justice

In 1873 the Judicature Act of that year was mainly concerned with the eradication of competition between various Courts. Ninety-seven years later, the Administration of Justice Act 1970 sought to solve the wholly different problem of Courts which had become the victims of their own complexity and were unable to serve the law which altering social attitudes had demanded should appear on the statute book. The Court was reorganised by that Act into three co-equal divisions. The Queen's Bench Division, the Chancery Division and the Family Division.[26] The judges of these three divisions all have equal authority and the Order of one judge has equal validity in the other two divisions.[27]

The judicial membership of the High Court includes the Lord Chief Justice, the President of the Family Division, the Vice Chancellor of the Chancery Division and technically the Lord Chancellor, although his sittings in the High Court are limited to one appearance a year, his normal forum being the House of Lords. In addition, the main body of work is executed by the Puisne Judges who are barristers of not less than 10 years standing and are appointed upon the recommendation of the Lord Chancellor.[28] With the exception of the Lord Chancellor all the Judges of the High Court hold office during good behaviour and can only be removed by a special parliamentary procedure.

The jurisdiction of the High Court is both original and appellate. In its original jurisdiction the Court is unlimited in amount and it extends to all causes of action. However, for the sake of convenience various types of action have been assigned to each of the divisions. For example, the Chancery Division deals with all those matters which were the province of the former Court of Chancery abolished in 1873.[29] Accordingly it now deals with contested matters concerning the administration of estates, partnership, actions relating to the redemption and foreclosure of mortgages, land charges, issues arising from contracts relating to land, and trusts.

The Queen's Bench Division's original jurisdiction now encompasses all matters of contract and tort[30] and some of the jurisdiction previously exercised by the Commercial Court and the Admiralty Court.[31]

The Family Division which arose from the previous Probate and Divorce Division, while it includes divorce and nullity amongst the matrimonial matters with which it deals, also entertains actions concerning wardship, adoption, guardianship of minors and the ancillary matters arising therefrom.

The appellate and supervisory jurisdictions of the High Court are exercised either by a Divisional Court of a particular division or by a single judge.

In the Divisional Court, either two or three judges sit together and may transact any business ordered by the Rules of the Court to be heard by a Divisional Court and can exercise any part of the jurisdiction of the High Court for this purpose.[32] But an important Divisional Court procedure is that carried out by the Queen's Bench Division which will entertain applications for Judicial Review by way of Order for Mandamus, Certiorari and Prohibition. By these Orders the Divisional Court supervises and controls inferior Tribunals and officials where a potential civil action or have failed to exercise, their legal powers. Even more important, is the power of the Court to issue the Writ of Habeas Corpus[33] whereby any individual can be required by the Court to deliver up to the Court any person alleged to be wrongfully detained. The Divisional Court of the Queen's

Bench also has the duty in certain circumstances to commit for contempt of Tribunals other than the High Court.[34]

The Queen's Bench Divisional Court also deals with appeals from Magistrates' Courts by way of case stated and hears appeals under certain enactments relating to professional disciplinary proceedings.[35]

The Divisional Court of the Chancery Division is far less prominent than that of the Queen's Bench Division and hears appeals in bankruptcy and land registration matters, amongst others.

In the Family Division, the Divisional Court has appellate jurisdiction where there is an appeal by way of case stated from the magistrates in, for example, affiliation or maintenance variation matters.[36]

The appellate jurisdiction of a single judge in the various divisions is as follows: in the Queen's Bench Division a single judge can hear appeals from Orders made by Masters of the Queen's Bench Division in Chambers, and in certain cases from Orders made by District Registrars,[37] and there is a similar appellate jurisdiction from decisions of the Secretary of State for Social Services under the Social Security Act 1975, appeals from Pension Appeals Tribunals,[38] some appeals from Industrial Tribunals[39] and finally from appeals from Taxing Masters on a further review of Crown Court taxation.

The single judge in the Chancery Division hears appeals in bankruptcy cases[40] and by way of case stated in relation to the registration of commons.[41]

In the Family Division, the single judge is mainly concerned with hearing appeals from registrars who make Orders particularly in relation to financial matters following a matrimonial order or divorce, nullity, etc. The single judge may also be required to adjudicate upon a case which would normally be dealt with by a Registrar of the Family Division but where the registrar has decided that it would be more appropriate, because of the importance of the matter, if a High Court Judge adjudicated upon it at once.

The Court of Appeal

While the Court of Appeal has power in exceptional circumstances to hear fresh evidence, and while technically all cases before the Court are 'by way of re-hearing', in fact the Court of Appeal deals with appeals upon the basis of the transcript of the evidence and judgment. Its jurisdiction is divided into two parts, the first civil and the second criminal.[42] Its composition in civil matters must be at least two judges on interlocutory issues, and in final matters there must be three judges. Appeals can be heard before five judges where it is considered to be an issue of exceptional importance. On appeals in criminal matters, there must be an uneven number of judges not less than three.[43] Those who are entitled to sit in the Court of Appeal are the Lord Chancellor, ex-Lord Chancellors, any Lord of Appeal in Ordinary who at the date of his appointment would have been qualified to be appointed as an ordinary Judge in the Court of Appeal or who was at that time a judge of that Court, the Lord Chief Justice, the Master of the Rolls, the President of the Family Division, and not less than eight nor more than 14 ordinary members of the Court, who are called Lord Justices of Appeal.[44] A Lord Justice of Appeal is appointed by the Crown by Letters Patent and all hold office during good behaviour subject to the power of removal by the Crown on an address of both Houses of Parliament.[45]

The civil jurisdiction of the Court of Appeal includes jurisdiction to hear appeals in certain cases from Masters of the Queen's Bench or Chancery Divisions, Registrars of the Family Division and District Registrars. Further, appeals can be heard in certain cases from judges in Chambers and in some cases an appeal lies from a Divisional Court.[46] Its principal work however is in hearing appeals from all divisions of the High Court and from the County Court.

In criminal matters the powers of the Court are dealt with under Part I and Part 2 of the Criminal Appeal Act 1968 and this provides for:

1. appeals by persons convicted in indictment by Crown Courts
   a. on any ground which involves a question of law alone,
   b. by leave of the Court of Appeal by Certificate of the judge who tried the case on a question of fact or of law or any ground which seems to the Court to be sufficient,

c. by leave of the Court of Appeal against any sentence (except one fixed by law) passed for the offence for which the appellant was convicted;

2. proceedings in certain cases before a Coroner's Court;

3. the Home Secretary may refer all or part of a case to the Court of Appeal in which a person has been convicted on indictment or found not guilty by reason of insanity or found by a jury to be under a disability.

The Court has power to quash convictions on the ground that the verdict was unsafe or unsatisfactory or that the direction of the trial judge was wrong in law or that there was a material irregularity in the course of the trial. The Court also has power to dismiss any appeal even if there has been an irregularity, if it is satisfied that no miscarriage of justice has actually occurred.

On appeals against sentence, the Court can quash any sentence which is the subject of appeal (other than a sentence fixed by law) and can pass such sentence or make such order as it thinks appropriate and as the Court below had power to pass when dealing with the appellant for the offence. However, this power must not be exercised so that the appellant is more severely dealt with than by the Court below. This means that the power which was previously exercised by the old Court of Criminal Appeal to increase sentences, where a prisoner had appealed against sentence, has now gone. The Court of Appeal Criminal Division can substitute a verdict for that in fact returned by the jury, and may vary sentence where the defendant was convicted properly only as to a part of the indictment or was convicted of the wrong offence. Where the conviction is quashed, only in the light of fresh evidence, the Court of Appeal has power to order a retrial.[47]

The House of Lords

The House of Lords is the ultimate Court of Appeal but it is one to which there is no automatic right of appeal. It can hear appeals from the Court of Appeal in England and Wales, but there has to be either leave of the Court of Appeal or of the House of Lords itself in criminal matters.[48] There

are further restrictions on appeals to the House of Lords for example under the Bankruptcy Act 1914, which limit the accessibility of this particular Court. A further limitation occurs by the practice of the House where at the time the case comes before them there is no live issue to be decided between the parties.[49] In such a case the House will refuse to hear the appeal.

Although Scottish law differs widely from that practised in England and Wales, the House of Lords will hear appeals from Scotland upon any judgment or order of any Court from which error or appeal lay before 1 November 1876, by common law or statute.[50]

Subject to various statutory restrictions, the House will also hear appeals from:

1. a decision of the High Court in England;[51]
2. any Order or judgment of the Court of Appeal in Northern Ireland by leave of that Court or of the House;[52]
3. direct from the decision of the High Court of Justice in Northern Ireland.[53]

In criminal matters, the rules of appeal differ. In general there must be either a certificate that a point of law of exceptional public importance is involved and that leave is granted. Such leave can be granted either by the Court of Appeal Criminal Division or if refused by the House of Lords.[54] The House will hear appeals from:

1. any decision of the Court of Appeal (Criminal Division) from an appeal to that Court;
2. any decision of the Divisional Court in a criminal cause or matter;[55]
3. any decision of the Courts Martial Appeal Court on an appeal to that Court;[56]
4. any decision of the High Court of Justice in Northern Ireland in a criminal cause or matter;[57]
5. any decision of the Court of Criminal Appeal in Northern Ireland on an appeal to that Court;[58]
6. any decision of the Court of Appeal in Northern Ireland in a criminal cause or matter on a case stated by a County Court or a Magistrates' Court.[59]

An appeal may not be heard unless not less than three Lords of Appeal are present and for this purpose a Lord of Appeal includes the Lord Chancellor, a Lord of Appeal in Ordinary, any Peer who holds or had held high judicial office (for example a previous Lord Chancellor or member of the Judicial Committee of the Privy Council), a Lord of Appeal in Ordinary, a Judge of the Supreme Court in England or Northern Ireland, or the Quarter Sessions in Scotland. The Lords of Appeal *in ordinary* are appointed by Letters Patent[60] and must have the qualifications of either having held high judicial office for not less than two years or having been for at least 15 years a practising barrister in England and Northern Ireland or a practising advocate in Scotland.

The House of Lords has authority to reconsider matters of fact except for the findings of fact by a Tribunals appeals from which are made final by statute. In practice however it is rare for the House of Lords to consider matters other than those purely of law. In considering matters of law the House has a duty to decide what ought to be done on the subject-matter of the appeal and this applies even when the appeal is by the 'leap frog' procedure whereby an appeal comes straight to the House of Lords from the High Court by consent of the parties, without being heard by the Court of Appeal.[61] In criminal appeals the jurisdiction of the House cannot be limited merely to determining the point of law of general public importance which is set out in the certificate of the Court below; the Court can also consider other matters of law which present themselves to the House on the hearing of the appeal.

The Judicial Committee of the Privy Council

Appeals to the Sovereign were at one time heard by the whole Privy Council. In practice now it is only the Judicial Committee of the Privy Council which entertains appeals. Membership of that Committee includes the Lord President of the Council, the Lord Chancellor, ex-Lord Presidents, Lords of Appeal in Ordinary and such other members of the Privy Council as from time to time hold or have held High Judicial office. Two other Privy Councillors may be appointed by the Sovereign by signed Manual. This body has been extended to include Privy Councillors being or having been Chief Justice or Justices of the High Court of Aus-

tralia, the Supreme Court of Canada, the Superior Court of a Canadian Province or the Superior Courts of New South Wales, Queensland, Southern Australia, Tasmania, Western Australia or any other Superior Court in the Dominions named by the Queen in Council.

The jurisdiction, which stemmed from the right of the Sovereign to entertain appeals from her Courts in the Dominions, has been extended so that appeals can be brought from any Court in any colony. However, with the diminution in the number of Colonies and, indeed, in the number of the countries in the Commonwealth who wish to have appeals heard by the Privy Council, the jurisdiction has considerably lessened in importance. It has always however been the case that the Judicial Committee of the Privy Council is not an English Court. It only sits in London for the sake of convenience. It does not apply English law to cases where that law would not be applicable in the Court from which the appeal comes.[62]

Appeals also lie from Colonial Courts of Admiralty and the Court of Admiralty of the Cinque Ports.[63]

It would be incorrect however to regard the Judicial Committee of the Privy Council purely as a Court of Appeal from the Dominions and Colonies. It has wide jurisdiction in relation to ecclesiastical appeals from England and Wales and it also hears appeals from a number of professional disciplinary bodies. For example, it hears appeals from the General Medical Council[64] where, inter alia, the Professional Conduct Committee of the GMC has given a direction or made an order that the name of a medical practitioner should be erased from the Medical Register or where that committee directs that a doctor be suspended or his period of suspension extended. The practitioner can appeal to the Queen in Council and the appeal is then heard by the Judicial Committee. This appeal is as of right.[65]

In the same way, the Judicial Committee of the Privy Council will hear appeals from the General Dental Disciplinary Committee ordering that a dentist's name may be erased from the Register;[66] Opticians[67] and veterinary surgeons[68] whose names have been erased from Registers of their professions, or who have been suspended, by the relevant Disciplinary Committee, have a similar right of appeal. With the claims of many paramedical practitioners to professional status it is not surprising that by the 'Professions Supplementary to Medicine Act 1960' and the 'Professions Supplementary to Medicines (Orthoptists Board) Order in Council 1966', a large number of paramedical disciplines ranging from chiropodists to remedial gymnasts now have a similar right of appeal when aggrieved by disciplinary proceedings which have resulted in their erasure or suspension by their professional body.

A little-used power in relation to the Judicial Committee is that the Crown can refer to the Committee any matter whatsoever by what is called 'a special reference'. Such divers matters as the privileges of the Jersey Bar and the law of piracy[69] have been the subject of such references.

THE CORONER'S COURT

Reference has previously been made to the basis of litigation of Courts in England and Wales as being the adversary system. The Coroner's Courts are an exception in that the entire proceedings are inquisitorial. There is no plaintiff or defendant, no prosecutor or accused, in a Coroner's Court. The Coroner is charged with a duty of establishing certain facts. He does this by means of inquiry and inquisition of witnesses. Both before and after the 'Broderick Report' on Coroner's Courts, both the jurisdiction and conduct of Coroner's Courts had been criticised and many proposals made for attenuation of the Courts' functions. It is somewhat surprising at a time when the setting up of private and public enquiries as fact finding procedures has grown, that at the same time one of the more effective Courts for elucidating facts on important issues should be in danger of emasculation if not extinction.

In order to qualify to be a coroner, or a deputy or assistant deputy coroner, the candidate must be a barrister or solicitor or legally qualified medical practitioner of not less than five years standing in his profession.[70] His jurisdiction is local in that he will be appointed for a particular area but provided a body is found dead within that area it is immaterial where the death actually occurred. The coroner's duty is:

1. to enquire into the death including the cause of death in certain circumstances either by inquest or post-mortem;
2. to hold inquests upon treasure trove;
3. to act on occasion in place of the sheriff.

Plainly, the most important aspect of this Court's jurisdiction is in relation to sudden and unnatural death. Where a coroner is informed that the dead body of a person is lying within his jurisdiction and there is reasonable cause to suspect that that person has died a violent or unnatural death, or has died a sudden death of which the cause is unknown, or that that person has died in prison, or in such place or in such circumstances as to require an inquest in pursuance of the Act, the coroner must hold such an inquest touching the death of that person.[71] However, where there is reasonable cause to believe that the person has died a sudden death of which the causes are unknown and the coroner is of the opinion that post-mortem examination may prove an inquest unnecessary, he may dispose of the case by a post-mortem examination without holding an inquest.

The coroner can sit with a jury but need not do so. It is the duty of the coroner or, where there is a jury, of the jury, to hear the evidence and to return a verdict setting forth as far as possible who the deceased was, how and when and where he came by his death, by murder, manslaughter or infanticide but cannot after 1 January 1978 find any person guilty of such offence.[71] The jury is permitted to make recommendations particularly in cases where a practice which has caused the death has been shown to be a dangerous one. It is not the role of the Coroner's Court to make any findings in relation to negligence or any other matters which might found a civil action, although it must be admitted that the calling of evidence soon after the event frequently provides the representatives of the personal representatives or administrators of the deceased's estate with valuable information in relation to the possibility or otherwise of bringing proceedings in the Civil Court against the person or persons who may have caused the death of the deceased.

TRIBUNALS

The development of Tribunals has been a prominent feature of the legal system during the twentieth century. There has been a conviction, whether justified or not, that the ordinary processes of the Civil and Criminal Courts are too cumbersome or are not designed to deal with the particular needs of an advancing industrial society. At the same time, there have been demands that particularly in the field of industrial law, the implementation of employment legislation requires specialised treatment which the legislature did not feel would be forthcoming at the hands of the usual Courts of Law. Accordingly, one finds that in fields concerning Industrial Relations, where there has been strong Trade Union pressure to resist submission of their proceedings to normal judicial process, specialised Tribunals have flourished. In other fields, also, the individual professions have sought to control their own affairs by seeking legislative sanction for disciplinary powers exercised by various committees over the members of that profession. So numerous are these Tribunals that it is impossible in the short space available to do more than mention in passing a few of the more important examples. Further, in various nationalised industries, for example the National Health Service, the nationalising statute has made provision for the Minister responsible for the particular service to set up either private or public enquiries into problems arising in that service or industry. Again, the frequency of such provisions is such that it would be fruitless to investigate each one here but there is no doubt that the creation of so many additional Tribunals and Enquiries has placed a great strain upon the available personnel who are adequately trained in judicial techniques and it is a matter of enquiry whether the standards of investigation of some Tribunals is not below that which the public has a right to expect.

Industrial Tribunals

Industrial Tribunals were originally established to hear appeals against assessments to levies under the Industrial Training Act 1964. The jurisdiction of the Industrial Tribunal has been considerably extended by various Acts of Parliament now consolidated by the Employment Protection (Consolidation) Act 1978. The establishment of Industrial Tribunals is now governed by S.123 of that Act and regulations made thereunder.

The Tribunal would normally consist of a chairman and two other members but the absence of one such member would not prevent the Tribunal being properly constituted provided the parties agreed. For certain interlocutory and formal matters, the chairman can act alone. At each hearing, the chairman must be either the president or a person selected from a panel of barristers or solicitors of not less than seven years standing, such panel appointments being made by the Lord Chancellor. Two of the members must be selected by the President from a panel of persons appearing to the Secretary of State to have knowledge or experience of employment in industry or commerce. The appointments are made by the Secretary of State after consultation with Trade Union and Employers' Organisation.

The jurisdiction of the Industrial Tribunal now encompasses the following:

1. hearing of complaints of unfair dismissal;
2. determination of questions of redundancy;
3. resolving issues as to the terms which ought to be included in the terms of employment;
4. determining any claim under the Equal Pay Act 1970 or under the Sex Discrimination Act 1975;
5. hearing appeals relating to Improvement Notices issued under the Health and Safety at Work Act 1974;
6. determining complaints under the Employment Protection (Consolidation) Act 1978.

The Employment Appeal Tribunal

This is a statutory tribunal which draws its powers as a Court of record from the Employment Protection (Consolidation) Act 1978 S.135.

The membership of the Tribunal is a High Court or Court of Appeal Judge nominated by the Lord Chancellor, at least one Court of Session Judge nominated by the Lord President of the Court, and such number of appointed members as the Queen may appoint on recommendation of the Lord Chancellor and the Secretary of State. Such appointed members must have a special knowledge of Industrial Relations as representatives either of employers or of workers.

The jurisdiction of the Employment Appeal Tribunal is mainly appellate and lies in respect of any question of law arising from any decision of, or rising in any proceedings before, an Industrial Tribunal under or by virtue of the following Acts:

1. a. the Equal Pay Act 1970,
   b. the Sex Discrimination Act 1975,
   c. the Employment Protection Act 1975,
   d. the Race Relations Act 1975,
   e. the Employment Protection (Consolidation) Act 1978.
2. On questions of law arising in any proceedings from any decision of the Certification Officer under certain provisions of the Trade Union Acts 1914–64.
3. On questions of law or fact arising under S.8 of the Trade Union and Labour Relations Act 1974 or S.8 of the Employment Protection Act 1975.

Further an appeal may lie to the Court of Appeal on any question of law arising from any decision or order of the Employment Appeal Tribunal with the leave of that tribunal or the Court of Appeal itself.

The Professional Conduct Committee of the General Medical Council

This committee is a useful example of a professional disciplinary committee which seeks to regulate the conduct of its members in the interests of the public. It derives its power from statute[72] and the General Medical Council is by statute empowered to make rules for the conduct of disciplinary matters.

It is the duty of the Professional Conduct Committee on behalf of the General Medical Council to investigate charges that practitioners have been guilty of criminal offences, usually when they have already been convicted of such offences, or have been guilty of serious professional misconduct. By S.7 of the Medical Act 1978 the Professional Conduct Committee, if satisfied of guilt, may if they think fit, direct that the name of a fully registered person be erased from the Register. Alternatively, a practitioner's registration may be suspended for a period specified, not exceeding 12 months, or such requirements may be imposed as the committee think fit for the protection of members of the public or in the practitioner's own interests. In this event the doctor's registration is conditional on his compliance with those requirements which may be imposed for a period of not exceeding three years. In the event of the Conduct Committee later making a finding that he has failed to comply with such conditions, his name may then be erased or registration suspended. The Conduct Committee may extend any period of suspension imposed in any case and indeed even on the expiry of a previous period of suspension provided the new period imposed does not exceed 12 months. Again, on considering whether to extend such period, the committee may exercise its powers of erasure and conditional registration. With regard to conditional registration any conditions imposed may be revoked or varied by the Conduct Committee. The Conduct Committee may also direct that the period of conditional registration already imposed be extended on the expiry of the initial period for a further period not exceeding 12 months. It should be noted that these provisions apply to any practitioner however registered.

The Professional Conduct Committee consists of a president and both elected and appointed members. Members of the committee, other than the president, are appointed by the General Medical Council. Before any case is considered by the Professional Conduct Committee, complaints are first scrutinised by the Preliminary Proceedings Committee which will refer cases thought to be worthy of further consideration by the Conduct Committee for enquiry.

A further area of jurisdiction is that exercisable by the General Medical Council itself under S.10 of the Act to investigate whether any entry in the Register has been fraudulently or incorrectly made. The penalty imposed in respect of such fraud or error is that of erasure.

A complaint to the Professional Conduct Committee is presented by either counsel or solicitors on behalf of the General Medical Council and the practitioner is entitled to be represented by solicitor or counsel. Evidence is taken on oath and the Committee has the benefit of the assistance of a legal assessor who is normally a Queen's Counsel. Appeals against the findings and directions of the Professional Conduct Committee with respect to erasure suspension and conditional registration or the finding of the General Council in respect of entry in the Register (see above) are heard by the Privy Council.

The Criminal Injuries Compensation Board

This Tribunal is atypical in that it is the result of a non-statutory scheme but otherwise it presents many of the features of the 'assessment board' type of Tribunal, so often set up under compensation legislation. The Chairman of the Board is usually a Queen's Counsel or a judge and is appointed by the Home Secretary and the Secretary of State for Scotland after consultation with the Lord Chancellor. Other members of the Tribunal are also legally qualified.[74]

The board considers applications for *ex gratia* payments of compensation where the applicant sustained personal injury which is directly attributable to either:

1. criminal violence;
2. the arrest or attempted arrest of an offender or suspected offender;
3. the prevention or attempted prevention of an offence;
4. the giving of help to any constable who is engaged in arresting or attempting to arrest an offender or suspected offender or preventing or attempting to prevent an offence.

Compensation is assessed upon the basis of common law damages and normally takes the form of a lump sum. The board has a discretion to make special arrangements for the administration of any sum by way of compensation which is awarded particularly in the case where the victim is a child or other person under a disability. The hearings are relatively informal and there is a greater tendency to accept written medical reports and to waive the necessity for calling a consultant to give evidence before the board than in a case in the High Court.

THE LEGAL PROFESSION

The profession can be divided into barristers and solicitors. Each has its own governing body, the Senate in the case of barristers and the Law Society in the case of solicitors. The entry to the profession, to the Inns of Court in the case of an intending barrister or into an articled clerkship with an established solicitor in the case of an entrant to that branch of the profession, must make his election at the outset. There is no immediate right to transfer from one branch of the profession to the other nor can anyone be at one and the same time both barrister and solicitor.

The relationship between barrister and solicitor is often likened to that which exists between the consultant and general practitioner. The solicitor will normally approach a barrister upon matters where he considers the expertise of the specialist advocate is necessary. In the area of advocacy, because of exclusive rights of audience in certain Courts, the solicitor is obliged to employ a barrister if he wishes his case to be presented on behalf of his client. Except in rare circumstances, a barrister can only accept work through a solicitor and may not approach a lay client direct.

The complaint is often made that this division of the profession which does not exist in continental jurisdictions is harmful in that it increases the costs to the public and is wasteful of time and manpower. There has been a singular lack of evidence to substantiate such claims and it is doubtful whether any continental lawyer would be willing to operate a legal aid scheme with the economy with which both branches of the profession manage to operate in England and Wales. On the other hand, the divided profession affords the lay client the inestimable advantage of having his advocate selected not by himself but by a solicitor who is trained in the estimation and selection of advocates.

After a barrister has been in practice for a number of years, he may apply to the Lord Chancellor for appointment as a Queen's Counsel. Until recently this meant that he could thereafter not go into Court unless he was accompanied by a junior (i.e., a barrister who was not a Queen's Counsel) but this practice together with other restrictions upon the activities of Queen's Counsel has now been abandoned. It is from the ranks of Queen's Counsel and senior juniors that most judicial appointments are made, although under the Courts Act 1971 solicitors may now be appointed to the Crown Court and the basis of appointments to judicial office has been widened recently by the appointment of persons who, though qualified as barristers or solicitors, are in effect Civil Servants but have been employed in Government Office for a number of years. It follows from this that there is in English law no separate profession for judicial appointments.

REFERENCES

1. It is debatable how far the Attorney General's reference to the Court of Appeal (Criminal Division) after an acquittal can be fairly described as an abstract question of law.
2. (a) Magistrates' Courts Act 1980, section 37.
   (b) Ibid., section 38.
3. Magistrates' Courts Act section 6.
4. *L.C.C. v. Betts* (1936) 1 K.B. 430.
5. *Trathan v. Trathan* (1955) 2 All E.R. 701 at 707.
6. Justice of the Peace Act 1979, sections 1–5.
7. Ibid., section 13, sub-section (1).
8. Ibid., section 13, sub-section (3).
9. Ibid., section 13.
10. County Courts Act 1959, as amended.
11. County Courts Act 1959, section 74; Administration of Justice Act 1969, section 6.
12. County Courts Act 1959, section 71.
13. County Courts Act 1959, section 45, section 54; Administration of Justice Act 1970, section 1, sub-section (6)(a), schedule 2, paragraph 22.
14. County Courts Act 1959, section 42; Administration of Justice Act 1970, section 1, sub-section (6)(a) schedule 2, paragraph 21.
15. Courts Act 1971, section 20, sub-section (1).
16. Administration of Justice Act 1977, section 12.
17. Courts Act 1971, section 20.
18. Courts Act 1971, section 21 (1).
19. Courts Act 1971, section 21, sub-section (3).
20. Courts Act 1971, section 6, sub-section (1).
21. Magistrates' Courts Act 1980, sections 37, 38.
22. Magistrates' Courts Act 1980, section 108, sub-section (1).
23. Affiliation Proceedings Act 1957, section 8, sub-section (1) Affiliation Proceedings Act 1972, section 1, sub-section (3).
24. Magistrates' Courts Act (Appeals from Binding Over Orders) 1956, section 1, sub-section (3); Magistrates' Courts Act 1980, section 154, schedule 7, paragraph 16.
25. Courts Act 1971, schedule 9 as amended.
26. Administration of Justice Act 1970, section 1.
27. Supreme Court of Judicature (Consolidation) Act 1925, section 4; Administration of Justice Act 1928, section 6.
28. Supreme Court of Judicature (Consolidation) Act 1925, section 9, sub-section (1).
29. Supreme Court of Judicature Act 1925, section 56, sub-section (1)(a).
30. Ibid., section 36.
31. Administration of Justice Act 1970, section 2, sub-section (1); section 3, sub-section (1).
32. Supreme Court of Judicature (Consolidation) Act 1925, section 63, sub-section (1); Administration of Justice Act 1977, section 9, schedule 5.
33. Rules of the Supreme Court (R.S.C.) Order 54, rule 1.
34. R.S.C. Order 52, rule 1.
35. R.S.C. Order 94, rule 6; see also, inter alia, Architects (Registration) Act 1931, section 9; Medicines Act 1968, section 82, sub-section (3), section 83, sub-section (2); Nurses, Midwives and Health Visitors Act 1979, section 13; Legal Aid Act 1974, section 12, sub-section (3); Administration of Justice Act 1977, schedule 1.
36. Domestic Proceedings and Magistrates' Courts Act 1978, section 29.
37. R.S.C. Order 58, rules 1, 4.
38. Pensions Appeals Tribunal Act 1943, section 6, sub-section (2); Social Security Act 1980, section 16.
39. Industrial Training Act 1964, section 12 as amended by the Employment Protection (Consolidation) Act 1978, section 159, schedule 16, paragraph 4.
40. Bankruptcy Act 1914, section 97, sub-section (2).
41. Commons Registration Act 1965, section 18.
42. Criminal Appeals Act 1966. section 1, sub-section (2); Criminal Appeals Act 1968, section 52, sub-section (1), schedule 5, part 1.
43. Administration of Justice Act 1970, section 9.
44. Supreme Court of Judicature (Consolidation) Act 1925, section 6, sub-section (2); Administration of Justice Act 1968, section 1 as amended.
45. Supreme Court of Judicature (Consolidation) Act 1925, section 12, sub-section (1).
46. Judicature Act 1925, section 24, section 31, sub-section (1)(f). See *R. v. Board of Visitors of Hull Prison*, ex parte St Germain, (1978) 1 W.L.R. 42 C.A.
47. Criminal Appeals Act 1968, section 7, sub-section (1); see also *R. v. Rose* (1982) 3 W.L.R. 192, 198.
48. Appellate Jurisdiction Act 1976, section 3, sub-section (1); Administration of Justice (Appeals) Act 1934, section 1, sub-section (1).
49. *Sun Life Assurance Co. of Canada v. Jervis* (1944) House of Lords A.C. 111.
50. Appellate Jurisdiction Act 1876, section 3, sub-section (2).
51. Administration of Justice Act 1969, part II, section 12–16 as amended.
52. Judicature (Northern Ireland) Act 1978, section 41.
53. Administration of Justice Act 1969, part II, section 36, sub-section (3).
54. Administration of Justice Act 1960, section 1, sub-section (2) as amended; Criminal Appeals Act 1968, section 33, sub-section (2).
55. Administration of Justice Act 1960, section 1, sub-section (1)(a) as amended.
56. Courts Martial (Appeals) Act 1968, section 39, sub-section (1).
57. Administration of Justice Act 1960, section 1, sub-section

(1)(a); section 18, sub-section (4) as amended.

58. Criminal Appeals (Northern Ireland) Act 1968, section 36; Judicature (Northern Ireland) Act 1978, section 40.

59. Administration of Justice Act 1960, section 1, sub-section (1)(a); section 18, sub-section (4), schedule 2, part II as amended.

60. Appellate Jurisdiction Act 1876, section 6; Statute Law (Repeals) Act 1973, section 1, sub-section (1), schedule 1.

61. Appellate Jurisdiction Act 1876, section 5; Administration of Justice Act 1969, section 14, sub-section (a).

62. *Hull v. McKenna* (1925) I.R. 402.

63. Colonial Courts of Admiralty Act 1890, section 6, sub-section (1).

64. Medical Act 1978, section 11.

65. Ibid., section 11, sub-section (3). The principles on which the committee will decide such appeals has been set forth in cases such as *Fox v. G.M.C.* (1960) 1 W.L.R. 1017; *Sivarajah v. G.M.C.* (1964) 1 W.L.R. 112; *Libman v. G.M.C.* (1972) A.C. 217.

66. Dentists Act 1957, section 22, section 25.

67. Opticians Act 1958, section 11, section 13

68. Veterinary Surgeons Act 1966, section 16.

69. *Re Piracy Jure Gentium* (1934) A.C. 586.

70. Coroners (Amendment) Act 1926, section 1, sub-section (1); Local Government Act 1972, section 272, schedule 30.

71. Criminal Law Act 1977, section 56, sub-section (1).

72. Medical Act 1956–78.

73. Medical Act 1978, section 7.

74. Criminal Injuries Compensation Scheme, paragraph 1.

3

Deaths

DIAGNOSIS OF DEATH

The increasing practice of organ transplantation, together with developments in resuscitation and artificial means for maintaining breathing and the circulation have introduced a new importance into the diagnosis of death. Death is a piecemeal process and many body tissues remain viable after the circulation has ceased. The crucial point is the decision that there is no prospect of the person functioning again as a whole organism. Removal of a liver or kidney for transplant must be performed as soon as possible; deterioration is rapid while the organ is still in the body after circulation has ceased, the period of warm ischaemia.

The diagnosis of death is a matter of clinical judgment. Even where legislation has been passed on this topic the ultimate decision has been deemed one for the medical practitioner. In Virginia, a statute requires that (1) respiratory and cardiac functions must have ceased and, in the opinion of a physician, because of the nature of the disease or the length of time since such functions ceased, could not be restored, or (2) a supporting opinion by a neurologist, neurosurgeon or specialist in electroencephalography states that spontaneous brain and respiratory functions are absent.[1] The above definition depends on medical opinion and does not take practice beyond that of other countries. It expresses the current view that irreversible cessation of brain function is the essential feature.

As regards clinical judgment a statute of Columbia concerned with human tissue enacts 'whenever any person is pronounced dead by a physician'.[2]

Breathing and the circulation may be maintained by life support systems but the quality of life without mental function is such that the patient cannot be regarded as being a whole person. In a Virginian case which led to the statute quoted above the judge advised the jury that they could accept the principle of cerebral death being final. In the United Kingdom a code of practice has been published by the Health Department which deals with the criteria for the removal of cadaveric organs for transplantation.[3] This code accepts the definition of death given by the Royal Colleges. The report runs to several pages, but it concludes that the identification of brain death means that the patient is dead, whether or not the function of some organs, such as a heart beat is maintained by artificial means. All the functions of the brain must have permanently and irreversibly ceased.

In day-to-day clinical practice diagnosis of death is seldom difficult. Presence of mortal disease, or severe injury, coupled with absence of reflexes, heart beat and respiration is sufficient to enable the doctor to pronounce life extinct. When there is doubt further examination may be made after an interval. When organs are to be taken for transplantation there is urgency and strict standards must be applied.

Diagnostic tests for the confirmation of brain death suggested by the Code of Practice require that all brain stem reflexes are absent.
(1) The pupils are fixed in diameter and do not respond to sharp changes in the intensity of incident light.
(2) There is no corneal reflex.
(3) The vestibulo-ocular reflexes are absent.
(4) No motor responses within the cranial nerve

distribution can be elicited by adequate stimulation of any somatic area.

(5) There is no gag reflex or reflex response to bronchial stimulation by a suction catheter passed down the trachea.

(6) No respiratory movements occur when the patient is disconnected from the mechanical ventilator for long enough to ensure that the arterial carbon dioxide level rises above the threshold for stimulation of respiration. The tests are qualified by a number of factors that must be taken into consideration, such as the presence of drugs and the temperature of the body. They have to be repeated before they can be accepted as conclusive.

Determination of death

When death is determined on the basis of brain death, the Code of Practice requires that a consultant, preferably the one in charge of the case, and another consultant or senior registrar clinically independent of the first shall assure themselves that the preconditions have been met before testing is carried out. Both should have expertise in that field and they should not be members of any proposed transplantation team that might utilise organs removed from the body.

ORGAN TRANSPLANTATION

Removal of parts of bodies for transplantation and other purposes is governed by the Human Tissue Act. If a person, orally or in writing in the presence of two or more witnesses during his last illness, has expressed a request that his body or part of his body be used for therapeutic or other medical purposes the person lawfully in possession of the body after death may authorise the removal of tissue.[4]

After death the person lawfully in possession of the body may authorise removal provided he has no reason to believe that the deceased would have objected or that the surviving spouse or other relative objects.[5] Doubt has been expressed as to whether the authority of a hospital in which a body is lying has lawful possession until the executors or relatives claim it. The Act states that it has such possession:[6]

In the case of a body lying in a hospital, nursing home or other institution, any authority under this section may be given on behalf of the person having the control and management thereof by any officer or other person designated by the first-mentioned person.

If a person has reason to believe that an inquest may be required to be held or a post-mortem examination directed by the coroner he shall not give authority or remove tissue without the coroner's consent.[7] The coroner has no power to authorise removal of tissue.

CERTIFICATION OF DEATH

Two persons may complete a certificate of cause of death—the medical practitioner in attendance on the last illness, and the coroner. The coroner's position will be considered later.

The medical practitioner has a legal duty to complete the certificate if his patient dies but he is advised to notify the coroner at the earliest opportunity if the death is violent or suspicious or if he has any reason to believe that the death is one that would eventually be referred to the coroner by the Registrar of Deaths.

The Act states:[8]

In the case of the death of a person who has been attended during his last illness by a registered medical practitioner, that practitioner shall sign a certificate in the prescribed form[9] stating to his knowledge and belief the cause of death and shall forthwith deliver that certificate to the registrar.

While 'attendance' has not been defined it should have been sufficient to enable the doctor to be reasonably sure of the cause of death. The practitioner is not required to see the body; he must write on the form the date on which he last saw the patient alive and he must state whether he saw the body after death.

To overcome the difficulty of defining attendance the Brodrick Committee recommended that the certifying practitioner must have attended the deceased at least once during the seven days prior to death. A proposed form of certificate requires the doctor to certify this fact, also that he has seen the body. If he is not sure of the cause of death or considers that there are suspicious circumstances or industrial disease he should notify the coroner direct.[10] Although the proposed certificate has not yet been introduced, the Industrial Diseases Notification Act 1981 enables the Registrar General to make some of the proposed changes.

REPORTS TO THE CORONER

The coroner should be informed in the following circumstances:

Abortion. Death after spontaneous abortion is so rare that interference should always be suspected.

Accident. Death thought to be due to an accident, at home, at work, while travelling or at sport; a common cause of accidental death is fracture of the neck of the femur in the elderly.

Alcoholism. Acute or chronic, alcoholic cirrhosis in which a frequent complication is haemorrhage from oesophageal varices.

Anaesthetics. Deaths associated with an anaesthetic, often hypoxic, require careful inquiry.

Drugs. Therapeutic, addictive or suicidal. Adverse drug reactions causing death.

Industrial disease or poisoning. Mesothelioma should arouse suspicion of asbestosis.

Medical mishaps. Deaths due to operative error, failure to tie blood vessels, perforation of a viscus during endoscopy and similar mishaps. It is recognised that surgery, and the use of potent drugs, carry risk. The coroner is unlikely to hold an inquest if a hazard has been fairly taken: the degree of care is the important point.

Murder, manslaughter or infanticide. Practitioners should bear in mind the possibility of child abuse.

Pensioners. Deaths of those in receipt of a disability pension.

Poisoning in any form.

Stillbirths. When there is doubt whether the child was born alive.

THE REGISTRAR OF DEATHS

The registrar must report a death to the coroner if there has been no medical attendance, if he has been unable to obtain a death certificate or where it appears that the deceased person was not seen by the certifying practitioner *either* after death *or* within *14 days* before death. He must also report if the cause of death is unknown, unnatural, violent, suspicious, due to abortion, operation or anaes-thetic or due to industrial disease or poisoning.[11]

By contrast with the medical practitioner, who has no statutory obligation to inform the coroner, although he may have one at common law, the registrar's duty is imposed by regulation.

DEATH IN PRISON

A death in prison must be notified to the coroner, whether or not it appears to be natural.[12] This also applies to the death of a prisoner in a hospital to which he has been sent for treatment. Deaths of prison officials are not subject to this rule. The governor normally makes the report.

REMOVAL OUT OF ENGLAND

A person intending to remove a body out of England must obtain the coroner's sanction. This affects removal to Scotland, Northern Ireland, the Isle of Man and the Channel Islands but not to Wales.[13]

POLICE

Many deaths are reported to coroners by the police. These are often violent—road accidents and criminal cases—but deaths of persons living alone and found dead from natural causes may also come from this source.

THE CORONER

The coroner is a barrister, solicitor or registered medical practitioner of at least five years standing in his profession.[14] Out of the 180 coroners in England and Wales, 22 are whole-time appointees. The part-time coroners are mostly solicitors, while some of the whole-time officers are qualified both in medicine and in law. Appointment is made by the County Council[15] and the coroner is assigned to a district, if any, of the county. He is paid by the county which has no power of direction over his duties. The number of deaths reported to coroners is rising while the death rate remains roughly static.

In 1969 131 639 deaths were reported to coroners out of a total of 579 378; 25 130 inquests were held. In 1980 170 207 deaths were reported out of a total of 593 019 with 22 963 inquests

DISPOSAL WITHOUT INQUEST

When a death is reported to a coroner a medical certificate of cause may be available. After inquiry from the certifying doctor the coroner may be satisfied that there is merely ambiguity in wording or he may be satisfied with an account of the death. In such a case he may notify the registrar that no inquest or post-mortem examination is indicated. Relatively few cases are concluded in this way.

VIOLENT OR UNNATURAL DEATH OR SUDDEN DEATH OF WHICH THE CAUSE IS UNKNOWN

The coroner has a duty to inquire into such deaths, and into deaths in prison. He also has jurisdiction in connection with treasure trove and may act on behalf of the sheriff.

Where a coroner is informed that the dead body of a person is lying within his jurisdiction, and there is reasonable cause to suspect that such person has died either a violent or an unnatural death, or has died a sudden death of which the cause is unknown, or that such person has died in prison, or in such place or under such circumstances as to require an inquest in pursuance of any Act, the coroner, whether the cause of death arose within his jurisdiction or not, shall as soon as practicable, issue his warrant for summoning not less than seven nor more than eleven good and lawful men to appear before him at a specified time and place, there to inquire as jurors touching the death of such person as aforesaid.[16]

Although enacted a century ago this section of the Coroner's Act still epitomises the coroner's function. Sudden death has not been defined but it might be interpreted as 'unexpected'. There have been two important modifications to this section— the power to dispose of a case after post-mortem examination without inquest and a great reduction in the kind of inquests in which a jury is required (see p. 23). The coroner can no longer find a person guilty of murder, manslaughter or infanticide and accordingly his inquisition may not name or charge a person with any of those offences.[17]

POST-MORTEM EXAMINATION WITHOUT INQUEST

If the coroner considers that a post-mortem examination may prove an inquest to be unnecessary he may direct its performance.[18] While in practice it can usually be anticipated whether or not a death is natural the autopsy may provide unexpected findings and should never be omitted. An inquest may be held without post-mortem examination but this is, and should be, an extreme rarity. The examination should be made by a pathologist with suitable qualifications and access to laboratory services.[19] If a charge of homicide is possible the coroner should consult the chief officer of police as to the selection of a pathologist.[20] In most areas there is a standing arrangement between the coroner and police of acceptable pathologists. Various persons may be represented by a medical practitioner at the autopsy,[21] relatives, the deceased's doctor or hospital in which he had been treated, the pneumoconiosis panel, factory or government departments and the chief officer of police. The examination, even in homicide cases, is made on behalf of the coroner who alone may direct its performance. The person making the post-mortem shall not supply a copy of his report to any person other than the coroner, who may authorise the supply of copies to other persons.[22]

THE MEDICO-LEGAL AUTOPSY

Examination of the dead body by an experienced forensic pathologist seldom fails to reveal important information, especially when backed by a well-equipped and staffed laboratory. The examination should be made as early as possible, before decomposition has set in, but it is never too late to examine what remains of the body. Bones, teeth and hair are minimally destructible and other organs may decay slowly; any of these may provide information. No one should refuse to make an examination on the ground that putrefaction is too far advanced. Special care should be taken in the case of a body believed to be Australia antigen positive.

An autopsy should never be performed in poor conditions. A properly lit and equipped post-mortem room is essential and a body may be removed out of a coroner's district if suitable arrangements cannot be made locally.[23] Notes must be made at the time and a tape recorder is often invaluable. Proper containers for specimens of blood, body fluids and hair should be at hand. The body should be identified by relatives or by the officer in charge of the case to the pathologist. Clothing should be removed with care, piece by piece, listed and laid aside or wrapped separately, not bundled together. An identifying police officer must always be present in suspected crime.

Records of body temperature, extent and position of hypostasis and rigor mortis should be made. External examination of the body is highly important and should be made with care. Scars and petechiae should be noted. Strangulation marks and injection sites are easily missed. Any injury which has special significance should be photographed with a scale laid alongside.

The dissection should be conducted according to circumstances but a standard routine will ensure that no part is omitted. If an operation has been performed precise details should be available. Fluids should be collected early, with all the necessary precautions to prevent contamination and to ensure preservation. Some may need special conditions of storage. No autopsy is complete until all parts of the body have been examined. If the naked eye examination of the body fails to reveal a cause of death, the pathologist should take all the specimens for histology and culture that he thinks may be required, in addition to those taken for toxicology. Although the Coroners (Amendment) Act 1926 requires the coroner to request any persons with special qualifications to perform these examinations, the coroner will obviously be advised as to the examinations needed.

In the cases of sudden deaths in infants or in deaths during or consequential upon childbirth, the assistance of a pathologist who specialises in these particular cases should be considered.

Poisoning

The nature of a death by poisoning is often apparent from the start, but if there is any uncertainty, the advice of a toxicologist should be obtained on the samples that need to be taken. This is particularly important in cases where minute quantities of drugs, such as LSD or the solvents of glue sniffing, are being sought. The standard screening for drugs, followed by the more specific routine tests may not detect such poisonings. It is too late to take urine and bile samples after the body has been dissected. Rapidly-acting and quickly metabolised drugs, such as barbiturates and tranquillisers may disappear before death so that analytical proof is not always feasible. The coroner should be informed that he must rely on circumstantial evidence and negative findings in reaching a decision. Every effort should be made to secure any samples that were taken by a hospital when the patient was first admitted, when the death has taken place later.

THE CORONER AND HOMICIDE

If the cause of death is unnatural the coroner is required to inquire into murder, manslaughter and infanticide. He may not record a criminal finding and may not name any person responsible. The inquisition should state, simply, that the deceased person was unlawfully killed.[24]

For example, if a woman is found stabbed and her husband is found poisoned with a suicide note expressing his intention, possible suspicion of living persons may be allayed by asking a police officer in court whether the person they wish to interview is dead. While the suspect may not be named in the inquisition there is no need, when the deaths are closely related in place and time, for the inquests to be artificially separated.[25]

No verdict shall be framed in such a way as to appear to determine any question of (1) criminal liability on the part of a named person, (2) civil liability.[26]

CHARGES OF HOMICIDE

If a coroner is informed that a person has been charged with murder, manslaughter or infanticide, causing death by reckless driving[27] or aiding or abetting suicide[28], he opens an inquest for the purpose of obtaining registrable particulars and adjourns until the conclusion of criminal proceedings.[29] If a coroner is informed by the Director of Public Prosecutions that some person has been charged before justices with an offence (whether or not involving the death of a person other than the deceased) alleged to have been committed in circumstances connected with the death of the deceased, not being a homicide he shall, if so requested, adjourn the inquest.[30]

There is provision for resuming an adjourned inquest after the conclusion of criminal proceedings; this is governed by strict legal safeguards and is practically never used. The progress of a prosecution through the criminal courts is notified to the coroner by the Court's administrators but these are administrative formalities which need not concern the medical jurist.

THE CORONER'S JURY

A person shall be qualified to serve as a juror at a coroner's inquest only if he is qualified to serve as a juror in other courts.[31,32] He must be on the electoral register, between the ages of 18 and 65 and fulfil the requirements as to residence. He must not be ineligible or disqualified. The coroner may appoint an appropriate officer to question any person summoned by the procedure used to obtain jurors for the other courts.[33,34] Penalties are prescribed for refusing to answer the questions or for making false representations.[35]

A jury is statutorily required in specified instances,[36] if there is reason to suspect:
1. that the death occurred in prison or in such place or in such circumstances as to require an inquest under any Act other than the Coroners Act 1887, or
2. that the death was caused by an accident, poisoning or disease, notice of which is required to be given to a government, under or in pursuance of any Act, or
3. that the death occurred in circumstances the continuance or possible recurrence of which is prejudicial to the health or safety of the public or any section of the public.
This last section was considered at length by the Court of Appeal in the case of Blair Peach. The judgement makes it difficult to hold an inquest without a jury if a jury is demanded.[37]

THE INQUEST

Every inquest shall be opened, adjourned and closed in a formal manner[38] and every inquest shall be held in public.[39] No inquest shall be held on a Sunday, Christmas Day, Good Friday or a bank holiday unless there are special reasons.[40]

Any properly interested person, as defined by the Coroner's Rules, shall be entitled to examine any witness either in person or by counsel or solicitor. The definition of a properly interested person is set out later.[41,42] No person may be asked a question the answer to which might show that he had committed an offence.[43]

The proceedings at an inquest shall be directed solely to ascertaining:
1. who the deceased was;
2. how, when and where the deceased came by his death;
3. the particulars for the time being required by the Registration Acts to be registered concerning the death.[44]

This restriction of the scope of the inquest, taken with the rule that no verdict shall appear to determine any question of criminal liability on the part of a named person or civil liability, does not mean that evidence concerning the death which discloses a potential civil action or a crime must be excluded. If evidence of certain serious crimes is disclosed, the inquest must be adjourned and the matter referred to the Director of Public Prosecutions. In all cases, it must be stressed that the inquest cannot inquire into allegations of negligence or of crimes that did *not* affect the cause of the death. Allegations of delay in diagnosing or treating a natural illness would not necessarily make the death an unnatural one and so bring it within the scope of an inquest. The correct procedure in these cases is to bring a civil action or to make a complaint to the Health Authority.

The coroner shall take notes of evidence at every inquest.[45] The duty to take depositions in murder or manslaughter no longer has effect.[46] Copies of notes of evidence may be supplied to any person who, in the opinion of the coroner, is a properly interested person. Proper interest is defined as a parent, spouse, child or personal representative of the deceased, an insurer or beneficiary of an insurance policy, a person whose act or omission may have caused the death and an employer of such a person,[47] a representative of a Trade Union to which the deceased belonged if he died as a result of his employment. (NB, This does not include a representative of a Trade Union representing a witness, only the deceased.) An inspector under the Health and Safety at Work etc. Act 1974. The Chief Officer of Police and any other person who is properly interested in the opinion of the coroner.

Coroners' jurisdiction

Subject to a Home Office direction (see below) a coroner could only hold an inquest upon a body that he had viewed in his jurisdiction. If it was thought that it would be more convenient to hold the inquest within the jurisdiction of another coroner, it may be necessary to transport the body to that area. The Coroners Act 1980 abolished this need for the view and enacted that the jurisdiction over the inquest could be transferred without moving the body. The second coroner had all the powers that would have been held by the coroner with possession of the body.

Where a coroner has reason to believe that a death has occurred in or near his jurisdiction and that the body has been destroyed or is irrecoverable, he may apply to the Secretary of State for directions to hold an inquest.[48]

DEATHS OVERSEAS

The duties of a coroner in connection with a body lying within his jurisdiction are not affected by the fact that the death took place overseas.[49] Save for certain provision, such as the Merchant Shipping Acts,[50] such a death cannot be registered in England. If the death is known to be due to a natural cause, such a death need not be referred to a coroner and the Registrar of Deaths may give a certificate of non-liability to register. The Home Office may give a certificate for cremation, when required.

DISPOSAL OF THE BODY

Burial

No body may be disposed of except by the authority of a Registrar of Death's Certificate for disposal

or by a coroner's order for burial, cremation or removal out of England. When a natural death has been certified by a registered medical practitioner the registrar supplies the informant with a certificate for disposal after registration.[51] If the registrar has received notice of the death he may, before registration, give a certificate for disposal before registration.

A registrar shall not give a certificate for disposal before registration except for the purpose of burial in England or Wales and then only:
1. where the death is not required to be reported to the coroner;
2. when the coroner has informed the registrar that he has completed his investigation and has not issued any order for disposal of the body.[52]

If the coroner is satisfied that no post-mortem or inquest is necessary he notifies the registrar on form 100 part A. If a post-mortem has been performed, but if there is to be no inquest, the coroner completes part B. From the colour these forms are generally known as pink form A or B. If an inquest is to be held the coroner issues an order for burial at any time; he need not have opened the inquest.[53] If pink form procedure is used the registrar issues the disposal order.

Cremation[54]

Cremation may only take place in a crematorium of which notice of opening has been given to the Secretary of State. Cremation of the remains of a person who has left a direction to the contrary, of an unidentified person and of a body which has been anatomically dissected is permissible. The registrar must have supplied a certificate for disposal after registration.

The person proposing to cremate, usually an executor or near relative, applies to the crematorium authority on form A. The circumstances of the death must be described and the possibility of violent or unnatural death mentioned. Names of doctors who have treated the deceased should be given.

The practitioner in attendance on the last illness completes form B. He must disclose any relationship or financial interest in the death. The history of the illness, mode of death, length of attendance and any operation must be described. He must examine the body and state the nature of the examination. He must give the names of nurses and other persons who attended the deceased, state any doubts which he has about the death and certify, provided it is so, that he has no reason to believe that it was violent or unnatural. The practitioner who completes from B has usually signed the certificate of cause of death; if not, he gives the name of the certifying doctor.

A confirmatory medical certificate must be given on form C by a registered medical practitioner of at least five years standing who is not a relative or partner of the doctor who signs form B. He must see the body. He should see and question the certifying practitioner and those who were about the deceased at the time of death. The documents are delivered to the medical referee of the cremation authority, usually by the funeral director.

Medical referee

The medical referee of a cremation authority is appointed by the Home Office; he is often, though not necessarily, a community physician. He must ensure that the death has been registered and that the applicant is a proper person to do so. The referee has power to direct a post-mortem examination and if this reveals a natural cause of death he issues certificate D. In these circumstances, or when a person licensed under the Anatomy Acts has signed form H after dissection, forms B and C may be omitted. Instead of directing a post-mortem himself the referee may inform the coroner. Form G is the register kept by the registrar of the cremation authority.

The coroner and cremation

When a death is reported to a coroner he assumes responsibility for authorising cremation although the medical referee must still add his approval. If the coroner is satisfied that neither post-mortem nor inquest is necessary he informs the registrar and form B and C procedure is followed. If, after post-mortem examination, he decides that an inquest is unnecessary, the coroner issues authority for cremation on form E; B and C certificates are not required. A coroner may also sign form E at any time after opening an inquest.

Anatomical dissection

The Home Secretary may grant a licence to practice anatomy to any person qualified by a University Faculty of Medicine or by a College of Physicians or Surgeons.[55] He also appoints Inspectors of Anatomy to supervise the suitability of places where anatomy is practised and to keep records of dead bodies supplied.[56] An executor or person lawfully in possession of a body may permit anatomical examination.[57] No body may be removed for 48 h after death from the place of death and 24 h notice must be given.[58] The person receiving the body for dissection must notify the Inspector of Anatomy within 24 h.[59] After dissection the body must be decently interred or cremated within two years;[60] the Secretary of State has power to vary this interval.[61]

Removal out of England

Every person intending to remove a body out of England must give notice of his intention to the coroner for the jurisdiction in which the body is lying; the registrar's or coroner's disposal, if any, must accompany the notice.[62] This ensures that two valid orders for disposal of the body do not exist at the same time. The coroner acknowledges the notice, informs the registrar of its receipt and returns to the registrar his disposal order.[63] The coroner must retain his own burial or cremation order unless it is intended to cremate in Scotland, Northern Ireland, the Channel Islands or the Isle of Man when he must endorse his cremation to that effect.[64]

The body may not be removed out of England until four days have elapsed since the receipt of notice by the coroner. This requirement may be, and usually is, waived by the coroner.[65]

Most countries receiving a body require a certificate of freedom from infection and that the body be sealed in a metal shell. The funeral director will obtain precise information on these points.

Burial at sea

Those who have followed a maritime career may leave instructions that their bodies shall be buried at sea. Removal out of England procedure should be followed.

EXHUMATION

In order to disinter a body from consecrated ground it is necessary to obtain a licence, or faculty, from the Diocesan Registry. Provided that the purpose is to rebury in consecrated ground no further authority is needed. In other circumstances, to exhume for cremation or to send the body out of the country, an order from the Secretary of State is required in addition to the faculty.[66] There are some exceptions under town and country planning which do not concern the medical jurist.

The coroner's exhumation

The coroner may order the exhumation of a body within his jurisdiction for the purpose of holding an inquest or discharging any other function of the coroner or for the purposes of any criminal proceedings connected with that person or some other person who died in connected circumstances. The old common law powers of the coroner have been abolished.[67]

Procedure at exhumation

An exhumation has news value and a senior police officer should make such statements to members of the press as he thinks desirable. Privacy should be preserved but absolute secrecy is seldom attained. Only those with a duty to perform should attend. These would include cemetery staff, a doctor who has attended the deceased, the pathologist, doctors representing a person under suspicion and funeral directors who may be able to identify the coffin.

The disinterment should take place in daylights; the tradition of carrying it out at dawn has no merits. Soil to within a few inches of the top of the coffin may be removed on the previous day. The cemetery superintendent locates the place of burial from his records and this may be confirmed by a gravedigger. As the coffin is raised the pathologist takes samples of earth and water from above and on each side and later from the bottom of the grave. The funeral director then identifies the coffin.

The coffin is taken to a mortuary before being opened. It is placed on trestles beside the autopsy table and the lid is raised. Although the body is seldom in a fit state for identification it should be viewed by those who placed it in the coffin and, if appropriate, by a friend or relative.

The post-mortem examination in no way differs from a regular medico-legal autopsy. Specimens should be taken and the containers carefully labelled. Before leaving the pathologist should ensure that he has all the material he requires, as there will be no good opportunity for coming back for more once the body is reburied.

A full report of the examination, together with detailed information about the identification, should be transmitted to the coroner and to the senior officer of police. No information should be given to the press or to any member of the public.

FURTHER READING

Anatomy Acts 1932 and 1971.
Births and Deaths Registration Act 1953.
Coroners Act 1887.
Coroners (Amendment) Act 1926.
Coroners Act 1980.
Coroners (Amendment) Rules 1977, SI 1977, No 1881.
Coroners Rules 1953, SI 1953, 2o 205.
Cremation Regulations 1930, SR & O 1930, No 1016, amended by SI 1965, No 1146.
Criminal Law Act 1977 (especially S 56).
Human Tissue Act 1961.
Polson, C. J. & Marshall, R. K. (1975) The Disposal of the Dead, 3rd edn. Sevenoaks: English Universities Press.
Purchase, W. B. & Wollaston, H. W. (1975) Jervis on Coroners, 9th edn. Sweet & Maxwell.
Registration (Births, Stillbirths and Deaths) (Prescription of forms) Regulations 1953.

Registration (Births, Stillbirths, Deaths and Marriages) Consolidated Regulations 1954, SI 1954, No 1596, amended by SI 1960, No 1604.
Removal of Bodies Regulations 1930, SR & O 1930, No 1016, amended by SI 1965, No 1146.
Report of the Committee on Death Certification and Coroners (The Brodrick Report), Cmnd 4810 (1971) London: Her Majesty's Stationery Office.
Russell Davies, M. R. (1965) The Law of Burial, Cremation and Exhumation, 3rd edn. London: Shaw & Sons.
The Removal of Cadaveric Organs for Transplantation. A Code of Practice (1983) London: DHSS.
Thurston, G. (1980) Coronership, 2nd edn. Chichester: Barry Rose.
Wolstenholme, G. E. W. & O'Conner, M. (1966) Ethics in Medical Practice. London: J. & A. Churchill.

REFERENCES

1. Code of Virginia 32–364. 3:1 effective on 1 June 1973.
2. Healing Arts Practice Act of the District of Columbia (45 Stat 1326; title 2, ch. 1, DC code 1951 ed.).
3. The Removal of Cadaveric Organs for Transplantation. A Code of Practice (1983) London: DHSS.
4. Human Tissue Act 1961, s 1 (1).
5. Ibid., s 1 (2).
6. Ibid., s 1 (7).
7. Human Tissue Act 1961, s 1 (5).
8. Births and Deaths Registration Act 1953, s 22.
9. Registration (Births, Stillbirths and Deaths) (Prescription of Forms) Regulations 1953, Reg 10 (1).
10. Report of the Committee on Death Certification and Coroners November 1971, Cmnd 481, paragraphs 5.12 and 7.06.
11. Registration of Births, Deaths and Marriages Regulations 1968, (51)(1).
12. Prison Rules 1964, SI 1964, No 338, Rule 19 (2): also see Coroners Act 1887, s 3 (1).
13. Removal of Bodies Regulations 1954, SI 1954, No 448 and SI 1971, No 1934.
14. Coroners (Amendment) Act 1926, s 1.
15. Local Government Act 1972, s 220 (1).
16. Coroners Act 1887, s 3 (1).
17. Criminal Law Act 1977, s 56 (1).
18. Coroners (Amendment) Act 1926, s 3 (1).
19. Coroners Rules 1953, SI 1953, No 205, rule 3 (a).
20. Ibid., rule 3 (b).
21. Ibid., rule 4 (2) & (3).
22. Ibid., rule 7.
23. Coroners (Amendment) Act 1926, s 24.
24. Criminal Law Act 1977, s 56 (1).
25. Home Office Circular 187/1977, p. 3, clause 11.
26. Coroners Rules 1953, SI 205 1953 as amended by Coroners (Amendment) Rules 1977, SI 1881 1977, rule 7.
27. Road Traffic Act 1972, s 1 (2).
28. Suicide Act 1961, s 2 (1).
29. Coroners (Amendment) Act 1926, s 26 1 (a) as amended by the Criminal Law Act 1977, schedule 10.
30. Ibid., s 20 (b).
31. Coroners Juries Act 1983 s 1.
32. Juries Act 1974 s 1.
33. Coroners Act 1887 s 3A (4) as amended by above Act
34. Ibid. s 3A (7).
35. Ibid. s 3A (6).
36. Coroners (Amendment) Act 1926, s 13 2, modified by Criminal Law Act 1977, s 56 2.
37. Ex Parte Peach 1980, 2 W.L.R. 496.
38. Coroners Rules 1953, SI 1953, No 205, rule 13.
39. Ibid., rule 14.
40. Ibid., rule 15.
41. Ibid., rule 16.
42. Coroners Rules 1980.
43. Ibid., rule 18.
44. Ibid., rule 26.
45. Coroners Rules 1953, SI 205 1953, rule 30.
46. Criminal Law Act 1977, schedule 12.
47. Coroners Rules 1953, SI 1953 205, rule 16.
48. Coroners (Amendment) Act 1926, s 18.
49. Ex Parte Smith. Times Law Report July 31 1982.
50. Merchant Shipping Acts 1970 and 1979.
51. Births and Deaths Registration Act 1953, s 24 (1).
52. Registration (Births, Stillbirths, Deaths and Marriages) Consolidated Regulations 1954, reg 88 (2).
53. Coroners Rules 1953, SI 1953 205, rule 11, third schedule.
54. This section gives an outline of the rules for cremation contained in the Cremation Regulations 1930, SR & O 1930, No 1016 amended by SI 1965, No 1146. The lettered forms are specified in the regulations.
55. Anatomy Act 1832, s 11.
56. Ibid., s 2.
57. Ibid., s 3; Human Tissue Act 1961, s 1 (4).
58. Anatomy Act 1932, s 9.
59. Anatomy Act 1932, s 11.
60. Ibid., s 13,; Anatomy Act 1871, s 2; Human Tissue Act 1961, s 3; Cremation Regulation 1930, SR & O 1930 1016, reg 8 (d); SI 1965, No 1146, reg 3; Anatomy (England and Wales) Order 1940, SR & O No 458.
61. Anatomy Act 1871, s 2.
62. Removal of Bodies Regulations 1954, SI 1954 448, reg 4.
63. Ibid., reg 5 (1).
64. Removal of Bodies (Amendment) Regulations 1971, No 1354, reg 3.
65. Removal of Bodies Regulations 1954, SI 1954 448, reg 6.
66. Burial Act 1857, s 25.
67. Coroners Act 1980, s 1(c) and 4(1).

4

Laws relating to medical practice

MEDICAL NEGLIGENCE

Medical negligence is a complicated subject and the liability of the doctor will always depend upon the circumstances of the particular case. The injury to the reputation of a member of the medical or dental profession resulting from a finding of negligence can be very serious indeed and this is appreciated by the Courts. In his summing up to the jury in the action of *Hatcher* v. *Black and others*,[1] the trial judge said:

In the case of an accident on the road, there ought not to be any accident if everyone used proper care and the same applies in a factory; but in a hospital, when a person goes in who is ill and is going to be treated, no matter what care you use there is always some risk. Every surgical operation involves risks. It would be wrong, and indeed bad law, to say that simply because a misadventure or mishap occurred, thereby the hospital and the doctors are liable. Indeed it would be disastrous to the community if it were so. It would mean that a doctor examining a patient, or a surgeon operating at a table, instead of getting on with his work, would for ever be looking over his shoulder to see if someone were coming up with a dagger. For an action for negligence against a doctor is for him like unto a dagger. His professional reputation is as dear to him as his body, perhaps more so, and an action for negligence can wound his reputation as severely as a dagger can his body. You must not, therefore, find him negligent simply because something happens to go wrong, as for instance, if one of the risks inherent in an operation actually takes place or because some complications ensue which lessen or take away the benefits that were hoped for, or because, in a matter of opinion, he makes an error of judgment. You should only find him guilty of negligence when he falls short of the standard of a reasonably skilful medical man. In short, when he is deserving of censure—for negligence in a medical man is deserving of censure.

In the case of *Roe and Woolley* v. *The Ministry of Health*[2] and an anaesthetist, which went to the Court of Appeal, it was held that neither the anaesthetist nor any other member of the hospital staff

had been guilty of negligence and when delivering his judgment Lord Justice Denning said:

It is so easy to be wise after the event and to condemn as negligence that which was only a misadventure. We ought always to be on our guard against it, especially in cases against hospitals and doctors. Medical science has conferred great benefits on mankind but these benefits are attended by unavoidable risks. Every surgical operation is attended by risks. We cannot take the benefits without taking the risks. Every advance in technique is also attended by risks. Doctors, like the rest of us, have to learn by experience; and experience often teaches in a hard way.

The doctor's legal obligation to his patient

It is the duty of every registered practitioner to bring to bear upon all his professional activities that standard of skill and knowledge which is to be expected of a practitioner of his experience and status and of comparable standing to him. It is also his duty to exercise reasonable care in his treatment of a patient. If the failure to exercise the necessary degree of skill or care results in injury to the patient he will have a right of action for damages. Whether reasonable skill or care has been exercised in a particular case is a matter which has to be considered in relation to the facts of each individual case but a number of conclusions from decisions of the Courts may be drawn.

The specialist is not necessarily expected to possess the highest degree of knowledge or to use the highest degree of skill. He would not be answerable in law merely because it could be established that some other specialist in his particular field might have shown greater skill or knowledge or might have handled the case differently. For instance, the degree of skill and knowledge to be expected of a surgical specialist practising in a remote country district would not be that which would be demanded from a consultant surgeon in a teaching hospital. Similarly, a general practitioner who, by virtue of an emergency and necessity, operates in a remote cottage hospital or in the patient's own home, would be judged only by what in the circumstances it was reasonable to expect of a general practitioner who did not profess to be a surgical specialist. He would not be liable unless it were shown that he had fallen short of what could reasonably have been expected of a practitioner acting outside his own normal sphere of work.

In the case of Hunter v. Hanley,[3] Lord President Clyde made the following observation: 'The true test for establishing negligence in diagnosis or treatment on the part of the doctor is whether he has been proved to be guilty of such failure as no doctor of ordinary skill would have been guilty of, if acting with reasonable care'. This is a concise and succinct definition of medical negligence.

Criminal negligence

In certain circumstances negligence may amount to a criminal offence and this goes beyond a mere matter of compensation. It involves an utter disregard for the life and safety of others and conduct deserving of punishment; consequently, the degree of negligence is a material factor.

The distinction between civil and criminal negligence was clearly drawn by Lord Hewart in the case of R. v. Bateman.[4] This was the memorable case in which Dr Bateman was charged with the manslaughter of a woman. During the course of the woman's labour Dr Bateman found it necessary to perform a version and, after delivering a stillborn child, he proceeded to do a manual removal of the placenta. Whilst removing the placenta he removed with it a portion of the uterus. The woman died and Dr Bateman was charged with manslaughter. Following his conviction he appealed to the Court of Criminal Appeal. His appeal was successful. During the course of his judgment Lord Hewart said that, in order to support a charge of manslaughter, the prosecution must satisfy the jury that the negligence of the accused showed such an utter disregard for the life and safety of others as to amount to a crime against the State and that the

accused's conduct must be so disgraceful as to warrant punishment.

Medical litigation

The medical malpractice problem in America, where doctors are covered by commercial insurance, has become so acute that in 1970 the President of the United States set up a special commission to consider the problem in all its aspects. Although doctors in Britain are only seldom charged with criminal negligence the number of civil actions against doctors based upon an allegation of negligence has increased considerably during the past three decades. Throughout the civilised world the public has become more and more compensation-minded and in recent years there has been a steady rise in the number of all classes of claims in which damages are sought for personal injuries whether they are sustained in road accidents, at work or otherwise. A claim may involve some other party and the damages may be apportioned according to the proportional responsibilities agreed upon or decided by the Court. There may, for example, be an apportionment of liability between a member of the hospital medical staff and a member of the nursing or laboratory staff.

In an action for negligence the Court has first of all to ascertain the facts. Often there is a direct conflict of evidence, for example, whether a particular examination was carried out. It is for the Court to determine whose evidence it will accept or reject. If the Court is not impressed by the evidence of the practitioner it will reject his version of the facts and the same applies to the evidence of the plaintiff or his witnesses. Only after it has ascertained the facts can the Court decide whether there has been negligence and, in reaching its conclusion, it is guided by the views of the expert witnesses who have been called to give evidence. If one expert supports the defendant and the Court is satisfied that his views represent that of a reputable school of thought it can find in favour of the defendant notwithstanding the contrary view held by another expert representing another school of thought. Whilst the law concerning the doctor's liability has not changed, its application by the Courts in recent individual cases has revealed a trend to the disadvantage of the practitioner. Those practising in this field of the law have noticed a 'swing of the pendulum' in the judicial approach to medical cases and in a number of these cases the Court has elected to disregard the school of thought which supports the defendant practitioner. When it is felt that the Court in finding negligence against a practitioner has reached the wrong conclusion the only valid criticism that can be made is that the Court preferred the evidence of the wrong expert and that it was misled by a practitioner who took the contrary view to the consensus of professional opinion on the facts of the particular case.

Although there has been an increase in litigation involving doctors practising in the United Kingdom, this has not been on the same scale as in the United States. It is generally believed that the increase in litigation against doctors and hospital authorities in the United Kingdom is due to two principal factors. The first is the impersonal element resulting from the introduction of the National Health Service Act in July 1948. The taking over of hospitals under the Act has brought about a radical change in the attitude and respect which patients had for their local hospitals and their staff. A good deal of this respect has now gone and with it an inherent unwillingness on the part of patients to institute proceedings against their local hospitals. The present attitude is that they are suing the 'State'. The general practitioner has also, to some extent, lost his status as the family friend and counsellor and his relationship with his patients has become, particularly in urban communities, more impersonal. This is especially so in large cities with a floating and non-indigenous population. The family doctor's relative immunity from malpractice claims has therefore diminished although the hospital authority and the hospital medical officer are still the more common targets.

The second factor arises from the operation of the Legal Aid and Advice Act 1949. This has made it possible for many members of the public who had hitherto not been able to afford to do so, to institute legal proceedings against a practitioner and/or a hospital authority for negligence. A person can hardly be blamed for instituting an action against a hospital authority in respect of personal injuries when he believes that he is suing the State at the State's expense! One of the features of the

legal aid scheme is that there are limitations upon those who have the right to claim the legal aid services. Eligibility for a legal aid certificate depends upon the applicant's capital and income and of a possession of 'disposable capital' or 'disposable income'. This means in effect that the applicant for a legal aid certificate has to undergo a 'means test'. Significant increases in the financial limits for legal aid have recently been made and the Lord Chancellor has estimated that 70% of average households are now eligible for legal aid. The legal aid scheme is administered by the legal profession and before a legal aid certificate is issued in a medical case the legal aid committee requires the applicant to provide a medical report from a doctor about his case. Legal aid committees consider each application on its merits and they will turn down an application for a legal aid certificate to sue a member of the medical profession or a hospital authority if they do not consider that the applicant has a *prima facie* cause for complaint.

When legal aid is not available the litigant is not necessarily forced to rely on his own resources. His trade union may feel disposed to give him financial support in respect of a personal injury claim and this may well involve a claim based upon an allegation of medical negligence.

Apportionment of liability in National Health Service hospitals

Shortly after the introduction of the National Health Service Act in 1948 the Ministry of Health informed hospital authorities[5] that, although they were authorised to go to the legal defence of other staff, they were not authorised to undertake the defence of any member of their medical or dental staff involved in an action for professional negligence. The Ministry issued instructions that, if it were sought to make the hospital authority responsible for the alleged negligence of a medical or dental practitioner on its staff, the authority should take such action as might be open to it to obtain a contribution or indemnity from the practitioner in respect of any damages and costs awarded against the hospital authority. As the result of this policy the defence organisations not infrequently saw the sorry spectacle of a practitioner appearing in court as a co-defendant with the governing body of the hospital, each seeking to blame the other for the injury sustained by the patient.

In 1954, as the result of the representations made by the medical defence organisations and the British Medical Association, this policy was modified.[6] The present policy is that where a practitioner is a member of a defence organisation and that organisation accepts responsibility for him, any payment made to the plaintiff is to be apportioned between the practitioner and the hospital authority as agreed privately by them. Failing agreement the practitioner's defence organisation and the hospital authority bear the damages in equal shares.

Accepted and approved practice

It is the normally accepted practice and standard of knowledge prevailing at the time of the act or omission complained of that must be applied when deciding whether the practitioner did or did not exercise reasonable skill or care. In the majority of cases a charge of negligence can be successfully resisted if the defendant practitioner can show that what he did was in accordance with current and approved practice. It is, however, for the Court and not the medical profession to determine whether or not negligence is established in a particular case. The Court will not be deterred from laying down that a particular practice was negligent if that practice had inherent and obvious risks. In the case of Urry v. Bierer[7] it was argued on behalf of the defendant—a consultant gynaecologist—that he had acted in accordance with an approved practice of a recognised school of opinion and that he had been justified in relying solely on the theatre sister's swab count. The action arose out of the retention of a surgical pack in the patient's abdominal cavity following the performance of a planned Caesarean section in a private nursing home. The trial judge concluded that both the gynaecologist and the theatre sister had been negligent and that the responsibility should be divided equally between them. The patient was awarded damages and an appeal was entered on behalf of the gynaecologist. At the Court of Appeal it was again argued that as the gynaecologist had followed a practice that was approved by many surgeons he should not be held to have been negligent and that the whole of the liability should fall upon the proprietors of the nursing home who had accepted the finding of negligence against the theatre sister. The appeal failed. The judgments of the trial judge and of the three judges of the Court of Appeal were to the effect that it was not sufficient for the surgeon to rely solely on the theatre sister's count but that he must himself take such additional precautions as are reasonable in the circumstances of the particular operation so as to minimise his dependence on the nurse's count.

Mistaken diagnosis

An erroneous diagnosis is negligent only if it implies an absence of skill or care. In the case of Whiteford v. Hunter[8] the plaintiff alleged that the defendant, a well-known surgeon, had been negligent in diagnosing as a cancer a condition which was in fact not cancer at all and that he had been negligent in not carrying out a cystoscopic examination and in not having performed a biopsy. The Court of first instance held that the surgeon had been negligent and the plaintiff was awarded damages. An appeal was entered on behalf of the surgeon and the case was taken to the House of Lords. Both the Court of Appeal and the House of Lords held that there had been no negligence on the part of the surgeon.

There have, of course, been numerous cases in which negligence in diagnosis has been established. In an action instituted against the Greenwich & Deptford Hospital Management Committee[9] the casualty officer was held to have been negligent in failing to diagnose acute appendicitis in an 11-year-old girl. She had been taken to hospital suffering from abdominal pain and vomiting. Following his examination of the girl's abdomen the casualty officer told the father that his daughter was suffering from a gastric upset and she was allowed to go home. Two days later the girl was seen by her general practitioner who had her admitted to hospital at once. An emergency laparotomy was carried out and this revealed generalised peritonitis due to a perforated gangrenous appendix. The girl died 36 h after the operation. In his summing up the judge stated that there was considerable onus on the court to ensure that persons did not obtain damages simply because a doctor had made a mistake. Nevertheless, he found that in this particular case the casualty officer had failed to exercise proper professional skill and care which all patients had a right to expect. The father, who had instituted the action in his capacity as administrator of the estate of his 11-year-old daughter, was awarded damages.

Clinical judgment

In 1970, after a trial of forceps and Caesarean section Stuart Whitehouse was born with severe brain damage. On his behalf his mother sued the obstetrician (at the time a senior registrar) alleging negligence and claiming damages for personal injury. After a trial lasting 11 days the trial judge found in favour of the infant plaintiff and awarded £100 000 damages. He found that the obstetrician at the trial of forceps had pulled too hard and too long so that the fetus became wedged or stuck and that in getting it wedged or stuck or unwedged or unstuck (prior to speedy delivery by Caesarean section, the obstetrician caused asphyxia which in turn caused the cerebral palsy.

By a majority decision the Court of Appeal reversed the decision and held that the obstetrician had not been negligent. In the appeal the difference between negligence and error of judgment was widely canvassed and the Master of the Rolls, Lord Denning, said: 'We must say, and say firmly, that in a professional man, an error of judgment is not negligent'.

This important statement was considered and expressly overruled when the case was reviewed on further appeal by the House of Lords[10] although the Court of Appeal judgment in favour of the obstetrician was upheld.

Dealing with the issue of clinical judgment, Lord Edmund-Davies said:

'The principal questions calling for decision are: (a) In what manner did Mr Jordan use the forceps, and (b) was that manner consistent with the degree of skill which a member of this profession is required by law to exercise?' Surprising though it is at this late state in the development of the law of negligence, counsel for Mr Jordan persisted in submitting that his client should be completely exculpated were the answer to question (b), 'Well, at worst he was guilty of an error of clinical judgment'. My Lords, it is high time that the unacceptability of such an answer be finally exposed. To say that a surgeon committed an error of clinical judgment is wholly ambiguous, for, while some such errors may be completely consistent with the due exercise of professional skill, other acts or omissions in the course of exercising 'clinical judgment' may be so glaringly below proper standards as to make the finding of negligence inevitable.

This view was re-enforced by Lord Fraser of Tullybelton in the following passage:

Having regard to the context, I think that the learned Master of the Rolls must have meant to say that an error of judgment 'is not necessarily "negligent"'. But in my respectful opinion, the statement as it stands is not an accurate statement of the law. Merely to describe something as an error of judgment tells us nothing about whether it is negligent or not. The true position is that an error of judgment may, or may not, be negligent; it depends on the nature of the error. If it is one that would not have been made by a reasonably competent professional man professing to have the standard and type of skill that the defendant held himself out as having, and acting with ordinary care, then it is negligent. If, on the other hand, it is an error that such a man, acting with ordinary care, might have made, then it is not negligent.

A supplementary but significant ruling emerged from this important case when Lord Wilberforce said:

I have to say that I feel some concern as to the manner in which part of the expert evidence called for the plaintiff came to be organised. . . . While some degree of consultation between experts and legal advisers is entirely proper, it is necessary that expert evidence presented to the court should be, and should be seen to be, the independent product of the expert, uninfluenced as to form or content by the exigencies of litigation. To the extent that it is not, the evidence is likely to be not only incorrect but self defeating.

In short doctors should write their own legal reports and not allow them to be written for them by lawyers.

Failure in communication

A failure in communication is a frequent cause of litigation against doctors and hospital authorities. If a patient's health is adversely affected or the treatment of an injury is jeopardised by a failure in communication it might well be difficult to resist the ensuing claim. During the past few years the defence organisations have been called upon to deal with several cases of this type. In the case of Chapman v. Rix[11] the trial judge held that, although the defendant's diagnosis had been clearly wrong, the evidence had not established that it had been a negligent diagnosis. The judge found, however, that the defendant had been negligent in respect of the allegation that he had failed to exercise reasonable care in not communicating with the patient's own doctor. The widow was awarded damages. An appeal was entered and the Court of Appeal reversed the decision and held that the defendant had not been guilty of negligence in failing to communicate directly with the patient's own doctor. The case was taken to the House of Lords which rejected the plaintiff's appeal and held that the defendant had not been negligent in failing to communicate directly with the patient's own practitioner. The basis for the decision of the Court of Appeal and of the House of Lords was that the defendant had acted in accordance with approved and current practice.

Failure to refer to consultant

In the case of Payne v. St Helier Group Hospital Management Committee[12] the trial judge held that the casualty officer's negligence consisted in failing to detain for examination by a consultant a man who had been kicked in the abdomen by a horse. On the day of his injury the man was seen in the hospital by the casualty officer and was allowed to go home. Several days later the man was found to be suffering from generalised peritonitis from which he eventually died. In his summing up the judge said that the casualty officer had not been justified in sending the man home but that he should have been detained in hospital for examination by a consultant.

What should a patient be told?

A 30-year-old freelance woman broadcaster was seen by a consultant physician at a teaching hospital. He concluded that she was suffering from a toxic goitre. She was told of the alternative forms of treatment and elected to undergo an operation. A consultant surgeon performed a subtotal thyroidectomy during the course of which the patient's left recurrent laryngeal nerve was injured. This resulted in paralysis of her left vocal cord which severely affected her voice. The patient brought an action[13] against the consultant physician, the consultant surgeon and the hospital authority. Against the physician she alleged that she had been negligently advised by him that the operation involved no risk to her voice, and against the surgeon she alleged that he had performed the operation negligently. The physician denied having told the

patient that there was no risk but the surgeon admitted that he had told her just that. In his summing up to the jury the trial judge said:

> What should a doctor tell a patient? The surgeon admitted that on the evening before the operation he told the patient that there was no risk to her voice although he was well aware that there was some slight risk but he did it for her own good because it was of vital importance that she should not worry . . . The law does not condemn a doctor when he only does what a prudent doctor so placed would do and none of the doctors called as witnesses have suggested that the surgeon was wrong. All the witnesses have agreed that it was a matter for the surgeon's own judgment. If they did not condemn him why should I? It is for you to say whether you think the physician told her that there was no risk whatever or he may have prevaricated to put her off as many a doctor would do rather than worry her, but even if you think that he did tell her that, is that a cause for censure?

The jury returned a verdict in favour of all three defendants.

Failure to X-ray

A common ground for a charge of negligence is failure to order an X-ray examination. The defence organisations deal with several claims on this ground every year. The Courts tend to assume that if a patient has an undiagnosed fracture or dislocation or if a foreign body in a wound was overlooked and no radiological examination was carried out the practitioner in attendance is *ipso facto* negligent. This is not good law. In the case of Sabapathi v. Huntley[14] the Judicial Committee of the Privy Council held that neither the defendant nor his assistant had been negligent because they had failed to recommend an immediate X-ray examination of the plaintiff's injuries sustained in a road accident. The Privy Council stated that the fact that the doctor attending a person injured in a road accident omitted to order an immediate radiological examination does not necessarily constitute negligence and that the advisability of such an examination must always depend upon the circumstances, including the condition of the patient, the nature of the injuries and the accessibility of the apparatus.

In the case of Braishaw v. Harefield & Northwood Hospital Management Committee,[15] the plaintiff alleged that the servants and/or agents of the hospital authority had been negligent in failing to order a radiological examination of his arm. The plaintiff had attended the casualty department stating that his arm had been 'knocked' by a piece of steel and this statement was recorded on the casualty card. He was found to have a laceration on his right upper arm. Examination of the wound revealed no evidence suggestive of any foreign body. No X-ray was taken and the wound was sutured. He made no complaint of any discomfort or pain when the sutures were removed. A few months later he developed pain in his right arm and was referred back to hospital. A radiological examination of his arm revealed the presence of a piece of metal which was removed without difficulty. The patient brought an action against the hospital authority alleging that his arm should have been X-rayed when he had first attended the casualty department. In view of the statement that the patient had made when he attended the hospital the Medical Defence Union felt that the casualty officer had been justified in assuming that there had been no high velocity penetration injury. The action was defended. In his summing up the judge said that as the plaintiff had stated that he had 'knocked' his arm the failure to order a radiological examination was not negligent and he dismissed the action. The plaintiff appealed. The appellant judge dismissed the appeal and said that this case showed that the Courts did not always find that there had been negligence because the patient had not been X-rayed and 'all such cases depended upon the circumstances of each particular case'.

In the case of McCormack v. Redpath,[16] a steel erector was hit on the head by a large spanner that had been accidentally dropped from a height of some 40 ft by a fellow workman. He was not rendered unconscious and was taken to hospital where he was seen by the casualty officer. His examination disclosed a laceration of the scalp but no apparent injury to the skull. The laceration was sutured and the patient was allowed to go home. He was off work for three weeks and during the next few months he complained of headache and dizziness. He was referred back to hospital and in due course was examined by a neurosurgeon. He found that the patient had a depressed fracture of the skull and that a piece of bone was protruding into the brain tissue. The piece of bone and a mass of scar tissue were removed. The patient subsequently suffered from epileptiform fits. He sued his employers, alleging negligence on the part of the workman who had dropped the spanner. The employers admitted this but claimed that all the plaintiff's injuries flowed from the negligence of the casualty officer in failing to diagnose the depressed fracture of the skull and to arrange for immediate surgical treatment. It was argued on behalf of the casualty officer that it was easy to be misled by an injury of this sort. The judge was unwilling to accept this defence and found that the casualty officer, whom he described as 'a most competent and careful young doctor', had in this particular instance fallen below the proper standard of skill and care in failing to arrange for an X-ray examination of the skull. The judge accepted, to a large extent, the submission put forward on behalf of the casualty officer that the plaintiff's injuries were attributable to the original accident and not to the casualty officer's failure to diagnose the fracture of the skull. The plaintiff was awarded damages against his employers but the casualty officer was ordered to contribute a substantial sum towards the damages.

The radiological examination of a patient following any sort of traumatic injury has nowadays become so much of a routine that it is quite likely that there would be a grave danger of a finding of negligence if no radiological examination was ordered in a case where the history was such as to suggest the possibility of a fracture or a dislocation or the presence of a foreign body in a wound.

Proof of negligence

The burden of proof in an action for negligence rests with the plaintiff and it follows therefore that in medical cases it is for the patient or his relatives to establish his claim and not for the medical practitioner to prove that he acted with due skill and care. In certain types of case the Court will accept that the nature of the occurrence complained of is such as to relieve the plaintiff from establishing that there was negligence and to place on the defendant the burden of proving the absence of negligence. In such cases the legal maxim res ipsa loquitur applies. An example of the application of this maxim was in the case of Cassidy v. Ministry of Health.[17] The plaintiff was operated upon for a Dupuytren's contracture of the third and fourth fingers of his left hand. After the operation the patient's left hand and forearm were bandaged to a splint which was kept in place for 14 days. During this period the patient complained of pain in his hand but apart from the administration of sedatives no other action was taken. When the bandage was removed it was discovered that all four fingers of the patient's hand were stiff and that the hand was to all intents and purposes useless. The Ministry denied negligence and liability for the surgeon under whose care the patient had been admitted. In the court of first instance judgment was given for the Ministry on the ground that the patient had failed to establish negligence on the part of the surgeon or of any other member of the hospital staff. The patient appealed. The Court of Appeal held that the mere proof of the facts would cause a reasonable layman to draw the inference that the injury could have been caused only by want of care on the part of the hospital staff and that it was sufficient to call for an explanation from the defendant. The appeal was successful and the plaintiff was awarded damages.

The British Courts are, however, somewhat reluctant to apply the doctrine of *res ipsa loquitur* in cases of alleged negligence in medical cases.

Degree of risk

Failure to take precautions to avoid a particular risk will only amount to negligence if the risk is of a substantial character. If the risk could be described as negligible then a failure to take precautions would be compatible with the exercise of proper skill and care. In 1935 an action[18] was reported which related to the death of a man aged 36 who had undergone an operation for the removal of 28 teeth. The man died from dental haemorrhage 24 h after the extractions. A post-mortem examination revealed that he had suffered from acute myeloid leukaemia. Proceedings were instituted by the widow against both the medical and the dental practitioner. The Court held that neither the doctor nor the dentist had been negligent in failing to examine the patient's blood before the extractions.

If the treatment or operation contemplated carries special risks which are known to the doctor but are probably unknown to the patient, the practitioner should, as a general rule, inform the patient of these risks and secure his consent to the treatment or operation. The doctor may, of course, in certain circumstances be justified in withholding or minimising the risk involved if he thinks it is necessary to do so in the interests of the patient.[19]

Gratuitous services

The legal duty which is imposed on the doctor to exercise due skill and care only arises where there is a doctor/patient relationship. If a doctor passes the scene of an accident in which some person has been injured and is in need of urgent medical attention he would not be held to have been negligent if he does not render assistance, as no doctor/patient relationship has been established and in consequence the doctor owes the patient no legal duty. If, however, the doctor goes to the assistance of a person who is injured in an accident a doctor/patient relationship is at once established. A doctor has a duty to exercise reasonable skill and care regardless of whether or not his services are being given gratuitously.

A National Health Service general practitioner is required by the terms and conditions of service to render emergency treatment to a person who applies for it whether or not he is on the doctor's list. If such a practitioner fails to attend an emergency call and a complaint is made against him it may well be that some disciplinary action will be taken against him by the health authority.

The good Samaritan

It is sometimes asserted that doctors are reluctant to render emergency aid at the scene of an accident because they fear that they will be sued for malpractice in the event of an unfortunate outcome. There is a widespread belief that many malpractice actions have resulted from such circumstances. In its report,[20] the Commission that was convened in the United States of America in 1970 to examine the medical malpractice problem in that country, exploded this myth. The Commission was aware of only one reported case in which a malpractice action was brought against a doctor in such circumstances and this was in Hawaii. Furthermore the Commission had no knowledge of any out-of-Court settlement of an action arising from that of a doctor rendering emergency treatment at the scene of an accident. The Medical Defence Union has never been involved in such an action. Though the fears of doctors about their potential liability for emergency aid may be real they appear to be based on little more than rumour or hearsay, generated and perpetuated in large part by the mass media. The legal risks involved are infinitesimal.

Inevitable accident

Where, during the course of treatment, an accident occurs which could not be avoided by any ordinary skill or care on the part of the doctor administering the treatment, the accident is said to be inevitable. The term 'inevitable accident' has been defined as an 'accident not avoidable by any such precautions as a reasonable man can be expected to take'. In the case of Gerber v. Pines[21] the plaintiff claimed damages against the defendant alleging that during the administration of a hypodermic injection the defendant left part of a broken needle in her buttock. The defendant denied liability and said that the breakage of the needle was due to a sudden muscular spasm and that no skill or care on his part could have prevented the fracture of the needle or the retention of the broken part in the plaintiff's body. The judge found that there had been no negligence on the part of the defendant in so far as the fracture of the needle was concerned. He found, however, that there had been a breach of duty on the part of the defendant in not informing the plaintiff or her husband that the needle had fractured and that a piece of it was still in her body. For this the judge awarded the plaintiff a small sum by way of damages.

In the case of Hatcher v. Black and Others[22] it was accepted by the Court that damage to the recurrent laryngeal nerve during the course of a thyroidectomy was an inherent risk of the operation and that such an injury could occur despite the adoption of all reasonable precautions.

Contributory negligence

The patient who ignores the advice of his doctor or fails to attend as requested for treatment might well lose his right, in part or in whole, to claim damages if harm ensues. There have been cases where the patient's own default was regarded as having been predominantly or at least partly responsible for the injury he suffered. By virtue of the Law Reform (Contributory Negligence) Act 1945 the Court is empowered to award damages proportionate to the defendant's share of the responsibility and this applies equally to actions for damages in respect of negligence leading to the death of any person. It is, however, only seldom that the Court will make a finding of contributory negligence against a patient. It would be only the more flagrant instances of stupidity or carelessness on the patient's part which might be held against him. It is often difficult to prove to the court's satisfaction that the injured person was also negligent and had therefore contributed to his own misfortune. A closely related defence in mitigation of damages is that the loss or injury was aggravated by the failure of the plaintiff to take reasonable steps to limit the effect of the defendant's negligence. It would be unreasonable, however, to expect a patient injured during the course of an operation to agree to undergo a further operation to remedy the injury if the additional operation itself entailed any serious risk.

In a recent American case[23] a Federal Trial Court ruled that the contributory negligence of the parents of a man who committed suicide after release from a veterans' hospital would debar them from recovering damages for the wrongful death of their son. The parents had brought a wrongful death action against the government claiming that the veterans' hospital had been negligent in releasing their son from custody when he had dangerous suicidal tendencies. The defence contended that the parents had been negligent in failing to have their son committed to another hospital after he had requested to leave the veterans's hospital which was not empowered to detain him against his will. The defence also argued that the parents had been negligent in failing to remove firearms from their home and in failing to inform the hospital of their son's dangerous suicidal tendencies. The Court held that the parents, who were the sole beneficiaries of their son's estate, could not be allowed to profit from their own negligence.

Competing techniques

'When there is more than one school of thought with competing techniques which have authoritative support a practitioner cannot be blamed for adopting either.' This pronouncement was made by the trial judge in the action of Moore v. Lewisham Group Hospital Management Committee.[24] The plaintiff, who developed a paralysis of the left leg following the administration of a spinal anaesthetic, alleged that the anaesthetist had been negligent simply because he had used a spinal anaesthetic for the purpose of a cholecystectomy. Conflicting views were expressed by the expert witnesses on the propriety of administering a spinal anaesthetic for a cholecystectomy. The judge held that the anaesthetist had not been negligent as he had followed a practice approved by many anaesthetists.

Negligence in anaesthesia

The administration of any kind of anaesthetic is a task calling for special knowledge and experience. Modern anaesthetic is complex and by no means free from danger. The responsibility of a doctor who administers an anaesthetic will, in the event of a disaster, be assessed with as much care as that of the surgeon. He must exercise due care throughout and his responsibility does not cease until the patient has recovered fully from the effects of the anaesthetic.

In the case of R. v. Gray,[25] the accused was found guilty of manslaughter at the Central Criminal Court and sentenced to 12 months' imprisonment. The accused, a consultant anaesthetist, was found to have been under the influence of the anaesthetic that he was administering to a two-year-old child. During the course of the operation—a herniorrhaphy—the surgeon observed that the child was pulseless and had ceased to breathe. The child died. It transpired that the accused was addicted to anaesthetic gases. The Court con-

cluded that his negligence was so inexcusable as to justify a finding of manslaughter.

CONSENT TO TREATMENT

No man of professional skill can justify the substitution of the will of the surgeon for that of his patient.[26]

A doctor has no right to do anything to a patient without his consent except in the case of an emergency when he must exercise his discretion. To do anything to the person of another is an assault, a wrong for which a doctor may have to pay damages even though he does no actual harm. When surgical operations are undertaken the patient's written consent should be obtained and as the full extent of the operation sometimes cannot be determined beforehand the surgeon should obtain a written authority to enable him to exercise his discretion when the exact nature of the condition has been ascertained. The patient's consent to an operation may be either express or implied; if express it may be either written or by word of mouth. Any one of these types of consent is equally effective as a means of defeating an action for assault. A written consent is preferable to an oral consent because it can more easily be proved to have been given. Where possible, it is advisable to have a witness present when an oral consent is given. The patient's written consent should invariably be obtained to any operation which requires a general anaesthetic and the form should include specific consent to the administration of a general anaesthetic. The nature of the operation should be entered on the form as precisely as is consistent with the best interests of the patient.

In the case of Breen v. Baker[27] the plaintiff alleged that the defendant—a consultant gynaecologist—had been guilty of an assault and negligence. The plaintiff was admitted to hospital suffering from a recurrence of excessive menstrual bleeding. During the course of the action she alleged that, although when she signed the consent form she had agreed to leave the nature and extent of the operation to the discretion of the gynaecologist, she had thought it was to be no more than a curettage but that she had not agreed to undergo a hysterectomy as she had hoped to have children.

She alleged that the hysterectomy to which she had been subjected had been unnecessary and that she had wantonly been deprived of the hope of having a child. The defendant's evidence was that there had been a full discussion with the plaintiff who had agreed that if at operation a hysterectomy was found to be necessary she would like this to be carried out at once. The defendant said that, as the result of the curettage, she had concluded that the bleeding was due to uterine fibrosis and that as she knew from experience that curettage would not be satisfactory she had proceeded with the hysterectomy.

In his summing up the judge said that the first issue to be decided was whether the operation had been performed with the plaintiff's consent. He had no hesitation, he said, in accepting the evidence of the defendant at this point. The second issue was whether the decision to perform the hysterectomy had been negligent. He said he had to decide whether the defendant had failed to exercise that degree of skill and care that a consultant gynaecologist should devote to a diagnostic problem during the course of an operation. He concluded that the defendant had not acted in any way improperly in performing a hysterectomy. He was satisfied that the defendant had diagnosed uterine fibrosis whilst carrying out the curettage; that it could not be said that there was negligence in removing the uterus of a woman aged 43 with uterine fibrosis and that the decision to perform a hysterectomy had been free from any taint of negligence. Accordingly he entered judgment for the defendant.

The age of consent

Section 8 of the Family Law Reform Act 1969 provides that the consent to medical, surgical or dental treatment of a minor who has attained the age of 16 years shall be effective consent and that in such cases it is not necessary to obtain the consent of the parent or guardian.

The need to obtain a fully-informed consent

The securing of a signature to a consent form should not be allowed to become an end in itself. The most important aspect of any consent procedure must always be the duty to explain to the patient or relative the nature and purpose of the proposed operation and thus to obtain a fully-informed consent.

The question of informed consent was considered by the High Court in Chatterton v. Gerson & Anor.[28] Miss Chatterton, aged 55, suffered intractable pain in the right groin following a herniotomy in which a nerve had been trapped. Normal analgesia failed to produce any relief and on two occasions she attended for treatment at a pain clinic established by Dr Gerson and the treatment administered consisted of intrathecal phenol injections. These did not cure the pain but caused neurological damage resulting in a loss of sensation in the right leg and foot.

In the action which Miss Chatterton brought against Dr Gerson she did not allege any fault in the treatment he had administered. She alleged, however, that her consent to the treatment was vitiated by a lack of explanation of what the procedure was and what were its implications so that she gave no informed consent and the operation was in law a trespass to her person and a battery. She further contended that the doctor was under a duty to give his patients such an explanation of the nature and implications of the proposed treatment that she could come to an informed decision on whether she wanted to have it or whether she would prefer to go on living with the pain which it was intended to relieve. In giving judgment for Dr Gerson, Bristow J. said:

It is clear law that in any context in which consent of the injured party is a defence to what would otherwise be a crime or a civil wrong, the consent must be real. In my judgment what the court has to do in each case is to look at all the circumstances and say 'Was there a real consent?' I think justice requires that in order to vitiate the reality of consent there must be a greater failure of communication between doctor and patient than that involved in a breach of duty if the claim is based on negligence. When the claim is based on negligence the plaintiff must prove not only the breach of duty to inform but that had the duty not been broken she would not have chosen to have the operation. Where the claim is based on trespass to the person, once it is shown that the consent is unreal, then what the plaintiff would have decided if she had been given the information which would have prevented vitiation of the reality of her consent is irrelevant.

In my judgment once the patient is informed in broad terms of the nature of the procedure which is intended, and gives her consent, that consent is real and the cause of the action on which to base a claim for failure to go into risks and implications is negligence, not trespass. Of course, if information is withheld in bad faith, the consent will be vitiated by fraud. But in my judgment it would be very much against the interests of justice if actions which are really based on a failure by the doctor to perform his duty adequately to inform were pleaded in trespass.

In this case, in my judgment, even taking Miss Chatterton's evidence at its face value, she was under no illusion as to the general nature of what an intrathecal injection of phenol solution nerve block would be, and in the case of each injection her consent was not unreal. I should add that getting the patient to sign a pro forma expressing consent to undergo the operation 'the effect and nature of which have been explained to me', as was done here in each case, should be a valuable reminder to everyone of the need for explanation and consent. But it would be no defence to an action based on trespass to the person if no explanation had in fact been given. The consent would have been expressed in form only, not in reality.

Consent for sterilisation

In 1973 the Minister of State, Department of Health and Social Security, was asked in the House of Lords whether 'it is a fact that under either English or Scottish law a woman must obtain her husband's permission for a sterilisation operation, but a man can have a vasectomy performed without the permission of his wife?'. He replied that he had been advised that there was no statutory requirement under either English or Scottish law that the consent of a spouse must be obtained to the sterilisation of the partner. It is debatable, however, whether in Common Law a man has a legal right to the opportunity of having children by his wife and whether, if deprived of that right without his agreement, he could claim damages against a surgeon. Accordingly doctors would be wise to continue to obtain the signatures of both spouses whenever possible until an actual Court case arises which would set a precedent under either English or Scottish law.

If the operation is to be carried out on therapeutic grounds it would not be necessary in law to obtain the consent of the spouse. If the patient is not living with his or her spouse the consent of the patient is all that is necessary.

Consent for abortion

The written consent of the patient who is to undergo a termination of pregnancy should always be obtained. If the patient is married and living with her husband the proposed operation should be discussed with him if time and circumstances permit. Every endeavour should be made to obtain his consent to the termination of the pregnancy unless the patient expressly forbids it. If the doctor in attendance honestly believes that the grounds for termination are reasonable despite an objection from the husband he need have little fear. If the patient is single, no consent is required from the putative father. It is not considered necessary in law to obtain the consent of the parents to terminate the pregnancy of an unmarried girl who has attained the age of 16. Prudence dictates, however, that the doctor should endeavour to obtain the consent of the parents of such a girl if she is living with them. The practitioner must obtain the girl's authority before he seeks the consent of her parents as her wishes must always be respected. If the girl is under 16 her parents should always be consulted even if she herself forbids the doctor to do so. In such cases the written consent of the parents should be obtained but their refusal should not be allowed to prevent a lawful termination to which the patient herself consents and which in the doctor's opinion is clinically necessary. A termination should never be carried out in opposition to the girl's wishes even if the parents demand it.

Jehovah's Witnesses

Children

It is generally accepted that the administration of a blood transfusion to a child in opposition to the wishes of the parents is an assault in law even if the child's life is in peril. The administration of a blood transfusion against the adamant refusal of the parents may lead to a Court action although it is doubtful if such an action would succeed. Although this is a matter for the practitioner himself to decide, he may feel that if the child's life is in danger a transfusion should be given despite the parents' opposition. When such a situation arises certain precautions should be taken. The doctor who is to administer the transfusion should discuss the position fully with the parents and explain as clearly as possible the purpose of the transfusion and the risks to the child if it is not given. This should be done in the presence of a medical colleague. If the parents still refuse they should be asked to sign a form acknowledging their refusal. If they refuse to do so a record should be made of their refusal in the clinical notes. If the practitioner should decide to administer the transfusion the parents' signed acknowledgement (or the note recording their refusal to sign it) will be evidence that they were warned of the dangers to their child. Equally, if the doctor should decide to be bound by the parents' refusal, there would be concrete evidence to show that the parents knowingly inhibited him from doing what he considered necessary.

In some cases when the child is in hospital advantage has been taken of the power given to magistrates by the Children and Young Persons Act 1969, to remove the child from the custody of the parents so that the necessary consent can be given by the person to whom the magistrates entrust the custody. The Department of Health and Social Security does not favour this procedure.

Adults

In so far as adults are concerned (in this context 'adult' means that the patient has attained the age of 16) the practitioner must appreciate that the adamant refusal of the patient to permit the administration of a blood transfusion in any circumstances places a restriction upon him. It must remain for the doctor in the exercise of his professional conscience to determine whether or not he will accept responsibility for the treatment of the patient under the limiting conditions imposed upon him. If the doctor should decide to accept these limiting conditions he should adopt the following procedure:

1. The patient should be interviewed in the presence of a witness. He should be given an unequivocal warning of the dangers that might arise as the result of his refusal to have a blood transfusion and an attempt should be made to make him change his mind.

2. If the patient remains adamant he should be asked to sign a form acknowledging the fact that, although he was warned that during the course of his treatment or operation he might require a blood transfusion, he was nevertheless unwilling to give his consent.

3. The patient's signature should be witnessed by the practitioner and by the witness who was present at the interview.

4. If the patient refuses to agree to a blood transfusion and also refuses to sign the form acknowledging this, the practitioner would be ill advised to accept any responsibility for the patient's treatment.

Statute of Limitations

The purpose of the Limitation Act 1939, as subsequently amended, is to protect defendants from stale claims and to encourage plaintiffs to institute proceedings within a reasonable period of time. Before 1963 the general position was that no action could be brought, where the damages claimed consisted of or included damages for personal injuries, after the expiration of three years from the date on which the incident which gave rise to the action occurred. 'Personal injuries' include 'any disease or any impairment of a person's physical or mental condition'. By virtue of the Limitation Act 1963 a plaintiff could sue for damages for personal injuries outside the normal three-year limitation period in certain circumstances if he obtained the leave of the court to do so. An application to the court was made *ex parte* and could not therefore be opposed by the prospective defendant. The Limitation Act 1975 does away with the need to obtain leave from the Court. Under this Act the three-year period runs from the date on which the cause of action accrued or the date (if later) of the 'plaintiff's knowledge'; this means knowledge that the injury was significant and that the injury was attributable wholly or partly to an act or omission of the defendant. A power is conferred on the Court (i.e. the Court in which the action is brought) to set aside a defence of limitation if, having regard to all the circumstances, it would be fair to do so as between the plaintiff and the defendant. If the injured person dies before the expiration of the three-year limitation period, the period—as respects the cause of action surviving for the estate of the deceased—runs from the date of death or, if later, the date of the personal representatives' knowledge.

Clinical notes

The importance of keeping accurate and contemporaneous clinical notes of findings on examination and all treatment administered cannot be overemphasised. Good notes are of inestimable value, not only when handing a patient over to another doctor but also in meeting any criticism that may arise. In many cases with which the medical defence societies have been concerned the notes have been found to be woefully inadequate. If a patient refuses to accept the advice of his doctor this fact should be recorded in writing. In such circumstances the doctor would be well advised to withdraw from the case and to inform the patient that he is not prepared to accept any further responsibility for his treatment. Those who teach students, housemen and assistants would render a great service to their profession if they insisted on proper note-taking during and subsequent to their training.

In the course of legal proceedings case notes are disclosable to the other side and many actions for alleged negligence have been imperilled because the notes did not tally with the evidence given by the doctor in the witness box. The omission of essential details from the notes may cast a doubt on the veracity of the witness. When there is a conflict of evidence the court will naturally attach importance to the notes written at the time. Good notes may, therefore, be of the greatest importance in supporting the doctor's evidence as against that of the plaintiff and his witnesses.

Summary

In the last resort the success or failure of every action for negligence against a practitioner depends upon the circumstances of the particular case. The vital question is always whether the practitioner exercised reasonable skill and care in the circumstances. The circumstances inevitably vary from case to case and a study of past decisions in medical negligence cases is indicative only of the manner in which the Courts apply the general laws of negligence to the facts of the particular case and of the kind of conduct which may amount to negligence.

GENERAL MEDICAL COUNCIL

The General Medical Council is, to all intents and purposes, the governing body of the medical profession. It was established by the Medical Act 1858. The Act was passed largely as a result of the initiative of the medical profession and the establishment of the Council was considered necessary to protect qualified medical practitioners from the competition of unqualified practitioners and for the protection of the public. The constitution and functions of the Council are regulated by the various Medical Acts. The preamble of the Medical Act 1858 began by stating that, 'It is expedient that persons requiring medical aid should be enabled to distinguish qualified from unqualified practitioners'. The general duty of the Council is to protect the public, in particular by keeping and publishing the Register of duly qualified doctors, by ensuring that the educational standard of entry to the Register is maintained and by taking disciplinary action against registered practitioners, if it appears by reason of their misconduct that they may be unfit to remain on the Register.

Constitution of the General Medical Council

The General Council consists of 93 members. Fifty of these are elected by a postal vote of the profession; 34 are appointed by universities with medical schools or by the Royal Colleges and Faculties and by the Society of Apothecaries of London; nine are nominated by the Crown on the advice of the Privy Council and the majority of these are required to be laymen. Because of the size of the Council much of its work has to be done by committees. The Council elects the President. He and the Registrar are responsible for directing the day-to-day work of the Council.

Quite apart from keeping and publishing the Register of duly qualified practitioners, one of the most important functions of the GMC relates to medical education. It is because of this function that the Council's membership includes representatives of nearly every university with a medical faculty and many of the Royal Colleges. The principal fields in which the Council's educational func-

tions are discharged include:
1. the undergraduate medical curriculum;
2. the pre-registration (house officer) year;
3. the recognition of overseas qualifications and internships;
4. the recognition of certain additional post-graduate qualifications.

A Royal Commission on Medical Education was appointed in 1965 and its report was published in 1968. In its report the Commission made no reference to the teaching of medical ethics or forensic medicine. In the joint memorandum submitted to the Royal Commission by the two English defence societies it was stated that in the interests of the patient, the doctor and the State, it was essential that adequate instruction should be given to students in both these subjects. The defence organisations recommended that students should be given guidance where ethical considerations conflict with their legal responsibilities and that the future doctor should be instructed in his legal and ethical conduct vis-à-vis his colleagues and his relationship with coroners, lawyers and the police. Although the National Health Service makes provision for the training of specialists, forensic medicine is excluded. Following the publication of the Royal Commission's report the British Academy of Forensic Sciences called a special meeting to discuss the place of medical ethics and forensic medicine in medical education. The meeting decided to make representations to certain medical members of both Houses of Parliament about these omissions from the Royal Commission's report. These representations were cited when the report came under scrutiny in the House of Lords in 1970 and subsequently in the House of Commons.

Privileges of registration

Registration confers a number of privileges. For example, only registered practitioners may hold medical appointments in the National Health Service or in the public services or in the armed forces. Furthermore, only registered medical practitioners may prescribe or supply dangerous drugs, issue statutory certificates and recover at law fees for medical advice and attendance. Registered practitioners may also claim exemption from jury service.

The use of the title 'doctor'

The use of the prefix 'doctor' is not controlled by any of the Medical Acts. Section 31 of the Medical Act 1956, whilst not forbidding the practice by the unqualified, enables the public to distinguish between qualified and unqualified practitioners. It prescribes penalties for the unlawful use of certain well-recognised titles including 'doctor of medicine' or any description implying that the user is registered under the Medical Act. The prefix doctor is not so included. The Medical Act 1956 raised the fine that might be imposed on a person for 'wilfully and falsely' holding himself out to be a registered medical practitioner from £20 to £500.

Annual retention fee

Until 1968 the Council had derived its income primarily from registration fees paid by doctors. In 1968 it had become clear to the Council that its income from this source was proving totally inadequate to finance its growing expenditure. In the circumstances the Council sought powers to charge an annual retention fee. These were conferred by the Medical Act 1969. The annual retention fee was initially fixed at £2 and is now £15. The annual fee may be claimed as an expense for income tax purposes.

Professional discipline

Statutory provisions

The disciplinary jurisdiction of the General Medical Council is regulated by sections 5–14 of the Medical Act 1978 and the Regulations made thereunder. This Act established three committees of the General Council known as the Professional Conduct Committee, the Health Committee and the Preliminary Proceedings Committee. The Act provides that where a fully registered person
1. is found by the Professional Conduct Committee to have been convicted (whether while so registered or not) in the United Kingdom or any of the Channel Islands or the Isle of Man of a criminal offence; or
2. is judged by the Professional Conduct Commit-

tee to have been (whether while so registered or not) guilty of serious professional misconduct, the Professional Conduct Committee may, if it thinks fit, direct that his name shall be erased from the Register or that his registration in the Register should be suspended (that is to say, shall not have effect) during such period not exceeding 12 months as the Committee may specify or that his registration shall be conditional on his compliance, during such period not exceeding three years as may be specified in the direction, with such requirements so specified as the Committee think fit to impose for the protection of members of the public or in his interests. The power of erasure applies also to practitioners with limited registration.

Convictions

The term 'conviction' applies only to a determination made by a Criminal Court in the British Isles. In considering convictions, the Professional Conduct Committee is bound to accept the findings of the Court as conclusive evidence that a doctor was guilty of the offence of which he was convicted. It is not open to a doctor to argue before the Committee that he was in fact innocent of an offence of which he has been convicted. It may, therefore, be unwise for a doctor to plead guilty in a Court of Law to a charge to which he believes that he has a defence. A conviction in itself gives the Committee jurisdiction even if the circumstances of the criminal offence did not involve professional misconduct. The Committee is, however, particularly concerned with convictions for offences which affect a doctor's fitness to practice.

The meaning of 'serious professional misconduct'

The expression 'serious professional misconduct' was substituted in 1969 for the phrase 'infamous conduct in a professional respect' which was sued in previous statutes. The phrase 'infamous conduct in a professional respect' was defined in 1894 by Lord Justice Lopes as follows:

If a medical man in the pursuit of his profession has done something with regard to it which will be reasonably regarded as disgraceful or dishonourable by his professional brethren of good repute and competency, then it is open to the General Medical Council, if that be shown, to say that he has been guilty of infamous conduct in a professional respect.[29]

In another judgment delivered in 1930 Lord Justice Scrutton stated that:

Infamous conduct in a professional respect means no more than serious misconduct judged according to the rules, written or unwritten, governing the profession.[30]

However, the venerable words of Lord Justice Lopes have been reviewed by the Judicial Committee of the Privy Council in two appeals from decisions of the Disciplinary Committee of the General Dental Council (where the same considerations apply).

In the first Lord Jenkins said:

Granted that ... the full derogatory force of the adjectives 'infamous' and 'disgraceful' ... must be qualified by the consideration that what is being judged is the conduct of a dentist in a professional respect which falls to be judged in relation to the accepted ethical standards of his profession, it appears to their Lordships that these two adjectives nevertheless remain as terms denoting conduct deserving of the strongest reprobation, and indeed, so heinous as to merit, when proved, the extreme professional penalty of striking off.[31]

In the second case Lord Edmund-Davies said:

For it has respectfully to be said that although prolonged veneration of the oft-quoted words of Lopes L. J. has clothed them with an authority approaching that of a statute, they are not particularly illuminating, it is for this reason that Lordships regard Lord Jenkins' exposition as so valuable that, without going so far as to say that his words should invariably be cited in every disciplinary case, they think that to do so would be a commendable course.[32]

The General Medical Council not only has the sole right of registering qualified practitioners but is also the only body that has the right to remove a doctor's name from the Register. This function is exercised by the Professional Conduct Committee which must hold a formal inquiry unless the request for the removal of his name emanates from the practitioner himself. The Committee is advised on questions of law by a legal assessor and normally sits in public. Witnesses may be subpoenad and evidence is given on oath. The Preliminary Proceedings Committee is a smaller committee which sits in private and, on the basis of written evidence and submissions, determines which cases shall be referred to the Professional Conduct Committee for inquiry. An inquiry by the Professional Conduct Committee is held in accordance with the procedure of a Court of law. The accusation against the doctor is formally presented and the facts have to be proved in accordance with the normal rules of evidence applicable in British Courts. The practitioner is entitled to be legally represented and is afforded all those safeguards against conviction which the law gives to those accused of having committed a crime.

At the conclusion of any inquiry in which a doctor has been proved to have been convicted of a criminal offence or is judged to have been guilty of serious professional misconduct, the Professional Conduct Committee must decide on one of the following alternative courses:

1. to admonish the doctor and conclude the case;
2. to place the doctor on probation by postponing judgment;
3. to direct that the doctor's registration be conditional on his compliance, for a period not exceeding three years, with such requirements as the Committee may think fit to impose for the protection of members of the public or in his interests;
4. to direct that the doctor's registration shall be suspended for a period not exceeding 12 months; or
5. to direct the erasure of the doctor's name from the Register.

Postponement of judgment

Where judgment is postponed the doctor's name remains on the Register during the period of postponement. When postponing judgment to a subsequent meeting the Committee normally intimates that the doctor will be expected, before his next appearance, to furnish the names of professional colleagues and other persons of standing to whom the Council may apply for information concerning the doctor's habits and conduct since the previous hearing. The replies received, together with any other evidence regarding the doctor's conduct, are then taken into account when the Committee resumes consideration of the case. If the information is satisfactory the case will then normally be concluded. If the evidence is not satisfactory judgment may be postponed for a further period or the Committee may direct suspension or erasure.

Suspension of registration

When a doctor's registration is suspended he ceases to be entitled to practise as a Registered Medical

Practitioner during that period. In such a case the Committee may, after notifying the doctor, resume consideration of his case before the end of the period of suspension and then, if it thinks fit, may extend the original period of suspension or order erasure. Before resuming consideration of the case in such circumstances the Committee may ask the doctor to give the names of referees from whom information may be sought regarding the doctor's habits and conduct in the interval. This information will be taken into account when the Committee resumes consideration of the case. Only if there is evidence that the doctor has not conducted himself properly, or if he is addicted to drink or drugs and has not responded to treatment, is the Committee likely to order further suspension or erasure.

Conditional registration

Examples of conditions which may be imposed are that the doctor should not engage in specified branches of medical practice or that he should practice only in a particular appointment or under supervision, or that he should not prescribe or possess controlled drugs.

When a doctor's registration is made subject to conditions the Committee may (after notifying the doctor) revoke the direction for condition registration, or revoke or vary any of the conditions, or it may extend the original period of conditional registration. If a doctor is judged by the Professional Conduct Committee to have failed to comply with any of the conditions of his registration, the Committee may direct suspension of his registration or erasure.

Erasure

Whereas suspension can be ordered only for a specified period, a direction to erase remains effective until the doctor makes a successful application for the restoration of his name to the Register. Such an application cannot be made until at least 10 months have elapsed since the original order took effect.

Appeal procedure

When the Professional Conduct Committee has

directed that a practitioner's name shall be erased or that his registration shall be suspended, the practitioner has 28 days in which to give notice of appeal from the direction to the Judicial Committee of the Privy Council. If he gives notice of appeal his registration is not affected unless the Professional Conduct Committee has made a separate order that the practitioner's registration shall be suspended forthwith. The Committee may make such an order if it is satisfied that to do so is necessary for the protection of the members of the public or would be in the best interests of the practitioner himself. There is a right of appeal against an order for immediate suspension to the High Court (in Scotland, the Court of Session) but such an appeal, whether successful or not, does not affect the right of appeal to the Judicial Committee of the Privy Council.

The more common type of offence and of professional misconduct which have in the past been regarded as grounds for formal inquiry by the Professional Conduct Committee are set out in the General Medical Council's booklet.[33]

Restoration to the Register after disciplinary erasure

Applications for restoration may be made at any time after 10 months from the date of erasure. If such an application is unsuccessful, a further period of at least 10 months must elapse before a further application may be made. An applicant may, and normally does, appear in person before the Professional Conduct Committee, and may be legally represented. The Committee determines every application on its merits, having regard among other considerations to the nature and gravity of the original offence, the length of time since erasure, and the conduct of the applicant in the interval.

Medical certificates

Doctors are constantly asked for certificates of various kinds and they should always be on their guard against carelessness in certifying. Careless or lax certification may result in a summons before the Professional Conduct Committee or, in a matter in which a National Health Service patient is involved, a 'fine' by the Department of Health. A medical certificate must always be regarded as a document of importance and the doctor should certify only what he is prepared to affirm on oath. He should not certify a statement which he does not personally know to be a fact. Many a doctor has been involved in a complaint because he relied on the patient's statements when issuing a certificate of incapacity for work without taking adequate steps to verify that they were accurate.

In the General Medical Council's booklet on 'Professional Conduct Discipline: Fitness to Practice, (1980), there appears the following sentence, 'Any doctor who in his professional capacity signs any certificate or similar document containing statements which are untrue, misleading or otherwise improper, renders himself liable to disciplinary proceedings'.

Several examples of the result of lax certification have been mentioned in the Annual Reports of the three British defence societies.

The Health Committee

The Medical Act 1978 also gives the Council jurisdiction where the fitness to practise of a doctor is seriously impaired by reason of his physical or mental condition. Where the Council receives information suggesting that the fitness to practise of a doctor may be seriously impaired, the information is first considered by the President or other preliminary screener. The doctor concerned may then be invited to undergo a medical examination to investigate his health. If he agrees, the medical examiners are asked to report on his fitness to engage in practice, either generally or on a limited basis, and on the management of his case which they recommend. The examiners' reports are communicated to the doctor. If he undertakes voluntarily to accept the recommendations of the medical examiners on the management of his case, including any limitations on his practice which they recommend, the preliminary screener normally requests a medical supervisor, who is often the doctor's own physician, to monitor the doctor's progress. Provided that the preliminary screener is satisfied that the doctor is implementing his undertaking, no further action is taken and the case is not referred to the Health Committee. If, however, a doctor refuses to be medically examined or fails after examination to undertake to follow the recommendations of the examiners, his case may be referred to the Health Committee. Cases may also be referred to the Health Committee by the Preliminary Proceedings Committee or by the Professional Conduct Committee, if evidence concerning a doctor's fitness to practise comes to light in the course of disciplinary proceedings. The Health Committee meets in private. The doctor whose case is being considered is entitled to be present and may be legally represented. If the Health Committee judge his fitness to practise to be seriously impaired by reason of his physical or mental condition, the Committee may attach conditions to his registration or suspend his registration. In 1981 the fitness to practise of 42 doctors was investigated. In nine cases the doctor was required to appear before the Health Committee and in six of these the Committee judged that the doctor's fitness to practise was seriously impaired: in one case they imposed conditions on his registration, and in the remaining five they directed that his registration should be suspended.[34]

GENERAL DENTAL COUNCIL

The Dentists Act 1921 was a most important landmark on the dental health of the nation. It restricted the practice of dentistry to registered dental practitioners and it set up the Dental Board and also provided for the supervision of the standard of dental education and for the exercise of professional discipline. The General Medical Council supervised the work of the Dental Board until the introduction of the Dentists Act 1957. This transferred the function of the Dental Board to the General Dental Council which became responsible for protecting the public, for maintaining a Register of Dentists and for removing dentists from the Register when they had shown themselves to be unfit to remain on it. It was also made responsible for the enrolment, training and behaviour of ancillary dental workers.

There are two standing committees that are responsible for the professional discipline of dentists. One is a small committee which sifts reports of the convictions of dentists and complaints of professional misconduct which appear to be frivol-

ous or vexatious in character. The other is a larger tribunal which considers each case in public in accordance with the rules of evidence applied in British Courts of law. The tribunal may hold an inquiry into the nature and circumstances of any conviction of a registered dental practitioner. It is bound by law to accept a conviction as conclusive evidence that the dental practitioner was in fact guilty of the offence. The tribunal may also hold an inquiry into an allegation that a registered dental practitioner has been guilty of serious professional misconduct for the purpose of determining whether or not the name of that dentist ought to be erased from the dentist's Register. The tribunal may find that the name of a dental practitioner ought to be erased on account of a conviction for an offence which is not directly concerned with his profession or practice. A dentist can appeal from a decision of the tribunal to the Judicial Committee of the Privy Council. Such an appeal must be lodged within 28 days of the service on the dentist of a notification by the tribunal of its decision to erase his name from the dentist's Register.

General Dental Council's warning notice

Every dentist should make himself acquainted with the Council's pronouncement on the subject of professional conduct and ensure that nothing that he does conflicts with the Council's notice which is sent periodically to every dental practitioner. These pronouncements relate to certain forms of conduct which may be held to be tantamount to 'serious professional misconduct' and may result in the erasure of the dentist's name from the Register. They include advertising and canvassing for the purpose of obtaining patients and the abuse of professional relationships.

MEDICAL ETHICS

From time to time attempts have been made to codify the standard of conduct of medical practitioners in the practice of their profession. The oath attributed to Hippocrates in the fifth century BC is the most honoured. This was intended to be affirmed by every practitioner on entry to the medical profession. Although only a few newly-qualified practitioners are now required to take the oath they nevertheless accept its spirit and intention as their ideal standard of professional behaviour.

An international code of ethics

The lapses from the Hippocratic ideal on the part of the medical profession in certain countries during the Second World War showed the need for a modern restatement of the Hippocratic oath and of the importance of reminding members of the profession of their ethical obligations. One of the first acts of the World Medical Association, which was established in 1947 on the initiative of the British Medical Association, was to produce a modern restatement of the Hippocratic oath. This became known as the Declaration of Geneva and in 1968 it was amended by the World Medical Assembly. The modern code of ethics is intended to apply both in times of peace and war and is set out in the British Medical Association's booklet.[35]

Professional secrecy

A great deal has been written about professional secrecy. The basis of the relationship between a doctor and his patient is that of absolute confidence, and the success of medical treatment depends to a large extent upon the confidence which the patient reposes in his medical attendant and this confidence in turn depends upon the doctor's discretion. Until recently it was generally believed that any information obtained by a doctor during the course of his professional relationship with a patient was sacrosanct and that, except under compulsion of law, such information could not be disclosed to a third party without the consent of the patient or, in the case of a child, without parental consent. It is now generally recognised that in the public interest there may be circumstances in which the doctor may feel that his duty to the community should override his ethical obligation to maintain professional secrecy. For instance, he may feel that he is under a moral and social obligation to disclose to the licensing authority the physical condition of a patient if his condition is such as to render him unsafe to drive a car, or to give information to the appropriate officer of the local children's authority or to the National Society for the Prevention of Cruelty to Children about a 'battered baby'. When a doctor feels that he is under a moral and social obligation to disclose confidential information to the appropriate authority, he must be guided by the dictates of his professional conscience.

The overriding consideration must always be the adoption of a line of conduct that will benefit the patient or protect his interests. If a police officer seeks information about a patient which the doctor can only disclose by a breach of professional confidence he should explain that to reveal the information would be to disclose facts that he has learnt during the course of his professional duties. It should be noted, however, that in 1974 the Lord Chief Justice ruled that a doctor had committed an offence by refusing to give a policeman information about a patient which might have led to the identification of a car driver who was suspected of having committed a motoring offence within section 168 of the Road Traffic Act 1972.[36]

Other third parties who frequently seek information from a doctor include employers who ask for reports on the medical condition of absent or sick employees and insurance companies who ask for particulars about the past medical history of proposers for life assurance or deceased policy holders. In all such cases where medical information is sought the doctor should make it a rule to refuse to give any information in the absence of the consent of the patient or the nearest competent relative.

If a solicitor should ask a practitioner for a medical report about one of his patients, and states in writing that he is acting for the patient, the practitioner would be justified in complying with the solicitor's request and provide him with a medical report. It should be noted, however, that the patient has the legal right to be provided with a copy of the practitioner's report. Where disclosure of information may have an adverse psychological effect upon the patient the practitioner who compiles the report should exercise his discretion about what he should include in his report.

If a practitioner is in any doubt about his course of action he should seek the advice of his defence organisation.

In the 1980 edition of the British Medical Association's booklet 'The Handbook of Medical Ethics' the principles of professional secrecy are set out in the following terms.

The nature of professional confidence varies according to the form of consultation or examination, but in each of the three forms of relationship the doctor is responsible to the patient or person with whom he is in a professional relationship for the security and confidentiality of information given to him.

A doctor must preserve secrecy on all he knows. There are five exceptions to this general principle:
1. the patient gives consent;
2. when it is undesirable on medical grounds to seek a patient's consent;
3. the doctor's overriding duty to society;
4. for the purposes of medical research, approved by the Chairman of the British Medical Association's Central Ethical Committee or his nominee;
5. the information is required by due legal process.

A doctor must be able to justify his decision to disclose information.

Abuse of professional confidence

Disciplinary proceedings may be taken against a doctor where it is alleged that he has improperly disclosed information which was obtained in confidence from or about a patient.

Furthermore, if a patient could show that his doctor had, by a breach of professional secrecy, brought upon him a loss that could be assessed in money, he might be entitled to damages. His plea would be that the understanding between him and the doctor had as one of its implied terms an obligation by the doctor to observe the universally recognised custom of professional secrecy. When a doctor is in doubt about a matter that may have legal implications he should consult his medical defence organisation.

The Criminal Law Act 1967

This Act abolishes the distinction between felonies and misdemeanours. The common law offence of misprision of felony, that is to say, of having knowledge of the commission of a felony but failing to inform the police, has disappeared. As the result

of this no doctor will be at risk of prosecution for simply not telling the police about an illegal abortion or an attempted abortion of which he may possibly have become aware during the course of his professional duties. If, however, for some consideration otherwise than allowed by section 5 of the Criminal Law Act 1967, anyone withholds information about the commission or the attempted commission of an arrestable offence he will be committing an offence.

Courts of law

A doctor is often required to give evidence in Court. He is not permitted to refuse to disclose in a Court of law information obtained during the course of his professional relationship with his patient. Unless he has the patient's consent, a medical witness who is asked a question which he can only answer by a breach of professional confidence should appeal to the judge or the presiding magistrate and ask if he is compelled to disclose the information. If he is directed to do so he must either obey or take the consequences which may be a fine or imprisonment or both.

The position of the medical witness and the attitude of the Court regarding his professional privilege was stated by Lord Denning, M. R. in A.G. v. Mulholland and A.G. v. Foster.[37] These two contempt cases were heard together in the Court of Appeal and concerned two journalists who were required to reveal a source of information to a statutory committee of inquiry. Lord Denning, in the course of his judgment, said:

The only profession that I know which is given a privilege from disclosing information to a Court of law is the legal profession and then it is not the privilege of the lawyer but of his client. Take the clergyman, the banker or the medical man. None of these is entitled to refuse to answer when directed to do so by a judge ... The judge will respect the confidences which each member of these honourable professions receives in the course of it, and will not direct him to answer unless not only it is relevant but also it is a proper and indeed necessary question in the course of justice to be put and unanswered. A judge is the person entrusted, on behalf of the community, to weigh these conflicting interests—to weigh on the one hand the respect due to confidence in the profession and on the other hand the ultimate interest of the community in justice being done ...

It should be appreciated, however, that the reference to the position of the doctor as a witness was not the subject of the two cases. Consequently what was said by Lord Denning about the position of the doctor would not be a binding authority. It was, however, substantially in line with what had for a very long time been understood to be the position.

The Criminal Justice Act 1967

This Act amends, *inter alia*, the law relating to the proceedings of Criminal Courts, including the law about the submission of evidence. Before the introduction of this Act doctors were often required to attend and testify at committal proceedings in the Magistrates' Court. Many committal proceedings are now conducted on documentary evidence only and the attendance of witnesses at such proceedings is hardly ever necessary. The evidence is submitted in the form of signed statements which are made available to both sides. The effect of this is that written evidence is permissible at such proceedings except in those cases where the accused raises an objection. In such a case the witness will be required to attend the proceedings and may be subjected to cross-examination.

Medical records

The Department of Health and Social Security, through various circulars to hospital authorities, has made it clear that the rights of patients to have their hospital medical records regarded as confidential must be respected. It has indicated that medical boards and medical appeal tribunals should not be provided with a patient's hospital medical records unless the written consent of the patient has been obtained. The Department has given the British Medical Association an assurance that, in the event of proceedings for defamation against a medical practitioner arising out of his entries in the medical records of a patient, the practitioner will be indemnified by the Department against any damages that may be recovered and against all reasonable costs that he may incur in defending the proceedings.

The administration of the Welfare State has brought practitioners into close contact with government departments and many other bodies composed partly or wholly of non-medical persons. The result of this is that requests are made by both medical and lay officials for clinical records or other information concerning patients. The exchange of medical details concerning patients should take place only between doctors, and the increasing tendency to exchange confidential medical details with lay officials is to be deplored. Medical records should be lent to medical officers employed by government departments only when written consent has been given by the patient himself or someone acting on his behalf.

Disclosure of documents

Before 1971 a doctor could not be compelled by law to produce his medical records concerning a patient unless a subpoena or a witness summons was issued and served upon him. Upon service of such an order the doctor named in the document had to appear in Court and produce his records. No privilege could be claimed by the doctor, although the Court might, at its discretion, allow that certain parts of the records be not disclosed in open court.

In 1970 the law, in so far as it related to claims for damages for personal injuries, was radically altered by the Administration of Justice Act and is now embodied in sections 33–35 of the Supreme Court Act 1981.

Section 33 provides that on the application, in accordance with the Rules of Court, of a person who appears to the High Court to be likely to be a party to subsequent proceedings in that Court in which a claim in respect of personal injuries to a person or in respect of a persons death, is likely to be made, the High Court shall, in such circumstances as may be specified in the Rules, have power to order a person who appears to the Court to be likely to be a party to the proceedings, and to be likely to have or have had in his possession custody or power any documents which are relevant to any issue arising or likely to arise out of that claim (1) to disclose those documents and (2) to produce them to the applicant or, on such conditions as the court may specify, (a) to the applicant's lawyers, or (b) to the applicant's lawyers and any medical or other professional adviser of the applicant or (c) if the applicant has no legal adviser, to any medical or other professional adviser of the applicant.

Section 34 gives the High Court a similar power

to order disclosure and production of relevant documents by a person who is not a party to the proceedings.

Section 35 provides that the court shall not make an order under either of the above sections if it considers that compliance with such an order would be likely to be injurious to the public interest.

In practice most claims concerning medical or surgical treatment start with an application for disclosure of the medical records either against the clinicians concerned or the health authority and if the applicant can satisfy the court that he may have reasonable grounds for advancing his claim an order for disclosure of the medical records will normally be made.

Records and computers

The responsibility of a doctor for the safe custody of his confidential records is the same whether they are kept in the conventional manner or in a computer. A doctor who commits confidential medical information to a computer or some other form of data-recording machine must bear in mind that he is responsible ultimately for the results of his decision. Before such information is recorded he must satisfy himself that disclosure will be possible only to the persons and to the extent that he has decided and that persons from whom he has the assurance of confidentiality are both competent and trustworthy. It would seem that there is urgent need for statutory sanctions to protect confidentiality of sophisticated methods of keeping medical records.

Clinical research

In 1964 the World Medical Association drew up a code of ethics on clinical research and human experimentation. The code, known as the Declaration of Helsinki,[38] has laid down certain principles for the guidance of doctors engaged in this field. Special problems arise regarding consent in relation to clinical research and human experimentation and any doctor who requires advice about this subject should seek the guidance of his medical defence organisation.

In the field of clinical research a fundamental distinction must be drawn between research in which the aim is essentially therapeutic in character

and research which is purely scientific and without therapeutic value to the person subjected to the research.

In the treatment of a sick person the doctor must be free to use a new therapeutic procedure if, in his judgment, it offers hope of saving life, re-establishing health or alleviating suffering.

If the experiment is being carried out on a person solely for the acquisition of knowledge and is of no direct benefit to the individual, this should be made clear to him and his written consent to the proposed investigation should be obtained. In order to safeguard his personal integrity the investigator carrying out research solely for acquiring knowledge must respect the right of each individual.

Euthanasia

In modern terminology the word euthanasia is generally understood to mean 'mercy killing', in other words, the deliberate termination of a life of a person suffering from a painful and incurable illness. The British Medical Association adheres firmly to its view that euthanasia should be condemned in all circumstances. It feels that euthanasia is contrary to the public interest and contrary to the spirit of the Declaration of Geneva.[39]

Attempts in Britain to introduce legislation to legalise euthanasia have been unsuccessful but further attempts will doubtless be made. Although the doctor's obligation is to preserve life this should not be taken to mean that life must necessarily be prolonged artificially when natural death is inevitable.

'Irreversible coma' which is regarded by many to be synonymous with death, should be accepted both from the legal and ethical aspects as a criterion for the discontinuance of further resuscitative measures.

Determination of moment of death

In 1968 the World Medical Association formulated a statement on death. This statement, known as the Declaration of Sydney, is set out in the British Medical Association's booklet on Medical Ethics.[40] The determination of the point of death of the person makes it not only ethically permissible to cease attempts at resuscitation but also, in countries where the law permits, to remove organs from the cadaver provided that the prevailing legal requirements have been fulfilled.

The medical profession in Britain expressed itself in the following resolution of the Representative Body of the British Medical Association in 1977:

That this Meeting affirms that the position of medical practitioners who are in conscience opposed to euthanasia must be fully protected in future legislation should it occur and that no legal obligation in this respect should be allowed to be imposed unilaterally on any member of the profession at any time.

Therapeutic abortion

In 1970 the World Medical Association drew up a statement on therapeutic abortion. The text of this statement, known as the Declaration of Oslo,[41] is as follows:

1. The first moral principal imposed upon the doctor is respect for human life as expressed in a clause of the Declaration of Geneva: 'I will maintain the utmost respect for human life from the time of conception'.
2. Circumstances which bring the vital interests of a mother into conflict with the vital interests of her unborn child create a dilemma and raise the question whether or not the pregnancy should be deliberately terminated.
3. Diversity of response to this situation results from the diversity of attitudes towards the life of the unborn child. This is a matter of individual conviction and conscience which must be respected.
4. It is not the role of the medical profession to determine the attitudes and rules of any particular state or community in this matter, but it is our duty to attempt both to ensure the protection of our patients and to safeguard the rights of the doctor within society.
5. Therefore, where the law allows therapeutic abortion to be performed, or legislation to that effect is contemplated, and this is not against the policy of the national medical association, and where the legislature desires or will accept the guidance of the medical profession the following principles are approved:
    (a) Abortion should be performed only as a therapeutic measure.
    (b) A decision to terminate pregnancy should normally be approved in writing by at least two doctors chosen for their professional competence.
    (c) The procedure should be performed by a doctor competent to do so in premises approved by the appropriate authority.
6. If the doctor considers that his convictions do not allow him to advise or perform an abortion, he may withdraw while ensuring the continuity of (medical) care by a qualified colleague.
7. This statement, while it is endorsed by the General Assembly of the World Medical Association, is not to be regarded as binding on any individual member association unless it is adopted by that member association.

Artificial feeding of prisoners

When the Council of the World Medical Association met in Tokyo in October 1975 it discussed the various aspects of forcible feeding and hunger-striking prisoners. The Council declared that forcible feeding in the case of a prisoner whose capacity for rational judgment was unimpaired was not only to be deplored but that it was also impermissible. This problem, vividly illustrated by recent events in Northern Ireland, is discussed in the British Medical Association Handbook on Medical Ethics in the following terms:

This categorical repudiation of forcible feeding of a prisoner who is lucid at the outset of a hunger strike overlooks some difficult medical and ethical problems. Whether all prisoners slowly dying of self-imposed starvation remain lucid to the moment of death seems questionable. The ethics of forcible feeding may be regarded as a special case of the much discussed question of 'the right to die'. In whatever context this problem may be considered, the physician is confronted by two conflicting ethical imperatives: his duty to do all in his power to preserve life, and his obligation to respect the right of a rational patient to refuse even a life-saving intervention. Different physicians might resolve this ethical dilemma in different ways, and might be influenced by such factors as the age, personality, and family status of prisoners, and the length of their prison sentence.

Discrimination in medicine

The Declaration of Geneva,[42] as amended by the World Medical Assembly in 1968, states, *inter alia*, that no member of the medical profession will permit considerations of religion, nationality, race, party politics or social standing to intervene between his duty and his patient. The Declaration applies both in times of peace and war.

In 1973 the World Medical Association vehemently condemned any form of discrimination in the training of medical practitioners, in the practice of medicine and in the provision of health services for the peoples of the world.

It is very difficult to believe that the World Medical Association will ever renounce these principles.

REFERENCES

1. *Hatcher v. Black and Others* (1954) The Times, 2 July; Br. Med. J., 2, 106.
2. *Roe and Woolley v. The Ministry of Health and Others* (1954) 2 Q.B. 66, W.L.R. 128; on appeal (1954) 2 All E.R. 131.
3. *Hunter v. Hanley*
4. *R. v. Bateman* (1925)L.J. (K.B.) 792; T.L.R. 557; 19 Cr.App. R8; 94 L.J.X. 791.
5. Paragraph 6 of Ministry of Health circular R.H.B.(49) 128.
6. Ministry of Health circular H.M.(54) 32.
7. *Urry v. Bierer* (1955) The Times, 16 March; on appeal The Times, 15 July.
8. *Whiteford v. Hunter* (1950) 94 S. Jo. 758 (H.L.); (1950) W.N. 533.
9. *Edler v. Greenwich & Deptford Hospital Management Committee* (1953) The Times, 7 March.
10. 1981, 1.267 H.L.
11. *Chapman v. Rix* (1958) The Times, 11 November; (1959) 19 November; (1960) 12 December.
12. *Payne v. St Helier Group Hospital Management Committee* (1952) C.L.Y. 2442, The Times, 12 November.
13. *Hatcher v. Black and Others* (1954) The Times, 2 July; Br. Med. J., 2, 106.
14. *Sabapathi v. Huntley* (1938) 1 W.W.R. 817; (1939) Med. Ann., 287.
15. *Braishaw v. Harefield & Northwood Hospital Management Committee* (1967) Ann. Rep. Med. Defence Union, p. 41.
16. *McCormack v. Redpath* (1961) The Times, 24 March; 3 C.L. 500.
17. *Cassidy v. Ministry of Health* (1951) 2 K.B. 343, All E.R. 574.
18. *Warren v. Greig and White* (1935) The Lancet, i, 330.
19. *Hatcher v. Black and Others* (1954) The Times, 2 July; Br. Med. J., 2, 106.
20. Report of the Secretary's Commission on Medical Malpractice (1973) Washington, DC; US Department of Health, Education and Welfare.
21. *Gerber v. Pines* (1935) 79 Sol. Jo., 13.
22. *Hatcher v. Black and Others* (1954) The Times, 2 July; Br. Med. J., 2, 106.
23. *Hall v. United States*, 381 F.Supp. 224 (D.C.,S.c., 9 Aug. 1974).
24. *Moore v. Lewisham Group Hospital Management Committee* (1959) The Times, 5 February.
25. *R. v. Gray* (1959) The Times, 21 February.
26. *Bennan v. Parsonnet* (1912) 83 A.948.
27. *Breen v. Baker* (1956) The Times, 27 January.
28. 1981, 1 All E.R. 257.
29. 1894, 1 Q.B. 750.
30. 1930, 1 K.B. 562.
31. 1962, All E.R. 391.
32. 1980, 1 All E.R. 461.
33. Professional Conduct and Discipline; Fitness to Practise (1980) London: General Medical Council, p. 9.
34. The General Medical Council Annual Report (1981), p. 22.
35. The Handbook of Medical Ethics (1980), p. 57.
36. Medical Defence Union Ann. Rep. (1974), p. 18.
37. *A.G. v. Mulholland*; *A.G. v. Foster* (1963) 2 Q.B. 477; (1963) 2 W.L.R. 658; (1963) 1 All E.R. 767 (C.A.).
38. The Handbook of Medical Ethics (1980), p. 59.
39. Ibid., p. 57.
40. Ibid., p. 66.
41. Ibid., p. 63.
42. Ibid., p. 59.

5

Medico-legal examination of the living

INTRODUCTION

In the reign of King Henry II, the principles involved in a prosecution for rape can be summarised thus:

The Victim must be of chaste character. She must go at once and while the deed is newly done, with hue and cry, to the neighbouring townships and there show the injury done to her to men of good repute—the blood, her clothing stained with blood, and her torn garments. And in the same way she ought to go to the Reeve of the hundred, the King's Sergeant, the Coroner and the Sheriff. And let her make her appeal at the first County Court, unless she can make her complaint directly to the Lord King or his Justices, where she will be told to sue at the County Court. Let her appeal be enrolled in the Coroner's Rolls, every word of her appeal, exactly as she makes it. A day will be given her at the coming of the Justices, at which let her again put forward her appeal before them, in the same words as she made at the County Court, from which she is not permitted to depart lest the appeal fail because of the variance.

Let the truth be ascertained by an examination of her body, made by four law-abiding women sworn to tell the truth as to whether she is virgin or defiled.

Thus wrote Henry of Bratton (Henry Bracton) in the thirteenth century describing the legal procedure to be followed by the victim of an alleged rape.

However barbarous the system, and however unfair to the woman victim, these principles included:
1. previous sexual experience of the victim;
2. early complaint;
3. detailed and consistent history;
4. physical signs of injury to corroborate the history;
5. physical examination to confirm that the offence has taken place.

In the twentieth century we should have moved away from some of the restrictions of Saxon law. The previous sexual history of the alleged victim is of importance only as to her veracity, and chastity is no longer a prerequisite for a rape victim. The 'four law-abiding women' of Saxon times should be replaced by one trained and experienced medical practitioner.

The principles of early complaint, detailed and consistent history, corroborative physical evidence, and physical examination of the person of the victim remain.

The offence of *rape* is a brutal, dirtying, demoralising assault on a woman, and if fully proven demands the most rigorous penalties allowed by law. Equally, the allegation of *rape* is easy to make, and the man accused falsely of the offence is in great peril.

Maybe the following chapter will go some way to ensure that the medical practitioners charged with the great responsibility of examining the alleged victims and the suspects in all cases of sexual assault will improve upon the standards of the 'four law-abiding women' of Norman times.

CLINICAL FORENSIC MEDICINE

Forensic medicine is defined as 'the medical specialty which applies the principles and practice of medicine to the elucidation of questions in judicial proceedings'.

If this definition is to be accepted, it follows that there must be as many specialties within the field of forensic medicine as there are in the entire field of medical practice. However, there is a marked tendency to consider forensic medicine as being synonymous with forensic pathology, and this synonymity can only be correct if pathology is interpreted as meaning the study of abnormal

64

conditions in their entirety—and not only in the findings after death.

It is an anomaly to view the entire subject of forensic medicine from the autopsy table. It is certainly true that the morbid anatomist has the advantage over the clinician in that the former's patients are in no position to object to, or hinder, his detailed examination. In general terms, conditions in the dead do not alter appreciably with the passage of a few hours, so the morbid anatomist has more time to complete his examination and can always 'go back' for a second examination should the circumstances require it or should he have omitted to take certain specimens. This is not the case in the examination of the living, for here the appearance of wounds and injuries is constantly changing, and the body's normal cleansing activities tend to destroy contaminants—be they alcohol or drugs in the blood, seminal traces in the vagina or rectum, or stains on the skin.

It is vital to understand the difference between the clinical examination of a living patient and the detailed examination of a dead patient performed by a forensic pathologist. In the latter case the detailed examination is performed in the calm atmosphere of a clean, quiet mortuary—with the assistance of the laboratory toxicologist and forensic scientist. In the former, the clinician is expected to carry out his entire examination in the not so peaceful environment of the patient's own home, the police station, or the emergency department of a hospital, and the calm and unemotional atmosphere is frequently complicated by weeping or aggressive relatives, bleeding victim, vomit, and eager police officers.

The difference between the two sets of circumstances is only too obvious, and it is therefore essential that any doctor called upon to examine a patient in what may become a 'medico-legal' situation must develop a routine that will enable him to perform a complete examination and to take all relevant specimens.

Basically there is no difference in the medicolegal examination of a patient compared with the 'normal' general clinical examination of a live patient seen for the first time in hospital or general medical practice. The routine examination falls automatically into several sections.[1]

1. A *full general history* must be taken in every case, and this must include such matters as past and present health; when last seen by a doctor and for what complaint; what, if any, medication is being taken and the last time that it was taken; past illness, operations and serious accidents; and the normal questions relating to such matters as occupation, hobbies, weight, sleeping habits, family history, bowel habits and micturition.

2. A *specific history* relating to the particular situation for which the examination is being undertaken should then be taken. It must be taken in great detail and should, if possible, always be taken from the patient rather than from any relative, police officer or other interested party. It must include detailed reference as to the exact nature of the incident; where the incident took place (indoors, in a field, etc.); details of all physical force used in any assault; location of all pain or discomfort mentioned; the quantity, time and nature of any food, medication or alcohol consumed; the time and date of the alleged incident or incidents.

3. A *complete general clinical examination* must follow, and this examination should be a complete 'top to toe' examination. It must include observation of height and weight; general build and appearance; skin of the entire body surface; all bodily systems. In many cases such a thorough medical examination may seem to be an unnecessary procedure, but it is a prudent step for the few extra minutes that such an examination demands may provide answers to what at first may seem to be quite irrelevant questions such as the presence of scarring or recent injury on distant parts of the body or pre-existing physical conditions. These matters may assume great importance at a later date. It is highly dangerous for the examining doctor to 'pounce' immediately on the specific part involved in any incident without first performing a full general examination.

4. A *special examination* of the specific areas involved should follow the full general examination. This special examination must include detailed description of any abnormality found; measurement and exact location of all injuries present; the taking of all valid and uncontaminated specimens for laboratory examination.

5. *Careful and full notes* must be made at each stage of the clinical examination, and these must

include an account of the general and specific history as given by the patient. When recording physical findings it is very unwise of the physician to use any form of abbreviation (such as the ubiquitous NAD of English medicine—'nothing abnormal disclosed') for such a notation can be interpreted by a lawyer as meaning any one of the following:

a. there was no abnormality present, *or*

b. the examining doctor failed to examine for any abnormality, *or*

c. the examining doctor was too dumb to recognise the abnormality that was present.

Notes that record fully the normal as well as the abnormal findings of an examination ensure that there can be no such doubt in interpretation, and are also of enormous assistance to any other doctor called upon to review the clinical findings at a later date.

Any specimens taken by the examining doctor during the course of his clinical examination must be clearly indicated in the notes, and special mention must be made of the manner in which the specimen was obtained and the identity of the person to whom it was later given. This simple precaution ensures the 'pedigree' of any specimen taken, and constitutes the first link in the 'chain of evidence' for the particular specimen.

6. A *clinical opinion* is given at the end of the clinical examination and before the results of any laboratory tests are available. This opinion must be based entirely upon the clinical findings during the examination—it may have to be modified at a later stage when the results of laboratory examinations are to hand.

The clinical opinion can only properly state that the examination findings are/are not consistent with the history given; the abnormal conditions found on examination and their possible cause; the immediate effects of the conditions found and their likely long-term effects. Medico-legal diagnosis depends upon finding abnormal conditions and assessing if the abnormal conditions found (or sometimes their absence) are consistent with the detailed history obtained. The vital importance of taking a detailed history before performing a thorough examination is therefore obvious.

7. A *detailed medical report* must be prepared as soon as possible after the examination has been concluded, and before the laboratory results are available. This report must include:

a. the identity of the patient examined;

b. the place, date and time of the examination;

c. the identity of the authority requesting the examination;

d. the fact that consent to examination and report was obtained;

e. the identity of all persons present during the examination;

f. the details of all the history, general examination and special examination performed;

g. the description of all specimens taken, and their disposal;

h. the clinical opinion formed during the examination;

i. the time spent in the examination.

A copy of this report should be retained by the examining doctor, and should be available, together with the original examination notes, should the matter come to Court.

Every practising doctor will develop his own technique of clinical examination, and as long as the essentials indicated previously are fulfilled, it is impossible to say that any one technique is any better than another.

A medico-legal situation varies from an ordinary clinical problem in one very important aspect. In 'ordinary' clinical practice the patient comes to the doctor for diagnosis and treatment. In medico-legal practice the patient is frequently brought to the physician by relatives, police or lawyers. Very often these 'interested parties' have already made up their minds as to diagnosis, and are merely asking the doctor to confirm the opinion that they have reached. The patient seen under the circumstances of a medico-legal situation may therefore have 'an axe to grind' and it is vital that the doctor bears this fact in mind throughout his history taking and his examination.

There are certain principles, therefore, that must be borne in mind by the examining doctor in a medico-legal situation, and he would be well advised to remember them throughout the history taking, examination and preparation of the report:

1. detail;

2. impartiality;

3. observation;

4. suspicion.

These are the essential principles of forensic medicine. The doctor who constantly remembers that 'things are not always what they seem to be at first glance' will avoid many of the pitfalls of the medico-legal situation.

Any doctor who gives a dogmatic opinion based upon inadequate clinical findings is of no value to his instructing solicitors or to the Courts. Such an opinion, unsupported by clinical evidence, could be taken to indicate extreme bias on the part of the doctor and could nullify the value of all his evidence.

INSTRUCTIONS AND PRE-TRIAL CONFERENCE

The doctor may find himself involved in legal medicine as either a professional witness, where he will be required to give evidence of fact arising out of his own examination of a patient, or as an expert witness, where he will be required to give evidence of opinion which may be based upon his own examination findings or on his interpretation of the examination findings of another doctor.

The responsibility for giving adequate instructions to an expert medical witness lies primarily with the instructing lawyer, and it is his duty to provide the doctor with all the information available, including information that at first glance may not be in the client's best interest. It is only by giving full and frank instructions that the lawyer can expect a valid opinion from his expert that will be maintained in the face of cross-examination in Court.

Incomplete instructions may lead to a complete volte-face by the doctor in the course of cross-examination when the full details of the situation may be put to him for the very first time by opposing counsel. Omission by instructing solicitors of even a small portion of the available information may cause the medical expert to reach a wrong conclusion which in itself may not be in the best interest of the client.

No doctor should be prepared to give an expert medico-legal opinion on inadequate instructions, and there should be no hesitation in informing the instructing lawyers of this fact.

Because of the pressures of work that now seem to exist, instructions and requests for opinions are often delayed until the very last moment. This applies particularly in criminal matters where the defence (and sometimes even the prosecution) suddenly become aware that they require a medico-legal opinion 'yesterday' and expect to obtain a full and carefully prepared report and opinion from a busy medico-legal practitioner within 24 h. The fact that such a report is often forthcoming within that very short period of time says much for the dedication and application of the medico-legal practitioners, but it is far from an ideal situation and carries with it the very real risk that some aspect of the case has not been considered by the doctor and that as a result his opinion is not as soundly based as it should be. The only guarantee of a sound, valid and supportable opinion from a correctly chosen medico-legal expert is full and early instructions.

Once the instructing lawyer has received the report and opinion from the doctor it is essential that there be some sort of conference between himself and the expert. The purpose of such a conference is not to persuade the doctor to change or omit some of his examination findings, but is to ensure that the lawyer is fully aware of the significance of the medical findings. It also serves to educate the doctor in the matters that the lawyer will attempt to emphasise during the course of his examination-in-chief.

The lawyer should ask the doctor whether there are any parts of his opinion and report which may be challenged by other experts in the field. Are the views expressed those that are commonly held in the medical profession? Can there be any other interpretation of the findings that may vary from those expressed by the doctor?

The lawyer must remember that the Courtroom is his normal environment, but that to many doctors it is a strange and hostile world. It is therefore advisable to warn the tiro medical witness of what is likely to happen to him in Court. He should be instructed briefly in the general scheme of examination-in-chief and cross-examination, and he should be warned that the bench may also intervene with questions if the judge has not fully grasped a point or if he feels that counsel has omitted to refer to some important matter.

It is often helpful if the lawyer explains to the

tiro medical witness that two potent weapons may be used by opposing counsel:
1. flattery—designed to persuade the medical witness to go slightly out of his own field of expertise and thereby to risk exposure to ridicule by a better qualified expert later in the hearing;
2. rudeness—designed to make the doctor lose his temper and thereby to give unconsidered and ill-advised answers.

To the practising lawyer these two ploys are perfectly legitimate weapons to use: to the tiro doctor they smell of treachery. If the medical witness has been forewarned of these and similar dangers he is less likely to be embarrassed in Court.

It is the lawyer's duty to ensure that the medical witness has his notes with him before he goes into Court, and also that any books or references that he may wish to make use of are available (Fig. 5.1).

THE TEN COMMANDMENTS
FOR THE MEDICAL WITNESS
Thou Shalt

I. Be always on time.

II. Be neat and tidy in thy person.

III. Stand upright, speak out, and look thine inquisitor in the eye.

IV. Take ye not sides: be fair, and never let thy bias show.

V. Never go ye out of thy field. Guess not, but say ye instead 'I know not'.

VI. Have all thy notes with thee—full notes and in a fair hand.

VII. Speak not in thine medical or technical tongue, but speak thou in the tongue of the common people.

VIII. Look not upon the judge, nor coroner, nor stipendiary, nor lawyer as a fool. Beware for they are wise unto the skills of medicine for they have heard many before you.

IX. Jest not thyself—but be ye always ready to laugh if his lordship maketh a quip however feeble that quip may be.

X. Ask thou a fair fee—based upon thy skill, experience, qualification, and true worth.

Fig. 5.1 Lecture notes of Dr Paul. Published in the Yale Journal of Biology and Medicine (1977).

The clinical examination in sexual offences

General

The reasons for a medical examination in cases of alleged sexual assault can be divided into the following:
1. so that emergency medical or surgical treatment can be given;
2. so that all the physical signs present at the time of the medical examination can be observed and recorded;
3. so that all relevant scientific specimens can be obtained and retained for laboratory investigation and identification.

In the context of this chapter, it is the second and third of the above reasons that are of importance. Attention to the first of the above reasons is of course of paramount importance when dealing with a live patient, but urgent medical treatment need in no way detract from the proper recording of physical signs and the taking of valid specimens.

From the medical-legal point of view, the doctor is expected to examine both the alleged victim and the alleged assailant in order to establish if any sexual assault has taken place, and if there is any medical evidence which may establish contact between the two parties. The problems encountered in attempting to answer these two questions will be dealt with in some detail under the specific offences.

Any situation involving an allegation of a sexual offence is unique in the degree of emotional tension generated in all the persons involved in such an allegation. The emotional tension extends to the alleged victim, the relatives of the victim, the person accused, and even the police officers involved in the investigation. The introduction of Rape Advisory Centres will add yet another organisation to the list of emotionally involved persons.

In this atmosphere of high emotional tension it behoves the clinician to remember the general principles of legal medicine referred to earlier in this chapter. As many of these examinations take place late at night or in the early hours of the morning, when the examining doctor is likely to be very tired, the value of a set routine is of great importance.

Rape: Indecent assault upon a female

Rape is defined as unlawful sexual intercourse by a man with a female other than his wife, without her consent. The merest penetration of the penis between the labia associated with the lack of consent is sufficient to constitute the offence.

The lack of consent may be the result of the female's failure to give a valid consent (under age of 16 years in the United Kingdom, severe mental subnormality or abnormality) or it may be as the result of force, fear, fraud, or as the result of stupefying drugs.

It has become the practice in the United Kingdom to consider acts of sexual intercourse with females below the age of 16 years and over the age of about 12 years, where there has been no objection to the act, as being the offence of unlawful sexual intercourse rather than that of rape. As in the majority of these cases there has not merely been lack of objection but enthusiastic co-operation by the young girl involved, it would seem quite correct to consider these acts of unlawful intercourse as less serious in general terms than the full offence of rape. In children of lesser age, and in all cases where there has been objection by the girl, or where the act has taken place when the girl has been the victim of general force, or has been under the influence of stupefying drugs or lack of objection has been obtained by fraud, the offence is considered to be rape.

Indecent assault is by definition any assault accompanied by circumstances of indecency on the part of the accused against the person assaulted. The essential ingredient is the lack of consent by the victim—and as in the case of rape, consent is not valid if given by a female under the age of 16 years, a woman suffering from severe mental subnormality or abnormality, or if given under duress, fraud or the effects of stupefying drugs (Fig. 5.2).

The type of assault may vary from the merest touching of thighs, breasts or buttocks to digital penetration of the vagina or anus, oro-genital contact.

The routine of examination of the alleged victim and accused should not vary for cases of rape or indecent assault. The examining doctor must plan his entire examination so that at the end he will

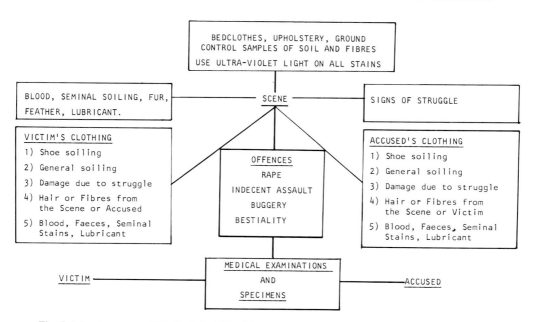

Fig. 5.2 Lecture notes of Dr Paul. Published in the Yale Journal of Biology and Medicine (1977).

be in a position to answer the following questions:
1. Is there medical evidence to confirm the allegation?
2. Has sexual intercourse taken place recently?
3. Is there evidence of previous sexual intercourse?
4. Are there physical signs present to confirm the use of force or of stupefying drugs?
5. Are the physical findings consistent with the history?
6. Have all the relevant specimens been taken to confirm the allegations and to assist in identifying the parties involved?

In many cases there are no signs of injury or intoxication by stupefying drugs, and the entire allegation of lack of consent is based on fear or on fraud. In such cases, where there has been no allegation of force or of intoxication, the evidential value of the negative examination findings is reduced, but that is no excuse for an inadequate medical examination.

False allegations of rape and of indecent assault are not uncommon, and may arise from many causes: the young girl out late at night and consenting to intercourse who later becomes fearful of parental wrath; the married woman involved in an extramarital affair who finds on her return home that her clothing is soiled or damaged; the fear of pregnancy; mental illness; spite or blackmail. These are only a few of the reasons for false allegations. It is essential that the examining doctor always remembers 'things are not always what they seem at first glance' and that his clinical opinion at the end of his examination must be based on his clinical findings being consistent with the history he has been given by the patient regarding the alleged incident.

Essentials in the medical examination of victims of rape and indecent assault[2]

Consent. Consent must be obtained by the examining doctor for his examination and for his subsequent report. This consent, in the case of an adult, should be obtained directly from the patient and need not be in writing. In the case of a minor, or of a female suffering from severe mental subnormality or abnormality, consent in writing should be obtained from a parent or guardian. The examination notes should record that consent was obtained, and any written consent form should be fastened to the original examination notes.

General history. A general history should be obtained from the patient herself, and must include details of all past illness, surgical operations and serious accidents. It must also include details of any recent medical attention, and details of any medication or alcoholic drink consumed during the preceding 24 h. In many cases, particularly if allegations of intoxication are being made, details of the amount and nature of any food taken during the preceding 24 h should also be noted.

Menstrual and obstetric history. It is important that the past menstrual history be explored, with special reference to the date of the last menstrual period, the type of menstrual protection normally used (pads, internal tampons) and the use of any hormonal or contraceptive medication.

The past obstetric history must be recorded, with special reference to the dates of birth of any children, and of any surgical involvement in delivery. Episiotomies or forceps deliveries may alter the normal genital anatomy and may have some relevance to the pattern of genital injury found.

Enquiry must be made as to past sexual experience, and the relevance of such enquiry is twofold. Firstly it is of relevance if prior virginity is being claimed by the complainant, for if the clinical findings are not consistent with such a claim the reliability of the complainant's evidence is immediately suspect. Apart from the claim of prior virginity, the complainant's previous sexual experience is of no evidential value and the doctor should not pursue this matter. Secondly, and of considerable scientific evidential value, all acts of consenting sexual intercourse within 14 days of the alleged offence must be explored by the examining doctor, and if any such acts have taken place the identity of the man must be established so that blood and saliva samples can be obtained from him in order to exclude his seminal fluid in subsequent laboratory examinations of the vaginal specimens from the alleged victim. Estimation of acid phosphatase activity using the modified Sigma method will also assist in excluding consenting partners in acts of intercourse more than 48 h prior to the obtaining of vaginal swabs.

Enquiry as to recent consenting intercourse is

obviously of the greatest importance when the alleged victim is a married woman or one who is cohabiting regularly with one partner, but may be of equal importance under other circumstances.

The specific history of the alleged incident must be very carefully taken and recorded, for it is this portion of the history that will be later found to be consistent or inconsistent with the examination findings. Specific questions must be asked by the examining doctor as to:

1. the date, time and place of the alleged acts;
2. the time of first complaint, and an explanation for any delay in this complaint;
3. what clothing was removed from the victim, and how and by whom it was removed;
4. what clothing was removed from the assailant, how and by whom;
5. was any general force used by the assailant and, if so, where and how;
6. was any pain experienced either at the time of the incident or subsequently;
7. what were the relative positions of victim and assailant during the acts complained of;
8. did ejaculation take place during the act, either within the vagina or outside;
9. what are the details of the act or acts alleged;
10. was any form of contraception used during the act;
11. did the victim struggle, scream or injure the assailant in any way;
12. has the victim changed clothes, or washed any of the clothes since the alleged assault;
13. has the victim bathed or washed any part of her body since the alleged assault.

General observation of the patient should be maintained by the doctor throughout the taking of the history. This observation must extend to the patient's demeanour and the examination notes must record if she is distressed, tearful, calm or aggressive. Women react in many ways to assaults, and it is dangerous to form any opinion based solely on the demeanour. Nevertheless, accurate observation of the behaviour is an essential part of the medical examination and it may play an important role when all the examination findings are weighed together.

The type of clothing worn, and the type and amount of make-up used should be carefully noted, as should any smudging or damage to the make-up.

The 15-year-old girl with heavy make-up, false eyelashes, grossly short mini-skirt and plunging neck line blouse seen at the time of the medical examination may be vastly different from the well scrubbed schoolgirl in gym-tunic who appears to give evidence at a criminal trial in a case of unlawful sexual intercourse. The examining doctor's observation as to her appearance and his assessment of her apparent age at the time of his examination may have very considerable bearing at the trial.

Smudged eye make-up can well be the result of previous crying, even if the patient presents a calm demeanour at the time of the medical examination. It is an unusual woman who repairs her damaged make-up before making an allegation of rape and, even if her behaviour is unemotional during the medical examination, disturbed make-up around the eye can indicate prior upset.

The clothing worn at the time of the offence should at least be inspected by the examining doctor. If the same clothing is being worn at the time of the medical examination it must not be removed by nursing staff but should be removed, garment by garment, by the patient and in the presence of the examining doctor.

It is vital that nothing which falls from the clothing in the course of its removal is lost, and to this end the patient should be made to stand upon a large clean sheet of paper so that anything that falls out of the clothing will fall on to the paper and can be preserved for laboratory investigation.

As each item of clothing is removed, the doctor should inspect it and note any areas of soiling or damage. After this inspection each item, if dry, should be placed by the doctor in a clean paper bag and should be identified by a number for subsequent delivery to the laboratory. If the garments are wet, it is better to hang them carefully in a safe place to dry, for packing wet garments may affect subsequent laboratory investigation.

The doctor should never attempt to remove any soiling from clothing. His duty is merely to observe and note soiled areas and to retain the garments for laboratory examination. In his inspection he should pay particular attention to the 'crutch' areas of tights and panties for it is here that blood and seminal soiling will frequently be found. The use of an ultraviolet lamp will assist in the location of areas of possible seminal soiling, for these will fluoresce.

When delicate clothing is forcibly removed it is usual for it to sustain damage, and to this end the doctor should look closely at the waistband of tights, panties and slips, and to the legs of tights and stockings, for it is here that such damage is likely to be seen. Blouse buttons and button-holes, and the fastenings of brassieres are also areas of likely damage in the forceful removal of clothing, particularly if against resistance, and should be inspected.

The lack of any damage to clothing is not consistent with a history of forceful removal, and this observation should be recorded in the examination notes.

General clinical examination must follow in every case, and this must include observation of the patient's height, weight and build, as well as a routine examination of all the bodily systems, and the recording of all the clinical findings both normal and abnormal. It is only by such a complete clinical examination that signs of pre-existing disease, injury or intoxication by alcohol or other drugs can be found. Such conditions may have a great bearing at a later stage in the case when the patient's overall behaviour is being considered.

The skin must be carefully examined from the top of the head to the soles of the feet, and during the examination all areas of skin soiling must be noted, with special reference to the hands, the backs of the legs and the buttocks, the abdomen and the tops of the thighs. Any soiled areas must be swabbed with plain cotton swabs, moistened with sterile water, and the swabs should be air dried before being placed in sterile containers for laboratory examination. The use of an ultraviolet lamp will reveal areas of fluorescence on the skin that may represent areas of seminal soiling and all such areas must also be swabbed.

A very careful search of the whole body surface must be made for signs of injury, and all injuries must be noted, including old injuries. Special attention must be given to signs of recent injury.

Bruises are often the most important corroborative sign of force, and the exact position, size and shape must be carefully noted. It is vital to remember that bruises undergo a colour change with age, and also that they may not appear on the skin surface for up to 24 h after the causal injury. For this latter reason it is important to re-examine the patient some 24 h later to confirm or deny the presence of bruising that was not apparent at the time of the initial examination in all cases of alleged rape by force. Early bruising may show merely as an area of redness, and the characteristic colour change to blue/purple may take several hours to develop. Yellow or green bruises are not consistent with recent injury of less than 4–7 days.[3]

Of particular importance are the small, roughly circular 'finger-tip' type of bruise, consistent with grasping injury, and almost invariably associated with an opposing bruise on the opposite side of the limb or neck caused by contralateral digital pressure. Such bruises are often found on the neck, hands, wrists, arms, inner surfaces of the thighs and knees, and the ankles. Often there is a more diffuse and larger area of bruising on the inner surfaces of the thighs or knees, and this is consistent with the victim's legs being forced apart by pressure from the knees of the assailant.

The ultraviolet lamp has a place in the examination for bruising: before colour changes are present at the skin, areas of extraversated blood beneath the skin can be seen if the area is illuminated by ultraviolet light. These areas of extraversated blood will present as darker areas under this form of illumination, even on heavily pigmented negroid skin.

Abrasions, although very minor injuries in themselves, may have a medico-legal importance quite out of keeping with their lack of severity. These injuries may be the result of fingernail scratch marks; of frictional movements against a hard floor or ground; of scratches by thorns, grasses or other foliage. Of great importance are the very superficial abrasions that are frequently found on the flanks when underclothing has been roughly pulled down by an assailant.

All abrasions must be carefully searched for, and their exact position, size, appearance and colour must be noted. Abrasions change in colour and appearance with the passage of time, from the pink and moist appearance of a very recent injury, to the brown and firmly scabbed abrasion of several days of age. The piling up of the superficial layers of the skin at the distal end of an abrasion will give some idea of the direction of the abrading force, and this observation can only be properly made if the injury is examined under a hand lens.

Lacerations and incised wounds are much more obvious than serious injuries, and are less likely to escape the attention of the examining doctor but, as with bruises and abrasions, their exact size, shape and location must be carefully noted. The use of anatomical landmarks, exact heel-injury or head-injury measurements, and simple line drawings are essential in noting the exact positions of all injuries.

During the examination of the skin, careful search must be made for any loose hairs or other foreign substance on the skin surface, and anything found must be removed and placed in a secure container for laboratory examination.

The lips must be carefully examined, both on their outer surface and on their inner surface, and it is the inner surface that is commonly injured by mild blows to the face, by the pressure of a hand across the mouth to prevent screaming, or by violent attempts to kiss the victim. Under all these circumstances the lip tends to be forced backwards to impact sharply against the teeth, and there is almost invariably a very small impact abrasion produced. This impact abrasion has in most cases an exact anatomical relationship to one or more specific teeth, and is not similar to the rather more diffuse area of swelling and abrasion that can occur as the result of enthusiastic and consenting kissing.

Injury to the lips can also occur where there has been forceful penetration or attempted penetration of the closed lips by the penis, and the mechanism is the same as that of the mild blow to the mouth in that the lips are forced back against the teeth. However, this is a rare injury, for in most cases where there has been oro-penile contact without consent it has been achieved through fear or by forcing the mouth open by pressure on the chin or at the corners of the mouth. Fear will leave no physical signs for the doctor to find, and pressure on the chin or to the corners of the mouth will leave signs of injury at those locations and not on the inner surfaces of the lips.[4]

The teeth may also show signs of damage such as looseness or chipping consistent with a blow to the mouth.

The fingernails must be examined for length,

and the presence of ragged or broken nails, and of chipping of nail varnish should be noted. Recent chips in varnish, and recent ragged tears of the nails are often the result of a struggle.

Bite marks on the skin surface must be carefully noted.[5] These tend to fall into two types: the love bite which is not really a bite at all but is an area of skin that has been subjected to a mixture of suction and tongue pressure against the upper teeth. It is present as an area of red/purple discoloration, of no precise shape, and often showing multiple tiny dots of red all over its surface consistent with tiny capillary haemorrhages. They are commonly found on the neck, breasts and chest wall, but they may be found on the lower abdomen and the tops of the thighs. They change colour quite quickly, and within two to three days are often no more than browny areas of discolouration. They are of course not indicative of lack of consent for they are very commonly found as a result of consenting love-making, but they can furnish evidence of contact between two persons if they are carefully swabbed with plain sterile cotton wool swabs, previously moistened in sterile water, and the contaminating saliva is grouped. If such swabs are taken, as they always should be, another area of uncontaminated skin should be swabbed in the same manner so that a control is provided for the laboratory.

True bite marks are also seen sometimes, and these are the result of strong apposition of the teeth leaving what is really an impact abrasion on the skin. Often there is a characteristic impression of the assailant's dentition left on the skin, and the opinion of a forensic odontologist or a dental surgeon should always be obtained in such cases. Bites of this type can be present on the same areas as the love bites previously described, and like the love bite they can also occur during consenting love-making. It is their severity that may be of significance, and bites such as these on the arms and hands have greater significance than those on the breasts, abdomen or thighs in relation to lack of consent. As with the love bite, swabbing may be of assistance in establishing the identity of the biter (Fig. 5.3).

The eyes must be carefully examined. The pupils and the reflex activity may give an indication of intoxication or concussion following a blow to the head. The presence of nystagmus is a further diag-

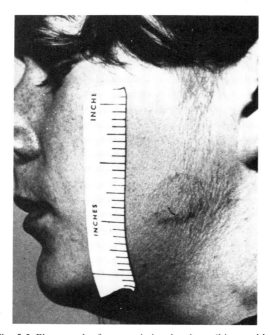

Fig. 5.3 Photograph of a rape victim showing a 'bite mark' on the cheek, and a 'love bite' on the side of the neck. The bite mark was a recent injury, demonstrating a red/purple colouration of the bruising at the time of examination: the love bite was an old lesion, demonstrating a brown/yellow colouration at the time of the examination. (With acknowledgement to The Chief Constable of Surrey Constabulary.)

nostic point in intoxication as well as in pre-existing disease of the central nervous system.

Redness and swelling of the eyelids and general suffusion of the conjunctivae are consistent with a history of previous crying: petechial haemorrhages on the conjunctivae, eyelids and skin of the face are strongly indicative of grasping pressure on the throat compressing the venous return. Frequently extensive subconjunctival haemorrhages are present, and even in the absence of petechiae these may indicate compression of the neck with an associated rise in venous and capillary pressure.

The presence of petechiae or subconjunctival haemorrhages, in association with finger-tip type bruising, abrasion or ligature marks on the neck provide very firm medical corroboration of any allegation of partial throttling. The production of petechiae in the skin and conjunctivae are almost certainly the result of increased intracapillary pressure due to obstruction of the venous return, rather than the result of increased capillary permiability

due to hypoxia. It therefore follows that petechiae occur even when the compression of the neck is not sufficient to obstruct the airway.

When petechiae are found during an examination, it is prudent to test for capillary fragility using a sphygmomanometer cuff on the arm of the patient, and inflating the cuff to between the systolic and diastolic pressures for about 5 min—the appearance of a petechial rash at the end of this period indicates an abnormal capillary fragility.

Petechiae and subconjunctival haemorrhages can occur following violent bouts of coughing, and violent episodes of vomiting or retching and these possible causes must be excluded before compression of the neck is corroborated as the cause.

Detailed examination of the genital area

This must follow the general medical examination, and must be carried out in a good light and with the patient in a comfortable position that allows full exposure of the entire genital area. It must follow a definite order to ensure that the risk of accidental contamination of any specimen taken is ruled out.

Firstly the pubic hair should be carefully inspected and any matted areas should be noted. The entire matted area should then be cut away as close to the skin surface as possible, and should be retained for laboratory examination.

Next the entire area of pubic hair should be combed with a clean and fine-toothed comb and the comb together with any loose hairs removed should be retained for laboratory examination.

To provide the laboratory with a sample of control hair for comparison purposes, one or two small bunches of pubic hair should be pulled out so that the root characteristics are available for comparison, and this sample must also be retained for laboratory examination.

The tops of the thighs, the labia and the perineum should next be inspected, and all areas of injury noted. Injury to the labia in an adult is not a common finding in rape or indecent assault, but fingernail scratches may be present at the tops of the thighs and on the labia, particularly the labia minora. Mere redness of the labia minora is not indicative of recent sexual activity and it may be no more than an indication of a lack of personal hygiene, especially in young girls. Swelling and tenderness of the labia minora may be indicative of sexual activity, but is certainly not indicative of lack of consent.

Swabs must be taken at this stage of the examination from the area of the introitus, the perineum and the anal margin, before any digital contact has been made by the examining doctor. Plain white cotton wool swabs, sterile, are the swabs of choice, and they should be air dried before being placed in their sterile containers.

The hymen should next be inspected, and the presence of any fresh hymenal injury must be noted. Bleeding from the genitals can come from recent injury to the hymen, from recent injury to the vagina, or as the result of a menstrual period. It is obviously vital for the examining doctor to differentiate between these causes.

Gentle swabbing of the hymenal area will reveal if the source of bleeding is from this site.

The anatomy of the hymen varies enormously from individual to individual. The membrane may be thin, very elastic, thick, rigid or a combination. In shape it may take the form of a very thin crescent with a large orifice; annular with small orifice; congenital frilly with a large orifice; strong midline bar only. Commonly the membrane is deficient anteriorly, and most pronounced posteriorly, and it follows that damage to the hymen occurs almost invariably in the posterior quadrant.

Rupture of the hymen on first penetration is of course very common but it is not inevitable, for the thin elastic hymen is quite capable of stretching to accommodate penetration even by an erect adult penis without frank rupture. Where there is hymenal tearing, the extent and position of the tear must be noted. Some authorities hold that hymenal tears due to digital penetration tend to be posterior in position, whilst tears due to penile penetration tend to be posterolateral. In the author's experience, it is merely a matter of chance as to the exact location of a tear, for in both types of penetration the main stretching force is taken on the posterior quadrant of the hymen. Tears due to digital penetration are frequently incomplete in that they do not extend to the margin of the hymen, and the same can be said for tears due to the insertion of tampons, while tears due to penile penetration are complete in that they extend to the margin, but even this situation is not constant, and digital tears

caused by 'full finger' penetration can extend to the hymenal margin and conversely penile tears with only limited penetration may be incomplete.

It is rare for tears due to either digital or penile penetration in an adult to extend beyond the margin of the hymen to the vaginal walls or the perineal body, but injuries of this type can occur in elderly adults, or if there is gross disproportion between the penetrating penis and the vagina, or in cases when large foreign bodies have been inserted into the vagina (large vibrators, sticks, dildos, etc.). Extended injury such as this is also found on both digital and penile penetration in the case of very young children, and may sometimes be found in adults when intercourse has been accomplished in the 'standing erect' posture.

Frequently, even in the absence of frank hymenal tearing, there is abrasion and bruising of the hymen and the vaginal orifice. Such a finding is certainly consistent with penetration of the hymenal orifice, but it is often difficult to differentiate between digital and penile penetration. The differential diagnosis must depend on the extent of the bruising, the elasticity of the hymen, and the size of the hymenal orifice.

After the hymen has been carefully inspected, and before any digital examination of the vagina is attempted, two further swabs at least must be taken. Firstly a low vaginal swab should be taken by gently separating the inner labia and passing a swab just into the vaginal canal without touching the labia or the perineum with the swab in transit. If these precautions are taken, any seminal traces subsequently found on the swab must have come from within the lowest part of the vaginal canal and could not have been introduced as a contaminant from the thighs, labia or perineum. Secondly, a small vaginal speculum should be gently introduced into the vagina and a high vaginal swab should be taken under direct vision through the speculum from a point well above the beak of the speculum. In this way it is ensured that any seminal traces subsequently identified by the laboratory arose from the vagina and were not introduced into the vagina as contaminants on the fingers of the examining doctor, or by contact of the swab with contaminated areas outside the vagina. It is vital that the low vaginal swab and the high vaginal swab are obtained before any digital examination of the vagina is attempted. Failure to obtain these swabs in that order will lead to the integrity of these swabs being suspect.

It may seem to be an unnecessarily painful procedure to introduce a speculum into a tender and possibly injured vagina in this way, but there is no other method of inspection of the interior vagina available, and it is impossible to exclude serious vaginal injury which may require surgical treatment without this investigation. In 26 years of practice the author has never failed to introduce a speculum with only minimal discomfort under these circumstances, and the knack lies in the selection of a speculum that is small enough to minimise pain whilst being large enough to afford a clear view of the interior of the vagina and the cervix. In cases of gross external injury, and in the case of very young children, resort to examination under an anaesthetic may be necessary, but the speculum examination should never be neglected.

Once the internal swabs have been obtained, and with the speculum still in situ, the interior of the vagina should be inspected for signs of bruising and abrasion as well as for the more serious but much rarer laceration of the vaginal vault or walls. At this stage a swab of the cervical mucus can also be taken should the local forensic science laboratory require one.

Bruising of the vagina is seen in its early stages as areas of darker red against the overall redness of the vaginal mucosa. It is more frequently seen on the anterior vaginal wall in the lower third, and on the posterior wall in the upper third. Bruising of this nature is more consistent with penile penetration than with digital penetration.

With the passage of time, vaginal bruising gradually takes on a darker hue, and normally within 24 h shows a deep red/purple hue. Because of the good blood supply and the comparative thinness of the overlying mucosa, vaginal bruises reveal themselves almost immediately and can be seen on examination within an hour of the injury. Abrasion of the vaginal mucosa can be the result of either digital or penile penetration, but is more frequently seen in the former.

Injuries of these types can occur during consenting sexual intercourse as well as during acts where there has been no consent, and it is almost impossible to differentiate between the two causes.

The degree of injury may be of some slight assistance in this matter, for local injury will tend to be more severe in situations where the normal lubrication of the vagina is lacking on first penetration. Thus in consenting intercourse, where there has been some preliminary lovemaking, there is normally considerable lubrication of the mucosa before penetration is attempted, and subsequent injury tends to be less severe. In rape or digital penetration without consent, where preliminary stimulation has not taken place, initial lubrication tends to be lacking and more severe local bruising or abrasion can result. Nevertheless, identical injury can result from consenting intercourse and intercourse without consent. It must also be remembered that the reaction of the vaginal mucosa to a penetrating foreign body is to lubricate, and therefore even in non-consenting intercourse there will be a certain amount of lubrication produced during the act, even if lubrication was lacking on initial penetration. The frequently repeated myth that the vagina will remain dry in non-consenting intercourse with the resulting production of serious abrasion and bruising is entirely untrue.

In the case of sexually experienced women, and those who have borne children, signs of even the most minor vaginal injury may well be absent.

Frank laceration of the vagina is rare following penile penetration in women of childbearing age, but it can occur in very young children and in the atrophic post-menopausal vagina. When present it does not indicate lack of consent. This may well be one explanation, but such injuries may also result from consenting intercourse where there has been considerable disproportion between the penetrating penis and the vagina; where there has been very active and enthusiastic copulation; and in cases where there has been complete abstinence from intercourse for a considerable length of time.[6]

Careful inspection of the vaginal mucosa with the speculum in situ may provide valuable information as to previous sexual experience. The vaginal rugae are well marked in the virginal vagina and in the vagina of women who are not used to sexual intercourse. They tend to become less well marked in women who are sexually experienced, and are almost obliterated in women who have borne children. It is impossible to be specific as to the number of acts of intercourse that will produce observable flattening of the rugae, for this is a subjective observation on the part of the examiner, but in the author's experience such a change is observable in most cases where there has been in excess of 12 acts of intercourse. Such a change does not result from the regular use of internal tampons, but will follow repeated use of a large vibrator or dildo, and this fact is well worth remembering in the face of the sexual climate that exists today.

Still with the vaginal speculum in situ, the vaginal portion of the cervix must be inspected in order to identify the possible source of any vaginal bleeding and to exclude any injury. Blood seen to be coming from the external cervical os is most likely to be of menstrual origin, but the cervix must be gently swabbed to ensure that the blood is coming from the os and not from an injury or abrasion of the cervix. Abrasion of the cervix is almost invariably the result of vaginal penetration, and is usually the result of digital rather than penile penetration, but it can be caused by the insertion of a tampon. Erosion of the cervix is not a result of penetration, but is always a pre-existing condition, even in the case of the young and previously virginal girl.

It is important to recall the types of cervical erosion in this respect:

1. Congenital erosion, due to a persistence of the columnar epithelium on to the vaginal portion of the cervix, so that the junction between the squamous epithelium of the vagina and the columnar epithelium of the cervical canal is situated outside the external cervical os. This type of erosion is common even in female infants, and frequently persists into adult life.

2. Acquired erosion, due to childbirth, injury or chronic infection.

3. Adenomatous erosion, due to the multiplication of the glands of the cervix during pregnancy and in any other state where there is an increase in oestrogenic hormones. In this type of glands increase both in size and in number, and rupture through the squamous epithelium producing a raw area on the vaginal portion of the cervix.

4. Hormonal erosion, due to a rise in oestrogens which cause a proliferation of the cervical columnar epithelium and the mucous secreting glands.

All these erosions are present as bright red areas on the overall redness of the cervix, and are usually situated around the external os with the exception of the adenomatous type that may appear at some distance from the portio vaginalis. They all have a sharply circumscribed margin, and many are sufficiently friable and vascular to bleed on contact.

It is sometimes difficult to differentiate between an abrasion of the cervix and an erosion, but as a general rule an erosion tends to be in the immediate vicinity of the external cervical os, and to have the sharply defined margin described above, while the abrasion is found away from the external os and has a much less clearly circumscribed margin.

When the careful visual inspection of the vagina has been completed, and the internal vaginal swabs have been taken, the speculum can be slowly withdrawn from the vagina under direct vision so that the vaginal mucosa is inspected throughout the withdrawal.

After the speculum has been removed further examination of the vagina is permitted. This further examination must consist of a digital examination, and may include an examination of the hymenal area with Glaister Keen rods or their modifications.

The original idea of the Glaister Keen rod was to examine the hymen so that the size of the hymenal orifice could be assessed in respect of the size of the rod accepted, and to inspect the hymenal membrane for recent and old tears. Unfortunately, the use of these instruments requires that the rod is introduced through the hymenal orifice, and is then partly withdrawn so that the illuminated knob on the end of the shaft is gently pulled back against the vaginal surface of the hymen. Such a manoeuvre is almost certain to introduce into the vaginal canal some contaminants from the introitus and the labia, and these contaminants may subsequently be recovered on the internal vaginal swabs. To obviate this risk, the introduction of such an instrument should be delayed until after the speculum examination has been completed and the internal swabs have been taken. If this is done, however, there may well be some distortion of hymenal tears which may have been extended by the passage of the speculum.

With increasing reliance being placed upon the scientific findings, the author has ceased using Glaister Keen rods in rape examinations, preferring to inspect the hymen as previously described. In cases where there has been no allegation of recent penile penetration, the Glaister Keen rod is a very valuable instrument for the inspection of the hymen, and may be used with complete confidence at the start of the examination of the genitalia and with no risk of carrying seminal contaminants into the vaginal canal.

During the digital examination, the examining doctor must assess the laxity of the vaginal orifice, the length of the vagina into the posterior fornix, the number of examining fingers that can be introduced through the hymenal orifice, and the areas and degree of tenderness complained of by the patient.

Frequently the question of prior virginity is raised in allegations of rape or unlawful sexual intercourse with a girl under the age of 16 years, and this question is of course of paramount importance in civil cases where issues of non-consummation are involved. It is a very difficult question for the doctor to answer, and in many cases the only possible answer is 'I do not know'.

The variable anatomy of the hymen has already been referred to, so the probative value of that ridiculous vestigial remnant is greatly reduced in assessment of prior virginity. Add to the variable anatomy the fact that the hymen can be stretched or torn by the regular use of tampons, by masturbation, or by digital penetration, and its value as a token of virginity is almost completely lost.

Severe hymenal lacerations may be indicative of first ever penile penetration, however, and the presence of a hymenal orifice that will not admit the tip of the examining finger is definite proof of virginity. Conversely, the thin, elastic hymen that allows two examining fingers to pass through the opening is no indication at all of lack of prior virginity.

The question of previous sexual experience is more easy to answer, for the vagina itself undergoes certain changes when it is exposed to fairly frequent sexual intercourse, and these changes do not take place as the result of regular use of internal tampons or of regular digital penetration and stimulation. The vaginal rugae tend to become less pronounced, and the vagina itself lengthens into the posterior fornix. In cases where the vaginal rugae have become smoothed out, and the vagina easily

accepts the full length of the examining finger into the posterior fornix, it is safe to give the opinion that the vagina is well used to sexual intercourse.[7] These changes can take place as the result of as few as six acts of intercourse, but more commonly some 20 acts are required to produce the 'well used' feel of the vagina. As the interpretation of these changes is a subjective one on the part of the examining doctor there can be no hard and fast rule, and there is no exact scientific measurement. In the present day situation there is the added complication that similar changes will be produced by the use of vibrators as masturbatory aids.

Genital herpes. The condition of genital herpes is sometimes considered to be indicative of venereal contact, and a brief consideration of this condition must be included in this chapter.

All types of genital herpes are not venereal in origin, and it is therefore quite wrong to assume that the mere presence of this condition is an automatic guarantee of sexual contact.

There are, in fact, two quite distinct viral strains that can produce herpetic eruptions on the genitalia. Herpes simplex Type 1 will produce herpetic infection without any venereal or sexual contact, and it is the strain that produces primary infection in children up to the age of about 10 years, with the peak between the ages of 1–6. It is most common in the area of the mouth, where it can affect the gums, mouth, lips and tongue, and from where it may be transmitted to the genitalia on the child's own fingers, producing the lesions of herpes genitalis. The condition is well recognised in female children, and is comparatively rare in male children.

The primary infection presents as an inflammation of the vulva and sometimes of the vagina, with the formation of small blisters associated with a moderate fever and some enlargement of the inguinal lymph glands. The blisters soon break to form flat whitish-yellow plaques which ulcerate within a few hours to produce typical 'punched out' ulcers. The whole condition settles down within 7–10 days, and it is only after this length of time that the patient shows any significant antibody response.

After the primary infection has subsided, some patients develop recurrent eruptions of herpes blisters at the site of the primary infection, and these secondary blisters are preceded by severe local irritation and pain, and quickly pass through to the healing stage without ulcer formation. Recurrent eruptions are commonly associated with non-specific factors, and may occur during any febrile illness, menstruation, gastric upsets and even emotional problems.

Primary infection in adults and adolescents however is very commonly due to sexual contact, and is caused by Herpes simplex Type 2.

It follows that before any opinion as to a venereal cause for a genital herpes can be substantiated, it is important that viral studies on swabs from the lesions are undertaken to identify the strain of herpes simplex, and that antibody studies are made on the blood of both parties involved. This question arises more frequently in the case of young girls below the age of 10 years, but it may arise in cases involving adolescents and even adults.

The opinion

By the end of his clinical examination the doctor should be in a position to answer the questions:
1. Could intercourse have taken place in that particular vagina?
2. Are there general signs of force or intoxication present?
3. The question 'has intercourse taken place recently?' is more difficult to answer.

Sexual intercourse without general force and not against resistance will show very little in the way of physical signs even if the patient is examined a short time afterwards. The pooling of seminal fluid in the vagina is obviously a sign of recent sexual intercourse, but this pooling may rapidly disappear if an upright posture is adopted soon after ejaculation has taken place when much of the seminal pool will drain out of the vagina. There will of course be no pooling at all if a condom has been worn or if ejaculation has not taken place within the vagina.

Some engorgement of the vaginal mucosa takes place during sexual intercourse, and this is associated with swelling and engorgement of the introitus, labia minora and clitoris, but this redness and swelling may persist only for a very short time, and medical examination within 1 h of the act may reveal very little abnormal. Mere redness of

the genitalia is no indication of recent sexual intercourse.

A patulous appearance of the vaginal orifice can sometimes be seen in women who have not borne children, but this sign is short-lived and very rarely persists for more than 1 h after intercourse. It is of no significance at all in the case of women who have borne children, and is only of very doubtful value in women who have regular sexual intercourse.

Some guide as to the time of ejaculation can be obtained if a few drops of the vaginal pool of secretion is examined under the microscope. In the living, the body reactions tend to cleanse the vagina of foreign proteins, and as a result the spermatozoa in the male ejaculate undergo changes within the vagina. Motility is maintained for 1–6 h after ejaculation into the vagina, with the number of motile spermatozoa gradually becoming less. Few motile sperm will be seen after about 6 h, but the persistence of motility is very variable depending upon the time in the menstrual cycle and the full effects of such hormonal preparations as the contraceptive pill upon sperm motility, which are not fully understood.

After motility has ceased, spermatozoa remain intact for as long as 48 h, and they then separate into heads and tails. In the living, identifiable portions of spermatozoa can be seen for up to four days after ejaculation into the vagina. In the rape–murder situation, where death has intervened before the natural vaginal cleansing process has proceeded, indentifiable spermatozoa or portions of spermatozoa can be found for many days if not many weeks after ejaculation (R. V. Christie).

It must follow that any opinion based upon the presence of motile spermatazoa cannot be precise to within 12 h.

Recently work has been undertaken at the Metropolitan Police Forensic Science Laboratory[8,9] in which p-nitrophenyl phosphate has been used to quantitate acid phosphatase activity on vaginal swabs. The method used was a modification of that outlined by the Sigma Chemical Company[10] for the determination of serum acid phosphatase activity. Acid phosphatase activity is determined on vaginal swabs obtained from the alleged victims of sexual assaults, and the activity is expressed in sigma units. Preliminary results indicate that levels of activity less than 20 sigma units on vaginal swabs indicate time intervals of at least 48 h between ejaculation and subsequent vaginal swabbing.

This method is of probable value in excluding semen of a consenting partner where the last act of consenting intercourse was 48 h or more prior to the incident under investigation.

Rape is not a medical diagnosis, it is a legal definition. No doctor can be expected to give an opinion regarding consent, for consent or the lack of it does not leave physical signs on medical examination. All that can be expected from the examining doctor are the results of his medical findings as to signs of general injury, intoxication, patient demeanour and genital findings as to penetration. The interpretation of these findings is for the Court.

There are no genital findings that *must* indicate lack of consent, other than the signs of penetration in females who are unable to give a valid consent. The genital signs can only indicate penetration and intercourse—sometimes they may indicate enthusiastic, vigorous and multiple acts of intercourse— but they can *never* indicate lack of consent. The examining doctor must avoid the pitfall of concluding that because certain sexual acts are repugnant to him they must have been committed without consent. Oro-genital contact, anal stimulation during normal heterosexual lovemaking, bondage and intercourse with a number of different partners (the so-termed 'Gang Bang') are rapidly becoming part of the 'sexual norm' and are indulged in with full consent and enthusiasm at the time, but may be the grounds for a delayed allegation of rape when the euphoria of the incident is replaced by self-disgust.

Specimens to be taken in cases of alleged rape and indecent assault

The object of taking specimens for the laboratory in cases of alleged sexual assault is threefold:
1. to obtain confirmation of the allegations;
2. to attempt to establish a link between the victim and the scene;
3. to attempt to establish a link between the victim and the assailant.[11]

The basis of the scientific investigation of sexual offences is found in Locard's principle of transfer of physical traces, and can be summarised as: 'Every contact leaves a trace'.

It is the examining doctor's duty to take all valid specimens so that the forensic science laboratories can identify these vital traces that will corroborate the various contacts that must arise during a sexual assault.

The choice of specimen will, of course, depend upon the allegations, and the following list is not exclusive, neither is it mandatory:

Blood. For grouping and for analysis for alcohol and drugs if the latter is indicated by the history or by the examination findings.

Urine. For routine testing for glucose and albumen, as well as for screening for drugs if the history indicates that this is needed.

Buccal swabs. For seminal testing if there has been any allegation of oro-penile contact. Seminal traces are quickly lost from the mouth of the live victim, but positive traces have been found up to 8 h after ejaculation within the mouth provided:
1. the victim has not cleaned her teeth nor taken a hot drink between the incident and swabbing, and,
2. careful swabbing has been done to both surfaces of the teeth.
'Deep throat' swabbing will give negative results even if the swabs are taken within about 1 h of ejaculation, and are therefore a waste of time—a negative result on such a swab cannot be taken to mean that no oro-penile ejaculation has taken place.

Saliva. To establish the secretor status of the victim.

Head hair. To be obtained either by combing or by avulsion, for comparison with hairs found at the scene or on the alleged assailant.

Soiling. So that the laboratory may attempt to identify its nature and compare it with material at the scene or from the assailant. All soiled areas on the body must be swabbed.

Bite marks. Must be swabbed so that possible saliva grouping of the biter can be established. If such marks are swabbed, a control swab must be taken from an uncontaminated area of skin for laboratory comparison.

Pubic hair. For comparison with any pubic hairs found at the scene and with the pubic hair of the alleged assailant. Samples should be obtained by combing with a fine toothed comb so that any loose and possible foreign hairs are recovered, and also by avulsion for comparison purposes.

Matted pubic hair. For identification of the contaminating substance. The entire matted area should be cut off as close to the skin as possible.

Fingernail samples. For identification of any soiling trapped below the nails. These samples may be taken by scraping the soiled material out from beneath the nails, or by clipping the nails. In either case, each nail or soiling must be placed in a separate container.

Genital swabs. For identification of seminal traces, infecting organisms. These specimens must be taken as described in the text so that the risk of accidental contamination is avoided (Figs 5.4A & 5.4B).

RAPID REFERENCE SHEET
EXAMINATION OF RAPE VICTIM

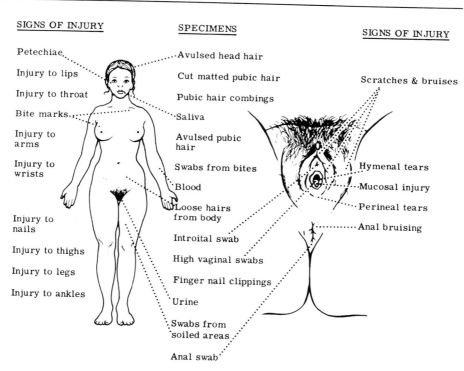

SIGNS OF INJURY

Petechiae
Injury to lips
Injury to throat
Bite marks
Injury to arms
Injury to wrists
Injury to nails
Injury to thighs
Injury to legs
Injury to ankles

SPECIMENS

Avulsed head hair
Cut matted pubic hair
Pubic hair combings
Saliva
Avulsed pubic hair
Swabs from bites
Blood
Loose hairs from body
Introital swab
High vaginal swabs
Finger nail clippings
Urine
Swabs from soiled areas
Anal swab

SIGNS OF INJURY

Scratches & bruises
Hymenal tears
Mucosal injury
Perineal tears
Anal bruising

ROUTINE
1. Obtain consent to examination and report.
2. Take detailed general history.
3. Take detailed menstrual history, and obstetrical history.
4. Take detailed history of event.
5. Observe - behaviour, distress, cosmetics, etc.
6. Examine clothing - retain for laboratory examination.
7. Full general clinical examination - record all findings.
8. Detailed genital examination - swab first.
9. Take all relevant specimens. Establish chain of evidence.
10. Give opinion - medical findings consistent or not with history given.

Fig. 5.4A Department of Medical Illustration, Guy's Hospital. Lecture notes of Dr Paul. Published in the Legal Medicine Annual (1977).

SPECIMENS IN RAPE AND INDECENT ASSAULT

TO PROVIDE CORROBORATIVE EVIDENCE SPECIMENS MUST BE TAKEN AND STORED WITH CARE.

ALWAYS MAINTAIN THE CHAIN OF EVIDENCE

1) Identify the specimen.

2) Label the specimen, and sign the label.

3) Record the disposal of the specimen.

THE VICTIM	THE ACCUSED
Avulsed Head Hair	Avulsed Head Hair
Pubic Hair Combings	Pubic Hair Combings
Avulsed Pubic Hair	Avulsed Pubic Hair
Finger Nail Scrapings	Finger Nail Scrapings
Swabs from any Bite Marks	Swabs from any Bite Marks
Introital Swab	Penile Shaft Swab
Perineal Swab	Coronal Sulcus Swab
High Vaginal Swab	Urethral Swab
Anal Swab (if Buggery alleged)	
Buccal Swab if oro-penile contact within 8 hr. of examination	
Saliva, for Secretor Grouping	Saliva, for Secretor Grouping
Blood, for Group, Alcohol & Drugs	Blood, for Group, Alcohol & Drugs
Urine, for Alcohol & Drugs	Urine, for Alcohol & Drugs
Swabs from all soiled areas	Swabs from all soiled areas

OBTAIN BLOOD AND SALIVA FROM ANY PERSON WHO HAS HAD CONSENTING INTERCOURSE WITHIN THE PREVIOUS 14 DAYS WITH THE VICTIM.

Fig. 5.4B Lecture notes of Dr Paul.

The clinical examination in cases of incest

It is uncommon for complaints of this offence to be made early. In the majority of cases the complaint is made to police, welfare services, or school only after the offences have been going on for some considerable time. The complainant is frequently the mother or sister of the 'victim', or it is the victim herself who makes the complaint because the incestuous activities are damaging her social activities or because she feels that she is being unfairly punished.

The examining doctor's role in most cases is merely to establish whether sexual intercourse has ever taken place, and the same routine examination as has been detailed previously should be undertaken.

Because of the almost invariable delay in the reporting of this offence, there is little point in tak-

ing the many specimens that should be the norm in the medical examination of rape victims. However, if the last episode of incestuous sexual intercourse is alleged to have taken place within 14 days of the medical examination, all the routine genital swabs, blood and saliva must be taken as in a case of alleged rape. These specimens could provide the corroborative evidence of identity of the partner involved.

The medical examination in sexual offences against children

The routine of clinical examination of the young child victim of a sexual assault varies little from the routine already described in detail in this chapter, but there are some special problems that may arise in the very young age group.

Sex of victim

Child victims can be of either sex. The offence of rape is obviously restricted to female infants, but the more common offences of indecent assault and buggery may involve children of both sexes.

Sex of assailant

The term 'pseudo-sexual' would be better applied to some of these assaults, for in some cases of alleged sexual assaults upon very young children the offence is not strictly sexual in that they do not take place to satisfy an overwhelming sexual urge on the part of the assailant.

These cases arise as an extension of the 'non accidental injury to children' and indeed take place in the same type of age group. The assault arises as an expression of anger, sometimes against the child because of bed-wetting or fouling, sometimes as an expression of anger or jealousy against another adult. Whatever the psychiatric explanation of the assault, the possible pseudo-sexual nature of the offence must cast doubt on the sex of the assailant.

Vaginal injury following digital penetration in an infant may have been caused by either a male or a female finger. Similarly an injury following digital penetration may have been produced by an assailant of either sex. In these cases the examining doctor must always be aware of these possibilities, and it is a prudent step to obtain relevant samples from all adults, of both sexes, who had possible contact with the assaulted infant, i.e. fingernail clippings and scrapings.

History of assault

It is obviously impossible to obtain a detailed history from a very young child, and the examining doctor is compelled to accept an account of the incident from relatives, neighbours, other children or police officers. Such accounts are rarely accurate and must be viewed with great suspicion, for in the main the history will relate only to the finding of the injured child.

As the age of the victim increases, so does the amount of detail available on direct questioning. By the age of four or five years a reasonable history can be obtained by the doctor from the child if the doc-tor is prepared to spend considerable time and patience, and to use a child's vocabulary in his questioning. Much patience and time is required if the doctor is going to obtain any sort of history from a hurt and frightened child, but the expenditure is worth while.

Anatomical

The very small size of the infant genitalia will obviously present difficulties during the examination and in many cases examination under an anaesthetic is the only way in which proper inspection of the vagina can be carried out. Such a procedure must be used if there is any doubt at all regarding the extent of the injuries, or if any surgical repair is required, or even if the child is very frightened.

In all cases involving children it should be obvious that special paediatric instruments must be used.

Anal and rectal examination does not normally present the same degree of difficulty as vaginal examination, and most children will tolerate such an examination well. However, if there is any doubt as to the extent of injury, or if the child is very frightened, resort to examination under anaesthesia should be made.

Genital tract injury

The pattern of injury to the genital tract will vary with the following factors:
1. the nature and size of the penetrating object;
2. the size of the pelvic outlet and the vagina of the victim;
3. the force with which penetration is attempted.

Pelvic outlet and vagina

The pelvic outlet of a female infant is irregular in shape but is approximately 'heart shaped' with the narrowest part situated at the front. Exact measurements are very difficult to make, for the bony margins are very flexible. The pelvic outlet accommodates the urethra, vagina and anal canal.

In view of the diameter of the stool that can be passed by an infant of one year of age, there can be no doubt that an object the size of an adult erect penis can pass through the pelvic outlet, but in so doing it will seriously compress all the structures that lie between it and the anterior and lateral margins of the outlet. It is this compression of the soft tissues against the bony margins of the pelvic outlet that dictates the pattern of injury found on attempted or achieved penile penetration.

At the commencement of penetration, the penis tends to compress the labia both anteriorly and laterally, producing bruising of both the labia minora and the labia majora for in the infant there is only poor separation between the labia. The amount of bruising will depend upon the force used in attempting penetration.

Further attempts at penetration force the penis backwards, for anterior movement is prevented by the symphysis pubis, and the hymen is torn. The resultant tear is directed at the area of maximum roominess (i.e., backwards) and the penis then advances into the vagina, putting additional pressure on to the anterior and lateral structures and extending the hymenal tear into or through the perineal body and often involving the anterior wall of the ano–rectal canal.

The smaller and younger the infant, the more widespread the injuries that will result from attempted or complete penile penetration. Bruising of the labia with extensive haematoma production affecting particularly the anterior half is very common. Circumferential tears of the mucosa of the vestibule, and posterior linear tears of the hymen extending up the posterior vaginal wall and downwards to involve the skin of the perineum and the perineal body are frequent. The circumferential mucosal tears are indicative of attempted penetration by an object the size of an erect adult penis.[12,13]

Full penile penetration will usually show, in addition to the preceding signs, bruising of the vaginal walls associated frequently with tears which may involve both the anterior and posterior vaginal wall. Anterior tears can involve the bladder and the peritoneal reflections; posterior tears can involve the ano–rectal canal; rupture of the vaginal vault can occur, with resulting vaginal hernation of abdominal viscera.

The pattern of injury will tend to become less marked as the age and size of the infant increases, but the characteristic circumferential tears of the vestibular mucosa are constant findings, in the author's experience, up to the age of six years, and are frequent findings beyond that age.[14]

Digital penetration of the infant vagina produces less compression of the soft tissues, and the pattern of injury is different. There is frequently some scratching or bruising of the labia and vestibule, but because the compression of the soft tissues is largely absent there is little shearing force applied to the mucosa and the characteristic circumferential tears are absent.

The commonest pattern of injury is a linear tear of the hymen, usually situated in the posterior or posterolateral quadrant. The tear may extend for a short distance upwards into the posterior vaginal wall and downwards on to the skin of the perineum where it may involve the perineal body. Involvement of the ano-rectal canal is rare. There is frequently bruising in the margins of the tear, and vaginal wall bruising on the anterior wall but vaginal vault injury is rare.

If the size of the penetrating object approximates to the dimensions of a penis, the resultant pattern of injury will approach that found on penile penetration or attempted penetration.

Effects of genital injury

Both the nerve and blood supply to the area of the genitals is very good, and it follows that injury to that area will almost invariably produce a marked response by the infant victim.

Pain response will be almost immediate, and will consist of loud screams at the moment the injury is sustained. This response is most marked in infants up to about four years of age. Above that age the crying response to the accidental 'splits' type of injury will be greatly reduced and may even be absent. The immediate cry will not be sustained, and in many cases of non-accidental injury to children under four years, crying ceases soon after the injury has been sustained with the child becoming apathetic, shocked or cowed. The degree of shock is directly related to the severity of the injury sustained. It is as though the child has become 'numbed' to pain soon after the injury is inflicted, and in many cases the child will not cry even during the subsequent medical examination.

Bleeding response to genital injury is again brisk

and almost immediate, although there may be a few seconds delay before overt bleeding is visible. This delay may be sufficient to prevent blood soiling of the penetrating object if prompt withdrawal is accomplished. Bleeding will be brisk from the skin and mucosa, but may only be slight from the perineal body. It normally ceases within 5–10 min, but may be re-started if the infant moves or if the wound margins are wiped.

Other genital signs

In addition to the signs of overt genital injury, other less specific signs may be present and may cause some confusion.

Redness of the mucosa is often seen and is frequently interpreted as being indicative of sexual assault. This is an incorrect interpretation for the infantile mucosa is normally much more red than that of the post-pubescent merely because the epithelium is much thinner.[15] This overall redness is not the same as the more localised redness due to bruising or abrasion.

Excoriation of the skin of the vulval and perineal areas, and of the skin of the natal cleft, is sometimes interpreted as being due to sexual assault, and this is again an incorrect interpretation for excoriation of this type is common in young children as a result of poor local hygiene, scratching due to worm infestation, or maceration following the exclusion of air by waterproof panties.

On occasions a frank vulvo–vaginitis may be found of the Monilia type following a course of oral antibiotics, and there may be the local lesions of a Herpes simplex infection. The examining doctor must be very careful in his interpretation of these genital findings, and must differentiate between these common and naturally occurring conditions and the injuries of sexual assault.

Accidental genital injury

There is no doubt that accidental injury to the genital area of female infants does take place. The mechanism of such accidental injury can be divided into two main groups:

Penetrating injuries where the injury results from a fall on to a pointed object, and where it is very rare indeed for the penetration to take place through the hymen. Commonly in these types of injury the hymen is intact and penetration has taken place through the lateral margins of the labia, with the wound entering the vagina through its walls.[16]

Stretching or 'splits' injuries can occur when the legs are violently abducted such as if the child slips on a slippery surface.[17] In these cases a tear can be produced which can involve the skin of the perineum, the perineal body and the hymen. Such tears are never associated with abrasion and bruising of the tear margins, and this lack of marginal injury enables the differential diagnosis to be made.

Deliberate forceful abduction of an infant's legs can also produce an identical injury to the perineum as can the accidental stretch, but under these circumstances there will almost invariably be the characteristic 'grasping' type of injury at the ankles, legs, knees or thighs, which will assist in the differential diagnosis of cause.

General signs of injury

The younger the child, the less able it is to resist its assailant, and the fewer signs of general injury that will be found on the body.

A full 'head to toe' examination is of course vital, and in the older child typical 'grasping' injuries and bruises resulting from blows may be found.

All signs of injury tend to be absent in cases where the sexual assailant is one of the parents, or is a person well known to the child.

Specimens

As in the case of the adult victim, it is the examining doctor's duty to take all relevant specimens at the time of his initial examination, and the list of specimens is identical to that for an adult.

Clothing worn at the time of the assault or put on immediately afterwards must be inspected and retained for laboratory examination, and this must include nappies. It is on these items that traces of semen, lubricant and blood may be found as well as on and in the body of the victim.

Examination of the suspected assailant

The general scheme for the medical examination of

a person suspected of a sexual assault is detailed later in this chapter, but there are some extra factors to look for in the case of a child's assailant.

Because of the pseudo-sexual nature of many of the assaults against very young infants, the examining doctor must advise the investigating authority that the sex of the assailant does not have to be male. All adults who had possible access to the child over the time interval when the offence is thought to have been committed must be examined, with particular search for contamination of the fingernails. Penile penetration into the vagina or the anus of a small child cannot be accomplished without considerable force, and this will very frequently result in some injury to the penis of the assailant.

The type of injury will vary, and the examining doctor should look carefully for abrasion of the glans penis and for tears of the frenulum in the uncircumcised. Swabbing from the coronal sulcus beneath the prepuce will often reveal blood or faecal traces even if the assailant has washed his genitalia after the assault. In cases of anal penetration the penis of the assailant may show an identical pattern of injury, and penile swabs may show the presence of lubricant traces. The penile swabs should never be omitted if the assailant is examined within 24 h of the alleged assault.

Essentials of medical examination of a man suspected of rape or indecent assault

The doctor will find himself confronted with the alleged victim of a sexual assault far more frequently than with the suspect. This is not a surprising state of affairs, for it is the victim who is first brought to the notice of the police, and whose medical examination is the first to be performed. In many cases it is only after the initial medical examination of the victim has been completed that the search for the perpetrator commences. There is nearly always a delay, varying from a few hours to many days, before the suspect is produced for medical examination. In many cases the suspect is never found.

In those cases where the suspect is available for medical examination, the same doctor should undertake the examination as examined the victim. In this way there should be better correlation between the injuries found on the female (bite marks, finger-tip bruises, comparison of size and build) and the physical features of the suspect man. Obviously there will be occasions when it is impossible for the same doctor to be involved in both examinations, and it is because of this fact that every doctor involved in medico-legal examinations of this type should follow a similar routine that embraces all the essential points of examination and specimen gathering. Ideally, a different examination room should be used for each of the examinations, so that the risk of accidental contamination of specimens is negated.

The clinical examination of the suspect male is to all intents a 'mirror image' of the examination performed upon the victim.

Consent. Consent to the examination and to any subsequent report should be obtained by the doctor from the accused man himself. It need not be in writing, but the fact that it was obtained should be recorded in the notes. In the case of a minor, or of a man unable to give a valid consent, written consent must be obtained from a parent or guardian and the parent or guardian is entitled to be present throughout the examination if they so wish.

General history. A general medical history should be taken from the patient, and this must include details of all past illnesses, surgical operations and serious accidents. It must also include details of all recent medical attention, medication and consumption of alcoholic drinks.

Specific history. It is here that the routines may vary between the examination of an alleged victim and a suspect man. In most cases of this type, the man is already under a 'caution' at the time of the medical examination, and it is no part of the examining doctor's duty to 'play the policeman'. It is therefore unwise for the doctor to attempt to obtain any history of the specific incident and he should restrict his questions to such matters as:

1. has the man been informed of the reason for the medical examination?
2. has consenting intercourse taken place with any person within the previous 24 h?
3. when was the last bath or wash?
4. when was the last change of clothing?
5. what are the explanations for any marks or injury found?

In the author's opinion it is wrong to read any statement said to have been made by the suspect male to police officers *before* the medical examination is complete. Such a statement may well influence the examining doctor, and affect the vital principle of impartiality previously referred to.

General observation of the patient should be maintained throughout the history taking and examination, and this extends to such matters as the patient's demeanour. Is he distressed or calm, co-operative or aggressive, dazed or shocked, intoxicated or in command of his senses?

The clothing worn at the time of the alleged offence should be carefully examined and, if being worn at the time of the medical examination, should be removed garment by garment with identical precautions as in the case of the alleged victim.

Frequently the original clothing will have been discarded, however, and the clothing being worn at the time of the medical examination will be of no significance. If the original clothing is available, the examining doctor should inspect it for areas of soiling and damage in the same way that he should inspect the clothing of the victim.

Certain garments require particular inspection: shoes often retain particles of earth or fibre trapped between the uppers and soles at the welt, and these particles may well identify the suspect with the scene; trousers will often show soiling at the knees from grass and earth, and the inside of the crutch and fly area may reveal seminal soiling under ultra-violet light; the zip fly is often the repository for loose hairs which may have originated from the victim; blood and seminal soiling will often be present on the inside of the trouser fly, the inside of the underpants and on the inner surface of the front shirt tail.

General clinical examination must follow in every case and, as in the case of the victim, this must include a record of the patient's height, weight and build, as well as routine examination of all bodily systems.

Special attention must be given to all visible signs of injury of whatever age. Fingernail injuries are the most common, and tend to be found on the face and neck, the hands and wrists, and only very rarely indeed on the genitals. The characteristic fingernail injury commences with a curved indentation, and then tails off both in width and depth,

often with visible 'piling up' of superficial tissue at the distal end.

Slapping marks can sometimes be seen if the examination takes place soon after the event, and there may be signs of superficial injury to the inner surface of the lips following even mild blows to the mouth.

Bite marks can be found as signs of resistance by the victim, and such marks tend to be on the hands, arms or face. This is not the case where sexual biting occurs during consenting lovemaking.

The entire body must be carefully searched for any loose hairs or other foreign objects, and anything found must be retained for laboratory examination.

Detailed examination of the genital area

This must follow the general examination, and again must follow a definite order to ensure that no possible contamination of any specimen can take place.

Firstly the pubic hair should be carefully examined and any matted areas must be noted. The entire matted area should then be cut away as close to the skin as possible, and the entire mat should be retained for laboratory examination.

Next, the entire pubic area should be combed with a sterile fine-toothed comb and the comb, together with any loose hairs, should be retained for laboratory examination.

A sample of pubic hair should next be avulsed to provide the laboratory with a control sample of hair.

The penis should be carefully examined, and any abnormality that could interfere with erection or ejaculation should be noted as must all injuries.

Penetration into a very tight hymenal orifice, even with consent, may produce injury to the foreskin, frenulum or glans penis. Such injury is of course not indicative of lack of consent, but may be due to great disparity in size between erect penis and hymenal orifice. It is indicative of penetration only.[18]

The testicles must be examined for any abnormality including non-descent, large scrotal herniae or testicular atrophy, and the skin of the scrotum should be inspected for abrasion or injury.

Obviously, if there has been a long delay

between the alleged offence and the medical examination, the value of the detailed examination is greatly reduced and certain aspects may in some cases be left out.

Even if the suspect is examined within a very short time of an alleged offence there are few clinical signs that can safely be interpreted as being indicative of recent sexual intercourse. Detumescence is rapid and is rarely incomplete within a time interval as short as even a few minutes; redness of the glans penis, prepuce or penile shaft is too unreliable a sign to have any specific significance; the presence of seminal traces at the urethral orifice does not survive the first attempt at micturition and anyway is not conclusive of recent sexual activity.

Specimens to be taken from the suspect in cases of alleged rape and indecent assault

Samples must be taken from the suspect in an alleged case of rape or indecent assault for the same reason as samples are taken from the female victim:
1. to confirm the allegations;
2. to attempt to establish a link between the suspect and the scene;
3. to attempt to establish a link between the suspect and the victim.

The time interval between the alleged offence and the medical examination will, to a certain extent, dictate the samples that may be relevant. In every case, whatever the time interval between the examination of the female victim and the suspect, the following samples should be taken:

1. *Blood* for grouping, for the blood group will be unchanged whatever the time interval, and will still be relevant for comparison with any blood stains, seminal swabs etc., found during the examination of the victim, victim's clothes, or scene. If the time interval is short, analysis of the blood for alcohol or drugs should be carried out if there are clinical signs to suggest intoxication.

2. *Saliva* for secretor grouping, for this will also be unchanged by any time interval, and examination of the saliva will be relevant for comparison with saliva traces found on bite marks on the victim, and for secretor comparison with any seminal traces found on clothing or within the victim.

3. *Head hair* for comparison with any loose hairs found on the victim or at the scene.

4. *Avulsed pubic hair* for comparison with any loose pubic hairs found among the pubic hair combings of the victim, or at the scene. If the time interval is short, pubic hair combings should also be taken as described in the text.

When the suspect is examined within a few hours of the alleged offence (24 h) or if he has not washed or bathed since the offence, the following specimens should be taken:

1. *Urine* for analysis for alcohol or drugs if there are clinical signs of intoxication present.

2. *Bite marks* must be swabbed and a control swab must be taken from an uncontaminated area of skin.

3. *Soiled areas* of the body must be swabbed.

4. *Fingernail samples*, either by scraping the nails or by clipping them, must be taken so that any foreign material trapped beneath them can be examined by the laboratory.

5. *Matted pubic hair* should be taken as described in the text.

6. *Penile swabs*, taken from the coronal sulcus, the prepuce and the urethral orifice should be taken, for these swabs may reveal infecting organisms or blood that may also be present on the victim's swabs. Penile shaft swabs should also be taken, for these may reveal saliva traces in cases of alleged oro-penal contact. Shaft swabs may also reveal mucosal epithelial cells which the forensic science laboratories may be able to identify as vaginal debris (Fig. 5.5).

There is no single clinical finding on examination of either the female or the male that points conclusively to a diagnosis of rape. The most that any examining doctor can be expected to state is that his examination findings are consistent with the detailed history he obtained from the victim. Any doctor who attempts to go further than that is doing a gross disservice to his profession, his patient and the Courts.

Anal intercourse and acts of gross indecency

In the United Kingdom, acts of anal intercourse are no longer criminal offences if they take place between consenting adult males (over the age of 21

RAPID REFERENCE SHEET
EXAMINATION OF MALE ACCUSED OF RAPE

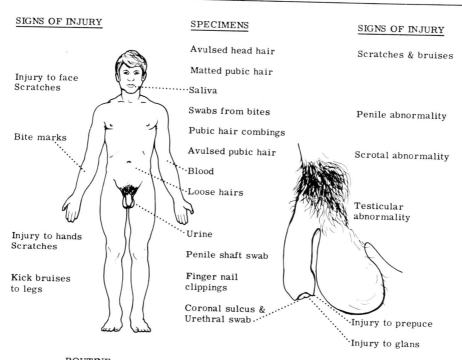

SIGNS OF INJURY

Injury to face
Scratches

Bite marks

Injury to hands
Scratches

Kick bruises
to legs

SPECIMENS

Avulsed head hair

Matted pubic hair

Saliva

Swabs from bites

Pubic hair combings

Avulsed pubic hair

Blood

Loose hairs

Urine

Penile shaft swab

Finger nail
clippings

Coronal sulcus &
Urethral swab

SIGNS OF INJURY

Scratches & bruises

Penile abnormality

Scrotal abnormality

Testicular
abnormality

Injury to prepuce

Injury to glans

ROUTINE

1. Obtain consent to examination and report.
2. Take detailed general history.
3. Observe - behaviour, state of dress, etc.
4. Examine clothing - blood and seminal stains. Retain for laboratory.
5. Full general clinical examination - record all findings.
6. Detailed genital examination - take swabs.
7. Take all relevant specimens. Establish chain of evidence.

Fig. 5.5 Department of Medical Illustration, Guy's Hospital. Lecture notes of Dr Paul. Published in the Legal Medicine Annual (1977).

years) in private. They are still criminal offences if one of the partners is below 21 years of age, if the act takes place in the Merchant Navy when on board ship, or if one of the partners is female.

The offence consists of penetration by the penis into the anus, and the merest penetration suffices to establish the offence. Proof of ejaculation is not necessary for conviction.

A doctor may be called upon to perform a clinical examination in cases where one of the partners is below the age of 21 years; where the act is alleged to have occurred in other than a private place (public lavatory etc.); where there has been no valid consent (severe mental abnormality or subnormality); or when the passive partner is female.

As in the case of alleged rape and indecent assault upon a female, a medical examination is essential on both the passive and the active partner, and the reasons for these examinations are identical.

1. So that emergency medical or surgical treatment can be given.

2. So that all physical signs present at the time of the medical examination can be observed and recorded.

3. So that all relevant scientific specimens can be obtained and retained for laboratory investigation and identification.

In the United Kingdom since the Sexual Offences Act of 1967 the requests for medical examination in respect of anal intercourse have been greatly reduced, and the changes in the marital laws have also resulted in a great reduction in the number of cases where anal intercourse during the marriage has been used as grounds for a divorce.

It is important to remember that in many parts of the world, heterosexual anal intercourse, although illegal, is a socially acceptable sexual variation and often takes the place of contraception, and in some countries heterosexual anal intercourse with the preservation of vaginal virginity is quite a widespread courtship activity.

Essentials in the medical examination of the passive partner

The routine medical examination of the passive partner of alleged anal intercourse follows a similar pattern to the medical examination of the alleged victim of rape: the examining doctor should plan his entire examination so that at its conclusion he will be able to answer the following questions:

1. Could penile penetration have taken place in this anus?
2. Has penile penetration taken place recently?
3. Are there signs that indicate that this anus is well used to penile penetration?
4. Are there physical signs to indicate that general force or stupefying drugs have been involved?
5. Have all the relevant specimens been taken to confirm the allegations and to assist in identifying the parties involved?

Unlike the situation in rape, consent is rarely an issue in cases of alleged anal intercourse.

Consent to the medical examination and subsequent report is required, and must be obtained by the examining doctor directly from the patient or from a parent or guardian in the case of a minor or a patient unable to give valid consent.

A general medical history must be taken, preferably from the patient. In the case of very young children, where a history may be impossible to obtain, the doctor should take the medical history from parent or guardian and this may be taken either at the commencement of the examination or after the physical examination has been completed.

The general history must include all details of past illnesses, surgical operations and serious accidents. It must also include details of recent medication and of intoxicating drinks consumed over the previous 24 h.

Special attention must be given to questions relating to the patient's bowel habits, including previous constipation, the regular use of laxatives, enemata or suppositories, and details of any surgical operation or instrumentation of the bowel. In the case of a female passive partner, details of previous childbirth and the extent of any perineal laceration and repair must be noted, for these circumstances can alter the normal anatomy of the anal verge and perineum.

Enquiry should be made regarding any previous acts of anal intercourse, and a note should be made of any such previous act and the frequency of such acts in the past.

The specific history of the incident under investigation must be taken, preferably from the patient. In the case of very young children it will be necessary for the doctor to use great patience if he is to obtain any proper story from the child victim, and in many cases the doctor may have to obtain some sort of history from the 'first finder'.

Special reference must be made to the following matters:

1. the date, time and place of the alleged act or acts;
2. the position in which penile penetration was achieved;
3. the use of general violence;
4. the use of any lubricant;
5. did ejaculation take place?
6. was pain experienced—at the time of penetration, during the act of anal intercourse, immediately after withdrawal of the penis, for some time after withdrawal, on the subsequent acts of defaecation after the alleged act or acts?
7. was any bleeding noted after the alleged act or after any subsequent act of defaecation?
8. has the patient defaecated since the alleged act and before the medical examination?

9. has there been any change of clothing since the alleged act and prior to the medical examination?

10. has the patient bathed or washed the anal area since the alleged act and prior to the medical examination?

11. have the parents or guardians noticed any sudden change in the bowel habits of the patient, or any soiling of underclothes since the date of the alleged incident?

General observation by the examining doctor should be maintained throughout the history taking and the medical examination, and the patient's demeanour should be noted.

The clothing worn at the time of the alleged incident should be inspected if possible. In many cases, however, there is a delay of weeks between the alleged offence and the medical examination, and in those cases there is nothing to be gained by an inspection of the clothing. If it is a recent complaint, and the clothing worn at the time of the medical examination is the same clothing worn at the time of the alleged offence, then the clothing must be removed item by item as in the case of a rape examination, and each garment must be inspected and retained for laboratory examination.

Particular attention must be given to the crutch area of underpants and trousers for the presence of seminal, blood or faecal soiling. The fly area of the trousers is not likely to be contaminated in the case of the passive partner.

General clinical examination must follow in every case, with careful inspection of the skin for injury, areas of soiling and loose hairs. Loose hairs may be found on either the front or back of the body for anal penetration can be accomplished in a variety of positions. In the clinical experience of the author, anal penetration from a posterior position is more common between adult males. Posterior and anterior positions are found in cases involving male and female, and in cases involving children.

Detailed examination of anal area and genitalia

This follows the full general examination and, as in the case of the examination of a rape victim, it must follow a definite order to ensure that the risk of accidental contamination of any specimen is obviated.

Firstly the pubic hair should be examined, and

any matted areas should be noted. The entire matted area should be cut away as close to the skin as possible, and retained for laboratory examination.

The penis should be carefully examined, for in many cases oro-penile contact is either a preliminary to anal intercourse or is actually the entire extent of the sexual contact. This applies in both the passive adult male partner and in the child victim.

Swabs must be taken from the penile shaft and the glans penis for the presence of saliva traces, and control swabs should be taken from an area of skin likely to be uncontaminated, such as the skin of the upper chest or shoulder. Any undue redness of the penis, and any obvious injury, must be noted.

The entire area of the perineum must be carefully inspected in good light, and particular attention must be given to the anal verge. Before any digital contact is made by the examining fingers, swabs must be taken from the anal verge and the skin of the perineum, and these swabs should be examined by the laboratory for seminal and lubricant traces.

The appearance of the anal verge must be carefully noted. Normally the anal orifice is slit-like running anteroposteriorly, and the surrounding skin of the anal verge shows marked natural folds, due to the act of the corrugator cutis ani muscle, radiating from the anal orifice.

In cases where anal intercourse has taken place there are commonly changes in the normal anatomy, and the degree of such changes is dependent upon the frequency of the acts of anal intercourse, the time interval between the last act of intercourse and the medical examination, the age and size of the patient.

First ever anal intercourse tends to produce a wide variety of anatomical changes in the appearance of the anal verge. There is very commonly some sign of injury, and this may vary from overt tearing of the anal skin and underlying sphincter muscle, through splitting of the skin and the production of anal fissure or the shearing of subcutaneous blood vessels and the production of local haematomata, to the merest abrasion of the anal verge skin.

In the most general terms, the younger the passive partner the more likely are the chances of serious injury to the anal verge. The use of effective lubrication tends to reduce the severity of local injury.

Local anal verge signs of penetration

Acute. Abrasions may frequently be seen, and these are very superficial and may be present at any part of the circumference of the anal verge. They can be caused by moderate frictional shearing by the penetrating penis, but may also be caused by fingernails in the course of digital anal penetration. Effective lubrication will tend to reduce the production of these abrasions.

Haematomata are very frequently seen, and these may take the form of an 'all over' swelling of the anal verge, with obliteration of the normal anal skin folds, or they may take the form of a localised 'peri-anal haematoma' presenting as a tense plum-coloured swelling at one particular part of the circumference. The mechanism of haematoma formation is simple to explain. The blood vessels immediately beneath the anal skin are poorly supported, and become ruptured as the overlying skin is moved by the shearing force of penetration. If the rupture is purely local the localised peri-anal haematoma results. If more general the overall swelling of the anal verge is produced. The use of an effective lubricant can reduce the frictional shearing forces, and under these circumstances haematomata formation can be avoided. It is important to remember that similar haematoma are frequently produced by the passage of a constipated motion passing from within the anal canal—outwards, and that haematomata are therefore not indicative of anal penetration from without—inwards.

Anal fissures are splits in the skin of the anal verge, and they may be restricted to the external skin only, or they may extend within the anal canal to the mucocutaneous junction which is situated in adults some $\frac{3}{4}$–1 inch within the anal canal. They are produced by overstretching of the anal skin which then gives way almost invariably in one place only. The situation of an anal fissure is dictated by the muscular support of the skin of the anal verge, and this tends to be weakest at the posterior quadrant with the result that the fissure is most frequently observed in that area. In the case of women who have had children, however, the support is reduced anteriorly as well, and anterior fissuring may take place.[19]

An anal fissure is therefore almost invariably solitary, and any additional overstretching of the anal verge skin merely results in the solitary fissure enlarging, and does not as a rule result in the formation of additional fissures. The weakest area of skin, i.e., the site of the first fissure, gives way and enlarges, rather than another area of unsplit skin breaking. A fissure is always roughly wedge shaped, with the wider portion being situated laterally, and the point of the wedge being directed radially towards the anal canal. This shape is dictated by the actions of the muscles underlying the anal verge—fibres of the sphincter ani externus and the corrugator cutis ani—and the shape of a fissure therefore gives no indications as to whether it was produced by the passage of an object from outside into the anal canal, or by the passage of an object from inside the anal canal to the outside.

Fissures are nowadays invariably caused by injury, but this injury may well be the passage of a constipated motion outwards from the bowel as well as, and indeed more frequently than, by the passage of some object inwards into the anal canal. The fissure of venereal disease and of tuberculosis is only rarely seen in practice in the United Kingdom, but still does exist in certain other parts of the world.

The main characteristic symptom of a fissure is pain—usually of a very severe type. This pain will be first noted at the moment of production of the fissure, when it will have a 'tearing' character, and the pain will always persist after the stretching has ceased. When no stretching of the injured verge is present, the pain becomes a constant dull ache, but quickly reverts to the severe tearing type if further stretching is applied to the anal verge. Thus further acts of penetration or attempted penetration, or the passage of a motion, will always result in an acute exacerbation of the pain, and in children may lead to a dramatic change in bowel habits with the previously 'potty trained' child refusing to sit on the lavatory pan, and screaming when having its bowels opened.

Anal sphincter spasm will invariably accompany any significant injury to the anal verge as long as the sphincter itself is intact, for violent contraction of the sphincter is the reflex response to injury at the anal verge. This response may be immediate or may be delayed for an hour or so, and when present makes detailed examination of the interior of the anal canal and lower rectum difficult. In children over the age of about six years, and in adults, the sphincter may seem lax if examined within an hour of penetration or it may be in marked spasm immediately.

Tearing of the sphincter muscle is rare in the case of adults and older children, but can take place in the case of young children, and in cases where this has taken place there will be considerable laxity of the anal orifice, sometimes with frank gaping.

The acute signs of first anal penetration are only transient, and the smoothness of the anal verge skin, spasm of the anal sphincter, and the fresh appearance of abrasions may all have disappeared within 24–48 h. If a fissure has been produced it will remain visible for many days, sometimes extending into weeks, and some degree of sphincter spasm will persist as will a history of sharp pain on defaecation; a peri-anal haematoma will take as long as 7–10 days to become absorbed. It follows that if medical examination is delayed for over 10 days after first ever anal penetration there may be very little to find on medical examination. Healing or healed fissures may be all that is present. If the sphincter has not been damaged, normal sphincter tone will have been restored and all signs of sphincter spasm will have gone.

Once the anal verge has been inspected and the verge and perineal swabs have been taken, the internal examination of the anal canal and lower rectum should be commenced. In all cases a small and unlubricated proctoscope should be passed. This is a vital step in the examination, and one that is frequently omitted. It is vital for several reasons:

1. It is impossible to exclude the possibility of serious injury to the anal canal or lower rectum without visualising the lumen;
2. It is impossible to obtain specimens from the anal canal or lower rectum with no risk of contamination of the swabs as they pass through the anal margin unless the swab is protected from any such contact with the anal margin, and this can only be guaranteed by passing them through the lumen of a proctoscope;
3. It is impossible to observe any changes in the lining of the anal canal without visualising the lumen and the mucosa.

If there is severe spasm of the sphincter so that even a very small proctoscope cannot be introduced without causing severe pain, further examination should be postponed until an anaesthetic can be administered. The author can only recall one case in an adult where he has been unable to pass a small proctoscope, and only a mere handful of cases in children above the age of 10 years where he has had to resort to examination under anaesthesia.

With the proctoscope in situ, swabs should be taken through the lumen of the instrument, both of the lower rectum and of the anal canal, and these swabs must be retained for laboratory examination for seminal traces and for lubricant.

After the swabs have been taken, the entire lower rectum and anal canal must be carefully inspected through the proctoscope, and any area of injury or of abnormality of the mucosal lining must be noted. Bruising of the mucosa will be seen as darker red areas against the all over redness of the background. Habitual and repeated acts of anal intercourse can produce a smoothing of the anal columns.

Signs of habitual anal intercourse. Most of the signs of habitual or repeated anal intercourse will be found at the anal margin and in the area of the anal sphincter. These signs appear only gradually, and very many acts of anal intercourse are required to produce them. The normal folds at the anal verge tend to be lost so that the anal margins appear much smoother than normal. Associated with this smoothing out of the skin folds, there is thickening of the skin at the anal margin extending up into the anal canal to the mucocutaneous junction, and sometimes well into the mucous membrane of the upper anal canal and lower rectum. The scars of healed fissures will be visible if carefully searched for, and this search may require the use of a hand lens for healed fissures present as small pale scars and are easily missed on cursory examination.

In very extreme cases of habitual anal intercourse over many years, the anus itself has the appearance of being 'deep set' so that the anal area looks as though it is situated in a funnel shaped depression, but it must be emphasised that this is a very rare finding, and is indicative of repeated and regular anal intercourse over many years.

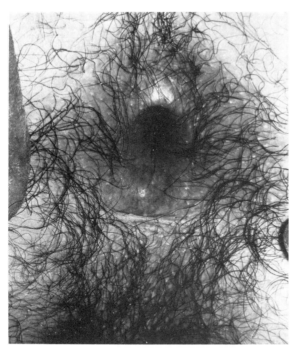

Fig. 5.6 Anus of an habitual 'passive partner'. Note the smoothing of the anal skin folds, and the thickening of the anal verge skin. This patient also demonstrated a 'positive' bilateral buttock traction test. Department of Medical Illustration, Guy's Hospital. Dr Paul's case book, 1968.

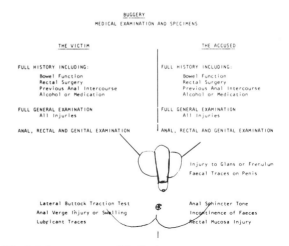

Fig. 5.7 Lecture notes of Dr Paul.

The anal sphincter itself, in life, very rarely demonstrates the gross laxity seen frequently on the post-mortem table. Digital examination in patients well used to anal intercourse may well extend to an easy three or four finger examination, and the sphincter may easily stretch to accommodate the examining fingers without any complaint of discomfort from the patient, but some 'grip' on the examining fingers can be demonstrated and when the fingers are withdrawn the sphincter will close down although there may be some reduction of the tone of the muscle (Fig. 5.6).

The classical, grossly dilated and keratinised anal orifice claimed to be indicative of the 'habitual homosexual' is only very rarely seen in live patients, although it is reported with some frequency by pathologists during their post-mortem examinations. It is likely that the relaxation of the anal sphincter after death is responsible for this frequently reported artefact.

A useful guide as to a patient's habituation to anal intercourse is the 'lateral buttock traction test' in which a thumb is placed on the buttock cheeks on either side of the anus, and gentle lateral traction is applied. In patients who are not accustomed to anal penetration (penile or instrumental) the gentle lateral traction results in a reflex constriction of the anal sphincter. Patients who are well used to anal penetration react to the gentle lateral traction by a relaxation of the anal sphincter. Some authorities hold that this relaxation of the sphincter is absolutely characteristic of anal intercourse over a considerable period of time. In the author's experience it is no more than a possible guide to the diagnosis, for patients with a history of anal surgery or repeated anal medical instrumentation will also react in this way. Additionally, in some cases of first ever anal intercourse where the anal sphincter has been severely damaged, pseudo-relaxation of the sphincter on gentle lateral traction can be demonstrated. This is due to severe loss of the contractile power of the damaged muscle but can be misinterpreted as being indicative of habitual anal intercourse. The differential diagnosis is made by testing the anal sphincter tone by requesting the patient to 'grip' on to an examining finger inserted into the anal canal (Fig. 5.7).

Infants and young children

The anal sphincter of an infant will always allow the penetration of at least one, and in most cases two, examining fingers without sustaining any injury, and this applies even to the newborn. It follows therefore that, because the anus of an infant admits a lubricated examining finger, it does not mean that anal virginity has been lost. Of greater significance is the presence of localised injury to the skin of the anal margin, the mucosa of the upper anal canal, and to the muscles of the anal sphincter.

Digital penetration of the anus by one finger may result in no injury of any kind, even in infants of less than one year. In some cases there may be some abrasion of the anal verge caused by the assailant's fingernail. Frank tearing of the anal verge is rare, as is sphincter damage.

Anal penetration by two or more fingers or by objects as large may produce signs of injury that are similar to those of penile penetration.

The signs of penile penetration will vary depending upon the use of a lubricant, the force used and the number of times that such an act has taken place. First ever penile penetration in a young child almost invariably results in some degree of injury even if a lubricant has been used, and the resultant injury varies from mere swelling of the anal verge with the loss of the normal puckered appearance, to gross tearing of the skin and underlying sphincter.

If the child is examined within 2–4 h of the assault there may be general laxity of the sphincter with gaping of the anus, but after this period of time an undamaged sphincter reacts in the normal manner to anal verge injury and goes into spasm. If the sphincter is ruptured the laxity will persist until repair is performed.

The general swelling of the anal verge persists for about two days and then gradually resolves over the subsequent five to seven days with the re-establishment of the normal anal skin folds.

The presence of a fresh, moist, pink-coloured anal fissure may support an allegation of penile penetration, but it must be remembered that infants can and do develop anal fissures following the passage of a constipated motion and a careful history must be obtained from parent or guardian regarding the bowel habits of the child, and particularly any change in those habits.

In general terms, the younger the child the more severe the injuries likely to occur. Frank tearing of the peri-anal skin, rupture of the anal sphincter, tearing of the walls of the ano-rectal canal, are all definite indications of anal penetration by some object approximating to the size of an erect penis.

Complete rupture of the anal sphincter will result in a lax and patulous appearance of the anus, with total loss of sphincter muscle tone. Partial rupture may not present with gross laxity of the anus, but sphincter tone will be found to be greatly reduced with weak 'gripping' of the examining finger.

When there has not been rupture of many fibres of the sphincter, tone is not reduced and spasm rather than laxity will be found. The spasm is frequently so severe that digital examination is very difficult. Gentle lateral buttock traction in such cases will reveal the traumatised anal verge and will allow the external parts of a fissure or abrasion to be seen.

In every case, where there are external signs of significant injury, the clinical examination must include proctoscopy of the anal canal and lower rectum to exclude tearing of the bowel. If the sphincter spasm is severe, then examination under anaesthesia is indicated.

Any child who has been the victim of anal penile penetration will experience pain on defaecation for some time afterwards, and this pain will persist for two weeks or so if there is a fissure present. So specific is this finding that the doctor should view with great suspicion any case where there is no history of pain or of problems of defaecation following such an alleged incident. Sudden change in bowel habit, sudden soiling of underclothes, the presence of small amounts of blood soiling of underclothes, are all consistent with anal verge injury.

As in all cases of supected sexual assault, specimens must be taken from the child victim so that laboratory examination can provide the necessary corroborative evidence. The nature of the specimens does not vary from those required in the case of the adult passive partner.

Specimens to be taken in cases of alleged anal intercourse

As in the medical investigation in cases of rape, the taking of valid specimens is the responsibility of the examining doctor. The choice of specimens will of course vary with the details of the allegations and with the time interval that has elapsed between the alleged incident and the medical examination. The following list is neither exclusive nor is it mandatory, and it must be remembered that seminal traces within the bowel are difficult to identify if more than 24 h have passed since the alleged act, and are also lost in the majority of cases if there has been a bowel action between the time of the alleged incident and the medical examination. Wiping or washing of the anal verge will also tend to destroy any anal verge contamination by semen or lubricant.

1. *Blood*: for grouping and also for alcohol or drug analysis if the history or examination indicates the use of intoxicants.

2. *Urine*: for routine testing and also as a screening substance for alcohol or drugs if indicated.

3. *Buccal swabs*: for seminal traces if there has been any allegation of oro-penile contact within 8 h of the medical examination, and there has been no cleaning of the teeth nor consumption of hot drinks. Swabbing must be of both surfaces of the teeth for it is here that seminal traces persist for the longest time in the live victim, and such swabs will frequently reveal seminal traces when 'deep throat' swabs give negative results.

4. *Saliva*: to establish the secretor status of the patient.

5. *Head hair*: to be obtained by either combing or avulsion, for comparison with any hairs found at the scene or on the suspected assailant.

6. *Soiling*: taken from all soiled areas of the body, so that the laboratory can identify its origin and compare it with material found at the scene or on the person of the suspect.

7. *Pubic hair*: for comparison with any pubic hairs found at the scene and on the assailant. Both combed and avulsed samples should be obtained.

8. *Penile swabs*: from the glans penis and penile shaft, for possible saliva traces.

SPECIMENS IN BUGGERY

TO PROVIDE CORROBORATIVE EVIDENCE SPECIMENS MUST BE TAKEN & STORED WITH CARE

ALWAYS MAINTAIN THE CHAIN OF EVIDENCE

1) Identify the specimen
2) Label the specimen and sign the label
3) Record the disposal of the specimen

THE VICTIM	THE ACCUSED
Avulsed Head Hair	Avulsed Head Hair
Pubic Hair Combings	Pubic Hair Combings
Avulsed Pubic Hair	Avulsed Pubic Hair
Anal Verge Swab	Anal Verge Swab
Anal Canal Swab	Anal Canal Swab
Perineal Swab	Perineal Swab
Buccal Swab if Oro-Penile Contact within 8 hr. of examination	Buccal Swab if Oro-Penile Contact within 1 hr. of examination
Penile Swab	Penile Swab
Urethral Swab	Urethral Swab
Coronal Sulcus Swab	Coronal Sulcus Swab
Finger Nail Scrapings	Finger Nail Scrapings
Blood: Grouping, Alcohol & Drugs	Blood: Grouping, Alcohol & Drugs
Swabs from any Bite Marks	Swabs from any Bite Marks
Saliva	Saliva
Urine, Alcohol & Drugs	Urine, Alcohol & Drugs

Fig. 5.8

9. *Anal and perineal swabs*: taken as indicated in the text so that accidental contamination is excluded, for laboratory examination for semen, lubricant and blood (Fig. 5.8).

Examination of the alleged active partner or assailant in anal intercourse

As in the case of alleged rape, the doctor will find himself confronted with the alleged passive partner of alleged buggery far more frequently than with the alleged active partner, and for the same reasons. Indeed in cases of alleged anal intercourse delay in 'first complaint' is much more common than in cases of alleged rape, with the inevitable result that the delay in the medical examination of both passive and active partner tends to be much greater.

There are many cases, therefore, when examination of the alleged active partner is of very limited value. Nevertheless it must be remembered that even very late medical examination of the suspect will produce some scientific evidence that will be of value in establishing possible contact between the two parties involved, for such matters as blood grouping and secretor status do not change with the passage of time. Laboratory comparison of seminal grouping, saliva grouping, and hair samples found on examination of the passive partner with samples taken many months later from a suspected active partner can still furnish evidence of corroboration.

The extent of the medical examination will vary with the time interval between the alleged incident and the medical examination of the suspected active partner. In those cases where there has been early 'first complaint' and prompt production of the suspect for medical examination, the medical takes the form of a 'mirror image' of the examination previously performed on the passive partner. In these cases the examining doctor should plan his entire examination so that at its conclusion he will be able to answer the following questions:

1. Are there any general signs of injury consistent with resistance?
2. Are there clinical signs of intoxication by alcohol or by drugs?
3. Are there any signs of injury or soiling of the penis that are consistent with recent anal penetration?

4. Have all the relevant specimens been taken to confirm the allegations and to assist in laboratory identification of the parties involved?
5. Are there any signs that are consistent with the active partner suspect having also been the 'passive partner' in acts of regular anal intercourse?
6. Are there any abnormalities of the genitals that could prevent erection or ejaculation?

In those cases where there has been long delay (beyond 48 h) between the alleged incident and the medical examination, the examining doctor may only be able to answer those questions under (4), (5) and (6) above. A medical examination even under circumstances of long delay is nevertheless a prudent step in the investigation of an alleged incident of buggery.

The medical examination must follow the same routine as has previously been described for the examinations of the victims and suspects in the rape situation, and for the passive partner in the buggery situation. It must include:

Consent to the examination and subsequent report;

Full general history encompassing the past medical history, use of medication and intoxicants, past surgical operations and bowel habits.

The specific history should follow the same lines as that in the case of the suspect of rape, and because of the probable 'caution' previously given to the suspect the doctor should refrain from asking specific and detailed questions of the incident under investigation. His questions should be restricted to such matters as:

1. Has the suspect been informed of the reason for the medical examination?
2. Has there been consenting anal intercourse or vaginal intercourse with any person within the previous 24 h?
3. When did he last bathe or wash, and change his clothing?
4. What is his explanation for all marks or injury found?

General observation of the patient should be maintained throughout the history taking and examination for general demeanour, signs of intoxication, etc.

The clothing, if unwashed and the same as that worn at the time of the alleged incident, should be inspected. Of particular importance are the trousers and underpants for these, together with the shirt or vest, are the most likely to bear soiling from faeces, lubricant or seminal fluid. This soiling tends to become deposited on the inner surface of the trousers and pants near to the 'fly' and 'crutch' areas and on the inner surface of the shirt front and vest front, during the process of detumescence after intercourse, and in the hours following. All clothing worn at the time of the alleged incident must be retained for laboratory examination.

General clinical examination must follow in every case, if only to establish the presence or absence of any general condition that would prevent the alleged acts from having been performed by the patient. All signs of injury must be noted, and all systems examined.

Detailed examination of the genitals

This must follow, and great care must be taken to ensure that any specimens taken from this area have not been accidentally contaminated whilst being obtained.

It is prudent to wear sterile gloves whilst handling the genitals, and before any manipulation of the foreskin is attempted the following specimens should be taken in every early examination:
1. pubic hair—both combed and avulsed specimens, as well as any matted area;
2. penile shaft swab and control swab from a distant area of skin. Many cases where there is an allegation of anal intercourse also involve an allegation of oro-genital contact where the passive partner has been required to suck the penis of the active partner, and it follows that saliva traces from the penis may be of great importance. Anal intercourse is not the commonest form of homosexual activity, and in many cases of gross indecency between males the acts have been restricted to mutual oral stimulation only (fellatio).

The foreskin should be gently retracted in the uncircumcised and, in those cases as well as in the circumcised, swabs from the coronal sulcus behind the glans penis, and from the urethral orifice must be taken. Faecal soiling, blood and foreign hairs are most likely to become trapped in the area of the coronal sulcus, particularly in the uncircumcised even if there has been an attempt to wash the genitals after the act. The urethral swab may reveal

faecal material which can corroborate anal penetration, and may also reveal organisms similar to those that may be identified on the anal verge swabs from the passive partner.

The foreskin and the glans penis must be carefully examined for injury. Damage to the frenulum of the foreskin can occur during penetration into a 'virgin anus' especially if no form of lubrication has been employed. Superficial abrasion of the glans penis can also occur, although this is a rarer type of injury.

The penis, testicles and scrotum must be examined to exclude any condition that may have prevented erection or ejaculation.

Examination of the anal area should be performed in every case to try to determine if anal intercourse has taken place. In a significant number of cases there will be physical signs to indicate that the patient has also played the 'passive' role on previous occasions. Anal and rectal swabs should be taken in the same way as they are in the case of the 'passive' victim if the history of the alleged incident indicates that there has been mutual penetration.

Specimens must be taken in every case—in early examination situations these must include the penile swabs detailed above, but in *all* cases samples of pubic hair, blood and saliva should be taken, no matter how long the delay.

Aspermia

With the increasing use of vasectomy as a method of contraception there are an increasing number of cases where laboratory examination of vaginal specimens following intercourse and ejaculation fails to reveal any spermatozoa. The examining physician must bear in mind that such an absence does not exclude ejaculation, and that laboratory tests for seminal fluid are not dependant upon the identification of spermatozoa but rely upon the identification of prostatic acid phosphatase, which is always present in ejaculate even after vasectomy. There are other causes of aspermia as well, and it is the doctor's duty in the course of his history taking to establish prior vasectomy, severe testicular mumps, venereal disease, urethritis or prostatis, or if the patient has indulged in repeated sexual activity associated with multiple ejaculation over the previous 24 h.

Bestiality

The Offences against the Person Act 1861, defines buggery as 'Carnal knowledge committed against the order of nature by man with man or in the same unnatural manner by man with woman, or by man or woman in any manner with beast'.

In the preceding section of this chapter the offence of anal intercourse or sodomy has been dealt with in detail, and it is this offence that goes to make up the first part of the definition of the offence of buggery.

Bestiality, the last portion of the definition of buggery according to the statute, again requires proof of 'carnal knowledge' but the identity of the orifice penetrated is not specified. Thus the offence is complete if there is proof of the merest penetration by a man of the anus or vagina of a mammal, or of the cloaca of a fowl, as long as the penetration is penile. Similarly the offence is complete if there is proof of the merest penetration by the penis of an animal into the anus or vagina of a woman.

It is a rare offence, and in 26 years of fairly wide medico-legal experience the author has only been invited to examine in three cases, all involving men as the 'active partner' and all taking place in rural communities.

Because of the rarity of the *reported* offence, and because of the natural revulsion such an offence engenders, it is essential that the clinician resorts to a set routine for examination should he ever be requested to examine in such a case. The reasons for medical examination are identical to those in any case of alleged sexual assault:

1. so that emergency medical or surgical treatment can be given to the human participant if required.
2. so that all physical signs present at the time of the medical examination can be observed and recorded.
3. so that all relevant scientific specimens can be obtained for laboratory investigation and identification.

Routine

The identical routine of history taking and physical examination after consent has been obtained applies here in regard to the human participant as to any person suspected of a sexual assault. Careful general history, history of alcohol or medication, and careful examination of all clothing worn at the time of the alleged offence, with retention of all clothing for subsequent laboratory examination. Full 'top to toe' medical examination, with special reference to any soiled areas of the body and any injury. Careful examination of the genitalia, noting any injury.

Specimens

Routine specimens are taken as in any sexual offence, with special reference to any loose hairs or feathers, matted or soiled areas of pubic hair, faecal or blood soiling.

Examination and specimens from the animal involved

In many cases of alleged bestiality, the police will have seized the animal suspected of being involved; in other cases they will know the herd or flock from which the animal is thought to have come.

Unless the doctor prides himself on his expertise in animal husbandry he would be well advised to decline any invitation to examine the animal and to obtain relevant specimens. A competent veterinary surgeon should be invited to examine the suspect animal, and the physician should content himself with advising on the type of swab required (blood sample, anal, vaginal, cloacal, seminal, etc.) and prudence dictates that this advice is given from a safe distance.

In the cases involving fowls, it is often more convenient for the bird to be killed and for the entire carcass to be sent to the forensic laboratory.

In cases involving women, the veterinary surgeon should be asked to take particular care to secure swabs from the penis, sheath (prepuce) and urethral orifice of the animal concerned. Sometimes it is of help if a sample of the animal's semen can be obtained.

In every case the forensic science laboratory *must* be fully informed as to the nature of the alleged offence, and the species of animal thought to be involved.

Diagnosis of pregnancy

There are cases where the diagnosis of pregnancy

is of great medico-legal importance, and the examining doctor will be required to form an opinion as to the possible pregnancy of his patient.

The only 100% certain sign of pregnancy from the medico-legal point of view is the presence of fetal parts on X-ray of the patient. Obviously this absolutely reliable diagnostic aid requires the passage of a considerable length of time before it can be demonstrated safely, and earlier diagnosis is required in most medico-legal situations.

The early diagnosis must depend on: history; physical signs; laboratory investigation.

History

1. Amenorrhoea, particularly in a patient whose periods have previously been regular. The single missed period may be significant, the second missed period is of even greater importance.
2. Nausea, the traditional 'morning sickness' sometimes occurring even before the first missed period, may be significant. The nausea of early pregnancy is not, of course, restricted to the morning but can occur at any time of the day, and frequently presents in the evening when the patient is tired.
3. Fatigue is often a presenting symptom, frequently unassociated with heavy activity.
4. Frequency of micturition is a common symptom in early and late pregnancy. In early pregnancy, when the enlargement of the uterus within the pelvic cavity produces pressure on the bladder—in late pregnancy when the engagement of the presenting part again produces pressure on the bladder. In the middle months of pregnancy there may be no increased frequency of micturition.
5. Breast enlargement, associated with a feeling of 'fullness' and a 'pricking' sensation is a common symptom as early as four weeks of pregnancy.
6. Constipation is a common symptom and, if it is of sudden onset in a woman of previously regular bowel habit, is of significance.
7. Increased size of abdomen, with complaint that the waist bands of skirts, trousers, panties, etc., are uncomfortable, is an obvious symptom that can present as early as eight weeks and is due in part to the very slight enlargement of the uterus, but mainly to the increase in the amount of abdominal fat.

8. Fetal movements (quickening) are frequently experienced as early as the 18th week of pregnancy, with the patient noticing a faint 'fluttering' in the abdomen. Primagravidae are less likely to appreciate this symptom early, but almost all pregnant women can recognise fetal movements by 22 weeks although the full significance of the flutter may not be appreciated. Young girls tend to think that they have flatus. Multigravid women certainly recognise the fluttering movements for what they really are.

Physical signs

These vary as the pregnancy becomes more advanced. The very early signs are unreliable and no firm diagnosis can be based upon them. The later signs such as the palpation of fetal parts and the hearing of a fetal heart are diagnostic when observed by an experienced obstetrician but are not as reliable in the hands of a doctor who is inexperienced in obstetrics.

1. Breasts feel 'shotty' and are enlarged. Montgomery's tubercles within the areola are enlarged, and the entire area of the areola and nipple is more heavily pigmented than normal. The increase in pigmentation of the areola and the development of a pigmented line running from the umbilicus to the pubes (linea nigra) is much more obvious in dark complexioned women than it is in the fair-skinned blonde, and it is worth remembering that a similar pigmented line is seen in some dark complexioned women who are not pregnant.

In primagravida a secondary areola develops as an outer zone of less marked pigmentation surrounding the true areola, and this presents as a well defined reticulum consisting of a tesselated arrangement of pale, oval shaped areas enclosed in the meshes of a pigmented web.

There is increased blood supply to the breast which shows itself in the presence of dilated veins beneath the skin. There is frequently some secretion which can be expressed from the nipple. In early pregnancy it is of a thin and straw-coloured appearance, but later in the pregnancy it becomes thicker and an opaque yellow.

In primagravid women these changes indicative of breast activity can often be seen as early as the 6th week, and are almost invariably present by the 8th week. In multigravid women the early signs of activity, including the development of Montgomery's tubercles and increased breast pigmentation can seldom be found to be significant, for once established during a first pregnancy these changes tend to persist.

In the later weeks of pregnancy the skin of the breast itself becomes markedly stretched and small areas of the cutis vera become thinned, commonly giving rise to the striae or stretch marks.

2. Skin changes also occur, partly resulting from mechanical factors such as stretching, and partly resulting from biological factors such as pigmentation. Striae, known as striae gravidarium and similar to the striae of the breasts, appear on the abdominal wall below the umbilicus and also on the buttocks and thighs. They are caused by the stretching of the skin and their appearance depends upon the individual resistance of the skin to stretching forces. This individual capacity of skin resistance varies from one patient to another, with the result that striae are not the invariable concomitant of pregnancy. When due to pregnancy they are not normally present before the 6th or 7th month. Initially they are pearly or pink in colour and linear in shape but as the pregnancy advances they become more irregular in shape and a deeper pink in colour. It must be remembered that the mere presence of striae on the abdominal wall, thighs and buttocks is not indicative of pregnancy, for identical stretch marks may result from other causes of abdominal distension such as obesity, ovarian cyst, etc.

Pigmentation has already been referred to in relation to the areola of the breasts and the linea nigra of the abdomen. Other areas of increased pigmentation may sometimes be seen on the face, where they are most marked on the forehead, the sides of the nose and the upper lip. These areas of pigmentation go to make up the so-called 'pregnancy mask' or chloasma.

3. The abdomen will obviously show changes as the uterus increases in size and rises out of the pelvis. Normally the fundus of the uterus cannot be palpated above the pelvic rim until the 12th week of pregnancy. Thereafter it gradually enlarges upwards until by the 20th week it reaches the level of the umbilicus. By the 32nd week it reaches approximately to the midpoint between umbilicus and ensiform cartilage. By the 36th week it reaches

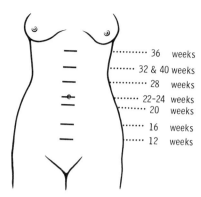

Fig. 5.9 Diagram of fundal heights during pregnancy. After Eden & Holland, Manual of Obstetrics, 10th edn.

its maximum height at the ensiform cartilage, and then between the 36th and 40th weeks it drops slightly to approximately the 32-week height as the presenting part engages in the pelvis (Fig. 5.9).

By the 24th week of pregnancy the uterus is markedly piriform in shape on abdominal palpation, and commonly extends further to the right than to the left of the mesial plane—a condition known as right lateral obliquity. Occasionally the obliquity is to the left, but the pregnant uterus is only very rarely medial. The fetus can be felt to be floating within the uterus—the sign of external ballottement—in which the external examining hands can recognise a momentary contact with a freely movable body within the uterus. In addition to this sign, by 24 weeks palpable fetal movements can be felt through the uterine wall on abdominal palpation. From about 20 weeks onwards a soft, blowing, systolic murmur, synchronous with the maternal pulse, is frequently heard on auscultation of the uterus near the lower and lateral borders. This uterine souffle is due to the greatly enlarged uterine arteries of pregnancy, but this same sign is also present in some cases of large uterine fibroids.

Careful auscultation from about the 24th week onwards can reveal fetal heart sounds, which can be distinguished from the maternal pulse because their rate is somewhere between 140 and 160 per min. As pregnancy advances towards term the fetal heart sounds become much more definite, and at term the rate of the fetal pulse is of the order of 120–140 per min. By 36 weeks of pregnancy fetal parts can be identified by abdominal palpation in most cases. Certainly the head, back and some of the limbs can be located in almost all reasonably lean women.

4. Pelvic examination will provide a guide to the diagnosis of pregnancy. Within the first 12 weeks some softening of the cervix may be noted, and speculum examination will reveal a deep violet colouration of the vaginal mucosa resulting from its increased vascularity.

Palmer's sign depends upon recognising the faint, regular and rhythmic contractions of the uterus which are known to occur from as early as the 4th week of pregnancy, and are most marked up to the 8th week. To elicit this sign the uterus is gently 'cupped' between two fingers of the right hand inserted into the vagina with the patient lying on her back, and the examining doctor should place his left hand gently on the abdomen. An experienced obstetrician may feel rhythmic contractions of the uterus, each contraction lasting about 30 s. and occurring about every 30 s. As pregnancy advances the interval between contractions lengthens, so that at about 10 weeks it is 90 s. At 12 weeks it has extended to 3 min, and by 16 weeks the interval has extended to some 8 min or more. A. C. Palmer, in first describing this sign in 1949, stated that although the time interval between contractions extended as the pregnancy advanced, the actual duration of each contraction remained at 30 s, and that by 20 weeks the interval could be as long as 20–30 min. It must be emphasised that recognition of these uterine contractions depends upon the experience of the examining physician, and in the hands of the inexperienced this sign is of little practical value in diagnosis—a negative Palmer's sign under those circumstances being of little diagnostic value.

Hegar's sign depends upon recognising the variation in consistency of the three portions of the uterus: the firm cervix; the soft and empty lower segment; and the enlarged and slightly globular upper part of the body of the uterus. To elicit this sign two examining fingers must be introduced into the anterior vaginal fornix and must be pushed upwards so that they almost meet the downwards and backwards pressure of the other hand, which is placed suprapubically on the abdomen. The experienced obstetrician can identify the three portions of the pregnant uterus between the 6th and 10th week of gestation. Present day thinking, how-

ever, indicates that there is considerable risk of causing an abortion unless this examination is carried out with extreme gentleness, and for this reason examination for Hegar's sign is only rarely performed.

Internal ballottement consists of detecting within the uterine cavity a solid movable body surrounded by fluid. During a vaginal examination the fetus sometimes comes to lie on the lower portion of the anterior uterine wall, and movement of the examining fingers in the anterior fornix may cause the fetus to become displaced upwards and float away in the amniotic fluid. The sensation of its displacement can sometimes be appreciated. If the examining fingers are allowed to remain in the anterior fornix a very slight impact can sometimes be appreciated by an experienced examiner, as the fetus returns to its position. Internal ballottement cannot be found if the fetus occupies a position high in the uterus, so its absence is not diagnostic.

Laboratory investigation

Laboratory tests to diagnose pregnancy depend on the presence of gonadotrophic hormones in the urine, and involve either biological tests in live laboratory animals or immunological tests based on antigens to human gonadotrophin.

The biological tests are believed to give positive results in some 97% of cases from within 12–14 days after the first missed menstrual period. They are, however, expensive tests to perform and the possibility of a false negative is present. The common biological tests are:

1. Ascheim-Zondek using mice, in which some four to five days are required for a result;
2. Friedman test using young female rabbits, in which ovulation is caused within 24–48 h after intravenous injection of urine containing gonadotrophic hormones;
3. Hogben test, using a female toad, in which ovulation can be caused within 12–24 h;
4. Mianini test in which spermatozoa can be made to appear in the urine of a male toad (*Bufo bufo*) in 2–4 h.

In the immunologically based tests (Prepurin, Pregnosticon) sheep red blood cells specially primed to serve as antigen carriers are used as indicators, and in other tests the antigen is linked to latex particles and these are used as indicators (Ortho Pregnancy Test). These tests have the advantage of being very much cheaper than the biological tests, and can give reasonable results within a couple of hours. Again they are thought to give positive results in over 90% of cases as early as the 21st day after the first missed period, but there is the real possibility of a false negative.

For a while the deliberate production of withdrawal bleeding in the non-pregnant by the administration of ethisterone, ethinyloestradiol, or orethisterone (Amenorone Forte, Primodos, etc.) were in vogue in the United Kingdom as convenient and cheap forms of pregnancy testing, but the risk of producing fetal abnormalities has resulted in this form of pregnancy testing being abandoned.

X-ray examination provides the earliest and most reliable diagnostic signs of pregnancy. Certainly by the 16th week the fetal skeleton can be clearly seen on a single A.P. film, and in many cases parts of the skeleton can be seen even earlier. The risk of damage to the mother or the fetus during the very short exposure of a single film is so small as to be negligible. Uterine scan now provides a safer method of investigating uterine contents, and can also indicate the maturity of any fetus contained within the uterus with reasonable accuracy.

Differential diagnosis of pregnancy

Pregnancy must be differentiated from any other condition which can produce abdominal swelling, but within the scope of this chapter only a few of the more common alternatives will be considered.

1. Abdominal obesity, which may be associated with amenorrhoea. Abdominal palpation can be extremely difficult to perform, but the differential diagnosis can be made on the absence of any signs of breast activity; no increase in size of the uterus and no associated softening of the cervix and engorgement of the vaginal mucosa; no increase in pigmentation of the areola or linea nigra. Abdominal striae may well be present as may striae on the breasts. In cases where a vaginal examination is difficult (small hymenal orifice, etc.), X-ray will fail to show any fetal skeleton after 16 weeks of amenorrhoea, and pregnancy tests will be repeatedly negative.

It must be borne in mind that conception can take place without full sexual intercourse and deep vaginal penetration, so the mere presence of a hymen with a very small hymenal orifice is no guarantee against a pregnancy being present.

2. Retention of urine from any cause can produce a distended bladder and considerable lower abdominal distension. Once again there will be no signs of breast activity or of pigmentation. Vaginal examination is often difficult under these circumstances, but rectal examination is usually possible and a normal sized uterus can be palpated through the anterior rectal wall. Catheterisation will confirm the over full bladder, and the disappearance of the abdominal distension after the bladder has been emptied in this manner will make the diagnosis. Some caution must be exercised, however, for some cases of retention of urine are caused by a retroverted gravid uterus, and in these cases all the abdominal distension will not disappear after catheterisation, and signs of breast activity, pigmentation and enlargement of the uterus must be carefully sought.

3. Constipation can produce considerable abdominal distension, and is most commonly seen under these medico-legal situations in the mentally subnormal or abnormal victims of sexual assaults. Breast activity is absent, the abdominal distension is not restricted to near the mesial plane, the vaginal mucosa is of normal colour without the purple hue of pregnancy engorgement and there is no softening of the cervix. Abdominal palpation will reveal the 'loaded' colon, with most of the mass palpable on the left side of the abdomen, and rectal examination will in most cases confirm the presence of a mass of faeces. Again some caution must be exercised, for constipation may well be one of the presenting symptoms of early pregnancy.

4. Fibroids can produce enlargement of the abdomen, but although they may be associated with amenorrhoea they are far more frequently associated with menorrhagia. The breasts show no sign of activity, the vaginal mucosa is of normal colour, and the cervix shows no sign of softening. The uterus is not uniformly enlarged but tends to have an irregular shape, and its increase in size is much slower than in pregnancy. The fetal heart is not heard, and no fetal movements are palpable—neither is there any internal ballottement. Uterine souffle can be heard in some cases of very large

fibroids. Pregnancy tests are repeatedly negative, and X-ray after 16 weeks of amenorrhoea does not show any fetal skeleton. Uterine scan is negative.

5. Ovarian cysts can produce considerable abdominal enlargement, and can also result in amenorrhoea and some breast activity including enlargement and secretion. On careful bimanual examination the uterus may be felt to be separate from the swelling of the cyst. There is no uterine souffle, fetal heart sounds cannot be heard, and there are no fetal movements. X-ray after 16 weeks amenorrhoea fails to show any fetal skeleton.

6. The menopause can be associated with abdominal distension and with amenorrhoea. Flatulence may cause nausea or even morning sickness, and distension of the large bowel by gas can cause violent borborygmi which may be interpreted by the patient as being fetal movements. In women who have borne children signs of breast activity are difficult to determine with accuracy. Vaginal examination should reveal no enlargement of the uterus consistent with the duration of the amenorrhoea, but there may be some uterine enlargement due to other causes. The vaginal mucosa will be of normal hue, however, and the cervix will not be soft. Repeated pregnancy tests will remain negative, and X-ray after 16 weeks of amenorrhoea will fail to reveal any fetal skeleton.

7. Pseudocyesis or 'phantom pregnancy' is moderately rare, and tends to occur in patients who desperately want a child. This condition can be associated with amenorrhoea, morning sickness, enlargement of the breasts and enlargement of the abdomen. There is not usually any increase in pigmentation, and vaginal examination reveals no softening of the cervix or enlargement of the uterus. Fetal heart sounds are absent, fetal parts can never be palpated, and of course X-ray examination fails to reveal any fetal skeleton. Repeated pregnancy tests are negative. The abdominal enlargement is due to a contraction of the diaphragm pushing forward the entire abdominal wall.

Signs of recent childbirth

There are circumstances where a doctor will be required to examine a woman to determine if she has recently been delivered of a child. Obviously, as in all medico-legal situations, the doctor is expected to perform a full and complete medical examination and there are some specific signs that will assist him to reach a diagnosis of recent childbirth.

Breasts

The increased pigmentation of the areola, and the presence of Montgomery's tubercles will persist for some considerable time after pregnancy (indeed may well remain permanently) and the general engorgement of the breast with dilatation of the subcutaneous veins will survive for at least two weeks after delivery, even if lactation has not become fully established. Milky secretions can be expressed from the nipples for many days after childbirth, even when lactation has been supressed.

Vulva and perineum

The vulva and perineum may show signs of injury such as abrasion of the fourchette or labia, of frank perineal lacerations which may be sutured if delivery was attended by a doctor, or will be unsutured if the delivery was unattended by professionals. Signs of perineal laceration will be clearly visible for many weeks, and where the tear has been extensive a permanent scar will be produced.

Vagina

The vagina will continue to show the purple hue of increased vascularity for several days after delivery, and in addition the vaginal mucosa will frequently show abrasion, bruising or tearing even in the absence of perineal lacerations.

Cervix

The cervix will show a patulous external os for some days after delivery, and there may be cervical tears present. Lochial discharge will be seen coming from the cervical os for three to four weeks after delivery.

Lochia

This is the name given to the discharge from the uterus after delivery. For the first three or four days after delivery it is markedly bloody, normally fluid but sometimes with small clots. Over the following days it becomes thinner but remains red for a few days, and then becomes brownish, yellow or green, and finally loses all colour and becomes white or merely turbid. The average duration of coloured lochia is in the region of 20 days, and this time interval seems to be constant in the face of age, parity, or subinvolution, but can be extended if lactation has been suppressed by the administration of oestrogens.

Lochia contains red blood cells, leucocytes, decidual debris, vaginal epithelium, peptones and cholestrin crystals and, after the early two or three days, numerous non-pathogenic bacteria. In the normal puerperium the lochia fresh from the uterine cavity is alkaline in reaction—that found in the vagina is acid.

Uterine involution

This commences immediately after delivery and continues for some six to eight weeks. Initially it is very rapid, for the first 10 days, with the uterus losing some 50% of its weight within the first week after delivery, and reducing from its post-delivery weight of about 2 lb to its normal non-gravid weight of about 2 oz within the six to eight-week period after delivery.

Immediately after delivery the uterus forms a firm pyriform swelling reaching up out of the pelvis to the level of the umbilicus, and it is freely movable. The actual height of the uterus over the next two weeks is affected by the state of fullness of the rectum and the bladder, both of which can push the uterus up out of the pelvis if they are full.

On average, and with an empty bladder and rectum, the uterine height on the 1st day of the puerperium is $5\frac{1}{2}$ inches above the pelvic brim, by the 6th day it is $3\frac{1}{2}$ inches, and by the 12th day it is 2

inches. Normally by the 14th day the fundus of the uterus is at the level of the pubes, but sometimes this stage is delayed until after three weeks. Multiparity increases the time taken for involution and, after four or five pregnancies, the interval may be considerably prolonged.

Pyrexia

This is a physiological reaction to labour and, immediately after labour, the temperature may rise to 100°F. During the first 24 h, especially in primagravidae, temperatures of 100–101°F are common, and this is believed to be due to 'reaction' from the severe muscular fatigue of labour. It is most probably due to a mild toxaemia resulting from absorbtion of the waste products of extreme muscular activity, and is never prolonged beyond 24 h.

Anaemia

Even in patients who were not anaemic before labour, this is a common finding, with haemoglobin levels falling to 10 G very frequently. In women who have not had any ante-natal care, severe degrees of anaemia are commonly present after delivery.

Hormonal levels in urine

These are of no practical value in determining recent delivery: pregnanediol shows no significant rise in urine after delivery; oestriol shows a rise for only the first two days; and oestrone for the first day only after delivery; H C G shows a rise in only 1% of patients for as long as 10 days after delivery, and after a short interval of only six days after delivery some 94% of women show no significant rise.[20]

REFERENCES

1. Paul, D. M. (1975) Med.-Legal Bull. Commonwealth Virginia, **24**.
2. Paul, D. M. (1972) Oklahoma J. For. Med., **1**.
3. Paul, D. M. (1975) Med.-Legal Bull. Commonwealth Virginia, **24**.
4. Paul, D. M. (1977) Police Surg., no. 11.

5. Cameron, J. M. & Sim, B. G. (1974) Forensic Dentistry. Edinburgh: Churchill Livingstone.
6. Frith, K. (1970) Br. J. Hosp. Med., **4**.
7. Frith, K. (1976) In: Gradwohl's Legal Medicine, 3rd edn. Bristol: John Wright & Sons.
8. Davies, A. (1978) Med. Sci. Law, **18**.

9. Allard, J. & Davies, A. (1979) Med. Sci. Law, **19**.
10. Sigma Technical Bulletin, no. 104 (revised August 1975).
11. Paul, D. M. (1975) Med. Sci. Law, **15**.
12. Huffman, J. W. (1960) Clin. Obstet. Gynecol., **3** 154.
13. Snyder, L. (1967) In: Homicide Investigation, 2nd edn. Springfield. Ill.: Charles Thomas, pp. 354, 358.
14. Paul, D. M. (1977) Med. Sci. Law, 17.
15. Frith, K. (1976) In: Gradwohl's Legal Medicine, 3rd edn. Bristol: John Wright & Sons, p. 397.
16. Huffman, J. W. (1958) Pediatr. Clin. North Am., **X**, 35.
17. Frith, K. (1970) Br. J. Hosp. Med., **4**, 765.
18. Paul, D. M. (1977) In: Wecht, ed. Legal Medicine Annual. New York: Appleton-Century Crofts.
19. Goligher, X. (1975) Surgery of the Anus, Rectum and Colon, 3rd edn.
20. Lorraine, X. & Bell, X. (1966) Hormonal Assays and their Clinical Application.

6

Blood tests in cases of disputed paternity

Blood group evidence has been accepted by the Courts in cases of disputed paternity for more than 50 years but it is only in the last few years that a legal framework has existed within which blood tests are performed. Part III of the Family Law Reform Act (1969) became operational in 1972 and gave the Courts the power to direct blood tests if one of the parties involved in the proceedings made an application. The Court cannot order blood tests as the taking of blood constitutes an assault in the absence of consent. To prevent parties refusing to comply with a direction as a matter of tactics, the Court is allowed to draw any inference from this failure if it thinks right to do so in the circumstances. The putative father will usually be advised by his solicitor to apply for blood tests if he wishes to defend an application by denial of paternity.

The Family Law Reform Act (1969) does not preclude blood tests being agreed by the parties concerned prior to any Court hearing and, in our experience, this course of action is taken by a large number of parties probably to avoid any unpleasantness that might result from a Court direction.

Following a Court direction it is the Clerk of the Court who is responsible for arranging the tests and he issues forms of identification for each of the parties which are then forwarded to the person taking the samples. Any qualified medical practitioner may take samples but the testing can only be carried out by one of a panel of testers appointed by the Home Secretary. This restriction of testing to a selected group of experts is intended to ensure that a minimum range of tests is performed that will give a falsely accused man a reasonable chance of exclusion. The present system does suffer from the disadvantage of a standard fee based on this

minimum range of tests, so any serologist who wishes to provide more does so at his own expense.

On completion of the tests, a report is sent to the Court listing the blood groups of the parties concerned and indicating whether the range of tests applied has shown non-paternity. Where no exclusion has been shown the likelihood of paternity is indicated.

EXCLUSION OF PATERNITY

Exclusions of paternity fall into two classes:

First-order exclusion

Where the child possesses a blood group gene that is absent in both the mother and the putative father, e.g. Table 6.1. In this example, the B blood group gene present in the child cannot have come from either the mother or the putative father, so he is excluded from paternity.

Table 6.1

Mother	Child	Putative father
O	B	O

Second-order exclusion

Where the putative father is homozygous for a blood group gene, which he must pass on to all his children, but the gene is not present in the child in question, e.g. Table 6.2. In this example, the putative father has only N genes to give, but the child has no N gene, so non-paternity is indicated.

Table 6.2

Mother	Child	Putative father
MM	MM	NN

No problems arise with first-order exclusions but unsupported second-order exclusions can pose problems as very occasionally persons have been found who lack any representation at one or other of the blood group loci. Thus the absence of both known Duffy alleles, Fy^a and Fy^b, is not uncommon in Africans, so here the finding of child Fy(a+ b−) and putative father Fy(a− b+) or vice versa is not even suggestive of non-paternity. The occurrence of these so-called 'silent alleles' has been described in a number of blood group systems but in Western Europeans they are so unusual that they can be considered as rare mutants. The Family Law Reform Act (1969) recognises the need to disregard the minute possibility of error through the unpredictable occurrence of mutation and defines excluded as 'excluded subject to mutation'. Apart from cases involving African subjects we have not encountered an apparent second-order exclusion of maternity other than where there was a possibility of an interchange of babies.

NON-EXCLUSION OF PATERNITY

Where no exclusion of paternity is obtained it is of value to the Court to be provided with some indication as to the likelihood of paternity. Great care must be taken with such evidence as false conclusions can easily be reached if a blood relative of the alleged father is involved or the parties come from an isolated community in which inbreeding may have occurred, resulting in a gene uncommon in the general population being more frequent. Any statistical approach to this problem may be misleading. The method most acceptable estimates the likelihood that the mother has named by chance a man who is not excluded and where the blood groups fit this or that well with paternity. Taking the case where it is shown that the alleged father, together with say 10% of men in the community, could be the father, then although this represents

a large number of possible fathers in the community, the mother stood a 90% chance of being shown to be wrong if the man she was naming were not the actual father. With the present range of tests over 90% of falsely accused men will be excluded from paternity so that a non-exclusion result in itself must be of some positive evidential value to the mother. Even where the proportion of other possible fathers is shown to be large, the case of the mother is not weakened, as this means only that the child has received common blood groups from its father rather than a rare group or rare combination of groups that would strongly support her case.

The method most widely accepted in this country is called the 'percentage method' which measures the usefulness of the tests employed in relation to the particular case being investigated. The calculation shows the percentage of men in the community who have blood groups compatible with paternity, a figure of say, less than 4% could be taken as pointing to actual paternity. The basis of the calculation is the frequency of the various blood groups in the population so it is essential that the ethnic origin of the parties be known as blood group frequencies can vary markedly between different populations. In the case of certain populations very limited data is available so no calculation should be attempted. It is our practice to limit such calculations to Western Europeans in which the gene frequencies are well established.

BLOOD GROUP SYSTEMS USED IN PATERNITY CASES

As stated by Race & Sanger[1], before any blood group system can be employed in the investigation of paternity problems, certain criteria must be met:
1. The blood group must be simply inherited and the mode of inheritance known with certainty.
2. It must be adequately developed at birth or soon after.
3. It must be permanent throughout life.
4. It must be unaffected by climate, age, disease or by any other environmental or genetical condition.

Other considerations include the stability of the

blood group in the blood sample, the relative usefulness of the system, the availability and cost of the necessary reagents to perform the test and the amount of blood required to allow testing. This last requirement applies to small babies in particular, as the amount of blood that can be taken easily is usually limited to about 1 ml.

The blood group systems currently employed can be listed under four major headings:

1. red cell antigens;
2. serum protein polymorphisms;
3. red cell enzyme polymorphisms;
4. HLA system.

Red cell antigens

The grouping of antigens present on the red cell is the oldest of the techniques used by the serologist and until about 25 years ago only these tests were available for use in paternity problems. The range of tests has remained roughly the same and normally includes the following systems: ABO, MNSs, Rhesus, Kell, Duffy, Lutheran and Kidd.

Serum protein polymorphisms

Since the discovery in 1955 by Smithies & Walker[2] of a genetic variation in the α_2 globulin fraction of human serum, which they called haptoglobins, a number of other serum proteins have been shown to be genetically polymorphic. Of these the group specific component, Gc, also found in the α_2 globulin fraction, the Gm and Km antigens located on the immunoglobulins and the Ag antigens found on the beta-lipoproteins are routinely tested. Two other systems, the third component of complement, C'3, and a recently discovered transferrin polymorphism, TfC, are not yet used routinely but are available for use in difficult cases.

Red cell enzyme polymorphisms

A large number of enzymes are present in the red cells and have been investigated for genetically inherited variation. This has proved to be the most rewarding field of study in the last 20 years and numerous polymorphic red cell enzymes have been discovered. They are usually demonstrated by the technique of starch gel electrophoresis, the same technique that Smithies[3] used to distinguish the haptoglobin types. A haemolysate is prepared from the red cells and subjected to electrophoresis. After separation of the enzyme proteins, according to their electrical charge, the bands of enzyme activity are located by applying to the surface of the gel a reaction mixture containing those substances required for the enzyme catalysed reaction to proceeo ano a stain that will reveal the regions of enzyme activity. A list of the red cell enzyme polymorphisms currently used is shown in Table 6.3.

A relatively new technique is isoelectric focusing. Here the enzyme proteins are separated according to their isoelectric points in a pH gradient established by applying an electric field to a mixture of amphoteric buffer substances. This has revealed further variants in the phosphoglucomutase system. Using the conventional starch-gel electrophoretic method, three phenotypes can be demonstrated; this number is increased to 10 when isoelectric focusing is used, thereby increasing the chance of exclusion by this system from 14.5 to 24.5%. The examination of other red cell enzymes and serum proteins by isoelectric focusing will probably reveal further variants in systems currently used and new polymorphisms may be discovered.

HLA system

The HLA system consists of a series of antigens present on the lymphocytes. The chance of excluding a falsely accused man using a comprehensive range of HLA genetic markers is 96%. This high exclusion rate makes it a most attractive system for use in paternity problems but a number of practical difficulties limit its usefulness. Quite a large sample of blood (approximately 5 ml) is needed in order to isolate a suitable lymphocyte fraction, which would prevent testing on many samples obtained from small babies. Another drawback is the short life span of the lymphocytes so that many samples received by post are unsuitable for testing. The initial cost of acquiring the necessary antisera and ancillary equipment is high, and to ensure accurate results the investigator must have a wide experience of HLA testing.

Table 6.3 Chance of exclusion of non-fathers

System	% Individual chance of exclusion	% Combined chance of exclusion
Red cell antigens		
ABO	17.6	17.6
MNSs	32.1	44.1
Rhesus	28.0	59.8
Kell	3.3	61.1
Duffy	4.8	63.0
Lutheran	3.3	64.2
Kidd	4.5	65.8
Serum proteins		
Haptoglobins (Hp)	18.1	72.0
Group specific components (Gc)	15.9	76.5
Ag	14.2	79.8
$Gm^1 Gm^2$	7.8	81.4
Km^1	4.1	82.2
Red cell enzymes		
Phosphoglucomutase (PGM)	24.5	86.6
Red cell acid phosphatase (EAP)	21.0	89.4
Glutamate pyruvate transaminase (GPT)	18.7	91.4
Esterase D (EsD)	9.0	92.1
Adenosine deaminase (ADA)	4.5	92.5
Adenylate kinase (AK)	4.2	92.8
Glyoxalase 1 (GLO)	18.0	94.1
Total combined chance of exclusion		
	94.1	

CHANCES OF EXCLUSION

Table 6.3 shows the average chance the non-father has of being excluded by routine tests employed by a specialist laboratory. This figure of 94% shows that the non-father would be unlucky not to be excluded, but there is a considerable element of chance. There are cases in which it is accepted that one of two men is the father, but neither is excluded.

Between 1969 and 1979, nine additional systems were added to the range of systems investigated but, as is shown in Table 6.4, the percentage of men shown not to be the father did not increase but the proportion of cases in which other possible fathers was shown to be below 4% increased from 9 to 39%. No range of tests will exclude all non-fathers but these figures suggest that the present range of tests approaches what can usefully be employed to be cost-effective.

Table 6.4

	1969	1979
% Cases showing exclusion	25	22
Average number of exclusions per case	2.1	2.6
% Cases showing non-exclusion	75	78
% Cases where non-excluded possible fathers were 4% or less of the population	9.2	38.5

REFERENCES

1. Race, R. R. & Sanger, R. (1968) Blood Groups in Man. 5th Ed. Blackwell, Oxford.
2. Smithies, O. & Walker, N. F. (1955) Genetic control of some serum proteins in normal humans. Nature (Lond.) **176**, 1265.
3. Smithies, O. (1955) Zone electrophoresis in starch cells. Group variations in the serum proteins of normal human adults. Biochem. J. **61**, 629.

7

Deaths due to sudden or unexpected natural causes

Under the coroner's system all sudden or unexpected deaths must be referred to the coroner so that he may make such investigations as he thinks necessary to establish the cause of death. These cases include all those who have not been seen by a doctor in the 14 days preceding death. The phrase 'been seen by a doctor' is to be construed to mean that the doctor had seen the deceased on a professional basis and should not be taken to cover those cases where the doctor knew the deceased socially but has not recently examined him.

In the majority of cases in England and Wales the coroner will order an autopsy, and the coroner's officer will obtain as much relevant medical history as he can from the deceased's spouse, close relative or other person who knew the deceased. The pathologist who performs the autopsy should constantly bear in mind the limitations of such a medical history. Many people will not inform even their spouses of severe symptoms and will, for instance, stoically suffer crushing chest pains without complaint either because they do not wish to unduly alarm others or because they are frightened that they have some fatal condition and try to blot it out of their minds. On the other hand it should be remembered that although the deceased has suffered from severe symptoms these are not necessarily related to the cause of death and a full autopsy must be performed. The pathologist should guard against making a final diagnosis on the basis of the history, and then looking at the organs to confirm this diagnosis. He should always bear in mind that what from the history appears to be a myocardial infarct may in fact be some other natural disease, or that a person who has suffered from an infarct from which he would have recovered, may have taken an overdose of sleeping tablets.

There is absolutely no justification for performing a limited autopsy. Rather, the medico-legal autopsy should be performed with the same high standard of care taken in a routine case. Indeed the standard of care taken should be, desirably, even higher as issues of greater weight are possibly involved. There are those who advocate that the pathologist should perform the autopsy before he reads the history and should then review the history in the light of his post-mortem findings. This procedure is probably not necessary if the medico-legal pathologist trains himself to keep an open mind and to guard against making a hasty decision. At the end of every autopsy all the facts, history and findings should be reviewed to see whether they fit together. If they do not then one is not entitled to say that one has made a firm diagnosis. Further studies such as histology, toxicology, bacteriology, etc., should be performed and pathologists should not allow themselves to be forced to make a diagnosis that they do not feel they have sufficient facts to make. On the other hand they should always remember that there are others, such as relatives, who have an interest in the body and should not delay matters longer than they can help. As an instance of this may be cited the case of a person who has obviously died of widespread metastases but the primary is not immediately obvious and can only be determined, if at all, by histology. One should immediately say that the cause of death is carcinomatosis and ask the coroner's officer to mark the special box on the death certificate which says that further information will be available later for statistical purposes. This enables the relatives to go ahead with their funeral arrangements, prevents the coroner from opening an unnecessary inquest but at the same time ensures that the statistics of deaths compiled by the Registrar General are as complete and as accurate as it is possible to make them.

The purpose of a medico-legal autopsy is to establish the cause of death and to decide whether it is due to natural or unnatural causes. It must be remembered that the 'cause of death' eventually recorded should be that condition which led to the death of the person. Death certificates and their associated statistics are not, and were never intended to be, a catalogue of all the disease processes suffered by the deceased and they should not be taken to indicate the prevalence of a certain pathological condition in a community. Only if a condition contributed to death should it appear on the death certificate. For example, the statistics of death due to coronary artery disease do not give any direct information as to its prevalence amongst the population. They only reveal what percentage of the population die from it. Many of those who die of other causes have severe coronary artery disease. If people desire to know the prevalence of a disease process they must look somewhere other than at death statistics. Too many pathologists include too much detail on a death certificate, particularly under Part II of the cause of death, and this leads to confusion as to the actual cause of death.

Pathology embraces all disease and every pathologist must do his utmost to keep up to date with advances in all fields of medicine as it is only by doing so that he will be able to recognise any disease process that comes his way. Medico-legal pathologists should in particular not allow themselves to get bogged down in one small corner. It is only too easy to think that as they do not treat patients they have no need to know anything about therapeutics but the side-effects of modern drugs sometimes play a large part in the cause of death and therefore, as far as possible, they should be aware of what these side-effects may be.

Another trap for the unwary is to forget that in certain cases death is a final outcome of a process that started many years previously, which process is not usually seen today because of modern therapy. Syphilis, for instance, is at the moment a comparatively rare disease (although it seems to be making a comeback) and most cases are easily treated with penicillin. This, however, has not always been so and a person may die of syphilitic aortitis having caught the original infection at a time when there was less public awareness of the disease and less success with treatment.

MORBID ANATOMY

Although sudden natural death may be due to a disease process in almost any organ, the majority are due to some affliction either of the heart, lungs or brain. The figures shown in Table 7.1 were compiled from the records of Southwark Coroner's Court, London (and are published by kind permission of Dr A. G. Davies, H. M. Coroner). They are of 1938 natural deaths dealt with by that office in the period January–June inclusive 1973. They include all natural deaths except those which occurred in a postoperative period even if it was considered that death was due to natural causes. The cases of bronchopneumonia are mainly due to chronic bronchitis and emphysema which are very common in London. An attempt has been made to put cases where bronchopneumonia was the terminal event of some other condition such as cerebral infarction into the category of the other condition. Each case has been placed in only one category. Thus, for instance, a person dying from massive haemorrhage due to a malignancy of the stomach would appear only under the heading of 'malignancy' and would not also appear under the heading 'gastro-intestinal haemorrhage'.

The cases dealt with by the coroner are a highly selected series and bear little relationship to the causes of death in the community in general.

CARDIOVASCULAR SYSTEM

In the Western World diseases of this system account for the largest number of sudden natural deaths. This is primarily because the diet and stresses of Western life predispose to the development of atheroma but is also because infectious diseases have been to a large extent eradicated by antibiotic therapy and improvements in hygiene

Table 7.1

Cause of death	Males		Females		Combined totals	
	Number	%	Number	%	Number	%
Myocardial infarction Coronary artery disease	525	48.4	319	37.4	844	43.6
Essential hypertension (Cardiac deaths)	40	3.7	35	4.1	75	3.9
Senile myocardial degeneration	6	0.6	31	3.6	37	1.9
Valvular disease	27	2.5	23	2.7	50	2.6
Dissecting aortic aneurysm	9	0.8	13	1.5	22	1.1
Atheromatous aneurysm	30	2.8	12	1.4	42	2.2
Syphilitic aortitis	1	0.1	2	0.2	3	0.2
Cardiomyopathy	5	0.5	5	0.6	10	0.5
Mesenteric thrombosis	2	0.2	6	0.7	8	0.4
Pulmonary embolus	30	2.8	47	5.5	77	4.0
Cor pulmonale	36	3.3	20	2.3	56	2.9
Bronchopneumonia	95	8.8	64	7.5	159	8.2
Lobar pneumonia	10	0.9	11	1.3	21	1.1
Intracranial haemorrhage	36	3.3	55	6.4	91	4.7
Cerebral infarction	27	2.5	27	3.2	54	2.8
Meningitis	2	0.2	4	0.5	6	0.3
Renal causes	6	0.6	20	2.3	26	1.3
Peritonitis	16	1.5	18	2.1	34	1.8
Gastro-intestinal haemorrhage	14	1.3	5	0.6	19	1.0
Acute intestinal obstruction	2	0.2	12	1.4	14	0.7
Hepatic (including bleeding varices)	9	0.8	6	0.7	15	0.8
All malignancies	89	8.2	74	8.7	163	8.4
Sudden unexpected death in infancy	5	0.5	1	0.1	6	0.3
Status asthmaticus	3	0.3	4	0.5	7	0.4
Miscellaneous	59	5.4	40	4.7	99	5.1
Totals	1084	100.2	854	100.0	1938	100.2

and people are now living to an age at which degenerative diseases can make themselves felt.

In death due to heart disease there is often a dramatically sudden fall in blood pressure so that the person may fall and injure himself. These injuries must be evaluated with extreme care as in most cases they are not contributory to death but are merely incidental to the dying process. They are, however, usually readily visible to relatives and compensation claims or allegations of homicide may be initiated although there is no factual basis.

A more difficult question to deal with is the part played by stress and energetic activity in contributing to death. A heart that has been damaged is not a normal heart even though that damage may have healed. Its functional reserve may be perfectly adequate for the ordinary day to day activities but it may lack sufficient reserve to cope with unusual exertion. One has, however, no way of testing the adequacy of the reserve and must be wary of saying that a person who has severe heart disease and had died during a fight, has died because of the fight.

All one can say is that such a fight, statistically speaking, cannot but have had an untoward effect on the heart condition.

Coronary artery disease

This is by far the greatest single cause of death in Great Britain. Atheroma is a condition which despite a great deal of research is still little understood. Many factors are associated with its development. These include diet, stress, exercise and sex. For reasons that are not known, women during the reproductive period of life do not develop it at the same rate as men of similar age. This is not true of post-menopausal women so that eventually the severity of the condition in women approaches that in men or it may be that those men who, for other reasons, are developing atheroma at a slower rate manage to survive to a greater age than their less fortunate brothers.

Atheroma affects the larger arteries of the body leading to a gradual narrowing of the lumen. It is in the smaller of these arteries that its most severe effects are usually felt as blood flow in a vessel is proportional to the fourth power of the radius.

The heart receives its blood supply from two arteries which arise from the aortic sinuses. The left arises from the left aortic sinus and divides after a short distance into two vessels: (1) the anterior interventricular which supplies the anterior surface and anterior half of the septum; (2) the circumflex which runs in the left atrioventricular groove and supplies the lateral border. The right arises from the right aortic sinus, passing in the right atrioventricular groove to become the posterior interventricular artery. It supplies the inferior (or posterior) surface of the heart and the posterior half of the septum. This is the usual arrangement but variability in the areas supplied by the right and left circumflex is very common and one of the arteries may be completely dominant. It is said that the coronary arteries are end arteries and do not form effective anastomoses with each other. This may be true of normal coronary arteries but is certainly not so in those affected by atheroma where every possible anastomosis has been opened up. Because of this one can get paradoxical infarction. If, for example, the circumflex artery is very narrowed and the lateral border of the heart is relying on the right artery for most of its blood supply, then partial occlusion of the right artery by thrombus may lead to lateral infarction although sufficient blood is still flowing to prevent inferior infarction.

The incidence of blockage, whether by atheroma or thrombus, is greatest in the anterior interventricular, followed by the right, the circumflex and lastly the left main trunk. The area of blockage is usually in the first 1–2 cm of the artery but it may be very small and cuts should be made with a sharp scalpel at 1–2 mm intervals. Scissors must never be used as they have a crushing as well as a cutting action and produce so much distortion that any thrombus is obscured. After death blood clots and then reliquifies. This latter is not true of the 'red tail' beyond a thrombus, and any such 'red tail' found in a coronary artery should be traced back towards the ostium to see if there is a thrombus at its head. All vessels should be cut across; they should not be opened along their length with a pair of coronary artery scissors as the point of the advancing blade can easily dislodge a small thrombus and its presence may be missed.

Occlusion of a coronary artery may come about in a number of ways.

Occlusion by atheroma

There is a slow build up of atheroma with fibrosis and possibly dystrophic calcification. This may affect the whole circumference of the vessel wall so that the lumen is narrowed to a pin point or it may only affect part of the wall. In the latter case the still relatively elastic part of the wall may contract down post-mortem so that the lumen appears narrower than it would have been in life when the vessel was distended by the pressure of blood in it. Heavily calcified vessels, even if of very good calibre, do not seem to perform their function as efficiently as the pliable vessels of young people so that in these cases infarction is possible even though the lumen may be perfectly adequate.

Thrombosis

The presence of atheroma in the wall of a vessel leads to disturbance of the intima and turbulence in the blood flow. Both of these predispose to the formation of thrombus and this may either completely block the vessel or further compromise an already inadequate blood flow. One of the theories of atheroma formation, the 'encrustation theory', states that atheroma is built up by degeneration of platelets that are continually being deposited on the intima, so that, if the theory is correct, a coronary thrombosis is merely the final stage in a process that has been going on for many years.

Coronary embolism

This is usually due to small platelet thrombi being carried down a coronary artery. It is a rare occurrence and even when it does occur, is not easy to prove by either macroscopic or microscopic means. Possible sites of origin of the embolus are the left atrial appendage, a mural infarct or vegetations on either the mitral or aortic valves.

Haemorrhage into an atheromatous plaque

The haemorrhage arises as the result of: (1) rupture

of the wall of one of the vasa vasorum; (2) an edge of the plaque lifting and letting blood in underneath. Some people refer to this condition as 'dissecting aneurysm of the coronary artery' but this term should be avoided. A dissecting aneurysm is caused by a defect of the media and the cavity is bounded on both sides by media. In haemorrhage into an atheromatous plaque the cavity is bounded, in part at least, by the plaque itself. True dissecting aneurysms of the coronary arteries do occur but they are exceedingly rare. The raising of the plaque may produce narrowing of the lumen or the plaque may tear away at one edge and pivot across the vessel causing complete obstruction.

Syphilis

This may produce fibrosis and narrowing of the coronary ostia which can be overlooked unless special care is taken. The condition is often further aggravated by the concommittent aortic incompetence which produces a lowering of the diastolic blood pressure and also leads to left ventricular hypertrophy which necessitates a greater blood supply.

Results of coronary artery obstruction

Cardiac arrhythmia

A ventricle which is overworked and undernourished may suddenly go into ventricular fibrillation or asystole and unless immediate steps are taken to correct the condition the patient will die. This can occur even if the arteries are not completely blocked and is often precipitated by a sudden demand for an increased cardiac output by running for a bus or becoming involved in a fight. At autopsy no changes, apart from severe narrowing of the arteries, will be seen and in these cases an accurate history of the events immediately preceding death is of paramount importance.

Progressive fibrosis

The oxygen requirements of fibrous tissue is lower than that of muscle and therefore there may be slow replacement of muscle fibres, one by one, by fibrous tissue without any signs of infarction either

to the naked eye or under the microscope. A heart so affected slowly loses its functional reserve and will fail as the foci of fibrosis act as 'areas of irritation' and trigger off a bout of arrhythmia. If the conducting system of the heart is affected by fibrosis then there may be history of bundle branch block or even complete heart block.

Myocardial infarction

In this a greater or lesser area of the myocardium is suddenly deprived of its blood supply and dies. Because of its greater oxygen requirements infarcts usually occur in the left ventricle but right ventricular infarcts are sometimes seen although they are rather rare. The post-mortem appearance of infarction is described below but it must be remembered that these are often considerably modified by previous heart damage and by the inability of the heart to repair itself in the face of a compromised blood supply. In younger people infarction is usually accompanied by severe crushing chest pain and signs of shock but in old people these are often absent. The reasons for this are not clear but the 'silent coronary' is a well recognised clinical entity.

Macroscopic appearance. Authorities differ considerably in their opinions as to how quickly changes occur following infarction but the author has found the following time schedule to be helpful.

12–24 h. Up to this time there may be no signs or possibly a slight pallor of the muscle fibres. This pallor is partly due to the cutting off of the blood supply and partly due to oedema of the fibres.

1–3 days. The muscle fibres become necrotic and change from their normal brown colour to a yellow colour. Blood vessels in the area of infarction will also become necrotic and the haemoglobin will diffuse into the surrounding necrotic muscle giving it a reddish or greenish hue. This may be a very patchy process so that there may be the appearance of many small punctate haemorrhages. At the same time an acute inflammatory reaction occurs in the surviving muscle so that the infarct is surrounded by an area of hyperaemia.

3–10 days. Progressive lysis and removal of the dead muscle leads to softening and thinning of the area of infarction, this process being maximal by about the 10th day. It is classically on the 10th day that rupture of the heart occurs.

10 days onwards. During this time the process of fibrous repair predominates and the infarct is slowly converted to a fibrous scar. By three months the scar has settled down and one can then only say that it is over three months old: there is no way of telling by its appearance how old it actually is.

Microscopic appearances. These are often very subtle and considerable experience is needed for their interpretation. Post-mortem autolysis may make the picture even more complicated and this is of particular importance in forensic medicine as many people who die suddenly are not found for some hours or even days.

One of the earliest changes is eosinophilia of the muscle cytoplasm which begins to occur some 6 h after infarction. Along with this goes swelling of the fibres and a granular appearance of the cytoplasm. Later the cell outlines become indistinct and polymorphs and macrophages may move in between the muscle fibres but it must be stressed that despite the classical descriptions of acute inflammation such a cellular infiltrate may not be seen at all. As the infarct ages the cells begin to lyse, their outlines disappear and their nuclei disintegrate and disappear. Even later granulation tissue and fibrosis occurs. These changes can be seen on standard haematoxylin and eosin preparations but certain special stains such as phosphotungstic acid-haematoxylin may make the picture clearer. Macro and microtechniques for the visualisation of early infarcts have been developed and reference should be made to histological textbooks for the methods.

Following an infarct the patient may die immediately or he may survive the initial episode only to succumb some days or weeks later.

Results of myocardial infarction

Cardiac failure

If the infarct is large enough, insufficient muscle will be left to carry the burden of maintaining the circulation and sooner or later the person will go into cardiac failure. The final stages may be rapid and the person may die very suddenly.

Mural thrombus

If the infarct affects the endocardial surface of the heart, thrombosis may occur. Pieces of thrombus sometimes break off and are carried away by the blood stream. Those arising in the right ventricle will end in the lungs and those from the left ventricle in any part of the systemic circulation. It is possible for pieces to embolise down the coronary arteries producing further myocardial damage.

Ruptured myocardium

If the process of repair does not keep pace with the rate at which dead tissue is being removed, then the heart may rupture. This occurs classically on the 10th day following an infarct but may of course occur at other times. The rupture is usually into the pericardial sac which is consequently filled with blood and the heart is unable to fill with blood during diastole. On rare occasions the rupture may occur through the interventricular septum causing a left to right shunt of blood.

Ruptured papillary muscle

The cusps of the mitral valve are prevented from being turned inside out by their attachment to the papillary muscles via the chordae tendineae. These papillary muscles are particularly prone to infarction as their tips are the furthest part of the myocardium from the ostia of the coronary arteries. Despite this, rupture of a papillary muscle is a comparatively rare event but when it does occur it leads to mitral incompetence and heart failure.

Cardiac aneurysm

Although fibrous tissue is an exceedingly strong tissue it will, if subjected to strain, gradually elongate. This sometimes occurs in the heart where each beat of the heart stretches the fibrous scar and it does not quite return to its previous length each time. Over a period of weeks the fibrous tissue is ballooned out into a cardiac aneurysm. At each beat of the heart a proportion of the cardiac output ebbs and flows uselessly into the aneurysmal cavity putting a strain on the surviving muscle. The final outcome is heart failure which may occur with dramatic suddenness: it is exceedingly rare for the fibrous tissue scar to rupture.

Valvular disease of the heart

Congenital

The most common cause of sudden death due to congenital valvular disease is seen in those cases where there is fusion of the cusps with consequent stenosis. Nowadays these lesions are usually diagnosed during life and some are amenable to surgical treatment. Occasionally only two cusps develop in the aortic valve instead of the normal three. Such a valve is liable to become the seat of bacterial endocarditis and this can lead to sudden death.

Aortic valve

Rheumatic fever is a disease which has been said to 'lick the heart but bite the valves'. It follows a streptococcal sore throat and although it affects all parts of the heart, it is because of its damage to the delicate, but vital, valves that its main effects are seen. It causes inflammation and fibrosis of the valve. When the fibrous tissue later contracts the valve becomes stenosed and distortion of the cusps leads to incompetence. Over and above this the inflammation may cause adhesions between the free edges of the cusps particularly at the commissures thus leading to a greater degree of stenosis. The stenosis and incompetence will put a strain on the left ventricle causing hypertrophy and at the same time the interference with the blood flow in the aorta will be reflected in the flow in the coronary arteries. A heart so affected is in a precarious position and sudden decompensation may occur at any moment. A previously damaged valve is always liable to be affected by subacute bacterial endocarditis which either leads to further damage in the form of more fibrosis or causes incompetence by destroying one or more of the cusps. There is always the possibility that pieces of the vegetations from the endocarditis will break off and embolise into the coronary arteries.

Calcific aortic stenosis is a condition of uncertain aetiology in which the aortic valve becomes fibrosed and calcified. This causes rigidity of the cusps with consequent stenosis. Usually there is little or no aortic incompetence. This condition affects only the aortic valve although areas of calcification are sometimes found beneath and behind the posterior mitral valve leaflet. This latter rarely causes any functional disturbance of the heart.

Syphilis has a twofold action on the aortic valve. It attacks the valve ring causing replacement of the elastic tissue by fibrous tissue which under the constant pounding from the heart slowly stretches; and at the same time affects the cusps causing the free edges to become rolled back upon themselves. Both these lead to incompetence.

Mitral valve

As with the aortic valve the mitral valve may be affected in rheumatic fever. The inflammation is followed by narrowing of the valve ring and adhesions between the leaflets lead to stenosis of the valves. At the same time inflammation of the chordae tendineae causes them to be shortened, thickened and fused. This means that the leaflets can no longer meet each other and mitral incompetence results. Like the aortic valve, a damaged mitral valve may become affected by subacute bacterial endocarditis. A very common sequel of mitral valvular disease is atrial fibrillation. This causes the atria to quiver instead of beating in a co-ordinated manner and the consequent disturbance of blood flow often predisposes to the formation of thrombus in the atrial appendage. If part of this thrombus in the left atrium breaks off it can become lodged in the stenosed mitral valve acting as a ball valve and leading to complete blockage of the circulation; or it may pass through the valve to become lodged in some other part of the system circulation, of which the cerebral arteries are the most important.

Aortic disease

Coarctation

This is a rare congenital anomaly in which a section of the aorta is markedly stenosed. It may lead to sudden death by obstructing the outflow of blood from the heart but more usually death is due to dissection of the aorta.

Atheroma

The deposition of atheroma leads to a loss of the muscle coats and elastic tissue and their replacement by fibrous tissue. The condition is usually more severe in the lower parts of the aorta, particularly below the origins of the renal arteries, but any part can be affected. The weakened wall is gradually bulged by the pounding of the heart beat and an aneurysm is produced. If the area of weakness is localised a saccular aneurysm is produced but more usually there is generalised weakness of a length of the vessel and a fusiform aneurysm results. Thrombosis of the aneurysmal cavity occurs but, unfortunately, this does not serve to strengthen the wall to any great extent and the aneurysm slowly grows till eventually the wall ruptures. If it is the abdominal aorta that is affected the blood usually spills into the retroperitoneal space. Thoracic aneurysms usually rupture into a pleural space, but may erode into the oesophagus, mediastinum, bronchus or trachea. Not all ruptures are sudden. They may be preceded by slow leaks which can give rise to symptoms such as abdominal pain. The final event, however, is shock due either to the loss of a large amount of blood from the circulation or to distension of the surrounding tissues by the blood. Very occasionally atheromatous aneurysms of other large arteries may occur and these too may rupture. The signs and symptoms will, of course, depend on the site of the aneurysm.

Syphilis

As well as producing changes in the coronary ostia and aortic valve syphilis can affect the rest of the aortic wall. It produces an arteritis of the vasa vasorum and leads to fibrous replacement of the elastic tissue. This may in turn lead to aneurysm formation. Syphilitic aneurysms are usually seen in the thoracic aorta as opposed to atheromatous aneurysms which usually occur in the abdominal aorta. Syphilitic aneurysms are often erosive and as well as rupturing internally may even

erode through the sternum and rupture outside the body.

Dissecting aneurysm

A dissecting aneurysm is due to a degenerative condition of the media in which small areas of mucopolysaccharides accumulate amongst the muscle fibres. It has no relationship to atheroma but as both conditions occur in older people they may co-exist. These areas of mucopolysaccharide develop insidiously causing no symptoms until the intima tears and blood tracks between this and layers of the media. The usual site of tearing of the intima is 2–3 cm above the aortic valve. The blood tracks in both directions and usually eventually bursts through the wall completely. Many walls rupture into the pericardial sac causing cardiac tamponade. Some rupture back into the aortic lumen causing a double-barrelled vessel. Such a vessel has a weakened wall and this usually ruptures at a later date although this may be some years later. The vessels that leave the aorta have to cross the cavity of the aneurysm and they may be severed or compressed by the outside pressure. If these vessels are supplying a vital structure then death will occur; the post-mortem findings will depend upon which vessels were affected.

Essential hypertension

This is a condition of unknown aetiology where the blood pressure is consistently raised above normal. Such a pressure puts a strain on the left ventricle and at the same time predisposes to the formation of atheroma. The heart is thus attacked from two angles and may fail at any moment. Usually such failure is gradual but may occur without any warning. The findings at autopsy are hypertrophy of the left ventricle with no obvious cause, increased amount of atheroma and possibly hypertensive changes in the kidneys. The heart muscle sometimes has a pale glassy appearance. If hypertension has been present for some years the pressure may be reflected back through the lungs causing right ventricular hypertrophy. The ventricular cavities may or may not be dilated. It must be appreciated that none of these findings is pathognomonic of hypertension and could be caused by other conditions but taken together, particularly if the deceased had a history of high blood pressure, usually enables the diagnosis to be made without too much difficulty.

Senile myocardial degeneration

Ageing is a process that is very ill-understood but there is no doubt that as the body mechanism gets older it becomes less capable of performing its functions. In the heart this is seen as flabbiness and softening of the muscle with accumulation of lipofuscin in the fibres. Such an accumulation of pigment changes the colour from its normal healthy red brown to an entirely different brown colour which defies description but is immediately recognisable when seen at autopsy. This is known as brown atrophy. Because of the softening a finger can easily be pushed through the wall and one is surprised that such a heart managed to function as long as it did.

Pulmonary embolism

Pulmonary embolism is a condition in which thrombi are formed on the walls of the pelvic and leg veins and such thrombi break away and embolise to the lungs. The veins themselves are usually normal and the condition is referred to as phlebothrombosis in contradistinction to thrombophlebitis where thrombosis occurs in a vein which is already inflamed. In this latter case embolism is much less likely to occur as the inflammation anchors the thrombus to the vessel wall. Although the thrombosis is the primary event the embolus itself usually consists of a tube of thrombus with a central core of clotted blood. When it reaches the lung its effects depend on its size. Small ones are carried to the periphery of the lung where they cause pulmonary infarcts but large ones straddle the bifurcation of the pulmonary artery completely blocking the blood circulation. Spasm of the pulmonary arteries around the thrombus only helps to make matters worse. The cause of the thrombosis is thought to be damage to the vessel wall by slowing of the blood flow and pulmonary embolism frequently causes death in people who are confined to

bed, particularly in the postoperative period. It has even been observed in people confined to an aeroplane seat on long journeys such as the flight to America.

Cardiomyopathies

As well as being secondarily affected by damage to its blood supply, hypertension, etc., the heart muscle may be primarily affected. This group of conditions is known collectively as the cardiomyopathies. Although they are comparatively rare they often come into the field of the forensic pathologist as the sufferer suddenly drops dead without any warning.

The following classification is taken from Robbins's textbook of pathology[1] to which further reference should be made for greater details.

Congenital

These are exceedingly rare. Some are familial and in these cases the history should give a good lead. Others such as those associated with Marfan's syndrome or muscular dystrophy should cause little trouble as other signs of these conditions will be apparent.

Inflammatory

The autopsy findings are those of a flabby dilated heart with patchy pallor of the myocardium. Histologically there is a varying degree of muscle fibre necrosis with interstitial oedema and a cellular infiltrate. The nature of the infiltrate will depend on the type of organism causing the condition but in general bacterial infections cause a neutrophil reaction, viruses a small round cell or lymphocyte reaction and parasites an eosinophil reaction. Occasionally a giant cell type of reaction is seen. None of these is specific and attempts to isolate the causative organism have not usually been successful. A great deal of care is needed in the interpretation of the findings as isolated foci of round cell infiltration are fairly often seen in hearts. In one famous case such foci were seen in the myocardium of an airline pilot whose aircraft crashed with many fatalities but it was subsequently shown that the cause of the crash was an instrument failure.

Toxic

Many substances have a toxic effect on the heart. The action of the halogenated hydrocarbons, some of which are used as anaesthetic agents, is well known. Cobalt salts which at one time were used to stabilise the head on beer have caused sudden death in people who consumed large quantities over a long period. Certain bacterial toxins of which diphtheria is the best known may affect the heart.

Sensitivity

In rheumatic fever, lupus erythematosis and similar collagen disease the heart may be affected. Some people show a hypersensitivity to certain drugs.

Metabolic

Of these amyloidosis, occasionally occurring as a condition localised to the heart rather than a generalised condition, is the most common unless one includes the disturbances in electrolytes which are seen in many diseases.

Nutritional

Lack of vitamins may have a direct detrimental effect on the heart such as thiamine deficiency leading to beri-beri. A more difficult problem is encountered in people with excessive alcohol intake. These people suffer from heart damage but it is not known whether this is due to lack of vitamins or other essential substances or whether it is due to a direct action of alcohol on the heart. It could also be due to other constituents of the alcoholic beverage.

Endocrine

Thyrotoxicosis may lead to heart failure and hypothyroidism to increased coronary artery disease.

Idiopathic

Apart from the different causes listed above there remain some cases where no known cause exists. These are rare but it should be remembered that at autopsy it is not usually possible to find the cause of a cardiomyopathy as the histology is not specific and post-mortem blood chemistry has been little investigated.

RESPIRATORY SYSTEM

Obstruction of major airways

Although this is usually due to blockage by inhaled foreign bodies and is therefore not 'natural' it can arise as a consequence of natural disease. Occasionally it is due to a neoplasm but because these grow fairly slowly they usually give rise to symptoms and the patient does not die unexpectedly. More acute forms are seen in acute glottic oedema due to allergy or local inflammation. The membrane formed in diphtheria can block the trachea but luckily this disease is now rare in developed countries due to the policy of immunisation of all infants.

Pneumonia

In theory this should not give rise to sudden death but it is surprising how often severe widespread pneumonia is found in people who have suddenly died without any signs or symptoms. Pneumonia is divided into two main types—lobar and bronchopneumonia. If bronchopneumonia becomes very widespread it may affect the whole of one lobe and some authorities call this lobar pneumonia; but it is better to refer to it as confluent bronchopneumonia affecting a whole lobe and to reserve the term lobar pneumonia to the specific disease caused by *Streptococcus pneumoniae*. It must be remembered that antibiotic therapy has considerably modified the course of infection and the classical pictures are not often seen. One must not forget that patients often do not take a complete course of antibiotics and so may have some tablets available for self medication when they next get an infection. Do not be led into thinking that, because they have not recently been seen by a doctor, they have not had any treatment.

Lobar pneumonia

Lobar pneumonia is a condition that affects the

whole of one or more lobes of a lung at the same time, so that in every piece of lung examined the disease is at the same stage of development. It is caused by *Strep. pneumoniae*, more usually called the pneumococcus. The pneumonia develops quite suddenly and at first there is an outpouring of red cells and fibrin into the alveoli but later these are replaced by polymorphs and macrophages. These two processes make the lung look red and grey, respectively, and give it a solid appearance. From their fanciful resemblance to liver they are called red and grey hepatisation. Lobar pneumonia may attack a previously normal lung and if the person recovers it usually leaves no damage.

Bronchopneumonia

This is an entirely different process from lobar pneumonia and usually develops in lungs which have been previously damaged. It can be caused by a wide variety of organisms. In Great Britain chronic bronchitis is a very frequent condition and the damage produced by this often proceeds bronchopneumonia. In chronic bronchitis there is an increase in the number of mucus secreting cells, an increase in the amount of mucus secreted by each cell, and an extension of area of distribution of the mucus cells so that they lie in those parts of the lung beyond the reach of the cilia. Moreover people who suffer from chronic bronchitis are frequently smokers and this has the effect of paralysing the cilia. All these lead to the retention of mucus which provides a suitable medium for the growth of bacteria. If infection gets a foothold it may spread out into the surrounding lung causing bronchopneumonia. As the infection spreads out it causes red and grey hepatisation although these are not nearly so clearly demarcated as in lobar pneumonia. A typical focus of bronchopneumonia seen under the microscope shows a small bronchus full of pus surrounded by a ring of grey hepatisation which in turn is surrounded by a ring of red hepatisation. If the areas spread far enough they may coalesce forming confluent bronchopneumonia. Healing of this process produces damage in the lung which will predispose to further bouts of bronchopneumonia. Death, which can be very sudden, is due to 'toxic' products absorbed from the areas of infection. In old people who have a tenuous hold on life,

death may occur before the infection has spread into the lung tissue and is still confined to the bronchioles. This condition is usually referred to as purulent bronchiolitis.

Other conditions may precede bronchopneumonia, the most important of which are viral infections. These damage the lung and enable the bacteria which are always present to get a foothold. An interesting condition exists in which the primary damage is by the influenza virus and the secondary invader is *Staphylococcus aureus*. These have a synergistic action and lead to the outpouring of copious quantities of heavily blood-stained fluid into the aveoli so that the patient literally drowns in his own secretions. It strikes with lightning rapidity and a person can be well in the morning and dead by tea-time. Autopsy shows extremely congested lungs from which large quantities of bloody fluid can be expressed and culture of this fluid will show *Staph. aureus*. The demonstration of virus post-mortem is not particularly easy but if facilities are available should always be undertaken.

Bronchopneumonia may progress to the state where lung tissue begins to break down and an abscess develops. If this ruptures, sufficient pus can be aspirated into the other air passages to cause mechanical asphyxia. Rupture of an area of tuberculosis may lead to tuberculous bronchopneumonia. The cavity left after such a rupture may contain in its walls, or even be crossed by, large vessels. If these burst there may be a fatal haemorrhage but luckily most of the vessels in areas like this undergo a progressive obliteration of their lumina due to endarteritis obliterans and catastrophic haemorrhages are not as common as they would otherwise be.

Carcinoma

As mentioned above carcinoma of the larynx may cause mechanical blockage of the airway either by direct growth but more usually by a combination of direct growth and swelling due to concommittant tissue break down and infection.

Carcinoma of the bronchus is a disease that is increasing amongst the population due to the increase in cigarette smoking. It is less common amongst women than men but this is probably related to the fact that there must be a long history of smoking and it is only comparatively recently that cigarette smoking has been a socially acceptable activity for a woman. If present trends continue it is to be expected that the incidence of carcinoma of the bronchus amongst women will come to rival that seen amongst men. There are, of course, factors other than smoking which are concerned in the aetiology but at the moment they remain largely unknown. Indeed primary bronchial carcinoma is divided into four main categories: squamous cell, oat cell, anaplastic and adenocarcinoma; smoking is an aetiological factor in the development of the first three but not of the last. Carcinoma kills in many ways. It may spread generally through the body to cause carcinomatosis but it must be admitted that the actual mechanism of such deaths is very ill understood. It may dam back secretions by partially or completely blocking a bronchus and such secretions are always liable to become infected, giving rise to bronchopneumonia or a pulmonary abscess. It may spread locally into surrounding tissue and erode into a major blood vessel, usually one of the pulmonary arteries but on occasions the aorta. If it erodes through into the oesophagus food material will get into the air passages and cause bronchopneumonia.

Cor pulmonale

Unless some right to left shunt exists the whole of the cardiac output has to pass through the lungs. In disease such as chronic bronchitis and emphysema there is a gradual reduction in the number of capillaries in the lung due to loss of alveolar walls and this means that it is less easy for the heart to force the blood through the lungs. This in turn leads to hypertrophy of the right ventricle. Such a heart under strain may fail quite suddenly. At autopsy right ventricular hypertrophy will be found as well as atheroma of the pulmonary arteries due to the increased pressure in this side of the circuit. It is a personal observation that people dying in this way very frequently show little atheroma of their coronary arteries but whether this is due to some direct action or whether it is due to the fact that people with good coronary arteries survive to die of their cor pulmonale is not known. Infections of the lung put a greater strain on the right ventricle and in people suffering from cor pulmonale this may be sufficient to tip the balance.

Bronchial asthma

This is to be distinguished from cardiac asthma which is the term used to describe an attack of left ventricular failure causing breathlessness by back pressure of blood on the lungs. Bronchial asthma is due to spasm of the bronchial muscles leading to narrowing of the air passages. It is an allergic condition but psychological factors are often very important. The asthmatic has even greater difficulty in breathing out than breathing in as the negative pressure in the chest on inspiration tends to dilate the bronchi. The lungs of asthmatics at autopsy are therefore ballooned out. For reasons which are not readily understood asthmatics die because of strain on the right side of the heart. They do not simply asphyxiate as might be thought. Recently concern has been expressed that some of the deaths are due to the propellants in the aerosol inhalers used in the treatment of asthma. It was thought that these propellants had a cardiotoxic effect but research on healthy volunteers showed that following the inhalation of large doses the levels in the plasma never reached high enough amounts to have an effect on the heart. The autopsy findings are ballooning of the lungs with congestion and signs of right ventricular failure. There may or may not be plugging of the bronchioles by viscid mucus. Under the microscope the findings are those of emphysema, bronchiolar plugging with mucus, peribronchiolar muscle hypertrophy, basement membrane thickening and submucosal infiltration with eosinophils. It must, however, be stressed that on occasions any or all of these findings may be absent and a good history is a great help in the diagnosis of asthma.

Pneumothorax

In young healthy people a pneumothorax, unless it is of the rather rare tension pneumothorax variety, is a non-fatal condition. In people who have already got chronic lung disease such as emphysema any reduction in respiratory capacity may be fatal. In most cases of pneumothorax the site of rupture is not easily found but sometimes it is an emphysematous bulla that bursts and the rupture site can be shown. Producing death by a similar mechanism except that air does not get into the pleural cavity are those cases where a bulla 'grows' to such an enormous size that it occupies a significant portion of the chest cavity.

CENTRAL NERVOUS SYSTEM

Most of the causes of sudden natural death associated with the central nervous system are due to disturbances of its blood supply by one means or another.

Cerebral haemorrhage

As its name indicates this is due to bleeding into the brain substance itself. The usual site is into the basal ganglia due to rupture of one of the lenticulostriate arteries. It is frequently associated with systemic hypertension and it has been shown that in this condition microaneurysms develop in these arteries. These microaneurysms cause no symptoms until they rupture. Death may or may not be sudden: it may be preceded by a period of coma. At autopsy a large area of haemorrhage will be found destroying the basal ganglia. The site of rupture can never be found as the vessels are very small and are destroyed by the haemorrhage. If the blood ruptures through into the lateral ventricles it may spread by way of the aqueduct of Silvius and fourth ventricle into the subarachnoid space or more rarely it may rupture outwards through the cortex straight into the subarachnoid space. There is rarely any difficulty in distinguishing between a cerebral haemorrhage which has thus spread and true subarachnoid harmorrhage. Death is usually due to raised intracranial pressure affecting the vital respiratory and cardiac control centres of the the brain but if the person survives the initial episode he may succumb to bronchopneumonia or pulmonary embolism which frequently complicate unconsciousness. Because the haemorrhage is on one side of the brain, the whole brain may be twisted and this frequently gives rise to secondary haemorrhages in the pons and brain stem. Although these are usually small, they are in intimate association with the vital respiratory and cardiovascular centres and are probably responsible

for a large number of the deaths. These secondary pontine haemorrhages are also seen in association with head injuries and care must be taken to differentiate between the two sorts.

Spontaneous haemorrhages can also occur in the cerebellum and midbrain but are much rarer than primary intracerebral haemorrhage. If in the cerebellum, death is usually rapid as the raised pressure is below the tentorium and its effects are readily felt on the brain stem which is also below the tentorium. At autopsy there may be marked coning of the cerebellar tonsils through the foramen magnum. It is very important in these cases not to perform a diagnostic lumbar puncture as lowering the pressure of the cerebrospinal fluid in the spinal canal may lead to even greater coning and the patient may die because of the procedure. Unfortunately it is in just such cases that the pressure is not communicated above the tentorium so that papilloedema does not develop. A careful evaluation of the patient's signs and symptoms will normally prevent a tragedy.

Primary pontine haemorrhage may produce pressure on the vital centres or even destroy them. Frequently it affects the heat regulation centre and hyperpyrexia is often seen. Pin point pupils may produce confusion with morphine overdosage. Rarely haemorrhages into brain tissue are associated with angiomata. Whether these can be found at autopsy or not depends on the amount of damage produced by the high pressure blood tearing up the brain substance. Frequently the haemorrhage destroys all trace of the underlying condition.

Subarachnoid haemorrhage

This is due in the majority of cases to rupture of a berry aneurysm. These are small saccular aneurysms located between the branches of the arteries of the Circle of Willis or of the major vessels leading off the Circle. Because of their size, shape and colour they have a fanciful resemblance to small berries: hence their name. They develop at their characteristic sites because in all people there is a gap in the arterial muscle coat and the pressure of the blood can balloon out the wall at this point of weakness. They are therefore more common in people with hypertension and in older people. In certain cases they grow to very large size, completely distorting the vessels from which they arise. They are sometimes multiple. The most common type of haemorrhage which results from rupture of such an aneurysm is subarachnoid haemorrhage. In this there is diffuse bleeding into the subarachnoid space but especially into the area around the Circle of Willis and down the brain stem. Death is often rapid due to pressure on vital centres. Sometimes, however, these aneurysms leak slightly before the final catastrophic rupture and there may be a history of headaches. If the aneurysm grows large enough it may 'erode' into the brain tissue itself and subsequent rupture will cause bleeding which may be confused with cerebral haemorrhage. At autopsy a careful search should be made for the aneurysm by washing away the blood clot, aided if necessary by careful dissection with some blunt instrument such as the 'wrong' end of a scalpel. When the aneurysm is found it is often collapsed but the site of rupture can usually be demonstrated by passing a probe along the artery into the aneurysmal cavity. Great care must be taken with this procedure as it is very easy to produce a false rupture. Many cases of subarachnoid haemorrhage occur in association with a raised blood alcohol level and it is thought that the generalised vascular dilatation caused by the alcohol puts a strain on the aneurysm wall leading to rupture. Not all subarachnoid haemorrhages are natural but those associated with direct trauma to the head should cause no difficulty as other signs of such trauma are usually present. It has recently become recognised, however, that these haemorrhages may be the result of karate type chops to the neck. This causes rupture of the vertebral artery as it lies in the vertebral canal and the haemorrhage tracks upwards through the foramen magnum in to the skull. Demonstration of the ruptured vertebral artery can usually be readily made by injection of the artery with a radio-opaque material followed by X-rays of the neck. If X-ray facilities are not available in the mortuary the cervical vertebrae may be removed *en masse* and the injection and X-raying performed later. This does not invalidate the procedure but care must be taken to differentiate between the site of rupture and leakage from vessels which have been cut during the removal of the vertebrae.

Spinal cord haemorrhages

These are said to be rare but as the cord is not routinely examined at autopsy some may well have been missed.

Haemorrhage into a tumour

Cerebral tumours themselves, whether primary or secondary, are rarely a cause of sudden death. However, haemorrhage may occur into a tumour because of necrosis of the tumour centre or because of direct invasion of the walls of the vessels running in the tumour. The malformed walls of vascular tumours such as haemangiomata may also rupture.

Cerebral thrombosis and infarction

These are rarely the cause of sudden death: death is usually preceded by a period of coma with signs of upper motor neurone lesions. However, in cerebral infarction due to an embolus death may be very rapid. This is particularly so in old people where the collateral circulation is already impeded by atheroma or previous thrombosis. The embolus may arise from atrial thrombus in auricular fibrillation, mural thrombus in myocardial infarction, vegetations or heart valves or thrombus on an atheromatous plaque in the vessels leading to the brain. Very rarely the embolus may arise from the veins of the pelvis and legs, being carried to the cerebral circulation as a paradoxical embolus through a patent foramen ovale or a septal defect in the heart.

Meningitis and brain abscess

These are rare causes of sudden death but are occasionally encountered. The meningitis may be caused by a variety of organisms but it is in those cases caused by the meningococcus that the most fulminating effects are seen. This organism produces a septicaemia as well as meningitis and it may cause death particularly by its effects on the adrenal glands. It produces massive haemorrhages into these glands, a condition known as the Waterhouse Friedericksen syndrome.

Epilepsy

This disease produces great difficulty in post-mortem diagnosis as there are usually no lesions in the brain. The cause of death is often stated to be due to asphyxia but it is more probably due to anoxia and strain on the heart. Sometimes bite marks are seen on the tongue but these are not of course diagnostic. There is no substitute for an adequate history in helping to sort out these cases. If a history of treated epilepsy is obtained, the blood should be examined for anti-epileptic drugs as the absence of these indicates that the patient has failed to take his therapy. Occasionally an organic lesion of the brain such as parasitic cysts or post-traumatic changes may be the cause of the epilepsy. A careful search should be made for these, as, particularly in the case of post-traumatic changes, there may be claims for compensation later.

GASTRO-INTESTINAL SYSTEM

Oesophagus

Lesions in the oesophagus are not often the cause of sudden death as they usually produce symptoms which will cause the person to seek medical help. Carcinomata of surrounding structures may invade the oesophagus causing fatal haemorrhage or may produce a tracheo-oesophageal fistula leading to bronchopneumonia. On rare occasions an aortic aneurysm ruptures into the oesophagus. By far the largest cause of massive oesophageal haemorrhage is oesophageal varices. These are caused by blockage of the portal circulation, usually by hepatic cirrhosis. The blood then has to find other ways back to the heart, the chief of these being the veins at the lower end of the oesophagus where there are anastomoses between the portal and system circulations. These oesophageal veins are thus distended rather like varicose veins in the leg and because of their superficial submucosal position they are poorly supported and are exposed to the trauma of passing food particles. If oeseophageal varices are suspected, the oesophagus and stomach should be removed in one piece at autopsy since cutting across the oesophago–gastric junction will cause

them to collapse making their demonstration exceedingly difficult or even impossible.

Lacerations of the oesophagus are rare but one, the Mallory Weiss syndrome, deserves special mention. Normally in vomiting there is a relaxation of the oesophagus which precedes contraction of the stomach and abdominal muscles. In bouts of prolonged vomiting in which the Mallory-Weiss syndrome is seen, it is thought that such a relaxation fails to occur. The gastric contents are forced into the lower part of the oesophagus from which there is no escape producing linear lacerations. The usual cause of death is a massive haemorrhage but spilling of gastric contents into the mediastinum may produce shock and thus lead to death.

Stomach and duodenum

One of the commonest sites of massive gastro-intestinal haemorrhage is from a peptic ulcer situated either in the stomach or the duodenum. Although these usually cause symptoms during life one is often surprised to find at autopsy huge ulcers which apparently have caused no symptoms. As an ulcer gets larger it comes to affect more major blood vessels. These tend to become progressively obliterated by endarteritis obliterans and if this keeps pace with the destruction of the outside of the artery, the whole vessel can be eroded away without haemorrhage. If, however, the lumen is breached before it has been obliterated then the endarteritis merely serves to make matters worse by acting as a splint and preventing the arteries contracting down to arrest the bleeding. Gastric carcinomata may also cause massive haemorrhage. Perforation of an ulcer into the peritoneal cavity will cause peritonitis.

Intestines

In babies gastro-enteritis may lead to rapid death. This can also occur in the elderly but is rare between these two extremes.

Peritonitis is still a fairly common cause of death despite modern advances in therapy. In elderly people it is often completely symptom-free and death may occur without any warning signs or symptoms. The usual causes of peritonitis are perforation of a viscus, appendicitis, interference with the blood supply to the gut or acute pancreatitis. It is also seen in cases of intestinal obstruction caused by such things as a volvulus, abdominal adhesions or intussusception. Peritonitis itself leads to intestinal obstruction by causing failure of the normal peristalsis (paralytic ileus). The intestines become dilated by a thin watery fluid which is rich in potassium and death is due to an upset in the body chemistry. A special form of colonic ulceration and perforation is sometimes seen in the elderly. This is stercoral ulceration and is thought to be because as old people eat little and are often constipated, the small hard faeces press on the colon well producing ulcers. It should be remembered that bacteria may get through the wall into the peritoneal cavity even in the absence of an actual perforation.

Acute pancreatitis is often associated with hypothermia or may develop in alcoholics.

HEPATIC SYSTEM

Diseases of the liver rarely cause sudden death except when cirrhosis is complicated by oesophageal varices as described above. Blockage of the common bile duct can lead to an ascending cholangitis. If the blockage is intermittent, as is sometimes seen with a stone acting as a ball valve, there may not be any history of jaundice.

URINARY TRACT

Diseases of this system rarely cause sudden death. One exception is renal infection, particularly in the elderly where large parts of the kidney can be affected with abscess formation without the person apparently suffering any symptoms. The cause of death is due to the absorption of toxic substances from the renal tissue and not due to progressive renal failure. Renal tract infections are more common in women as the urethra is much shorter than in men, allowing bacteria easy access to the bladder and thence ascending via the ureters to the kidneys. Any obstruction to the outflow of urine will predispose to renal tract infection and such obstructions should be sought at autopsy. As well as

leading to infection, urinary obstruction also causes progressive renal failure. Although this usually causes symptoms the patient may not seek medical aid and may apparently die suddenly.

Polycystic disease of the kidney can cause sudden death. This is a condition in which multiple cysts develop in the kidneys causing pressure atrophy of normal renal tissue. This is a very slow process and although starting in utero may be compatible with life until the fifth or sixth decade. Because of its insidious nature the person and his relatives may not realise he is ill until he suddenly drops dead due to either renal-induced hypertension or because infection overwhelms the already severely compromised renal function.

GENITAL SYSTEM

Diseases of the male genital system are almost never responsible for sudden death but this is not so for the female genital tract. Pedunculated subserous fibroids or ovarian cysts may undergo torsion producing shock. It is however complications of pregnancy that produce the most dramatic pictures.

Ruptured ectopic pregnancy

If the fertilised ovum is prevented from reaching the uterus as, for example, by intra-tubal adhesions due to previous infection, it may implant in the wall of the fallopian tube. As it grows it produces no symptoms until it eventually ruptures the tube producing shock which may kill.

Toxaemia of pregnancy and eclampsia

This is a condition of unknown aetiology which occurs during the later months of pregnancy. In most cases it is preceded by warning signs of hypertension, albuminuria and oedema of the ankles. Rest in bed at this stage usually prevents the process from becoming worse and good antenatal care has done much to prevent the mortality that used to be associated with this condition. However in some cases eclampsia may occur with little warning causing death in convulsions. Examples have been seen in which the deceased was apparently well at the ante-natal clinic a few days before death but was found dead or in convulsions by the husband when he returned from work.

It must be remembered that young unmarried girls who become pregnant are often, because of their good abdominal musculature, able to conceal the pregnancy even from their mothers and do not attend ante-natal clinics. Such girls are in real danger of eclampsia as the premonitory signs will not be recognised. It is to be hoped that the availability of contraceptives and changes in the social climate will help to prevent these tragedies.

Apart from the pregnancy there may be minimal findings at autopsy and toxicological examination of the blood should be made to exclude drugs which may produce convulsions.

SUDDEN UNEXPECTED DEATH IN INFANCY

No one condition causes more problems to the forensic pathologist than sudden unexpected death in infancy (SUD). That it is a pathological entity no one doubts but so far the cause remains undiscovered. It typically occurs during the 3rd and 4th months of life and shows a peak incidence during the winter months. It is rarely observed after the 11th month of life. Depending on the series studied there is either a male preponderance (up to 70% boys) or equality of the sexes. The majority are bottle rather than breast fed infants. Although the condition is given the adjectives 'sudden' and 'unexpected' careful questioning of parents has revealed that in a large number of cases the baby showed signs of general malaise, such as irritability or refusing feeds on the day before death. There is often a history of a mild upper respiratory tract type of illness. These symptoms are rarely sufficiently severe to cause the parents to summon a doctor. Apart from these mild symptoms the usual history obtained is that the baby was well when placed in its cot or when the parents looked in before going to bed themselves, but was dead in the morning. The infant is often found lying face downwards and it was thought that perhaps it had suffocated, this being aided by the use of a soft pillow which could obstruct the mouth and nose. This is now thought to be extremely unlikely as abandoning the use of pillows has had no effect on the SUD statistics and even when found face downwards the position of the post-mortem livor usually shows that there has been no mechanical asphyxia. It is important that parents are made aware of this fact as many unnecessarily blame themselves for the death of the child.

The findings at gross autopsy are minimal but there are usually petechial haemorrhages of the thoracic viscera (not associated with petechiae of the face and conjunctivae) and congestion of the lungs with areas of collapse alternating with areas of emphysema. The histological findings have been the cause of much dispute but it is generally accepted that desquamation of the bronchiolar epithelium, slight peribronchiolar cellular infiltration with lymphocytes and plasma cells and some changes in the spleen are fairly typical findings. Bacteriological and virological studies have been of no help.

Many theories have been advanced amongst which may be cited: allergy to cow's milk, hypogammaglobulinaemia, overwhelming bacterial or viral infection, inborn errors of metabolism and disorders of electrolyte balance. None of these has found general acceptance and the debate continues.

REFERENCE

1. Robbins S. L. (1967) Pathology, 3rd ed. London: W. B. Saunders, p. 554

8

Post-mortem changes

DEFINITION

The older definitions of death which, in the main, depended on the cessation of respiratory movement and detectable heart beat will no longer work for the anaesthetist or surgeon who today may deliberately arrest both these natural functions and substitute artificial alternatives. They are maintaining life, and it is immaterial that the means should be artificial.

There is still life so long as a circulation of oxygenated blood is being maintained to *live* vital centres, for instance the brain stem. The word 'live' is important for one can circulate useful blood to a dead centre. Pathologists encounter frequent instances today where it is clear from autopsy that 'brain death' had occurred several days before the artificial support systems were withdrawn. In these cases the brain is softened, the cerebral sinuses thrombosed and the spinal cord frequently autolysed and in a liquid state. The hypostatic lividity may be pink due to good oxygenation of blood and there is no post-mortem change present in the other viscera.

IMMEDIATE SIGNS OF DEATH. POST-MORTEM CHANGES

Insensibility and loss of voluntary power

These signs are concomitants of death but may obviously be found in cases where death is merely apparent. Thus not only are they found in the apparently drowned, but perceptible heart beats or respiratory movements are also absent for a time in cases that ultimately recover entirely, a fact calling for sustained efforts at resuscitation.

Table 8.1 Signs of death

IMMEDIATE	
Insensibility and loss of EEG rhythms	Somatic death
Cessation of circulation (i.e., ECG rhythms)	
Cessation of respiration	
Cadaveric spasm	
EARLY	
Cooling	Cellular death
Skin changes	
Eye changes	
Blood changes	
Hypostasis	
Fibrinolysis	
Post-mortem bleeding	
Chemical changes in body fluids	
Muscular changes—rigor mortis	
LATE	
Putrefaction	Decomposition and
In air	decay
In water	
In earth	
Adipocere formation	
Mummification	
Larval infestation	

Insensibility and loss of power to move also occur in prolonged fainting attacks in vagal inhibitory phenomena, in epilepsy, trance and catalepsy, in narcosis, in electrocution and during the therapeutic use of muscle relaxants such as curare. In fact these two signs of death have been given undue weight without attention being paid to other more certain signs.

A remarkable but credible account has survived of the tardy relinquishment of life in the case of a lady from Cologne.

La femme d'un Consul de cette ville aiant été enterre l'an 1571 avec une bague de prix. Le fossoieur ouvrit le tombeau le nuit suivant pour voler la bague. Je laisse á penser s'il fut bien etonnée quand il se sentit serrer la main et quand la bonne dame l'empoigne pour se tirer du cercueil. Il s'en dépêtra pourtant, et s'enfuit sans autre conversation.[1]

There are numerous other accounts in the earlier medico-legal textbooks of premature pronouncement of death and even of premature burial. In order to prevent this occurrence, at one time in Germany bodies were placed in a room under observation for 48 h before burial was allowed. Today, with the almost universal provision of refrigeration for the dead, any premature certification of the fact of death may be irrevocable.

If the observation of *cessation of circulation* can be made with sufficient accuracy by stethoscope and over a sufficiently prolonged period, failure of heart beat is acceptable evidence of death. It is, however, an important decision, not to be made lightly.

In 1950 one of the former authors was at work in a London mortuary when the body of a woman aged 75 was brought in, stripped and laid on the table for autopsy. She had been found, lying on a common, cold and apparently lifeless, some 20 min previously. On her arrival at hospital a doctor had got into the ambulance, placed a hand on her chest and, finding it cold and feeling no pulse, pronounced her dead. Some 4 or 5 min after she had been placed on the mortuary table she was seen to swallow twice. She was found to be breathing and to have heart beats. She died of coronary thrombosis and myocardial infarction $2\frac{1}{4}$ h later.

In 1957 a 78-year-old solicitor's widow was found in Walsall apparently lifeless in bed. An empty box of sleeping tablets and several letters indicating suicide lay on the bedside table and a doctor certified her to be dead. Undertakers removed the body to a mortuary where 6 h later she was prepared for autopsy. A young police officer then noticed she was breathing. She was hurriedly removed to hospital where she died early next morning. The doctor had only 'felt both cheeks and touched her eyes and neck'. She thought 'there was no sign of heart beat and that rigor mortis had set in'. She was wrong: the old lady survived 16 h.

In another case reported in 1956 from Melbourne, a 45-year-old woman sat up and spoke to the constable deputed to search the body in the mortuary to which she had been conveyed after being certified dead. She had collapsed whilst waiting for a train in a Melbourne suburb. She walked out of the hospital to which she was taken from the mortuary and survived.

In a case known to the author, a motor cyclist with a pillion passenger lost control whilst going downhill and crashed into a tree. A passing doctor certified both as dead and they were conveyed to the local hospital mortuary and undressed. In order to clean the bodies for identification they were hosed down to wash the blood and brain tissue from their heads. Whilst this was being done the pillion passenger sat up and asked where he was. He had been certified dead because the doctor had seen blood and brain tissue from the driver on his head.

In another case a doctor was informed by relatives that an elderly patient of his was dead. He was told that the house was open and requested to issue a certificate. He went to the house and saw the elderly gentleman in bed and, without examining him, wrote a death certificate which he left by the bed. On reflection he recalled that he should report the case to the coroner as he had not seen the elderly gentleman for several weeks. When the coroner's officer was informed, he went to the house and upstairs to the bedroom. He picked up the death certificate and, as he was reading it the deceased sat up in bed and asked what he was doing! The 'deceased' was seen by the coroner's officer walking around the village six months later.

Vagal inhibitory reflexes, electrical shock, narcotic poisoning and severe 'syncopal attacks' of various kinds are notoriously likely to cause conditions simulating death, and the greatest care may be necessary in order to avoid the calamity of premature certification. Mark Twain was able to extract humour from his, for he was in another place, alive and well, but the victims of careless certification are liable to be condemned to the undertaker or the public mortuary—or to the refrigerator.

Life is not incompatible with a temporary suspension of heart beat, but circulation must be speedily re-established or death is certain. The limit of tolerance of arrest of heart action will vary with the degree of oxygenation of the blood at the time of the suspension, on the general metabolic rate and on the body temperature. Operations which are undertaken when the body temperature has been artificially lowered (hypothermia) can be extended to an hour without heart beat, yet normal rhythm will return on warming. However, certain brain cells are especially susceptible to deprivation of oxygen and even if death does not occur they may be permanently damaged. Under normal circumstances longer than 3–5 min cessation of heart beat is irrecoverable.

The phenomena of hibernation in many animals can have no reference to this condition. It is natural for such animals to remain torpid during the winter season, living on a feeble respiration and circulation, but this would be an unnatural condition for a human being and inconsistent with the maintenance of life.

Anoxia in neonatal life is a separate problem.[2,3] The vitality of newborn children is commonly restored when no pulsation whatever could be discovered for a period of 10–15 min after birth. In one instance a child was revived after 20 min of apparent death by insufflation of the lungs, although during that time no pulsation could be heard or felt. Numerous cases of resuscitation by massage of the heart and by other means after the heart has stopped beating have been recorded. Temporary arrest during anaesthesia is common, and, provided there is a circulation, can be sustained artificially.

This blood flow, as in extracorporeal circulation, may be artificial. Surgical procedures under complete arrest for as long as 40–60 min have become commonplace. But these are artificial conditions, and we must concern ourselves with evidence of a natural circulation. Tests for blood flow are rather unsatisfactory.

A casualty officer, uncertain of the fact of death in a plethoric man who was intensely congested in the head and neck, made an incision into the scalp to see if active bleeding could be observed. The body, though dead, bled from the turgid scalp so freely as to require stitches to control the post-mortem bleeding.

The electrocardiogram will record any current accompanying the heart beat, even when this is too weak to be palpated or only fibrillatory: if the electrocardiogram fails to demonstrate the passage of any current after a period of several minutes, it must be assumed that death has occurred. This method, though superior to those described above, is obviously not practicable in most cases.

The practitioner must rely on his stethoscope.

Cessation of respiration, like cessation of the heart beat, must be complete and continuous to constitute proof of the reality of death. It may cease for a very short period without death ensuing in the following conditions, none of which is likely, however, to give rise to any difficulty in connection with real or apparent death:

1. As a purely voluntary act. Some 2 min seems here to be the outside limit, which experience shows cannot be exceeded; even expert sponge-divers, who have spent their lives at the occupation, cannot remain under water without artificial contrivances for any longer than some 2 min.

2. In the disturbance of respiration known as Cheyne–Stokes breathing the limit of the apnoeic interval seldom indeed exceeds some 15–20 s.

3. In the apparently drowned and new-born infants visible respiration is frequently absent for long periods, and doubts often occur as to whether life really remains in the body. It is likely that in some cases suspended animation passes into real death owing to the want of perseverance in artificial aids to establish natural breathing; the subject is more fully discussed elsewhere (see Chapter 13).

4. Electric shocks may cause every appearance of death, but continuous artificial respiration may cause natural breathing to commence after long periods.

These statements do not, of course, take into consideration the special conditions under which an anaesthetist may artificially maintain some useful kind of ventilation of the lung.

Tests for breathing

Very feeble movements or respiration can sometimes be overlooked. The stethoscope must be continuously applied to the upper part of the lungs in front or to the larynx itself, by which means very slight currents of air may be detected. This test alone is usually sufficient.

EARLY SIGNS OF DEATH AND POST-MORTEM CHANGES

After somatic death certain tissues, cells and enzymes in the body continue to live individually or collectively for a period of time depending to some extent on the cause of death, the condition of the cells or tissues before death, and their oxygen requirements. For instance, for periods up to 2 h voluntary muscles may be made to contract by mechanical or electrical stimulation. That the heart continues to beat or contract for a while after certain forms of violent death, e.g., judicial hanging, is well-known. These post-mortem muscle contractions have been mistaken for vital movements, and in cases where these have occurred after rapid interment and subsequent exhumation, changes in the position of the limbs have been assumed mistakenly to indicate premature burial. The pupil will react for varying periods to certain drugs.

Cooling of the body

When life ends, the body, after a very short interval, loses the heat which it possessed at the moment of death. The usual temperature of a healthy adult at rest is approximately 98.4°F (37°C) when taken by the mouth, whereas the temperature of the rectum at the same time and under the same conditions is about 99°F and in the axilla about 97°F. None of these temperatures is constant and there are individual and daily variations up to 1–1.5°F. The temperature varies according to the time of day and will be lowest in the morning between 2 and 6 a.m. and highest in the afternoon at 4–6 p.m. Mild exercise may cause a slight rise and heavy exercise a rise of greater extent which, however, drops to normal in 20–30 min.

Of all the changes that occur in a dead body, that of cooling to the temperature of its surroundings was the first to be used as an index of the time of death. The rate of loss of heat from a cadaver offers one of the more reliable methods of estimating the time which has elapsed since death up to a period of about 24 h, though the loss of heat does not obey physical laws, which apply to an inanimate object, as cellular metabolism continues after death.

Although the rate of heat loss can theoretically be precisely defined there are a great many factors to be taken into account and their importance can only be assessed within a range of approximation. It is for this reason that the very precise formulae devised by de Saram et al.,[4] and Marshall & Hoare[5] fail in their practical application, though of theoretical interest. The chief of many unknown factors while militate against accuracy is uncertainty as to the temperature of the body at the moment of death. In many cases, notably in asphyxial deaths, it is raised, in many others lowered, and, unless the death temperature is known, efforts to achieve accuracy in the estimation of temperature loss are of limited value. Nevertheless a recording is in itself often sufficient to provide the police who are investigating a crime with a useful guide to the time of death. It must be pointed out that the time of death is not always the same as the time the victim of an assault was injured: minutes may elapse before even severe bleeding becomes fatal, and hours may pass before head or other injuries cause death. But at least some approximation of the time of death is possible, and this is often of the greatest importance to the police in testing accounts of the movements of a suspect.

In *R. v. Heath* (C.C.C. 1946) the nude body of a woman was found bound, gagged and dead of asphyxia, in a Notting Hill Gate hotel. The rectal temperature at 6.30 p.m. on the day the body was found was 84°F (room 63°F). It was assumed by the investigating authority that the murder had taken place around midnight the previous night, for Heath had arrived at the hotel with the girl at about 12.15 a.m., and was heard to slam a door as he left at about 1.30 a.m. If the temperature of the body at the moment of death was 98.4°F it would mean that the body temperature had fallen only 14.4°F in about 18 h. The body, though in a closed room, was naked, and in this case it appeared reasonable to assume that the initial temperature was raised above the normal by the act of strangulation.

In *R. v. McKinstry* (C.C.C. 1942) a girl's body had been found at 8.30 a.m. on the foreshore of the Thames under a parapet of the newly constructed Waterloo Bridge. A police surgeon certified death and, after placing a hand on the body, expressed the view that death had occurred some four to seven days previously. In fact, on autopsy at the mortuary at 12.20 p.m., a rectal temperature of 47°F was measured (air 38°F, Thames river 31°F). McKinstry had been seen to leave a local public house with Peggy Richards, the murdered girl, at 11 p.m. and to walk towards the then deserted

Waterloo Bridge, and it was assumed that the murder had occurred about midnight the previous night. In this case, if the initial temperature is placed at 98.4°F, it would mean that 51.4°F of temperature were lost in about 12–13 h, that is about 4°F per hour, which in view of the fact that the river water was below freezing point is not specially rapid.

It cannot be assumed that the body temperature is normal at death. Indeed, in many cases of asphyxiation, of fat or air embolism and of other vascular conditions affecting the thermal control centres of the brain, it is well known that sharp rises in temperature occur.

In a case brought into Guy's Hospital at 8.10 a.m. following a vehicular street accident in which a bus had knocked down and pinned a cyclist beneath the chassis, pronounced traumatic asphyxial changes were present. The temperature at autopsy 5 h later was still 99°F. The casualty officer had been given a temperature of 106.4°F by the nurse who made routine observations of pulse, temperature and respirations on admission at 8.15 a.m.

In aspirin poisoning severe dehydration may occur and in the terminal stages hyperpyrexia of 106–108°F may occur.

The recorded temperature may even continue to rise after death for a period of an hour or two. This occurs in certain severe bacterial infections, and after haemorrhages into the brain stem.

Increase of temperature after death has been referred to under putrefaction; but it can occur soon after death, and before rigidity sets in. Some of the cases reported by Wilks & Taylor[7] also show that it may take place independently of putrefaction. Dowler has noticed it as a common occurrence, in a warm climate, in the bodies of persons who have died from yellow fever. When the maximum, which is variable in different bodies, has been attained, the body gradually undergoes the cooling process observed after death. In a death from epidemic cholera the dead body reached its maximum temperature of 109°F in about an hour and a half. These observations may serve to explain that in some exceptional instances a dead body may retain for many hours a temperature as high as, or higher than, that which is usually found in the living.

Among cases observed by Taylor[8] at Guy's Hospital it was remarked that in several a high temperature was retained by the viscera for a long period after death. In two instances a thermometer indicated a temperature of 76°F in the viscera, in one instance 17, and in the other 18 h after death, the temperature of the air being comparatively low (49°F), and the surface of the body cool. In a third instance, 10 h after death, while the surface of the abdomen had a temperature of 65°F the interior was 85°F.

In all observations on the temperature of the dead body a mechanical or electrical instrument, such as a thermometer recording from 32°F to 120°F (or a similar range centigrade) or a thermocouple, must be employed. The instrument should in all cases be introduced into the rectum or through a puncture in the abdominal wall into the cavity of the abdomen, and the temperature should be read whilst the instrument is in situ. Readings should be made at intervals in order to obtain the rate fall of temperature. Under no circumstances should the temperature be taken in the vagina in cases of suspected foul play, or near sites of injury which might thus be disturbed.

The principal factors involved in cooling are: *the difference in temperature between the body and the medium*. This is largely a physical phenomenon. The rate of cooling is roughly proportional to the difference in temperature between the body and its surroundings; the greater the difference between these the more rapid the rate of cooling.

The process is not, however, a simple physical one, as both Fiddes & Patten[5] and Marshall & Hoare[6] have pointed out. They devised precise formulae on which the loss of heat could be estimated: as with all such formulae, only an approximate timing of death can be indicated. de Saram et al.[4] seem to have borne in mind more than some investigators in this field the principal fallacy—the assumption that the temperature at death was normal.

James & Knight[9] recorded their errors in estimating the post-mortem interval in 110 cadavers where the time of death was known. Joseph & Schickle[10] reviewed the literature and carried out a number of tests using cylinders and concluded that the rectal temperature is unreliable and that temperature recordings should be taken from the centre of the cadaver. Simonson, Voigt & Jeffeson[11] took continous post-mortem temperature recordings in different organs of 20 cadavers where the time of death was known. The organs and areas where cooling time was recorded included the brain, liver, calf, rectum and axilla. Their results confirmed those of previous investigations that attempts to determine the time of death can never be more than a rough estimate.

In *R. v. Smith* (Lewes Assizes 1946) a body found lying in the snow in a yard at Hastings at 9.30 a.m. was left covered by a tarpaulin until the arrival of the investigating team at 6 p.m. The rectal temperature was still 55°F—though the man had been shot, it was subsequently proved by evidence in statements, somewhere between 6 and 8 p.m. the previous night. Death could not have taken place as long as 20 to 22 h previously, for the rate of fall could hardly have been as little as 2°F per hour on average during this period of exposure overnight in the snow. The air temperature during the day had been 32° to 36°F. The explanation lay in the nature of the wounds which were such that death would be likely to be delayed several hours: the extravasation of blood confirmed this. The time of injury is not necessarily the time of death.

It is accepted standard procedure in forensic practice that the post-mortem temperature of a cadaver be recorded in all cases of suspected crime, irrespective of the apparent irrelevence of such an undertaking, and even though a post-mortem temperature recording may seem superfluous when external factors, such as exposure to heat from a fire, may have raised the body temperature or where putrefaction has commenced.

In the Fisher Report on the death of Maxwell Confait and the trial of three persons upon charges arising from his death,[12] criticism was levelled at the pathologist who had not recorded the temperature of the deceased. There were several reasons why this had not been done, including a fire at the premises where the body lay, poor lighting and the possible disturbance of suspected evidence concerning recent homoxesual activities. In this case the time of death became a vital issue and it was later discovered that death had occurred sometime before the estimated time arrived at from the visual and tactile examinations by both the police surgeon and the pathologist.

The build of the cadaver. The relationship of mass to surface area

The rate of loss of heat is to some extent proportional to the weight of the body to its surface area; thus children and adults of small stature will cool more rapidly than the average adult although their actual heat loss per unit of time will be less over the same ranges of temperature.

The physique of the deceased

Fat is a bad conductor of heat, and therefore the greater the quantity and the more general the distribution of the body fat, the slower will be the rate of cooling. Young women commonly have more subcutaneous fat than young males. A thin or emaciated person will cool more rapidly owing to the absence of this subcutaneous fatty insulator.

The environment of the body

The environment of the body exercises a profound influence on the rate of cooling. A body in air loses heat by convection and radiation; some heat, however, will be lost by conduction through the material on which the body is lying. Anything which will increase the rate of radiation, conduction or convection will accelerate cooling. Thus a body lying exposed in a well ventilated room will cool more rapidly than one in a sealed room, as the freely circulating air will rapidly carry away the air warmed by the body. A body lying snugly in bed or sealed in a coffin will lose heat much more slowly than one lying on top of the bed or in a street, owing to the smaller volume of air present around the body and the lack of air-change. A body in a cool mortuary or on a cold slab cools quickly. A naked body immersed in cold water cools at about twice the rate of a body exposed to air, and movement of the water will tend to accelerate the process by carrying away more rapidly the water warmed by the body. Bodies found dead in baths may, on the contrary, have become initially warmed after death.

Bodies buried in earth will usually cool more rapidly than those in air but more slowly than those in water. However, this is by no means a general rule, much depending on the moisture of the soil;

a body, for instance, buried in dry soil will retain its heat for longer than a similar body exposed to air. If a body is buried in rotting material such as a dung-heap the body temperature will rise or fall to that of the dung-heap. The activities of maggots may raise the temperature to something near or even above that of normal body heat.

Coverings on or around the body

Clothing on a body, or bedclothes, substantially retard the rate of cooling. Generally speaking, clothing is a bad conductor of heat, the conducting properties depending to some extent on the nature of the clothing, e.g., wool, cotton or silk, but to a greater extent on its texture. The more minute air spaces within the clothing, the poorer its conducting properties, and the slower the rate of cooling.

Wet clothes will, in drying on the body, increase the rate of cooling. It is not uncommon for relatives to place hot water bottles in the beds of persons who are dying at home. Under these circumstances the body temperature may be raised after death, and the more advanced states of decomposition to be described later may develop after only a few hours.

Likewise a person dying upon a warm electric blanket may decompose rapidly. The decomposition will be more advanced in those parts of the body in contact with the heated blanket. If only part of the body is in contact with the blanket there may be a sharp line of demarcation between the decomposition caused by the blanket and the unheated areas of the body. In one case suspicion was aroused when a child, who had been alive the previous evening, was found dead in bed with advanced post-mortem changes below the mid-thorax due to an electric blanket. The upper part of the body was normal. The decomposition was mistaken for bruising and a full CID inquiry was initiated before the arrival of the pathologist.

It has been alleged that in death from haemorrhage the rate of cooling is accelerated owing to the loss of blood. This has no foundation in fact; the only physical difference created is that some heat has been lost in the extravasated blood, and though there is a reduction in the total amount of heat in the body no difference occurs in the rate of cooling.

A healthy man, aged 47, died suddenly from hae-morrhage. A ligature which had been placed on the axillary artery to control bleeding gave way, and about four pints of blood were lost. Four hours after death the shoulder, chest and abdomen of the deceased were quite warm. The skin of the abdomen had a temperature of 84°F; 8 h after death the temperature was 80°F, and the arms and legs were not rigid. The conditions under which this body was exposed were favourable to rapid cooling; it was placed in a shell with a shirt loosely over it, and the temperature of the mortuary was 38°F.

Cooling of the body is the most important real phenomenon in the estimation of the time of death and every factor in connection therewith must be recorded and carefully considered. Even when the body appears to be quite cold the rectal temperature must be recorded and also the temperature of the medium in which the body is found, repeating the observations at intervals in order to arrive at some estimate of the rate of change over a period of several hours.

It is obvious that when we have to consider so many variables it is quite impossible to devise an accurate formula to define the rate of heat loss. In temperate climates it has been suggested that for an average adult the overall heat loss in air may average 1.5°F per hour, and in tropical climates about 0.75°F. Such figures have to be used with great circumspection and looked upon merely as a broad generalisation.

In the case of *R*. v. *Whiteway* (C.C.C. 1953)[13] two girls were murdered on the Teddington tow-path and thrown into the river. The first body was recovered the next morning and the rectal temperature at that time was 68°F. The mortuary temperature was 60°F and the average water temperature of the Thames during the preceding 24 h was 64°F. It was estimated, bearing in mind the period of immersion in water and of cooling after recovery, that some $2\frac{1}{2}$–$3\frac{1}{2}$°F would have been an approximate rate of fall in temperature during the period of hours immediately following death. This gave the estimated time of death as somewhere between 9 p.m. on the previous night and 2 a.m. on the morning the body was found. This wide limit was later shown to embrace pretty squarely the time (11.30 p.m.) when the crime had been committed.

In personal practice over many years it has been

clear that the cooling curve evolved by Fiddes & Patten[5] gives the most accurate estimate of the post-mortem interval. Their method has the advantage that it compensates to some degree for all the external factors which may affect the cooling of the body but like all other methods assumes that the body temperature was normal at the time of death.

It might be argued that to have to admit a wide range is of little use when the police are seeking accuracy, but to set closer limits can only expose the pathologist to severe and damaging cross-examination and is unwise. This method of estimating the time of death may, however, be of the utmost value to the police in their investigations and though it is subject to so many variables should always be undertaken.

Changes in the skin

After death the skin may be observed to become unreactive owing to the failure of peripheral circulation. In some parts as the body cools it becomes tinted by livid discoloration (cadaveric hypostases). One of the most striking changes in the skin is its loss of elasticity. In the living body, if any part of the surface is compressed, the skin will gradually return to its original form on removing the pressure.

The 'cutis anserina' effect referred to by the public as gooseskin, often pronounced after death, is also commonly seen as a transient phenomenon in life. It must not be used as a sign either of death or of the mode of dying. It is due to contraction of the erector pilae muscles of the skin.

EYE CHANGES

Loss of corneal reflex

This is found in all forms of deep insensibility, e.g., general anaesthesia, epilepsy, narcotic poisoning, and cannot be considered to be a reliable sign of death.

Clouding of the cornea

This affords little stronger presumption of death, for it may occur in certain diseases before life is extinct; it is therefore unreliable.

The speed with which the cornea becomes opaque after death is due to drying, and is retarded if the lids are closed after death.

On exposure to air for a few hours after death the cornea develops a film of cell debris and mucus upon which dust steadily settles, and later on the corneal surface becomes wrinkled and brown where exposed between the eyelids.

Flaccidity of the eyeball

The intra-ocular tension falls rapidly after death, and the eyeballs tend to sink into the orbital fossa. This flaccidity is readily appreciated by simple palpation.

State of the pupil

The iris contains a large proportion of muscular tissue which in common with all muscles exhibits 'tone'. This 'tone' is rapidly lost after death and the iris relaxes into a condition of equilibrium.

The action of drugs—atropine, eserine—continues usually for a period of an hour or somewhat longer after death.

No conclusion can be drawn from the size of the pupils in death. This is of some practical importance in suspected narcotic poisoning.

Changes in the retinal vessels

After death the bloodstream in the retinal vessels rapidly becomes segmented. This change appears within minutes after death, and persists for an hour or so, after which the vessels are so contracted that details are difficult to observe. This condition of 'trucking' is considered a most reliable sign of death by many police surgeons who are regularly called to pronounce death in persons who have collapsed suddenly and unexpectedly.

Chemical changes in the vitreous

Jaffe,[14] and later Sturner,[15] studied the rise in potassium in the vitreous humor after death. The vitreous was chosen because it was accessible and remained free from infection. A steady rise was found to occur and K values were thought likely to provide a useful indication of the post-mortem interval. The range is, however, too wide to have a practical application.

Post-mortem hypostases

Post-mortem hypostasis or lividity is caused by the fact that while the blood is liquid it obeys the law of gravitation and settles into the lowest available parts. Furthermore, the heavier red corpuscles have a tendency to settle first, so imparting a deeper colour to the affected parts. This passive 'welling' of blood into the dependent or underlying parts of the body is prevented by pressure, notably in the skin where the constricting effect of collar, waistbands, garters and the like cause a sharply contrasting whitening of the skin.

Hypostasis may thus be of some importance in deciding the position in which a body has lain during the hours immediately following death. As seen by the naked eye it consists in the appearance in the skin of the body of discoloured patches—having the same colour as the blood and changing in tint with the development of decomposition. Many different names have been given to this change— post-mortem hypostasis, subcutaneous hypostasis, cadaveric lividity, suggilations, vibices, post-mortem stains. Of these names post-mortem hypostasis, or simply hypostasis, is the best, founded as it is on the accepted theory as to the method by which they are produced. These appearances have sometimes been mistaken for the effects of violence applied during life, and serious mistakes have thus arisen. Innocent persons have been accused of violence, and have been tried on charges afterwards proved to be groundless. Christison[16] refers to two cases, in one of which two persons were convicted, and in the other three narrowly escaped conviction, upon a mistake of this kind.

Hypostases generally start to form within an hour or so of death and under certain circumstances when the dying process is prolonged, or in narcotic poisoning, where the circulation becomes almost stagnant, they may actually be forming at the moment of death. If death has been taking place slowly over a period, early hypostases may be present before death has actually occurred, especially when the affected part is already engorged. At first hypostases form patchy or mottled areas,

but within about 12 h they are complete in their primary form by coalescence of the smaller areas. Clotting 'fixes' them.

The rate of development of hypostasis was an important part of the medical evidence in the case of Emmett–Dunne heard at Court Martial at Düsseldorf in 1954. It was a part of the case for the Crown that the victim, Sgt. Watters, found hanging in a barracks stairway, had livid stains pronounced over the face and chest front—though found, according to the accused's story, hanging. Emmett–Dunne later admitted striking Watters across the throat, leaving him slumped either in the car (head and shoulders down) or on the ground (after attempting to carry the body away) for a total period of something like 30 or 35 min. Was this long enough to cause lividity to become noticeable? The validity of much of Emmett–Dunne's statement was open to question, and this minimum time seemed also open to doubt, but medical evidence was led that hypostasis was not impossible in as little as the 30 to 35 min available—if the circumstances were, in fact, as stated. Accused's evidence was self-incriminating and he was found guilty.

In deaths from wasting disease, from profound anaemia or haemorrhage, the staining may be so slight as to be barely discernible. If the body is constantly moving its position, as after drowning in moving water, the change may never develop. It is important also to remember that hypostases occur in the viscera such as the lung or bowel as well as in the skin, a condition which is liable to be mistaken for congestion occurring during life, or attributed to some pathological condition responsible for death.

One of the former authors was called to Watford to examine the body of a man suspected to have been poisoned by his wife, with whom he was on bad terms. He had died suddenly after taking an evening meal prepared by her and the plum–coloured reddening of the loops of small bowel suggested to the local pathologist that a poison had been taken. The colour was undoubtedly due to hypostasis and further dissection of the coronary vessels revealed a fresh coronary thrombosis. Analysis, made for the sake of security, proved entirely negative.

Congestion without inflammation and simple hypostasis may be confused by one who is unaccustomed to making autopsies. After death the signs of active congestion are likely to diminish, and those of passive or simple filling of veins to increase; and it is the latter which may be difficult to distinguish from inflammation in certain viscera. Microscopy will settle the issue.

Hypostases may resemble marks of violence (bruises)

Doubt may arise on a superficial examination, but there are many definite points of distinction, which may be tabulated:

Several-day-old bruises will, of course, begin to changes in consequence; they may change in colour pared in any case of doubt and microscopic examination will resolve any difficulty.

A body recovered from the River Thames was found to have striking engorgement of the head above a linear constricting mark set around the neck at about midthyroid level. Suspicion of strangling arose, and the finding of a number of plum-coloured haemorrhagic areas in the soft tissues of the neck along the upper level of the mark —and of protrusion of the tongue between the teeth—heightened this. It was plain, however, that the intensity of engorgement and the deep-seated petechiae were due to tight constriction by the collar (which had been removed upon recovery of the body). The head, hanging low in water, had acquired the more pronounced lividity common to cases of immersion.

Circulatory stasis in the aged, and sometimes the effect of exposure to cold, may resemble the effects of violence. Such marks are, however, usually found on parts, such as the ear, the shins, the forearms and hands, where the circulation is comparatively poor and the skin is exposed. The livid stains in hypothermia are pink owing to the oxygenated state of the blood and hence should not be confused with injury.

When decomposition commences the blood shares in the process, and hypostases undergo some changes in consequence; they may change in colour to coppery red or light or olive green; and since the blood gradually lyses it permeates the tissues causing a general discoloration throughout. Hence it follows that as putrefaction advances it becomes progressively more difficult to distinguish between a bruise and a hypostasis, for the crucial test of finding blood actually effused from the vessels into the tissues becomes more difficult to appreciate. It is impossible without microscopy to give an opinion when the body is decomposed.

Inferences from livid staining

Hypostases, by definition, both in the dependent parts of the body and, according to the mode of dying, may become fixed or partly fixed within 4–12 h. It is thus possible to deduce that the position of the body has been moved after death provided it has lain in its original position long enough

Table 8.2

Bruise	Hypostasis
1. Lies under the epidermis in the interstices or deeper still. The epidermis has no blood-vessels	1. Lies in the cutis, as a simple stain confined to underlying engorged capillaries or later staining the tissues owing to haemolysis
2. Cuticle may be abraded by the same violence that produced the bruise	2. Cuticle uninjured because the hypostasis is a mere sinking of the blood
3. A bruise appears at the seat of and surrounding the injury. This may or may not be a dependent part	3. Always in a part, which for the time of formation, is ordained by gravity
4. Often swollen or turgid because the extravasated blood and oedema swell the tissues	4. Not swollen because either the blood is still in the vessels or, at most, has stained the tissues
5. Incision shows blood outside the vessels. No flow of blood occurs from a bruise.	5. Incision shows the blood in vessels; and if any oozing occurs it is from the cut mouths of the vessels
6. If the body happens to be constricted at, or supported on, a bruised place, the area of pressure may be a little lighter than the rest of the bruise	6. Pressure of any kind, even a simple support (the wrinkling of a shirt or necktie, garters, etc.) is sufficient to prevent livid staining. White lines or patches or pressure bordered by the dark colour of a hypostasis are thus produced

for the hypostasis to have become fixed or partly fixed. An observation of this nature may be valuable in verifying or otherwise the story of a potential accused person or in giving an indication of where the body has been lying after death.

In two recent personal cases the distribution of hypostasis when the body was first examined verified the statement of a man under suspicion in the first case and disproved the statement of a woman in the second case.

In the first case a woman of 21, a known drug addict, was found dead, lying supine, in the bed she shared with a boyfriend and yet the livid stains were distributed irregularly over the front of the body. In his statement the boyfriend said that they had been drinking heavily the night before and had come back and each had taken several capsules of a quick-acting barbiturate. He passed out at once on the bed. He awoke some hours later and noticed she was fully dressed and lying prone with her face in the pillow. He thought she looked uncomfortable, so he undressed her and turned her over on to her back. He then went off to sleep, waking at about 10 a.m., when he found her dead and raised the alarm. Autopsy revealed no suspicious injuries and toxicological examination of the blood and urine revealed a high blood alcohol and high blood barbiturate level, consistent with the statement of the man.

In the second case a mother reported finding her child dead lying face downwards, in its cot in the morning. She stated that she had fed it during the night and that it had appeared quite well. It was considered a cot death and the first post-mortem was not conducted for some four days. During this period the infant was lying supine in the mortuary refrigerator. The pathologist found a fractured skull. Ten days later at a second autopsy it was seen that the livid stains were completely fixed down the front of the body and that no blood whatsoever had gravitated to the back of the body. When the mother was later questioned by the police she admitted that she had not fed the baby since early the previous evening. She also admitted punching the child's head about the same time as it would not stop crying.

The hypostasis stains may exhibit numerous coarse or fine petechial haemorrhages. These petechial haemorrhages signify death during an anoxic state. They are very common in narcotic poisoning and in sudden collapse due to acute cardiac arrest and especially when the deceased collapses forwards they will be found in the skin of the face and upper chest. In hanging they are frequently present on the feet and lower legs.

The colour of the livid stains may also give a guide as to the cause of death. In deaths associated with severe terminal anoxia, they are deep blue. In carbon monoxide poisoning they are bright pink and in cyanide poisoning and hypothermia pinkish red due to the oxygenated state of the blood. Bodies which have been in a refrigerator, especially if they are moist when placed inside, will become pink due to surface oxygenation through the damp skin. In these cases, however, the nail beds will retain the cyanotic tint present when the body was first refrigerated.

Fibrinolysis

There has been a good deal of controversy about the conditions which lead to fluidity of the blood after death in certain cases. It used to be taught that in asphyxia the blood remained fluid for longer than normal, due it was supposed, to some change in the availability of calcium. Recent work has shown that fibrinolysin develops as a result of a wide variety of stimuli.[17] It has been assumed that fibrinolysin may cause lysis of a blood clot when absorbed on the surface of the clot but does not actively impede clot formation. The work of Mole[18] has clarified the mode of action of these ferments.

The following observations, obtained from in vitro and in mortuo investigations, provide a summary of recent knowledge.[19]

1. Blood is spontaneously coagulable in all cases of sudden death where the autopsy is carried out within an hour or so of death.

2. The spontaneous coagulability of blood may disappear as shortly as $1\frac{1}{2}$ h after death.

3. Fibrinogen is absent from post-mortem blood samples which have lost their power of spontaneous coagulation.

4. Fibrinolysin obtained from post-mortem blood acts only on fibrin and not on fibrinogen.

5. Fibrinolysin acts by becoming absorbed on to the clot as it is being formed, and it is later released

into solution when the clot lyses. It is not effective when added to a clot already formed.

6. Fibrinolysin is probably produced by the endothelial linings of the vascular channels and body cavities.

7. The concentration of fibrinolysin in the blood does not increase after death.

It is clear that uncoagulable fluid blood is normally present in the limb vessels and often in the heart of any healthy person who dies a sudden natural or unnatural death from almost any cause. The finding of fluid blood at autopsy does not in itself give any precise indication of the cause of death.

The cause of the liberation of fibrinolysin is not clear, but in all cases where a fibrinolysin was demonstrable a period of 'shock' or 'collapse' has most probably existed for a short time before death; it has been suggested that the liberation of fibrinolysin is due to some non-specific general reaction to injury.[20]

Post-mortem bleeding

After death, the heart having ceased to beat, the blood lies in the blood vessels in a stagnant condition, and, under normal circumstances, remains for a time in a fluid state. In these circumstances a blood vessel which has been opened after death may bleed post-mortem and give rise to suspicion that the wound was produced before death. Such an extravasation of blood, post-mortem, may, of course, spread into the tissue spaces or body cavities, especially where these have been loosened or stripped by the process of dissection, or where the dead body has been crushed or the limbs avulsed by running over.[21]

A police officer, thrown at night from his bicycle by a non-stop car, struck his head on the ground and lay unattended. A second car ran over the victim some few minutes later before the driver had time to avoid the body. Two groups of injuries could be detected:

1. Injuries to the right elbow, right shoulder and head from which there was considerable extravasation of blood including the inhalation of blood from the nose injury into the deepest recesses of the air passages.

2. Crushing injuries to the middle of the trunk caused by the passage of a wheel and resulting in

injuries to the mesentery and right kidney amongst other. None of these injuries were accompanied by bleeding to anything like the extent of the injuries in (1).

It was, therefore, obvious that death from the head injuries had taken place before the second car had run over the body.

One important area where post-mortem artefactual bruising may give cause for suspicion, if not recognised, is in the neck. If an autopsy is carried out within a few hours of death, or if the head and neck are congested owing to the position of the deceased after death, haemorrhage may occur into the spaces between the muscles of the neck whilst the structures are being dissected or removed. As these artefactual haemorrhages occur in the areas which become bruised during manual compression of the neck, special techniques should be employed to obviate these artefacts in every case where the possibility of manual compression of the neck exists. The method is simple. The brain is first removed, followed by the internal viscera below the neck structures. The head is then moved slowly up and down and allowed to drain of blood before the neck is opened to allow examination of the larynx and surrounding muscles. This technique has an added advantage that petechial haemorrhages in the skin of the face and eyes, which may not have been apparent earlier, now become pronounced.

Chemical changes in the body fluids

The uncertainties attaching to traditional means of establishing the lapse of time since death, loss of heat, lividity and rigor mortis, have directed attention to the chemical changes in body fluids—especially the cerebrospinal fluid and vitreous eye fluids which do not deteriorate early. Schourup[22] in Denmark first explored the changes in cerebrospinal K, lactic acid, non-protein nitrogen and various amino acids. He found a certain constancy of change but encountered difficulty owing to the presence of blood traces in the cerebrospinal fluid. This approach is therefore inapplicable in all cases of head injury.

Studies on the level of ascorbic acid in the vitreous[23] proved unsatisfactory and attention was concentrated on K levels, which appeared to offer an advance but has since been shown to be unreliable.[23]

Recent work[24] has shown that there is a post-mortem rise in ammonia concentration in the vitreous humor related to both the cause of death and the ambient temperature.

Muscular changes

Except where cadaveric spasm becomes instantly established, the first effect of death is in most cases a general relaxation of muscular tone. The lower jaw drops, the eyelids lose their tension, the muscles are soft and flabby and the joints are flexible. Within a few hours after death, and generally while body is cooling, the muscles of the eyelids and jaw begin to stiffen and contract followed by similar changes in the muscles of the trunk and limbs so that the whole body becomes rigid. This condition is known as cadaveric rigidity or rigor mortis.

Muscular tissue passes through three stages after death:

(1) it is flaccid but contractile, still possessing cellular life;

(2) it becomes rigid and incapable of contraction, being then dead; and

(3) it once more relaxes, never regaining its power of contractility.

Subsequently it may mummify, putrefy or be the subject of adipocerous change. The first stage defines the duration of post-mortem muscular irritability, the second stage that of cadaveric rigidity, and the third that of decay.

Rigor mortis

After the period of irritability has passed there is a gradual stiffening of the muscles together with a shortening of the fibres. Every muscle in the body, voluntary and involuntary, takes part in the process, including the musculature of the heart and vessels, the platysma of the neck, the erector pilae muscles (contraction of which leads to cutis anserina), and the dartos of the penis. The chemical changes which take place in muscle tissue during contraction and relaxation are complex and the series of changes by which carbohydrate is utilised for the production of energy is also highly compli-

cated. For details of these changes and the part which various enzymes, especially adenosine triphosphate (ATP), play in this muscle contraction the reader may consult current works on physiology. When sufficient oxygen is not available lactic acid tends to accumulate in the muscles together with inorganic phosphates. Finally all of the ATP becomes broken down, and the lactic acid accumulation reaches a level of about 0.3%, at which point the muscle goes into an irreversible state of contraction known as rigor mortis. In its initial phases the process is essentially similar to muscular contraction in life, but is not reversible.[25]

There are, in regard to its medico-legal relationships, several points to be considered, and these we shall take in the following order:

1. The time of onset of rigor mortis and of its disappearance.

2. The order of its appearance and disappearance in different muscles.

3. Rigor mortis in involuntary muscles.

4. Other forms of muscle spasm.

Time of onset and disappearance of rigor mortis. In sudden natural deaths occurring in a temperate climate during average seasonal conditions rigor mortis usually commences within 2 to 4 h of death. It reaches a peak in about 12 h and starts to disappear after another 12 h, the cadaver becoming limp some 36 h after death. These times are variable even under the conditions mentioned. There are, however, many extrinsic and intrinsic factors which may profoundly affect the onset and duration of rigor mortis. As some of these influencing factors are frequently associated with violent or unnatural deaths, the value of rigor mortis in assessing the post-mortem interval is limited and its use may be misleading.

The onset of rigor mortis is solely dependent upon the chemical changes which occur in the muscles themselves as the result of cellular activity and enzymic activity which continues after death. Division of nerves supplying the muscle groups or the removal of the brain does not influence its onset. Rigor mortis occurs in amputated limbs, whether amputated traumatically or surgically.

It is easy to understand why rigor develops slowly and uniformly in healthy muscular subjects who have died suddenly from whatever cause, provided they were not exercising or convulsing when they died. In these cases the blood has been circulating up to the time of death and therefore the muscles will hold no more than the normal amount of acid metabolites at the time of death.

If, however, immediately prior to death the deceased has been violently exercising, the onset of rigor will be determined by the increased amount of metabolites in his muscles at the time of death. If the exercise has been of a violent nature immediately prior to death, complete rigor mortis or instantaneous cadaveric rigidity may occur at the moment of death. This instantaneous rigor may be seen in hunted animals and deaths from convulsant poisonings such as strychnine.

The ambient temperature has a profound affect. In tropical climates rigor may be complete in 2 h. In North America wide variations exist.[26] Bodies found in the vicinity of fires may likewise develop rapid rigor.

The following cases illustrate how dangerous it may be to place too much emphasis on the degree of rigor mortis when attempting to estimate the post-mortem interval.

1. In the case of *R. v. Alcott* (Surrey Assizes 1952), a young man was stabbed to death in a railway booking office. He had put up a fight when attacked and the time of the death was known within 5 min. Two hours later rigor mortis was complete.

2. A young woman had taken a fatal overdose of aspirin unbeknown to her husband, who thought she was suffering some physical ailment on account of her sweating. Shortly before she died her temperature commenced to rise, and the husband phoned for an ambulance which arrived within minutes of her death. The ambulance men were suspicious because she was in a state of complete rigor mortis. A police surgeon was called and recorded a temperature of 106°F.

3. Dr Lawrence S. Harris (personal communication 1976), whilst Chief Medical Examiner of Vermont, examined a lady in her mid-seventies who died from coronary thrombosis during the act of sexual intercourse. He examined her some 20 min after death and she was in a state of complete rigor mortis.

4. In another case a housebreaker was disturbed by the unexpected return of the occupier of the house. A fight ensued during which the occupier

was receiving the major injuries. The housebreaker, however, suddenly collapsed from natural disease and called for water. A cup of water was placed in his hand at the moment of death. When I first saw the deceased 4 h later he had clearly gone into instantaneous rigor mortis. His extended arm was raised and the hand held the full cup of water some 10 inches above the ground and none had been spilt.[27]

Thus it is easy to understand that rigor mortis should come on slowly in healthy, muscular subjects who have died without convulsions, as, for instance, by decapitation, by sudden haemorrhage, by judicial or even other forms of hanging. In such cases the muscles have no more than the average amount of waste metabolites in them, and have their usual circulation at the moment of death, conditions favourable to the continuance of local life, of which rigor marks the end.

Ante-natal rigor mortis: two cases of this condition are reported.[28] The first case occurred in a quadripara, aged 35, in labour near term with a history of 12 h haemorrhage. Version was performed as soon as possible, and was rather difficult owing to the rigidity of the child. When extracted, the lower limbs were still slightly stiff, and the arms markedly flexed and rigid. The rigidity did not return. Fetal movements had ceased for 10 h. No attempt had been made to hear the fetal heart. The second case occurred in a primipara, aged 30, in labour at term. The labour was slow, and the membranes ruptured early, and 5 h later the fetal heart could not be heard. The fetus was extracted by forceps later on, and was in pronounced rigor mortis. There is no doubt that rigidity does interfere with delivery, in spite of statements to the contrary. Of the various obstetric conditions associated with ante-natal rigidity haemorrhage seems the commonest.

Rigor mortis is thus of no value as a sign of live-birth, though of course it does not indicate the contrary.

Flaccidity following rigor mortis is caused by the action of the alkaline liquids produced by putrefaction. There can be no doubt that those circumstances at death which tend to leave a muscle full of products from its own disintegration, presumably unstable organic bodies, tend to shorten the duration of rigor mortis and to hasten the onset of decomposition. These are precisely the conditions which, we have seen, hasten the onset of rigor, and from these facts the well-known rule follows as a matter of course, viz., the sooner rigidity sets in the more quickly it disappears and gives way to putrefactive processes.

On the other hand, myosin is soluble in acids, and the view has been put forward by Hermann[29] that the disappearance of rigidity is due to solution of myosin by excess of acid produced during the continuance of rigidity.

A third supposition is that in dead muscle enzymes are developed which have the power of dissolving myosin by a process of autodigestion.

Speaking in general terms, rigor mortis lasts from 16 to 24 h in sound, muscular subjects; it may, however, in apparently normal cases last from 24 to 36 h, and exceptionally it may continue for several days.

In a case in which Taylor[30] was consulted, a stout muscular man died suddenly from an attack of apoplexy. His body was exhumed and examined three weeks after death in the month of January. It was in a good state of preservation and the limbs were so rigid that it required a great degree of force to bend them. There was no doubt in this case that cold favoured the deferment of onset and caused continuance of rigidity. We have seen a body develop a state of rigidity eight days after death by immersion in Icelandic waters. The body had been recovered from the sea frozen, and had been kept so in transport.

Recent experimental work[31] on exercised and strychnine-poisoned rats has shown a marked decrease in muscle glycogen at the time of death.

Other work in the evolution of rigor mortis in different sized muscle groups in rats[32] showed that rigor mortis commenced simultaneously in all muscle groups, supporting the views of Shapiro[33], but was apparent first in the smaller muscle groups (forelimbs) although it reached maximum intensity in the fore and hindlimbs at the same time. Further work on the strength and evolution of rigor mortis following exercise[34] in rats showed that the intensity of rigor mortis was increased in its initial phases and although the maximum intensity of rigor mortis was reached in both exercised and controlled animals at the same time, the maximum intensity was significantly greater in the exercised animals. It was also shown that resolution was complete simultaneously in the same groups. These experimental observations do not conflict with the purely qualitative observations on the development of rigor (*vide infra*).

The influence of atmospheric conditions: atmospheric changes appear to modify considerably the duration of this state. Cold will cause it to persist and thus it is that during the winter season, especially in a frost, it is slow in disappearing, its mean duration being then from 24 to 36 h. If the air is warm it soon ceases. In the tropics, where the temperature ranges between 80° and 100°F, rigor may begin to disappear within 8 or 9 h of death.

Sommer[35] found that, other things being equal, bodies became rigid as quickly in an atmosphere of from 59° to 63°F as in one from 77° to 81°F; but that the bodies of strong persons continued rigid for eight or 10 days at a temperature of from 36° to 45°F, while rigidity disappeared in from four to six days when they were exposed to a temperature of from 65° to 86°F.

Bodies sunk in cold water will retain the rigidity for a long time. Cold water also tends to retard putrefaction.

The influence of the nature of the death: it has been observed that the bodies of those who are emaciated, or who die from debilitating diseases, pass rapidly into a state of rigidity, which is commonly of short duration. Brown-Séquard[36] observed that cadaveric rigidity appeared in cholera deaths late and lasted long in those patients who died quickly; and that those muscles which had been attacked with violent and frequent cramps became rigid very soon after death, and remained so only for a short time. It has been noticed that rigor mortis is frequently absent in the bodies of those who have died from septicaemia; and this has been the case especially in separate limbs which have been the seat of purulent inflammation of the muscles. This is a most striking phenomenon, owing to the contrast between rigid and flaccid muscles in the same body.

Influence of electrocution and lightning: it was at one time thought that rigor mortis did not occur after death from electric shock, but this idea is incorrect. Rigor mortis may occur quite normally after deaths from lightning or electrocution, but owing to the violent convulsions of the muscles which occur in deaths from these causes the rigor may develop rapidly and pass away early.

The order in which rigor appears. As a rule, cadaveric rigidity first appears in the muscles of the face, neck and trunk; it then takes place in the muscles of the upper extremities, and lastly in the legs. Shapiro[33], drawing attention to the physiochemical nature of the change, suggests that the process may start at about the same time everywhere, merely fixing the smaller muscle masses (e.g., of the face and jaw) before those of the limbs. This suggestion, however, does not explain why the small muscles of the fingers and toes should be the last to stiffen. In regard to its disappearance the muscles of the lower extremities will often be found rigid, while those of the trunk and upper extremities are again in a state of relaxation. It appears later and lasts longer in the lower extremities than in other parts of the body. It begins almost always in the neck and lower jaw. Sommer[35] found only one exception to this rule in examining 200 dead bodies. From the neck it passes in two directions: upwards to the muscles of the face and downwards to the muscles of the upper extremities and trunk, then attacking those of the lower extremities. In individual limbs, it commonly proceeds from above downwards, and it generally passes off in the same order. It always sets in, increases and decreases gradually, in which respect it differs strikingly from other forms of rigidity in muscle.

Rigor mortis in involuntary muscles. The involuntary as well as the voluntary muscles are subject to rigor and, by reason of either their small mass or of the more speedy loss of muscular irritability, it appears in them more rapidly. The heart commonly loses its irritability within an hour after death. The muscle becomes rigid and remains in that state for 10 or 12 h, sometimes for 24 or 36 h, then again becomes relaxed or flaccid.

Other forms of stiffening

Effect of freezing: when a body is frozen so rapidly after death that there has been insufficient time for acid metabolites to appear in the muscles the process of rigor mortis is suspended until thawing takes place. When the body thaws rigor mortis appears with great rapidity and passes off very rapidly.

A man lost overboard in freezing Arctic waters was recovered the same day dead and frozen stiff: the body was kept in ice packs until, eight days later, it was deposited for autopsy in a London mortuary. Rigor developed as the body thawed.

Effect of heat: all muscle protein in the body is coagulated at temperatures above 149°F. When a body is subjected to temperatures above the coagulation point of the muscle protein a rigidity is produced, which, if complete, is far more intense than that found in rigor mortis. Changes in posture, especially of the limbs, may follow upon muscle contractions, e.g., in burning cases. This heat stiffening cannot be broken down by extending the limbs as in rigor mortis, and it will persist until disintegration occurs. Heat stiffening may also follow high voltage electric shocks such as occur when a person grasps a high tension cable, for sufficient heat is often liberated at the point of contact with the cable to cause heat stiffening in addition to the spasm caused by the electric discharge.

Cadaveric spasm: this is a phenomenon which appears in its totality to lie outside the factors regulating ordinary rigor mortis, and yet is one of the most important phenomenon in legal medicine, owing to the certainty of the conclusions which may be drawn from it when it occurs. Ordinarily, immediately after death, the muscles relax, although they are still irritable and capable of being stimulated into contraction. This period of flaccidity does not occur in instantaneous rigor mortis (*vide supra*). In cadaveric spasm this instantaneous rigor affects a group of muscles which have been actively working at the moment of death and it is also evident that the deceased knew they were about to die or had good reason to believe so. There is sufficient understanding of instantaneous rigor mortis to understand why cadaveric spasm may occur but not why it continues after rigor mortis has passed and until putrefaction has set in. It is possible that an extension of Krompecher & Fryc's work[34] may provide an explanation.

Older textbooks on forensic medicine gave much space to cadaveric spasm, inferring that it was not an uncommon phenomenon. This is because cases of complete instantaneous rigor mortis or instantaneous rigor affecting certain groups of muscles or even the entire body were included under the same heading.

The importance of cadaveric spasm is that it cannot be artificially induced. A person who shoots himself may be found gripping the pistol in cadaveric spasm but it is quite impossible for a pistol to be placed in someone's hand and the contraction of rigor mortis made to appear as cadaveric spasm. There are records of buttons or pieces of clothing of an assailant being firmly gripped by the victim.

In practice it is most commonly seen in drowning—hence the 'dying man clutching at a straw'. In these cases twigs or vegetation may be firmly grasped in the hand even though rigor mortis itself has passed. It may be virtually impossible to extend the fingers when they are in cadaveric spasm.

In summary it may be said:

1. that instantaneous stiffening is more likely to be found when great muscular exertion has been made previous to death.

2. that it is more likely to appear in emotionally tense subjects, whether they are or are not exerting themselves powerfully at the time of death.

3. that sudden death is a predisposing factor.

4. that death due to violent disturbance of the nervous system (firearm wound of the head, etc.) may also be a powerful element in causation.

5. that the condition of affairs produced by it is easily distinguishable from that produced by simple rigor mortis in that an object grasped by the fingers is firmly gripped just as it would be during life, only that more force is required to extract it from the grip than would be necessary during life; whereas if held by rigor mortis alone the object can be released by 'undoing' the fingers, so to speak, there being no intensely tight grip.

6. That it is the strongest and most conclusive proof that the object so gripped was thus gripped at the moment of death.

It is for practical purposes impossible for the condition to be imitated. The reason for this is that if someone has a knowledge of the above facts sufficiently acute to lead him to try to imitate the condition after death he must find one of two conditions:

1. the muscles flaccid, in which case he must place the fingers round the weapon and fix them there in some way, and in this case there will be evidence of the pressure applied; or

2. the muscles stiff, in which case he must loosen them and again try to refix them. The renewed stiffening of the muscles will not take place.

The following cases collected by Taylor[37] are illustrative of the above conclusions.

In the case of Lord William Russell, who was murdered by Courvoisier in 1840, it was observed that one hand of the deceased firmly grasped the sheet of the bed, 'as if in a struggle against an assassin'. The position of the hand of the deceased furnished, among other circumstances, some evidence against the presumption of suicide.

In R. v. *Ellison* some of the prisoner's hair was found grasped in the victim's hand. The body of the deceased was found lying dead in a house, with injuries that made it clear that she must have been murdered. In her right hand was found a considerable quantity of brown hair, and in the other hand some grey hair, grasped evidently in the struggle for life. On the morning following the murder the prisoner went to a hairdresser's in the town, and desired to have his hair and whiskers cut. This man observed that the hair and beard had been recently cut, and evidently by someone unaccustomed to haircutting. There was a difference between the hair of the beard and that of the head, the former having turned grey. The hair found in the hands of the deceased was of the same colour and kind as the hair of the prisoner. This, with other corroborating circumstances, led to his conviction.

In R. v. *Gardner* a woman had died from several wounds in the throat which 'could not have been self-inflicted', and a common table-knife was found loosely in her right hand, with the back of the blade towards the palm of the hand, and the weapon in the direction of the length of the body. According to the evidence of the medical witnesses, the principal wound in the throat was of such a nature that it could not have been inflicted with the right hand. The knife, it was alleged, had been placed in the hand after death.

On this opinion, that there had been interference with the body after death, Taylor remarked:

On these occasions it may be suggested that a weapon, although grasped by an alleged suicide to inflict the death-wound, may either drop from the hand or be found loosely in it, as a result of the relaxation of the muscles in death. This must be admitted; hence the mere fact of a weapon being found loose should not be taken as evidence of murder, unless other circumstances—such as the nature of the wound, the freedom of the hand from blood, the position of the body, etc.—concur to prove that the act was not one of suicide.

Other circumstances may show that the weapon has been placed in the wrong hand, or that the blood-marks on it and on the hand do not correspond.

The difficulty of thus endeavouring to imitate an act of suicide, when the facts are properly observed and compared, will be apparent from the following case.

A woman was found dead in bed with her throat cut. The wound was 6 inches from right to left, extending across the throat to a point under the left ear; the upper portion of the windpipe was severed, and the jugular vein as well as the muscular branches of the carotid artery were divided. The doctors considered that the wound in the throat was not self-inflicted. It was such a wound as a *left-*handed person would have inflicted, and the hand inflicting it, as well as the weapon, could not have escaped being marked with blood. It appears that when the body was found there was a razor in the *right* hand, not tightly held. The arms were folded across the chest, the right hand resting on the left, the back of the razor being towards the body of the deceased. There was *no blood on the hands*, arms, or chest, and only one small spot on the razor. There was blood on the *underside* of a pillow, and a corresponding stain on the bolster, showing that this must have been turned over, and the head placed on the clean side after the wound had been inflicted. All the circumstances concurred in showing that an attempt had been made to simulate an act of suicide, while the facts were only consistent with homicide. The accused was convicted.

LATE SIGNS OF DEATH AND POST-MORTEM CHANGES

Putrefaction

This final stage in the changes following death is brought about largely by the action of bacterial enzymes, mostly from anaerobic organisms derived from the bowel. Aerobic fungi, insect larvae—many of which have proteolytic enzyme systems,[38] protozoa and adult insects[39] also take part. Lipolytic enzymes are less active, but hydrolytic break down starts early and goes on steadily until eventually little neutral fat remains, the residual tissue consisting largely of adipocere.

A large number of chemical substances may be present in the putrefying mass. Of these many have been chemically identified, such as formic, acetic, butyric, valerianic, palmitic, lactic, succinic and oxalic acids; amines and amino acids, such as leucin and tyrosin; and various aromatic substances like indol and skatol. Mercaptans are formed in anaerobic putrefaction.

We know also that when tissues die, as in cardiac infarction, there is a rise in certain enzyme levels, notably of glutamic oxalacetic transaminase. Enticknap[40] has studied the post-mortem rise in enzyme activity which he found started 3 or 4 h after death and rose fairly steadily for some 60 h (with transaminases) or longer (with lactic dehydrogenases).

Shortly after death, in cases where the process of dying has been slow, or where death has been accompanied by a bacteriaemia, especially in intestinal obstruction, anaerobic organisms pass in increasing numbers from the bowel into the blood vessels and spread rapidly throughout the body. Initially the bacteria recovered from post-mortem tissues are mixed, consisting of coliform organisms and anaerobic bacteria, but after a time the anaerobic organisms predominate.[41] Organs receiving the largest blood supply, and those nearest the source of bacteria, naturally receive most bacteria and normally putrefy first. The flanks of the abdomen will usually show the earliest colour change in about 36–48 h, the liver soon after.

Bacteria produce a large variety of enzymes and these break down the various tissues of the body, different enzymes acting on carbohydrates, fats and protein. One of the most important enzymes is the *lecithinase* produced by *Clostridium welchii*. This hydrolyses the lecithin which is present in all cell membranes including blood cells, and thus is responsible for the haemolysis of blood post mortem.

At and around the normal body temperature (98.4°F) *Cl. welchii* multiplies freely. The rate of multiplication, however, is slowed as the temperature falls, and below 70°F propagation is almost at a standstill, though most enzymes produced by bacteria will continue to act at much lower temperatures, even around freezing point. Thus the initial spread of putrefaction is largely influenced by two factors, (1) the cause of death and (2) the period of time that the internal temperature of the body remains above 70°F.

1. In cases where persons die from acute intestinal obstruction there is usually a frank bacteraemia before death so that organisms from the bowel are already spread throughout the body, and although the body temperature may fall rapidly putrefaction commences almost immediately. This state of affairs is accelerated when death is due to a gas-forming septicaemia, as in gas gangrene or postabortive clostridial infections.

Suspicion of phosphorous poisoning was raised by a resident medical officer at a Portsmouth hospital owing to (a) jaundice, (b) recurring vomiting and (c) purpuric skin patches developing in a woman of 22 who had been admitted for an incomplete abortion during the afternoon on the day of her death: she had been ill only 16 h in all when she lapsed into coma and died. Autopsy revealed a haemolysis of the blood in circulation, scanty gas formation, and a recently emptied uterus, enlarged to about three to three and a half months gestation size, the interior of which was remarkably dry looking: the wall crepitated and (together with a heart blood sample) gave a strong growth of *Cl. welchii*.

2. The period of time that the internal temperature of the body remains above 70°F is clearly of paramount importance. Any factor which delays the cooling of the body (see p. 131) will therefore hasten putrefaction processes.

Environment and posture may considerably alter the development and course of putrefaction and we must now consider certain points in this connection.

The site and colour of purefaction

The first visible sign of putrefaction in the cadaver is the appearance of a greenish discoloration of the skin in the right iliac fossa overlying the caecum (lower right anterior abdominal wall). This discoloration darkens to a coppery red and spreads across the abdomen and is rapidly followed by the appearance of blue or purplish red lines over the trunk, the root of the neck and upper arms and thighs. These lines are due to the decomposition and

haemolysis of blood in the veins. Owing to their appearance they are know as 'marbling'.

The time of onset of these putrefactive processes, except in cases of death associated with septicaemia, is dependent upon the environmental temperature. In temperate climates they may take from 36 h to five days to develop. In high summer or in the tropics they may appear within a few hours, whereas in a cold winter they may be delayed for several weeks.

The distribution of the putrefactive changes may be influenced by the position in which the deceased was lying after death. For instance, if a cadaver dies with his head in a dependent position, putrefactive changes will be advanced in the head and neck compared with the remainder of the body. Where a body is lying in water the head tends to lie lower than the trunk and upon recovery from the water the putrefactive processes are found to be more advanced in the head and neck.

A short period after the appearance of marbling, vesicles appear on the body. These usually make their appearance first on the abdomen. These vesicles enlarge, coalesce and rupture, freeing foul smelling fluid. The exposed subdermal tissue dries with a yellow parchment appearance. Changes also take place in the internal organs. The brain becomes soft and liquifies early especially in drowning. Blood vessels are stained by haemolysed blood and the colour changes observed externally take place in the internal organs and have been mistaken for pathological processes.

As putrefaction continues, gases of putrefaction are produced in the internal organs. The composition of the gases varies according to the post-mortem interval and environment of the body. In the early stages offensive gases are emitted and these frequently first call attention to the presence of a decomposing cadaver. After some weeks of earth burial ammonia is one of the most common gases.

Carbon monoxide may be found in the blood and more especially in the tissue fluids during putrefaction. The significance is not fully understood. Recent observations of the phenomenon have been recorded by Kojima et al.[42]

Blood rapidly leaves the general circulation after putrefaction has commenced. Post-mortem pleural effusions often form and these may be large following freshwater drowning. Ante-mortem haemorrhage into a body cavity will remain even when putrefaction is well advanced. Small fetuses rapidly disappear in putrefied blood in cases of ruptured ectopic pregnancy.

The gases of putrefaction produce certain changes, some of which could be mistaken for some other process. Gas forming in the blood vessels could be mistaken for air embolism especially if there has been a septic abortion or gaseous putrefaction has occurred early. The foamy liver of gas gangrene is closely mimicked in gaseous putrefaction.

Gas present in the subcutaneous tissues must not be mistaken for surgical emphysema.

As gas is evolved in the tissues where putrefaction occurs, these become swollen. The areas where swelling is most pronounced is in the face, especially after drowning, and in the abdomen. Limbs are sometimes relatively free of putrefaction in cadavers where the changes are very marked in the face and trunk.

The early putrefactive changes occurring in the face, especially when the head of the deceased is dependent, has not infrequently been mistaken for signs of strangulation especially when the exudation of fluid from the lungs commences. The writer has been frequently called out by the CID over the years to examine cadavers exhibiting these early putrefactive changes as the officer called to the scene has considered the changes to be suspicious.

The gases in the abdomen increase in pressure as the putrefactive processes advance and the lungs are forced upwards and decomposing blood escapes from the mouth and nostrils. The tongue may protrude from the mouth. Stomach contents may also be forced upwards into the mouth, and the rectum, bladder and pregnant uterus may be emptied by this internal pressure built up by the gases.

The extrusion of a fetus from a pregnant uterus requires further discussion as the possibility of illegal interference may be present. Keith Simpson[43] recorded the following case in an earlier edition.

A woman of 27, dying in hospital of 'septicaemia following abortion', was prepared by a nurse for transfer to the mortuary: she had not then any discharge or conception product visible in the vagina which, with the rectum, was plugged with wool in the usual manner. When seen 20 h later lying on the mortuary slab she was found to have a macerated three-months' fetus with shredded membranes lying external to the vulva: a slightly sanious, laked, discharge bubbled slowly from the vagina, and the uterus was found to contain the same kind of material together with a partly detached placenta from which the cord led to the fetus.

A similar case was reported by Gordon, Turner & Price in 1953.[44]

A native woman who died in childbirth, before the delivery of the infant, was exhumed some two weeks after burial. Marked putrefaction was then present, and the fetus, still attached by the cord, was found between the thighs.

It is obvious that in certain cases this condition might be used to cover and conceal a case of criminal abortion. The subject was once brought before the Medico-Legal Society of Paris by Pénard.[45] He was required to report on an alleged case of delivery 36 h after the death of a young woman under suspicious circumstances following eight days' illness. It was only just before her death that the doctor in attendance discovered that she was pregnant, and had probably reached the 5th month. He made no examination after death, and when the body was laid out there was no unusual appearance. When raised to be placed in a coffin, 36 h after death, a fetus fell from between the legs of the corpse. On examining the body, the uterus was found with the placenta attached, inverted, and extruded from the outlet.

Pénard came to the conclusion that, after the death of the woman, the uterus would not have the power of expelling the fetus and inverting itself by spontaneous muscular contraction, We should agree.

Floating of a body in water. The specific gravity of a cadaver is slightly greater than that of water, so a body either drowned or thrown into the water after death will sink unless certain mechanical factors operate which may prevent this. The body will remain submerged until sufficient gas is evolved to make it buoyant. The time taken is dependent upon the temperature of the water surrounding the cadaver. In deep lakes the upper layer of water will only become warmed in summer and below this heated layer of water the temperature is at a constant 39.2°F. Bodies which sink into this layer may remain submerged for several weeks, whereas in shallow water or rivers the body may float after a few hours in late summer.

Circumstances influencing the onset and progress of putrefaction

Since the essential processes of putrefaction are dependent upon the presence of organisms and their ferments, any factors which tend to accelerate or retard the multiplication or spread of these organisms will influence the process of putrefaction. Certain factors justify more detailed attention:
1. the temperature of the air to which the body is exposed;
2. the presence of moisture;
3. presence of clothing;
4. influence of access of air and of light;
5. the state of the body and cause of death;
6. immersion in water;
7. burial in earth.

The effects of temperature of the air. Putrefaction proceeds most rapidly when the body temperature encourages the growth of bacteria (an air temperature of between 70° and 100°F), provided other factors detrimental to the growth of bacteria are not present. When the organisms have been distributed about the body and have already liberated their enzymes, obvious putrefaction will commence, although delayed, at any temperature above 50°F. At 32°F (freezing point) decomposition appears to be wholly arrested; however, certain bacterial enzymes will continue to act slowly at that temperature. A dead body may thus be preserved indefinitely in refrigerators, snow, ice or in freezing soil.

Erman states that the body of Prince Menchikof, one of the favourites of Peter 1, was exhumed at Beresov, in 1821, after burial of 92 years in the frozen soil of Siberia. Although so long a time had elapsed the body had undergone but little change. The heart and some other parts, with a portion of the grave-clothes, were removed and sent to the descendants of the deceased.[46] A still more remarkable instance of the preservative power of cold is exhibited in the discovery in a mass of ice at the mouth of the River Lenz in Siberia, in 1805, of the body of an ancient elephant, the race of which was extinct before the historical period.[47]

In a high temperature, i.e., 120°F or over, the tissues rapidly dry, bacterial growth usually ceases, putrefaction is arrested, and mummification takes its place. At low temperatures, as in the mortuary refrigerator, the process can also be arrested.

The effect of the temperature of the air is strikingly seen in the influence of the seasons. Thus in summer a body may show more putrefactive changes in 12 h than a similar body under the same environmental conditions will show in 10–14 days in winter.

The influence of moisture. Putrefactive bacteria need water, and the body contains sufficient for their growth. In a human body weighing 150 lb there are about 100 lb of water. Hair, teeth and dense bone resist owing more to their structure.

Quekett[48] examined a portion of dried human skin with hair upon it which had been exposed for many centuries on a door of Worcester Cathedral, and also other portions taken from the church doors of Hadstock and Copford, in Essex. He found upon them some hairs which were proved under the microscope to be human, thus confirming the old tradition that the skins of persons who had committed sacrilege were nailed to the doors of the churches which they had robbed.

Holden[49] also found a remarkable state of preservation in the hairs of the effigies of royal persons in the historic collection from the Westminster Abbey museum—mostly dating from the fourteenth century. All were human except the eyebrow hairs of the effigy of Edward III. These were dog hairs, also well preserved.

If an organic substance is dried, putrefaction is arrested. Dehydration of food stuffs is now in everyday use as a means of preservation.

The presence of clothing. The effect of clothing on decomposition after burial or immersion in water is discussed under the respective headings, but mention should be made here of the effect of clothing on decomposition of bodies exposed to air. Clothing acts initially by hastening putrefaction by maintaining the body temperature above that at which putrefactive organisms multiply for a longer period. Tight clothing delays putrefaction owing to the pressure producing a degree of bloodlessness in the part. At a later stage clothing delays decomposition by protecting the body against the ravages of flies and insects. Fly larvae not only hasten the decomposition of a cadaver by directly attacking the soft tissues but also by generating heat which may raise the body temperature to a level well above that at which putrefactive organisms multiply.

In *R. v. Gribble* (Leicester Assizes 1944) the body of a murdered boy was found in a copse, very badly decomposed by putrefaction and maggot infestation in the entire head (which was uncovered) and nearly as badly in the chest and upper abdomen (covered only by a loose shirt). Below this a belt, thick trousers, socks and boots had preserved the body to a remarkable extent. The changes had taken place in nine days (in August) in a copse in the Midlands district of England.

The influence of air and light. Air influences decomposition mainly by (1) its temperature, (2) its moisture content (rain) and (3) flies.

Bacteria are normally present in the air but it is unlikely that these by themselves play any significant part in the process of putrefaction. Flies and their maggot larvae introduce supplementary processes which hasten decomposition to a remarkable extent (*vide supra*).

Light: this has no practical influence on the putrefactive processes, except that flies and other insects avoid those parts of the body exposed to direct light, tending to lay eggs in crevices like the eyelids.

The state of the body. The earlier stages of putrefaction are usually hastened when the body is fat or flabby. Dehydration tends to retard the course of decomposition throughout its course. Intestinal stasis promotes the process.

The bodies of newborn or still-born infants are normally sterile, and thus putrefaction can only occur by the invasion of the body by external organisms. As the body of a newborn child cools rapidly, putrefactive organisms can rarely gain a foothold and thus it is unusual for putrefaction, in the sense that it is applied to adults, to occur. When it is found in a newborn infant it constitutes some evidence of the child having breathed, inhaled (and also swallowed) organisms.

Care must be exercised when examining a body which has been dismembered at the time of death. In most instances the limbs will be devoid of putrefactive organisms and hence their decomposition

will be slow; the trunk, however, will putrefy as usual.

Disease: the bodies of persons who have died from acute diseases usually putrefy more readily than those persons who have died from wasting or chronic disease, except when intestinal stasis accompanies this. Where there has been a clostridial (e.g., *Cl. welchii*) infection before death, as in the bacteriaemias of some acute intestinal obstructions, in certain abortions and in gas-gangrene itself, putrefaction may develop with remarkable speed.

The body of a woman admitted to hospital the night of her death was noticed to be rapidly becoming 'dusky' and somewhat yellow as she spent her last 3 or 4 h. She was placed in the cool mortuary on her death at 8 a.m. and brought out for autopsy at 5.30 p.m. By this time she was developing blood-tinged blisters in the skin, had become purple, almost black in patches and was tense with gases. She had died of a clostridial gas-forming bacillary infected abortion with final septicaemia. The intima of the blood vessels was plum-coloured throughout, and the blood 'laked'. One would have judged her to be dead three to four days at that (September) season. She had a fulminating *Cl. welchii* septicaemia from a criminal abortion.

Deaths from poisons: conflicting statements have been made regarding the process of putrefaction in the bodies of those who die from certain poisons. There appears to be no foundation in fact for believing that any poison will constantly accelerate or retard decomposition. Traditionally arsenic is believed to preserve a body after interment but this traditional belief does not appear to have any sound basis.[50]

Influence of immersion in water. Certain factors influencing decomposition are peculiar to immersion. Still or running water, polluted water or seawater, all have their own influence on subsequent decomposition owing to their varying bacterial and animal content; salt water crustacea may remove all the soft tissues in a matter of two or three days. Unless the water is hot, bodies cool about twice as rapidly as in air and this delays the process.

After several hours' immersion the skin of the palms of the hands and the soles of the feet becomes wrinkled and sodden. If the water·is well oxygenated due to its shallowness, movement or temperature, oxygen exchange takes place through the wet skin. A recovered body may appear quite pink irrespective of the cause of death.

Owing to the more rapid cooling of the body in water, and since for the greater part of the year the temperature of the water remains below atmospheric temperature for the whole 24 h, decomposition *per se* tends to proceed more slowly than in air. When the water temperature is persistently below 40–45°F the body may show no appreciable decomposition after several weeks' immersion. At 50–70°F it may be expected after three to five days; above this decomposition may be found in two days or less according to the temperature. In the tropics, for example, it may be obvious in 18 to 24 h.

The order of the superficial appearance of the colours of decomposition is usually altered when a body is immersed in water, thus:

Table 8.3 Superficial appearance of the colours of decomposition are shown in order from above downwards

Water	Air
Face and neck, or sternum	Abdomen
	Chest
Shoulders	Face
Arms	Legs
Abdomen	Shoulders
Legs	Arms

Casper & Kanzler[51] described how, while the lower part of the body may be in a tolerably fresh condition, the face, head, neck and upper part of the chest may present a reddish colour passing into patches of a bluish green, first seen on the temples, ears and nape of the neck, thence spreading to the face, and afterwards to the throat and chest. These changes may be observed in the English summer when a body has remained in water from four to five days, in spring and autumn from eight to 10 days, and in winter for a longer period. The head of a drowned person is sometimes much discoloured from putrefaction when the rest of the body is in an apparently unchanged condition, owing to the fact that the head floats lower than the rest of the body and blood gravitates first to the head and neck.

The skin covering the palms of the hands and the soles of the feet is found thickened, white and sodden when the body has remained several days in water. Owing to this cause, ecchymoses resulting from violence during life are not always apparent on the body when it is removed from water. It is only when the skin has dried that ecchymoses and other marks of violence may be seen. Wiping away the outer cuticle will often reveal tattoos and scars.

The influence of air upon the skin of a body which has been for some days submerged is chiefly seen, after its removal from water, on the face and chest. In a few hours, if the temperature of the atmosphere is moderately high, the face may be found bloated, and either livid or black, afterwards changing to a deep green. The discolorations are not commonly found on surfaces which have been in close contact, as in the armpits and upper and lower limbs, where the arms have been closely applied to the sides of the body or the legs have remained close together. The stains are not commonly seen at the back of the body, or on those parts which have been closely wrapped in clothes, owing to the pressure excluding blood and preventing the accumulation of fluids.

Clothing protects the soft tissues from the ravages of fish, crustacea and other small animals. When a body becomes partly buried in mud or silt, the exposed skin of the face and hands is attacked by shrimps, crabs and or fish. Passing craft and the effect of tides may increase the amount of damage and disintegration. The damage that ensues must be carefully distinguished from ante-mortem injury or suspicion of crime will be raised without foundation.

When a body with incised wounds or lacerations is immersed in water shortly after the infliction of the injuries the water will lyse the blood in the wounds and this will then pass into the water so that the wounds may be indistinguishable from post-mortem wounds.

In warm weather a thick covering of algae may form over the exposed parts of the body. This matting of algae, if formed rapidly enough, will offer some protection to the body from the attacks of small animals, and will seal up the body orifices. This later phenomenon may be of great value.

In the case of *R*. v. *Whiteway*[52] the body of one of the victims was recovered from Thames water in midsummer five days after rape and murder; the vagina had been completely sealed by the algae and the vaginal contents were uncontaminated. Spermatozoa were readily recognisable on microscopic examination of the vaginal contents.

The algae attach themselves firmly to the surface of the skin and have to be gently scraped off before the examination of the body can begin. The superficial layer of the skin comes away with the algae and thus fine abrasions of the cuticle may disappear during the cleaning process.

The period of time required for a body to rise to the surface from gaseous putrefaction must depend on many circumstances but principally, of course, on the temperature of the water. In Europe in the height of the summer it is two to three days, and in the spring or autumn from three to five days after death from drowning (or from 8 to 9 days in deep seawater). In winter a body may not rise to the surface for up to six weeks if the water temperature is cold. In very deep water the bottom temperature remains constant at 39.2°F throughout summer and winter, and in these circumstances gaseous putrefaction will be no more rapid in summer provided the body sinks to the bottom; generally, however, the depth of water is insufficient to permit this state of affairs. Wind affects the distribution of cold and warm waters in deep lakes, and if the body is lying at the windward end of the lake the wind may alter the distribution of the warm layer so that the temperature of the body is raised to that in which bacteria can multiply rapidly. The facts connected with the buoyancy of the dead body became of great importance in the trial of Spencer Cowper[53] (1699) for the alleged murder of a woman. After some 12–14 days the skin of the fingers begins to become detached and may, in two to three weeks, be detached as a kind of glove, the nails loosening last. The hair becomes easily detachable—by mere wiping—in slightly shorter periods of time.

When several months have passed, the muscles become soft and discoloured, or the fatty parts may have been converted into adipocere. Ultimately the soft parts will be washed from the bones, and the skeleton separated.

The changes due to putrefaction in the drowned, or apparently drowned, even when comparatively slight, may, as Casper justly remarks, seriously affect the value of the medical evidence. The blood becomes decomposed, acquires a darker colour, and produces the appearance of congestion in the brain, lungs, right side of the heart and other parts of the body, so as to render it difficult to form a conclusion on death from asphyxia.[54]

After the occurrence of such changes from putrefaction in the drowned as those above described it is extremely difficult to restore the features. Mistakes have been made by persons relying upon the features as proof of identity in the drowned.

In *Hollis* v. *Turner* one William Turner, a person of restless, unsettled habits, wandering about the country, and in a state of great mental and bodily depression, walked into a house at Guildford. On the following day he left the place, and was never again seen alive. Ten days after his disappearance the body of a much decomposed man was found in the River Wey, near Guildford. At an inquest held on the same day, two men, named Etherington, claimed the body as that of their father, who was missing. Others who saw the body identified it as that of Turner. The body, however, was buried as that of Philip Etherington. Some months afterwards Etherington, sen., the supposed deceased, walked into his daughter's house. The body was undoubtedly that of Turner.

Burial in earth. The following factors influence the course of post-mortem changes.[55]

The state of the body at the time of death: in a temperate climate a well-covered body will decompose more slowly than one which is thin or emaciated if buried under the same conditions.

Time which has elapsed between death and burial, and the environment of the body during this period: the longer the body remains above ground before burial, the more advanced is likely to be the state of decomposition, especially if the body has been kept in a warm environment. This was quite clear from a series of exhumations carried out in Germany after the 1939–45 War in cases where bodies of aircraft crew, who had all been killed at the same time but buried at different intervals, although in the same cemetery under the same conditions. If a body is buried at greater depth immediately after death decomposition is greatly delayed.

The effect of a coffin: a well-sealed coffin, especially one which is lead lined, will delay decomposition, and under such circumstances the features may be recognisable after as long as 150 years' burial. A poor coffin, however, which readily admits water tends to hasten decomposition. This decomposition is further hastened in coffins where there is a considerable volume of air.

Clothing or other coverings: clothing or other coverings will delay decomposition when a body is buried in earth without a coffin. Also, under these circumstances adipocere will form more readily, the action of the clothing being twofold; it will afford some protection from insects, and will aid the formation of adipocere by keeping the body beneath it continually moist by absorbing moisture from the soil.

The depth at which the body is buried: generally speaking the greater the depth of the grave, the greater the degree of preservation. In shallow graves the soil is aerated, and the body itself will become the prey of a far greater variety of insects and animals; also in summer these shallow graves, and consequently the body, will become warmed by the sun.

Type of soil: the part played by various soils in altering the rate of decomposition must be considered in every case. In heavy clay soils the formation of adipocere is encouraged whereas sandy and porous soils, in general, are conducive to mummification.

The presence of chemicals around the body: when a body is buried in lime, decomposition is retarded, and soft tissues are largely preserved. The preservative effect of lime was well illustrated in the case of *R. v. Dobkin*[56] where sprinkling of lime over the tissues preserved the evidence of fracture of the thyroid by strangling during life: dried bruising around a fractured cornu was well preserved and permitted microscopy.

Access of air to the body after burial: the access of air to a body after burial, provided the body has not become mummified or converted to adipocere, considerably accelerates decomposition.

Mass graves: in cases where a number of bodies are buried in a common grave without coffins, those bodies lying in the centre of the grave may be better preserved than those at the periphery.

The basic facts may be set out briefly as follows:
1. Decomposition starts in the flanks of the abdomen, usually rather earlier on the right side, over the caecum; it spreads into the trunk, reaching out through the blood vessels into the tissues of the neck, face and head, arms and legs.

2. It is more pronounced (but not developed earlier) in vascular tissues and in parts where the blood has gravitated, e.g., in the head and neck in bodies floating in water, etc.

3. It develops, at any given season, about twice as fast in air as in water, and about a quarter the rate-in-air when the body is buried.

4. Sewage or decomposing organic matter will hasten the process appreciably. A stagnant environment is adjuvant.

5. Certain organs decompose early, other more tardily, as follows:

Table 8.4

Early	Late
Intestines and stomach	Lungs
Liver	Heart
Spleen	Kidneys
Brain	Bladder
	Prostate, testis
	Uterus, ovaries

With regard to the period after death at which these putrefactive changes are likely to become established, Table 8.5[57] will be found to fit the course of events at moderate temperatures such as apply to an average English spring or autumn—giving a usual range of 50° to 70°F—when no special accelerating or retarding conditions are present.

Broadly speaking, above 70°F the rate becomes doubled for every 15°F rise and below 50°F the rate becomes halved for every 15°F; below 35°F little putrefaction is likely to occur. Experience will show, however, that it is impossible to be didactic about such matters; such generalisations as are set out above can only act as a guide to what is well recognised to be one of the most difficult tasks in forensic pathology—that of estimating the lapse of time since death.

Adipocere formation

This substance, reputedly studied by Bacon, was first described as 'adipocire' by Fourcroy in 1789[58]

Table 8.5

Period	Land	Water
Days	*Putrefaction*	
2	Green staining in flanks	
2–3	Green and purple staining over abdomen and some distension	
3–4	Marbling of veins. Further spread of stains into neck and limbs	Discoloration at root of neck
5–6	Gaseous swelling and disruption internally. Skin blebs	Neck and face discoloured and swollen. Body floats in 6–10 days (period halved in hot weather). Decomposition well established in trunk, but little distension. Cutis peeling and hair loosening, easily pulled out. Nails pulled out with difficulty
Weeks		
2	Abdomen distended to tight tension. Swelling of body marked, and blebbing with purple transudate widespread. All organs disrupted by gas	
3	Vesicles bursting and tissues softening and disrupting. Eyes bulging. Organs and cavities bursting. Disfiguration to extreme	Face swelling and becoming discoloured
4	General slimy liquefaction and disruption of all soft tissues	Body greatly swollen with gases and organs crepitant. Hair easily wiped away. Nails (fingers easily, toes less easily) pulled out. Casts of hands and feet separate

during the removal of vast numbers of bodies from the Cimetière des Innocents in Paris. He gave it this name owing to its properties being intermediate between those of fat (adipo) and wax (cire). It is a condition which develops in fat as a result of enzyme and chemical changes usually some weeks after death.

Taylor gave an account of the appearance and physical properties of adipocere in earlier editions of this work.

Adipocere is formed by the hydrolysis and hydrogenation of body fats after death by the action of bacterial enzymes.[59] The main constituent of adipocere is palmitic acid. The introduction of modern sophisticated analytical procedures has made the analysis of adipocere a relatively simple investigation and several analyses have been published in recent years. Nanikawa[60] examined samples from various sources and more recently more specific studies have been made by Takatori & Yamaoka.[61,62]

Adipocere will form wherever there is any body fat. Older works on forensic medicine implied that it only formed in the subcutaneous tissues. This is untrue.

As adipocere is the product of hydrogenation and hydrolysis of fat, water is essential for its formation. The intact cadaver, however, will normally contain enough water to convert the fat to adipocere.[59] During this process the muscles and internal organs become dehydrated and mummified.

The rate of adipocere formation is extremely variable depending upon both the temperature and humidity of the environment. Its presence may be detected by analytical examination within a few days of death. It is not normally apparent to the eye for several months but under unusual climatic conditions it may appear within weeks. One such recent case is recorded by Simonsen.[63]

Adipocere is essentially composed of saturated fatty acids, glycerides being present in traces only. The hard waxy character of the mature substance is largely due to the presence of the two hydroxystearic acids. Calcium soaps, proteins, etc., are variable incidental components.

A close experimental study of adipocere formation by Mant[59] has shown that it is formed from pre-existing fat which gradually hardens as the other fats disappear. The hydrogenation of the unsaturated body fats into saturated firmer fats requires certain enzymes which are liberated from decomposing protein. Though it is possible that an ammoniacal soap may be formed in the early stages, this is not an essential change.

Distribution

Adipocere is usually first seen in the subcutaneous fat of the cheeks, the breasts, buttocks and the abdomen, but only because these parts are better padded with fat. The condition may develop wherever fat is present, so long as bacteria, their enzymes and water are also present. The latter may come from the body, from rain or running water or upon burial in moist soil—or from all of these sources. It has frequently been described in conditions of relatively dry environment after very long periods of interment.

Evans, studying a group of brick vault interments in London in which inhumation had been continuous for 103 to 127 years, found adipocere in 56% of cases.[64]

The formation of human adipocere is similar to the hydrogenation of vegetable fats in the manufacture of margarine, both consisting of the conversion of unsaturated fatty acids. Bacterial enzymes are probably essential for its formation. Water is certainly essential in the chemical changes which occur not only because it takes part in the synthesis but also because it helps to remove glycerine which is formed during hydrolysis of the fats.

Time required for adipocere formation

The rate of development of adipocere depends upon the temperature more than any other single factor. So long as the natural lipases of the body, those of the anaerobic bacilli and water—whether merely body fluid or extrinsic humidity, rain water, or burial in a wet soil—are present, adipocere will develop. In the cool North American and European climates five or six months may be necessary for adipocere to become obvious: in the height of a European summer it may be obvious in five or six weeks; in Egypt and India it is often seen in half this time. The local conditions are of great importance because of their bearing on the temperature.

In *R. v. Sangret*, a murdered girl's body was buried under a thin layer of wet turf on the higher part of an English heathland where the sun had access all day. Adipocere was present in the thighs and breasts in five and a half weeks of late summer rain and sunshine, with the day temperatures ranging between 65° and 75°F.[65]

In the case of the Loves a couple had lain under the waters of London dock for a period of four years, trapped in a submerged car. More or less uniform adipocere encased the trunk of the woman and avulsed or disintegrated arms and legs showed the same degree of change. Four summers and three winters had intervened.[66]

Laboratory analysis will plainly show the process to have commenced within two or three weeks of death—i.e., long before it has become obvious to the eye.[59]

Mummification

This is the dehydration of the body tissues. Deprived of moisture, putrefactive organisms do not proliferate and therefore a warm drying atmosphere, especially with a free circulation of air around the body, is ideal for mummification. These conditions are met with when burial occurs in the hot arid sands of a desert for there high temperature, dry air and the loose sand combine to produce rapid dehydration of the tissues.

The Egyptian mummy, encased in sarcophagi, is a chemically preserved, not merely dried body, and the well known Danish bog mummies are peat preserved at a low pH. Both are chemically aided—or inactivated—processes.

In this country mummification is unusual in adults, as the conditions necessary for it are rarely present. The mummification of infants, however, is common, for newly born infants are often concealed in warm, dry places, and as their tissues are usually free from organisms at birth they do not develop the normal putrefactive changes. Occasionally a body which shows evidence of mummification in certain parts may show adipocerous change in others. Thus there may be found some adipocere in the cheeks, abdomen and buttocks, and mummification of the arms and legs. This is in accordance with the observations above. It is frequently found during exhumations of bodies buried without coffins; it may, however, happen equally well in the open, as shown by the following cases.

Harry T., aged 42 years, was found hanging from a tree in a wood in late November, having been missing for nine weeks. All the internal organs had been liquefied by putrefaction and had run out of the body through the pelvis. Adipocere had formed over the chest and abdomen, and analysis showed that the adipocere contained 80% fatty acids. There was mummification of the lower arms and lower legs.

In *R. v. Sangret*[65] (Kingston Assizes 1943), the body of a girl, missing for five and a half weeks, was found buried in a shallow sand-and-gravel grave on a heath near Godalming. The right hand, which protruded slightly on the surface of the soil, was mummified, and adipocere was appreciably well advanced in its formation in both breasts and on the thighs. The late summer period when these changes had taken place had been marked by warm sun and intermittent rainfall.

REFERENCES

1. Bruhier, J. J. (1742) Dissertation sur l'incertitude des signes de la mort. Paris.
2. Barcroft, J. (1946) Researches on Pre-natal Life. Oxford: Blackwell.
3. Abramson, H. (1960) Resuscitation of the Newborn Infant. St Louis: C. V. Mosby.
4. de Saram, G. S. W., et al. (1855) J. Crim. Law Criminol., **46**, 562.
5. Fiddes, F. S. & Patten, T. D. (1958) J. For. Med., **5**, 2.
6. Marshall, T. K. & Hoare, P. E. (1962) J. For. Sci, **7**, 56.
7. Wilks, S. & Taylor A. S. (1863) Guy's Hosp. Rep. 184
8. Taylor, A. S. ibid.
9. James, W. R. L. & Knight, B. H. (1965) Med. Sci. Law, **5** 111.
10. Joseph, A. E. A. & Schickele, E. (1970) J. For. Sci., **15**, 364.
11. Simonsen, J., Voigt, J. & Jeffersen, N. (1977) Med. Sci. Law, **17**, 112.
12. Report of an Inquiry by the Hon. Sir Henry Fisher (1977) London: Her Majesty's Stationery Office, p. 60.
13. Mant, A. K. (1954) J. For. Med., **1**, 260.
14. Jaffe, F. A. (1962) J. For. Sci., **7**, 231.
15. Sturner, W. Q. (1963) Lancet, **1**, 807.
16. Christison. Taylor's Med. Jurisprudence.
17. Astrup, T. (1956) Lancet, **2**, 565.
18. Mole, R. H. (1948) H. Path. Bact., **64**, 413.
19. Mant, A. K. (1953) In: Simpson, K., ed. Modern Trends in Forensic Medicine. London: Butterworths.
20. Selye, H. (1946) J. Clin. Endocrinol., **6**, 117.
21. Prinsloo, I. & Gordon, I. (1951) S. Afr. Med. J., **25**, 358.
22. Schourup, K. (1951) Int. Crim. Police Rev., **51**, 279.
23. Schleyer, author. (1973) Z. Rechsmed., **71**, 281.
24. Van den Oever, author (1978) Z. Rechtsmed., **80**, 259.
25. Gyorgyi, S. (1947) Chemistry of Muscular Contraction. New York: Academic Press Inc.
26. Fisher, R. S. & Petty, C. S. (1977) Forensic Pathology. Washington: US Department of Justice, p. 57.
27. Mant, A. K. (1967) Med. Sci. Law, **7**, 135.
28. Paddock, C. E. (1903) Am. J. Obstet., **48**, 145.
29. Hermann. Taylor's Medical Jurisprudence 12th ed.
30. Taylor, A. S. ibid.
31. Krompecher, T. & Krompecher-Kiss, E. (1978) For. Sci. Irit., **12**, 89.
32. Krompecher, T, & Fryc, O. (1978) For. Sci. Int., **12**, 97.
33. Shapiro, H. A. (1950) Br. Med. J., **2**, 304.
34. Krompecher, T. & Fryc, O. (1978) For. Sci. Int, **12**, 103.
35. Sommer. Taylor's Med. Jurisprudence 12th ed.
36. Brown—Séquard. (1852) Amer. J. Med. Sci. 221.
37. Taylor, A. S. Med. Jurisprudence 12th ed.
38. Evans, W. E. D. (1963) The Chemistry of Death. Springfield, Ill.: Charles Thomas.
39. Megnin, A. (1894) La Faune des Cadavres. Paris:Gauthier-Villars et fils.
40. Enticknap, J. B. (1960) J. For. Med., **7**, 135.
41. Burn, C. G. (1934) J. Infect. Dis., **54**, 395.
42. Kojima, T., Nishiyama, Y., Yashiki, M. & Unei, author (1982) For. Sci. Int., **19**, 243.
43. Simpson, C. K. Taylor's Med. Jurisprudence 12th ed.
44. Gordon, I., Turner, R. & Price, T. W. (1953) Medical Jurisprudence, 3rd edn. Edinburgh: Livingstone, p. 427.
45. Penard. Taylor's Med. Jurisprudence 12th ed.
46. Erman, author Travels in Siberia, vol. 1, p. 462.
47. Erman, author (1820) Q. J. Sci., **8**, 95.
48. Quekett. Taylor's Medical Jurisprudence 12th ed.
49. Holden. ibid.
50. Copeman, P. R. & Bodenstein, J. C. (1955) J. For. Med., **2**, 196.
51. Casper & Kanzler.
52. Mant, A. K. (1954) J. For. Med., **1**, 260.
53. Famous Trials of History (1926) Birkenhead, p. 89.
54. Casper, J. L. (1861) Handbook of Forensic Medicine New. Syd. Soc., **1**, 219.
55. Mant, A. K. (1953) Modern Trends in Forensic Medicine, ch. IV. London: Butterworths.
56. Simpson, C. K. (1943) Med. Leg. J., **XI**, 132.
57. Simpson, C. K. (1974) Forensic Medicine, 7th edn. London: Arnold.
58. Fourcroy, A. F. (1789) Mem. R. Acad. Sci.
59. Mant, A. K. (1957) J. For. Med., **4**, 18.
60. Nanikawa, R. (1973) Z. Rechtsmed., **72**, 194.
61. Takatori, T. & Yamaoka, A. (1977) For. Sc., **9**, 63.
62. Takatori, T. & Yamaoka, A. (1977) For. Sc., **10**, 117.
63. Simonsen, J. (1977) Med. Sci. Law, **17**, 53.
64. Evans, W. E. D. (1963) Med. Sci. Law, **3**, 145.
65. Simpson, C. K. (1944) Police J., **17**, 212.
66. Simpson, C. K. (1961) Med. Leg. J., **29**, 39.

9

Identification of the living and dead

The identification of a dead person is commonplace in hospitals, mortuaries and in Coroner's and other Courts. Cases of mistaken identity arise from time to time, and these errors have usually arisen because of the traditional reliance which is placed upon simple visual identification by friends or relatives: this is often distasteful to relatives who may be too readily satisfied. Decomposition of the body, post-mortem mutilation, or sometimes the mode of dying may so alter the features and general appearances of the deceased that visual recognition even by the closest relatives may be uncertain or impossible. When this state of affairs is present, other means of identification, which have been developed principally during the last century, must be employed and it is often the sum total of the results of these various ancillary methods which permits identification to become established beyond reasonable doubt.

The problems associated with the identification of the recently dead are identical with those of the living if one excludes such functions as speech, handwriting, gait, etc., and this is not the place to deal with the identification of the living as a separate entity. With decomposition of a body the ordinary means of identification become difficult, being obscured by the natural putrefactive processes, and so one relies more and more upon the scientific methods available.

Problems of identification lie mainly in four groups, namely identification of

(1) recently dead persons,
(2) disintegrating and decomposing bodies,
(3) skeletal remains,
(4) fragmentary remains.

In practice some overlap is common among these categories.

Identity will be dealt with under the following headings:
1. Features.
2. Personal effects—pocket contents; clothing marks; jewellery.
3. Contact or occupational data.
4. Height or stature.
5. Sex (intersex)—sexing cells and remains.
6. Weight.
7. Developmental, congenital or acquired defects:
    a. Asymmetry and deformities.
    b. Injuries.
    c. Scars.
    d. Tattoos.
8. Age—perinatal; children; adults.
9. Handedness and reconstruction of features.
10. Fingerprints, palm prints and footprints.
11. Race.
12. Hair.
13. Anthropometry.
14. Fragmentary remains.
15. Duration of burial.
16. Cause of death.

LIKENESS OF FEATURES

During life the general expression of the face can be so readily altered that mistakes can easily be made. The notorious Charles Peace, who was executed in 1879, was so clever at disguising his features by voluntary movements that he was said to be able to converse without discovery with detectives who knew him. After death such voluntary alteration is, of course, impossible; but death so speedily alters expression that too much reliance must not be placed upon this mode of identification. Photography is a notoriously unreliable method of identification unless minute details are considered.

In the Luton 'sack murder' (*R. v. Manton*, Bedford Assizes 1944) it was admitted that when the profile photograph of the victim was flashed on the screen of the local cinema and placed in shop windows in efforts to identify her, even her own daughter of 17 failed to recognise the likeness of her mother. Thirty-nine identity visits were made to the body and nine people positively identified the victim as four different women of which she was not one.

The details of features are usually satisfactory as evidence of identity. The colour of the irides, possibly different in the two eyes, or with peculiar segments in them, the size of the ears and their lobes, the length of the nose, the shape of the chin, lend themselves to exact observation and measurement,

as in the Bertillon system, and may lead to definite identification. A photographer or artist is usually much better qualified than a medical person to speak of such details.

The identification of persons by sight alone leads to innumerable mistakes in ordinary life without any particular inconvenience, but such mistakes occasionally occur in connection with criminal identification with possibly serious results.

In 1953 the photograph of a man 'wanted for interview' by the police in connection with a murder in Kent was televised—for the first time in English police history. Scores of people 'saw Pettit' during the next few days, some simultaneously in places hundreds of miles apart. He was, in fact, already lying dead in bombed-out City premises. It is common experience that the average truthful witness is absolutely unreliable in the majority of cases when asked to identify a certain individual whom he is supposed to have seen. Nearly every person has seen others who are more or less like him, and occasionally this resemblance is so start-

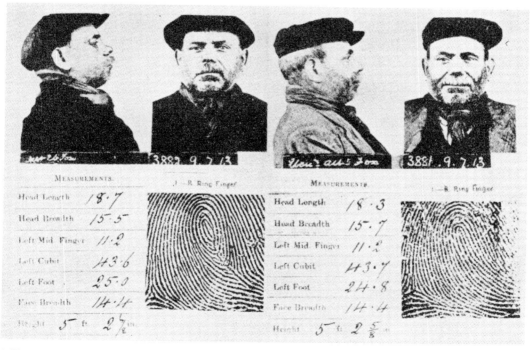

Fig. 9.1 The notorious Stevenage (Herts) twins, Albert Ebenezer (L) and Ebenezer Albert Fox (R). The former had a substantial criminal record, the latter playing a minor role, creating alibis by his similar appearance. The only secure means of distinguishing the two lay in their fingerprint record at Scotland Yard. (By courtesy of The Commissioner of Police in the Metropolis and The Editor, Police Journal.)

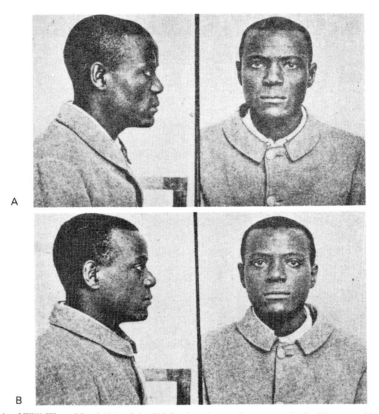

Fig. 9.2A Photograph of Will West, No. 3426, of the US Penitentiary at Leavenworth. B. Photograph of William West, No. 2646, of the same Penitentiary. These two men were in prison at the same time. Their fingerprints were, of course, different in innumerable respects. (After Wilder & Wentworth, 'Personal Identification'.)

ling that it is impossible to recognise the difference between the two people when seen apart. A good example of such resemblance is seen in the famous Fox twins, but a more remarkable case is that of two men quite unknown to one another and unrelated (Figs 9.1 and 9.2) who were in the same prison at the same time, bore the same name, and had practically the same Bertillon measurements.

These examples serve to show the great danger of sight recognition in criminal identification. In other instances the same individual may be completely changed by modifications in the trimming of the moustache or beard, or by shaving.

PERSONAL EFFECTS (Pocket contents, clothing and laundry marks, rings and other jewellery)

Clothing and pocket contents, papers, letters, keys,

etc., found on a deceased often provide the initial evidence which leads to positive identification. Even when attempts have been made to remove all marks of identity, laundry marks or the contents of a pocket are easily overlooked.

In the Love case the identity of a disintegrated headless torso was established beyond doubt by a laundry identity mark on the collar of a shirt that still clung to the body. Four years had elapsed.

In a series of exhumations of Allied war crime victims, following the Second World War,[1,2] over a third of the bodies identified were identified by laundry marks and personal effects, although in several cases every effort had been made to conceal the identity of the deceased.

Watches frequently have private marks inside the cases made by the watchmakers who have carried out repairs. All contents of pockets must be recorded and filed with great care.

In 1953 a man named Pettit, 'wanted' by the police in connection with a murder in southeast London, was found dead in bombed-out City premises, so decomposed that identity had to rest with clothing, papers therein, and teeth. A letter beside the body was identified as in his writing and a card bearing the wanted man's name was found in the jacket pocket: it referred to dental treatment at Guy's Hospital, giving a file number from which X-ray and other dental data exactly comparable with those of the dead man were obtained. They bore the name 'Pettit' (Fig. 9.3).

At an inquest held at Southwark in September 1953, a man's body recovered from the Thames was identified by:

1. Clothing including a shirt marked L. 254—a laundry mark similar to that of the landlady whose lodger the dead man was thought to be.

2. Underclothing similarly marked in the lodger's chest of drawers.

3. A key in the jacket pocket which fitted the lodger's door.

4. The general features of sex, age, height, hair and skin colouring. No distinguishing feature was

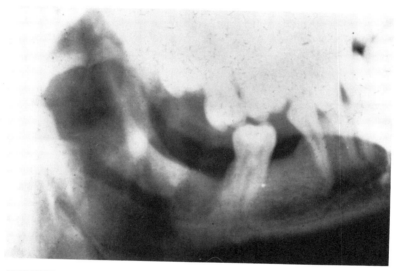

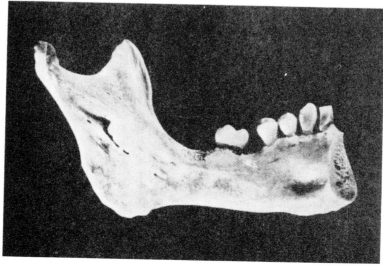

Fig. 9.3 Pettit—dental data.

present. A bank book, ration book, N I (national insurance) card and identity card still lay in his vacant room: they remained unclaimed.

Warning should be given against accepting laundry marks on small articles as evidence of identity; handkerchiefs, etc., are easily transferred or misplaced, and are unsafe clues.

Mistakes may also arise with second-hand clothing, or when letters and other personal papers are carried by someone other than the original owner.

In *R. v. Heath* (C. C. C. 1946) the ankles of the victim of a sadistic sex murder, Marjorie Gardner, were found to be tied with a handkerchief embroidered with the letter 'K' and laundry mark 'L. Kearns'. No one connected with the case had such a name.

CONTACT OR OCCUPATIONAL DATA

These are divisible into two groups:
1. recent and temporary;
2. permanent or semi-permanent.

Recent and temporary

In this group we include contact traces—the transference of some solid or liquid the man is working with on to his body or clothing. These contact traces may be found on the skin, beneath the nails, in the hair, the ears or on the clothing, and include paint spots on painters and decorators, grease on engineers and mechanics, flour on bakers and millers, dyes on dye workers, sawdust on those engaged in timber cutting, and so on.

An abortion victim of 21 lying dead in a block of flats where she was not known, having merely been brought to the address by her boyfriend for the 'operation', was noticed to have the rubber soles of her shoes smelling very strongly of petrol. Enquiry at local filling stations resulted in quick identification.

The microscopic examination of dust and debris on clothing, in the pockets and trouser turn-ups, under the fingernails and in the cerumen of the ears, is of prime importance as an aid in the identification of unknown bodies, possibly providing evidence of the occupation, or recent whereabouts,

or connecting the body with a specific locus where a crime was committed.

Nevertheless contact traces may be misleading. In 1977 the body of a partly clad, decomposing young woman was found in a woodland. The decomposition and depredation of fly larvae had rendered her features unrecognisable. On arrival at the mortuary all available material, including hair, was taken for examination. The hair was found to be contaminated with cornflour. A very intensive enquiry was conducted at all the biscuit factories using cornflour with negative results. Further examination of the cornflour revealed that this was of an exceptionally high quality used for dusting rubber gloves. The cornflour had therefore been transferred to the hair during the process of moving the body or of handling in the mortuary prior to the samples having been taken. The deceased was later identified.

Factual information may also be obtained concerning the deceased's habits and social status from study of the clothing, and of the care taken with the personal appearance.

Permanent or semi-permanent

Characteristic permanent or semi-permanent external marks on the body resulting from the deceased's occupation are occasionally distinctive. Forbes[3] carried out a limited survey of changes in the hands of persons following different occupations. He found that not all the workers in any one trade or industrial process necessarily had the occupational stigmata associated with their work, although in certain cases the presence of stigmata might be of value.

The irregular carbon tattooing of the face, arms and hands of a coal miner, the calloused hands of the manual labourer, and the callosities on the bricklayer's thumb, are some of the few distinctive occupational marks remaining in an age where the machine is superseding the craftsman.

HEIGHT OR STATURE

The height of a recently dead or partly decomposed and yet intact body may be estimated by direct measurement. The value of such measurements for identification depends upon the existence of a record of the deceased's height taken during life. Although the accuracy of the post-mortem measurement should not be in question, recordings of height taken in life may not be so accurate. Life recordings may have been just an estimate, or it may not be known as to whether the measurement was the actual height or the height in shoes, or inaccurately read. The age at which the recording or estimation was made is also pertinent, as height may lessen with advancing years due to atrophic changes occurring in disc cartilages or bones. The measured height of the deceased, therefore, might frequently vary an inch either side of the recorded height even in the absence of disease. This variation must always be considered in problems of identification.

The height of bodies that are found disarticulated, in a very advanced state of decomposition or as skeletal remains, cannot be measured directly with the accuracy possible with an intact body. In determining the stature from the measurement of the entire skeleton it is usual to add from 1 to $1\frac{1}{2}$ inches for the thickness of the soft parts (soles of the feet and the scalp). Even when the bones have become entirely disarticulated they should be laid out in their natural anatomical order and a rough estimate made.

When the skeleton is incomplete or severely disintegrated, the stature may be calculated by applying mathematical formulae to the length of the long bones (a small allowance must be made for the differences between wet and dry bones).

The estimation of stature from measurements of the long bones has engaged the attention of anatomists and anthropologists since the middle of the eighteenth century. Sue,[4] on a limited number of bodies of all ages, showed that before 14 years of age the trunk was longer than the lower limbs but after that age they were equal—that is after 14 years of age the symphysis pubis lies about halfway up the body. Sue was followed by Orfila, Beck, Thurnam, Humphry, Bedaloe, Dwight, Broca, Topinard, Rollet, Manouvrier, Pearson, Stevenson, Dupertuis and Hadden. These historical investigations were usually carried out upon relatively small numbers of skeletons with a predomi-

nance in the sixth decade. The work of these pioneers showed collectively that the weight-bearing bones, e.g., those of the lower limbs, provided the most accurate assessment of stature but there were distinct racial differences. The formulae of Rollet[5] and Pearson[6] were used in Great Britain for many years and their original tables have been published by Krogman.[7]

This historical work has now been superceded by that of Trotter & Gleser[8] who studied over 5000 skeletons from five ethnic groups. The majority of those studied were caucasian and negroid. They found that the equation based upon the combined lengths of the femur and tibia gave the most accurate results. Their series was largely aged between 18 and 30 years and their formulae are based upon this age group. For skeletons older than 30 years there is a simple correction formula. Trotter and Glesers' complete tables and formulae have been recently published by T. D. Stewart. There is no place in this volume for reproduction of the tables or details of the technique for measuring bones on an osteometric board. This information may be found in T. D. Stewart's *Essentials of Forensic Anthropology*.[9]

A comparatively recent case where both the older and more recent formulae were applied is of some interest. In *R. v. Christie*[10] (C. C. C. 1953) the stature estimations made from the four principal long bones (f h t r) and their separate sums (e.g., f + t) confirmed the existence of 'a systematic negative error' using the Pearson formulae (R. J. Harrison[10]). The Dupertuis & Hadden 'general formulae and the Trotter and Gleser formulae gave mean errors of 0.14 and 0.16 cm—negligible errors. A variance ratio test showed no significant error with the latter two methods at the 5% level. The actual height of Ruth Fuerst was 172.7 cm. Pearson's formulae gave a mean of 165 cm Dupertuis and Hadden 171.3 cm, Trotter and Gleser 172.2 cm. The same underestimation was evident in a re-examination of the Ruxton and Rogerson statures which Harrison made during the reconstructions of the Christie case.

Fetal bones

From measurements of the stature of 50 newly

born children and the subsequent measurements of the dried bones *without* articular cartilages (i.e., diaphyses only) the following ratios have been calculated:

Table 9.1 Stature of child

Femur	× 6.71	Radius	× 9.20
Tibia	× 7.63	Clavicle	× 11.30
Humerus	× 7.60	Lower jaw (symphysis to condylar surface)	× 10.00

SEX

The identification of the sex of an individual may also be important in legal medicine. Individuals of one sex carrying many of the secondary sexual characteristics of the other sex are not infrequent. Much rarer are those individuals who carry the primary sexual organs (testis and ovary) of both sexes.

Sex may require to be established positively in one direction or the other for the following reasons:
1. For the purpose of simple identification in a living or dead person.
2. For the purposes of deciding whether an individual can exercise certain civil rights reserved to one sex only.
3. For deciding questions relative to legitimacy, divorce, paternity, affiliation and also to some criminal offences.

Evidence of sex

This may ordinarily be divided into three categories:
1. Presumptive.
2. The highly probable.
3. The certain.

Presumptive evidence of sex

This is based upon the outward appearance of the individual, the features and general contours of the face, the presence and distribution of hair upon it or evidence of shaving, the clothes, the figure, the habits, the inclinations, the voice and many other almost intangible minutiae of everyday experience.

The fact that presumptive evidence may be unreliable is revealed occasionally when men who have been posing as women for many years are brought before our Courts. The adoption of male attire by females with strong secondary male characteristics is more common but less publicised, as this is no offence in law.

Highly probable evidence of sex

The possession of external sexual structures—in the female developed breasts, the appropriate distribution of body hair, muscular development, distribution of subcutaneous fat and the vagina—in the male the absence of breast tissue, the general male physical characteristics and a penis.

Certain identification of sex

The presence of ovaries in the female and testes in the male. Cell sex data (*vide infra*).

Intersex states

During recent years great advances have been made into the investigation of intersex states. Sex identification in a living intersex state is no longer within the competence of the pathologist but is now the domain of the skilled cytogenetecist.

Davidson[12] divides the congenital intersex states into four groups.

Gonadal agenesis

In this condition the sexual organs (testes or ovaries) have never developed. This abnormality is determined very early in fetal life. The nuclear sex (*vide infra*) in these cases is negative.

Gonadal dysgenesis

In gonadal dysgenesis the external sexual structures are present but at puberty the testes or the ovaries fail to develop. These conditions are known as Klinefelter's syndrome and Turner's syndrome. The former refers to the male type of dysgenesis and the latter to the female type. In cases of Klinefelter's syndrome, although the anatomical structure is entirely male the nuclear sexing is female (chromatin positive) and in Turner's syndrome the nuclear sexing is negative.

True hermaphroditism

This is a state of bisexuality. Both ovaries and testicular tissue are present. The nuclear sex is usually female.

Pseudo-hermaphroditism

Pseudo-hermaphrodites are classified as male or female according to the presence of testes or ovaries, and independent of anomalies of the external genitalia which may be the reverse of normal. With pseudo-hermaphrodites nuclear sexing will normally give the true sex.

Other forms of intersex

Types of intersex may develop in a normal individual owing to the development of hormone secreting tumours or after the exhibition of hormones and steroids.

Nuclear sexing

In 1949 Barr & Bertram[13] noticed a nodule in the nuclei of some cells of the female cat. Later investigations revealed that this nodule was normally found in a percentage of all normal women's cells. When nodules are found, the person is said to be chromatin positive. These nodules are absent in men but may appear in certain types of intersex where the sex appears at first sight to be male. The examination of cells from the lining of the mouth and the examination of the white cells in the blood has now become a routine procedure in the determination of true sex where the anatomical development is abnormal.

Re-registration in cases of sex error

In any case in which it becomes clear that an error has been made about the sex of a child, the following procedure is to be followed:

Application for the re-registration of the birth should be made to the Registrar-General accompanied by the particulars of the case by the medical practitioner who has examined the child.

If this is satisfactory the Registrar would be instructed to re-register the birth on the information of one of the parents or other informant qualified under the Births or Deaths Registration Acts. Should there be no qualified informant available, then the original entry would be corrected on the authority of a statutory declaration made by two persons cognizant of the facts, one of whom would be the medical practitioner.

Determination of sex from human remains

The normal non-pregnant uterus and the uterus containing non-degenerating fibroid tumours is more resistant to putrefactive processes than the remaining and more vascular internal organs. The non-pregnant uterus is, therefore, usually the last of the internal organs to become destroyed by decomposition. The presence of a uterus is, of course, proof of sex.

When the sexual organs have disappeared, sex can only be determined by the secondary sexual characteristics which have developed in the skeleton. In the case where there is a complete adult skeleton available, sexing is unlikely to pose a problem. Where, however, the skeleton is prepubertal or there is some degree of intersex, even the experienced anthropologist or anatomist may be unable to sex the remains accurately.

The anatomist can usually sex an adult bone by visual examination. For presentation of his conclusions in Court, however, some more objective evidence is required. The female pelvis, on account of its development for child bearing, has always been the principal and most reliable indicator of sex. However, many bones may be used with a lesser degree of accuracy. The male bones are in general of larger dimensions than those of the female. Tables have been compiled from the measurements of a certain area of particular bone from both sexes. These measurements when tabulated will show an overlap of measurements where the sex is indeterminate, but one side or the other of the overlap will be either male or female. An improvement on this method is to take two measurements at right angles and express the differences as a ratio. These readings are also tabulated and there will again be an overlap where sex is undetermined by this method. The most recent application of these measurements is known as the discriminant function where the sex is determined by groups of measurements from different bones.[14]

The bones, excluding the pelvis, which have been extensively studied for the purpose of sexing human skeletal remains include: the skull, the mandible, the clavicle, the sternum, the scapula, the humerus and the femur. Krogman[7] claims that his degree of accuracy achieved in sexing adult skeletal remains is as follows:

Table 9.2

	%
The entire skeleton	100
The skull alone	90
The pelvis alone	95
The long bones alone	80
The skull and pelvis	98

Other anatomists in the field do not claim 100% accuracy even where the whole skeleton is available.

Iordanidis[15] published a series of papers dealing with the sexing of individual bones, excluding the pelvis, from the study of 300 skeletons. He concludes in his final paper[16] that it is possible to determine the sex of individual or paired bones with the following degree of certainty:

Table 9.3

	%
The skull and femurs	97.35
The coccyx and sacrum	97.18
The coccyx	92.25
The complete skull	91.38
The skull less the mandible	86.29
The sternum	80.18
The scapula	61.72
The sacrum	41.10
The femur	39.64
The atlas and axis	31.18
The clavicle	28.08
The mandible	26.24
The humerus	21.08
The radius and ulna	18.62
The calcaneum	14.72
The astragalus	13.36

Eliakis & Iordanidis[17] describe a method for sexing long bones by use of the medullary index. Their work is based upon the examination of 110 skeletons of each sex varying in age from 25–84 years. They found that the humerus, radius, ulna and tibia were the most reliable bones for this deter-

mination. A full description of their technique and the tables they compiled for individual bones may be found by reference to their original paper.

WEIGHT

Weight is generally of little assistance in establishing identity. Tables of average weights for age and stature are available, but these are only averages and the variations within any one stature age group are considerable. The weight of a particular individual may also show marked variations from time to time, and many acute and chronic diseases may also cause rapid and marked variation in weight.

The dead body loses weight rapidly after the onset of putrefaction, and may, with vermin infestation, become virtually skeletal. The weight of the body is, therefore, only of relative value as indicating that a person of certain stature is either of average build, or above or below the mean.

DEVELOPMENTAL, CONGENITAL OR ACQUIRED DEFECTS

The presence of any defect on a body may be a valuable factor in identification. It is natural, of course, that the greater and more uncommon the defect the greater its aid in establishing positive identification. Abnormalities of soft tissues disappear with decomposition and therefore have a limited application unless their presence is reflected by changes in the underlying skeleton.

Asymmetry and deformities

These may be congenital or acquired. An individual may be born with a congenital defect or a birth injury to some part of his nervous system which will lead to permanent weakness and lack of development to that part of the body supplied by the injured nerves. Torticollis or wryneck will not only produce the characteristic asymmetry of the soft tissues but also skeletal changes.

Congenital deformities such as harelip, cleft palate, polydactylism and hammer toes are frequently treated surgically and are therefore losing some of their past importance. Deformities of the chest due to rickets and certain occupations, e.g., cobbler, are becoming very rare.

Diseases of bone may cause gross skeletal changes. The acute kyphosis (hump back) associated with localised tuberculosis of the spine is but one example.

In old age degenerative changes which develop may cause symmetrical and asymmetrical deformities. As these tend to develop slowly, relatives or friends may not notice changes which appear so gross and obvious to the outsider.

Acquired diseases of the nervous system such as poliomyelitis result in soft tissue and skeletal wasting. Injury or arthritis of one joint will lead to wasting of the surrounding muscles.

Damage to the brain by injury or natural disease (stroke) may result in unilateral wasting, sometimes confined to certain groups of muscles, e.g., the arm or a leg.

There are many congenital skin blemishes such as 'port wine' stains, moles, etc., which may be characteristic.

Injuries

Injuries involving full skin thickness or causing fractures of bone will leave permanent marks. Injury to bone is a valuable aid when soft tissue decomposition is advanced as healed fractures are almost invariably recognised, even when healing has occurred without deformity. Limbs may have been amputated. The more severe the resulting deformity, the greater its aid in identification.

Scars

Scars may be caused by trauma involving the whole skin thickness by any crushing or penetrating injury, by fire, burns or scalds, by corrosive acids, electricity or radiation. Scars due to corrosive acids, burns or radiation are particularly liable to cause disfigurement, and keloid may develop in the scar tissue. Scars contract in time and small scars may be difficult to identify. Unsightly scars may also be removed artificially, by surgery, being replaced by smaller scars.

Striae gravidarum is the term given to the scars which appear on a woman's abdomen during the later months of pregnancy. Similar scars may occur in obesity and certain other conditions such as gross ascites, Cushing's syndrome, and after the prolonged use of steroids.

During recent years surgical techniques of skin closure have improved to the extent that it may be virtually impossible to identify a surgical scar macroscopically, especially if it is lying in a natural skin fold.

In the trial of Dr Crippen (C. C. C. 1910) for the murder of Cora Crippen (Belle Elmore), the presence of a 4-inch scar on a piece of abdominal skin was an important factor in the identification of the remains as those of the missing woman. It was proved in evidence that Mrs Crippen had had an operation in that part just before the marriage.

Time required for scar formation

This will vary according to the nature, size and position of the wound, the presence or absence of sepsis, the method of healing and the vascularity of the part. This latter factor is influenced by age and pathological conditions of the blood vessels.

A clean surgical wound (incised wound) will heal firmly in five to six days and a definite reddish scar will be apparent in less than two weeks. This method of healing is known as healing by first intention or primary repair, and occurs only when the edges of the wound can be approximated and there is no sepsis.

Secondary repair occurs when the edges cannot be approximated or sepsis is present. Granulation tissue covered by a scab forms in the base of the wound; after a few days the edges of the wound contract and then fresh skin grows out from the edges of the wound to cover the granulation tissue.

If the wound is large the skin will be unable to grow more than about 1 cm from the edges and if skin grafting is not undertaken a chronic ulcer will result. The introduction of sepsis may considerably enlarge the original wound.

Depending, thus, upon the size of the wound and the presence of infection, a scar may be formed within a week, or not be seen for two to three weeks. It is well known also that, owing to the depth and nature of the initial damage, burns by fire, chemicals and electricity heal indolently, often requiring grafts.

Age of scars

When a scar is first formed it is reddish or bluish in colour and tender. With age it contracts and becomes more dense, white and shiny. The normal cuticular pattern will not return and no hair follicles are present. If friction is applied to the scars of some individuals, even years after their formation, they may become reddish or bluish and some may remain tender. Once a scar has become contracted, it is impossible to date it.

Tattoos

Tattoo marks are designs effected by multiple small puncture wounds made through the skin with needles or similar penetrating tools dipped in colouring matter. The permanency depends upon the manner of the operation and the type of dye used. The colours commonly employed are indigo, cobalt, finely divided carbon, China ink, cinnabar, vermilion and cadmium selenide. Techniques and dyes vary from country to country and may assist in determining the origin of the tattoo.

Although there are a number of standard tattoo patterns, the distribution of these patterns over the body and the initials or names of loved ones, which are frequently incorporated, strengthen their value in identification.

In the notorious German Concentration Camp at Auschwitz prisoners had their prison numbers tattooed upon their arms. Special tattoos are sometimes used to achieve identification with a specific society or cult. The bluebird design on the back of the hand between the bases of the thumb and forefinger is commonly used by homosexuals. Some persons have their blood groups tattooed on them.

Tattoos may be developed post-mortem in naturally pigmented skin or in a mummified part by treating the skin with 0.5% caustic potash.

Tattoo marks have always been a valuable means of identification subject to the limitations already referred to.

Natural disappearance of tattoo marks

If the pigment has been deposited below the epidermis it will very slowly become fainter and certain pigments such as vermilion, cinnabar and ultramarine may eventually disappear after a minimum of 10 years. Some authorities assert that when carbon is deposited at this depth it will never disappear. Even when the less persistent dyes have disappeared from the skin they may be found in the regional lymph glands.

Tattoos may be removed surgically. Other means such as cautery result in scarring.

On the occasion of the second trial of the claimant of the Tichborne estates the possibility of the effacement of tattoo marks became a prominent question. It was well known that the missing baronet had been tattooed along the whole length of the forearm. The claimant had no tattoo marks, nor any signs of tattooing; but above the left wrist there was a large scar, as if a piece of the skin had been cut or burned out. Ferguson and Holt stated that nothing would remove a tattoo mark short of the knife or a cautery. The man Orton was said to have had the letters 'A. O.' tattooed on his arm. Evidently a clumsy attempt had been made to obliterate the implicating letters 'A. O.' on the wrist.

One of the most remarkable cases of identification from a tattoo mark is the so-called Sydney shark case. A man called James Smith disappeared on 8 April 1935, and was never seen again. On 22 April a shark was caught off the beach at Coogee and was sold to the aquarium—where after three days it vomited up a quantity of material including a human arm. The arm, which belonged to an adult male, was in a fairly good state of preservation, and, according to the medical evidence, had been severed from a dead body, not by a shark bite, but by a clumsy incision with a sharp instrument. On the forearm there was a tattooed design of two men boxing.

Several men whose arms were tattooed were missing, and finally the search was narrowed to two men, of whom James Smith was one. Smith's wife and brother both definitely identified the arm as that of Smith and fingerprint experts were able to support the identification. An arrest was made of an associate of Smith, one Patrick Brady, who was tried for murder at the C. C. C. Sydney, in September 1935. Truly a unique series of coincidences which led to positive identification of the missing man.

AGE

The establishment of the age of an individual has so many medico-legal bearings that it must be fully discussed. Inasmuch as even the age of the earliest embryo may have a bearing on the chastity of a woman, it is necessary to commence at the time at which an embryo can be distinguished, although the early products of conception have more connection with evidences of pregnancy and abortion than with identity.

It is convenient to discuss the evidences of age in periods:

1. The age of an embryo up to seven months (the threshold of viability).
2. The age of a fetus between seven months' intra-uterine life and full term.
3. The age of a child recently born.
4. The age of a child which has survived birth more than a day or two.
5. The age of an adult.

Age of embryo up to seven months

First Month. At the end of the third week the diameter of an ovum is two-thirds of an inch, the length of the embryo one-sixth of an inch; the amnion is formed; the embryo's back is curved, and the enlargement of its cephalic extremity marked. At the end of the fourth week the greatest diameter of the ovum is about seven-eights of an inch, its weight about forty grains; the length of the embryo is about one-third of an inch; the eyes, the ears, and the visceral arches are distinguishable. Four bud-like processes mark the commencement of the limbs. The umbilical vesicle is manifest, but smaller than the embryo. The amnion is not much distended and separated by an interval from the chorion.

Second Month. At the end of the second month the ovum is about one inch and three-quarters in its greatest diameter, and the embryo three-quarters of an inch long. The umbilical vesicle is very small, and hangs by a thin thread. The limbs are more manifest, the hand has a human appearance. Points of ossification have appeared in the lower jaw and clavicle. The mouth and nose are manifest. The Wolffian bodies have atrophied, and the kidneys have appeared.

Third Month. At the end of the third month the ovum is about four inches long, the placenta is formed, and the rest of the chorion has to a marked extent lost its villosity. The cord has now become long relatively to the fetus, and already shows its spiral twist. The fetus is four to four and a half inches long, and weighs about 450 grains. The head is separated from the body by the neck, and the oral from the nasal cavity by the palate, and the mouth is closed by the lips. The sexual organs have appeared, but the penis and clitoris are scarcely distinguishable. The limbs are developed, including the fingers and toes, and a first appearance of formation of nails can be detected. Points of ossification have appeared in most of the bones.

Fourth Month. At the end of the fourth month the fetus is, on an average, about six inches long, and weighs about three ounces. The sex can now be distinctly recognized. The bones of the skull have partly ossified, but still have very wide fontanelles and sutures. There is a slight commencement of the formation of down on the skin. Movements of the limbs have commenced; but these may, however, be detected in a freshly expelled embryo even before the end of the third month. *X-ray of the mother's abdomen may now reveal the fetus.*

Fifth Month. The fetus is, on an average, nine to ten inches long, and weighs nearly eleven ounces. Hair has appeared upon the head, and lanugo or down over the whole body. The skin begins to be covered with vernix caseosa. There is a centre of ossification in the calcaneum.

Sixth Month. The fetus is, on an average, about twelve inches long, and weighs about 24 ounces. The eyebrows and eyelashes are beginning to form. Subcutaneous fat is commencing to be deposited, but only in small degree, so that the skin is still wrinkled. There is a yellowish material in the small intestine, and there may be a commencing appearance of the darker meconium in the large intestine. The hair on the head is longer and less like down. A centre of ossification appears in the manubrian sterni.

Seventh Month. The fetus is about 14 inches long and weighs some two and a half to three pounds. The eyelids are opening and the pupillary membrane undergoing atrophy. The skin is reddish and loose, but the hair thickening and darkening. Ossification centres are present in the talus and (three) in the upper two-thirds of the sternum—appearing successively from above down. The testis is descending within the abdomen and may have reached the inguinal ring.

For further particulars the reader is referred to special works on embryology.[18] The term 'ovum' signifies the embryo *and* its membranous coverings; the 'embryo' is the body which is afterwards converted into the fetus; 'fetus' is the name applied to the embryo after the 3rd month of gestation.

One great difficulty consists in determining the nature of the supposed ovum or embryo in aborted matter in the first two months. In making the examination the material should be placed in a dish of water, and all coagula gently washed away or removed by some blunt instrument. If the embryo cannot be found, the decidua and chorion, or portions of them, may be recognised, the former by its forming the outer investment, with its smooth internal and rough external or uterine surface, the latter by its villous or shaggy appearance. Between the 3rd and 4th months the fetus may be commonly identified without much difficulty. The ovum in many instances escapes first, leaving the decidua behind. When a semi-decomposed or dried mass of blood clot, etc., is presented for examination, it is often convenient to take an X-ray plate of the specimen. If the fetus is about the 3rd month onwards the ossified ribs and limb bones will be seen. It is important to remember that, in some states of the virgin, decidua-like structures are shed from the uterine mucous membrane which, when examined by the microscope, are like the true decidua. Both are constituted of the innermost portion of the uterine mucous membrane, and contain all its elements. It requires a skilled microscopist to distinguish placental tissue with certainty. Evidence of this nature formed the basis of the libel action *Kitson* v. *Playfair*, in which Dr Playfair threw doubts on the chastity of the plaintiff.

Such are the principal points we have for determining the age of the contents of the uterus in the early stages of pregnancy.

The points themselves are of such a nature that, while it is easy to give approximate estimations, it is quite impossible to draw hard and fast lines between say the 2nd and 3rd months and between the 3rd and 4th; and these are precisely the cases in which lawyers will attempt, in defence of a woman's chastity, to obtain an opinion when, for instance, the last possible date of connection is five months, and a fetus is born which might be of three, four or five months'development. The great variability in development renders it essential for the medical witness to fix reasonably wide limits and to leave the decision to other evidence and to the jury.

With regard to the question of live-birth in immature fetuses *vide* 'Live-birth (ch. 15). At seven months the fetus becomes 'viable', that is,

capable at law of a separate existence, but it may survive if born as early even as the 5th month.

Age between seven months and full term (10 lunar months)

The following description of the child between seven and nine months corresponds very closely with those in most text-books on midwifery:

Between the Seventh and Eighth Months. The child measures between 14 and 16 inches in length, and weighs from three to four pounds. The skin is thick, of a more decidedly fibrous structure, and covered with a white unctuous vernix caseosa which now first appears. Fat is deposited in the cellular tissues, whereby the body becomes plump; the skin previously to this is of a reddish colour, and commonly more or less shrivelled; the nails, which are fairly firm, do not quite reach to the extremities of the fingers; the hair becomes long, thick, and coloured; ossification advances throughout the skeleton; the talus shows a centre of ossification; valvulae conniventes appear in the small intestines; and meconium is found occupying the caecum and colon. The testicles in the male are considered about this period to make their descent, towards the scrotum. The time at which these organs change their situation is probably subject to variation; in the abdomen at the seventh, and in the scrotum at the ninth month, at the eighth month they will commonly be found in the inguinal canals. Its absence from the scrotum at birth does not necessarily indicate that the child is immature, because the organ sometimes does not reach the scrotum until after birth, and sometimes not at all.

Between the Eighth and Ninth Months. The child is from 16 to 18 inches in length, and weighs from four to five pounds. The membrane pupillares have disappeared. The quantity of fat deposited beneath the skin is increased, and the hair and nails are well developed. The surface of the brain is grooved or fissured but presents no regular convolutions. The meconium occupies almost entirely the large intestines; and the gall-bladder contains some traces of liquid resembling bile. The testicles in the male may be found occupying some part of the inguinal canal, or they may be in the scrotum. The left testicle is sometimes in the scrotum, while the right is situated about the external ring. A centre of ossification appears in the lower epiphysis of the femur.

Table 9.4

Age lunar month	Length(L)		Surface areas(S)	Weight(W)	
	cm	inch	sq cm	g	lb
Ovum	1/93	—	1/28 000	1/1 700 000	—
2	2.6	1.0	—	—	—
3	2.0	3.5	42	19	—
4	16.7	6.6	171	100	$\frac{1}{4}$
5	24.3	4.7	402	312	$\frac{3}{4}$
6	31.1	12.2	706	667	$1\frac{1}{2}$
7	37.1	14.5	1055	1151	$2\frac{1}{2}$
8	42.4	17.7	1430	1754	4
9	47.0	18.7	1809	2396	$5\frac{1}{4}$
10	51.0	20.0	2178	3087	7

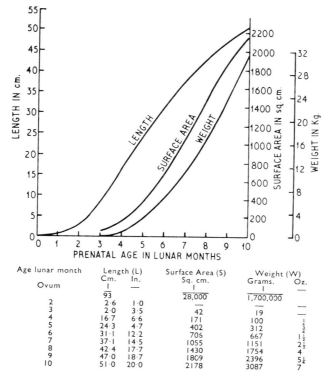

Age lunar month	Length (L) Cm.	Length (L) In.	Surface Area (S) Sq. cm.	Weight (W) Grams.	Weight (W) Oz.
Ovum	l	—	l	l	—
	93		28,000	1,700,000	—
2	2·6	1·0	—	19	—
3	2·0	3·5	42	100	—
4	16·7	6·6	171	312	$\frac{1}{4}$
5	24·3	4·7	402	667	$\frac{3}{4}$
6	31·1	12·2	706	1151	$1\frac{1}{2}$
7	37·1	14·5	1055	1754	$2\frac{1}{2}$
8	42·4	17·7	1430	2396	4
9	47·0	18·7	1809	3087	$5\frac{1}{4}$
10	51·0	20·0	2178		7

Fig. 9.4 After Edith Boyd, from Scammon in Morris' Human Anatomy.

Tenth Month: Signs of Maturity. At the tenth month the average length of the body is about 20 inches, and its weight from six to eight pounds [Fig. 9.4]. The male child is generally rather longer, and weighs rather more than the female. Considerable variation in length and weight occurs. Children are sometimes born mature and survive which weighs less than five pounds. On the other hand, records of the birth of a child weighing 18lb 5oz, and lengths of 24 and 32 inches also exist.

By the end of the 10th month the centre of ossification in the lower epiphysis of the femur measures about a $\frac{1}{4}$ in in diameter. Great stress is placed on the size at this point of ossification in the lower epiphysis of the thigh bone (femur) in its bearings upon the maturity of the fetus. This point usually makes its appearance at the 36–37th week; at the 37–38th week it is commonly about $\frac{1}{4}$ inch in diameter; and at the full period it is $\frac{1}{4}$ to $\frac{1}{3}$ inch in diameter. When the point of ossification has reached this size it may be confidently affirmed that the fetus has reached the full period, but the size of the centre is subject to some slight variation.

A centre of ossification is usually found in the head of the tibia and one in the cuboid bone of the foot in full-term well developed children.

At the full-term the head of a child forms nearly one-quarter of the whole length of the body. The cellular tissue is filled with fat, so as to give considerable plumpness to the whole form, while the limbs are firm, hard and rounded; the skin is pale; the hair is thick, long and somewhat abundant; the nails are fully developed, and reach to the ends of the fingers—an appearance, however, which may be sometimes simulated in a premature child by the shrinking of the skin after death. Ossification will be found to have advanced considerably throughout the skeleton. The surface of the brain presents convolutions, and the grey matter begins to show itself.

The characters given at the different stages of gestation must be regarded as representing an average statement. They are, it is well known, open to numerous exceptions. Twins are generally

Table 9.5

	6 months	7 months	8 months	9 months
Length	About 12 inches	About 14 inches	About 16 inches	18 to 20 inches
Weight	1½ to 2 lb	3 to 3½ lb	4 to 5 lb	6 to 8 lb
Skin	Red and wrinkled	Paler and smoother	Sebaceous matter forming	Copious vernix
Fat	No subcutaneous fat	Fat beginning to be deposited	Child plump	
Scrotum	Empty	—	Corrugated	Occupied by testes
Testes	On psoas muscle	Near the internal ring	In canal (L before R)	In scrotum (L before R)
Sex	Well differentiated			
Hair	Lanugo	Scalp 'downy' with lanugo	—	Hair on scalp 1 inch long
Nails	—	Nearing finger-tips	Reach end of fingers	Project over fingers. Reach end of toes
Eyelids	Adherent	Non-adherent eyelashes present	Well formed	
Brain	Sylvian fissure formed			
Intestine	Meconium in small intestine	Meconium in large intestine		
Centres of ossification appear	Manubrium and os calcis	Astragalus (talus)	Lower epiphysis of femur	Cuboid, upper epiphysis of tibia
Placenta weight	9 to 10 oz	12 to 13 oz	About 15 oz	16 to 18 oz

smaller and less developed than single children; the average weight of a twin child is not often more than 6 lb, and is very often below this. The safest rule to follow in endeavouring to determine the intra-uterine age of a child is to rely upon a majority of the characters which it presents. That child only can be regarded as mature which presents the greater number of the characters found at the ninth month of gestation.

It is convenient to remember that the length of the child in inches during the later stages of pregnancy is about double the intra-uterine age in months. Hesse's rule[19] states that the square of the number of months gestation gives the length of the fetus in centimetres.

The age of a child recently born

We have now to deal with a different class of age data from those we have hitherto considered. We have to consider for how long the child has lived, and we assume that there is definite evidence of some duration of life. Under 'infanticide' will be found a full discussion of the evidence bearing upon this assumption (*vide* ch. 15).

Changes in the lungs

Whether gross or microscopic, and changes in the fetal circulation will not be of much assistance, though they may be of great importance in deciding whether the child was born alive (*vide* Live-birth). We have mainly to rely upon changes in the umbilical cord, changes in weight and stature, and the progressive disappearance of the 'fetal' form of haemoglobin during the first six months in endeavouring to determine the age of a newborn child, and it must be admitted that none of them yields very decisive indications.

Changes in the umbilical cord

These are the most trustworthy of any data we have, for the changes are due to vital processes, and are dictated by conditions of atrophy and healing which pursue a fairly regular course. Thus when the cord is tied and severed in the usual way the portion left adherent to the body begins to dry up in from 12 to 24 h, and in about 24 h from birth a ring of inflammation makes its appearance round the site of its insertion. This inflammatory redness must not be mistaken for the thin red circle which is almost constantly present at birth. About the 3rd or 4th day the drying of the cord is complete, and the dried portion separates from the navel on about the 4th or 5th day, leaving a raw area which takes from seven to 12 days to heal completely. Hence if a child is found with well-marked inflammation or a raw area at the umbilicus a very reasonable approximation may be made to the time that it lived after birth, though even here the different rates at which wounds heal in healthy and unhealthy children must render the judgement somewhat tentative.

It was formerly stated that if a child had lived two or three days, long enough, that is, for the cord appreciably to mummify, no amount of soaking in water would cause a *restitutio ad integrum* in the dried parts, but this statement is much too positive. A dried cord swells up, and, except that it may be a little darker, it is difficult to distinguish from a cord which has not become dry before soaking. Children's bodies at this stage are frequently thrown into water, and in bodies thus recovered a dried piece of cord suggests two or three days' exposure to air before immersion.

Weight

If we consider the extreme limits for the weights of newborn children and then remember that we have no means of knowing what the weight of a child was at birth, it can be seen that the absolute weight of a child found dead is of no use in estimating how long it lived—when it is probable from other reasons that it was a few days or weeks old.

The body of an infant found in an attaché case at Ashford was too dry to give its weight any significance. The length and the size of the lower femoral and upper tibial ossification centres suggested it was 'somewhere about two months old'. The mother, when traced, said it was four months old: further questioning elicited the important fact that birth was two months premature. To her it was four months old, but its development was that of an infant of about half that age. Ageing could only be approximate.

Height

Precisely the same reasoning applies to the length of a newborn child. The birth length is too variable, and therefore the initial basis for comparison is not available.

The following may be taken as a summary of the appearances observable in the body of a child that has survived its birth for the undermentioned periods:

After 24h. The skin is firm and less red than soon after birth. The umbilical cord is somewhat shrivelled, although it remains soft and bluish-coloured from the point where it is secured by a ligature to its insertion in the skin of the abdomen. The meconium may be discharged, but a green-coloured mucus is found in the large intestines. The lungs may be more or less distended with air, but it should be remembered that though, when these organs are fully and perfectly distended, the inference is that the child has probably survived some hours, the converse of this proposition is not always correct. When the lungs contain a small quantity of air it does not follow that the child must have died immediately after it was born.

From the 2nd to the 3rd day. The skin has a yellowish tinge; the cuticle sometimes appears cracked, a change which precedes its separation in scales. The umbilical cord is brown and dry between the ligature and the abdomen: its vessels are thrombosed.

From the 3rd to the 4th day. The skin is more yellow, and there is an evident separation of the cuticle from the skin of the chest and abdomen. The umbilical cord is of a brownish-red colour, flattened, semi-transparent and twisted. The skin in contact with the dried portion presents a ring of vascularity or redness, gradually shaded off towards the abdomen. The colon is by now free from any traces of green mucus.

From the 4th to the 6th day. The cuticle in various parts of the body is found separating in the form of minute scales or a fine powder. The umbilical cord separates from the abdomen usually about the 5th day, but sometimes not until the 8th or 10th day. If the umbilical aperture is cicatrised and healed, it is probable that the child lived for three weeks to a month after birth. The ductus arteriosus may be found contracted both in length and diameter.

From the 6th to the 12th day. The cuticle will be found separating from the skin of the limbs. If the umbilical cord was small, cicatrisation will have taken place before the 10th day after birth; if large, a seropurulent discharge may sometimes continue to escape from it for 25 to 30 days. The ductus arteriosus may become entirely closed during this period, but this is open to exceptions, which are pointed out elsewhere. The body rapidly increases in size and weight when the child has enjoyed active existence and adequate feeding.

On the whole, it can be seen that the signs of survival for short periods after birth are not very distinct, and it is in some respects fortunate that great precision in assigning the time of survival is rarely demanded of medical witnesses. It is sufficient in law that a child did, in fact, achieve a separate existence.

It is expected, however, that a medical person will be able to distinguish between a newborn child and one which has been born for several days; evidence on this subject is occasionally required in reference to supposititious children. Those who attempt a fraud of this kind have sometimes been compelled to substitute a child two or three days old for one just born. A medical person called into a woman after an alleged delivery in the presence of a nurse (perhaps an accomplice) is bound to exercise great caution. In the event of litigation at a subsequent date, he is expected to be able to inform a Court of the condition of the child when first seen by him and of the probable date of its birth. He will not be allowed to throw the blame for a mistake upon others. Success or failure in penetrating a fraud of this kind will depend upon the doctor's alertness.

R. v. Ward was a case of some difficulty respecting the identity of a child alleged to have been murdered. The dead body of a child which had survived its birth was found wrapped in clothing and concealed near a highroad by which the woman charged with murder had been seen to pass on a certain day. The doctor who examined the body thought that from its state the child had been dead a month, and that it was some 10 days old at death. The child of the accused had disappeared when it was about a fortnight old.

The defence was that the child whose body was found was not that of the accused. The child found, as well also as that of the woman, was male, and had light hair but the age created doubt and, upon this evidence, the accused was acquitted.

This old case serves as a warning of the legitimate limits of medical evidence. When the body of a child has been lying putrefying for a month, it is difficult to suppose that it could yield evidence on so fine a point as to whether it were 10 or 14 days old.

Estimation of age in a child which has survived birth for a longer period

In the absence of documentary proof, the estimation of the age of a living child can be only approximate until it arrives at the time when dentition commences. The height and weight may afford some little assistance, but it must be remembered that there is a difference in the rapidity of growth not only in children of a different sex, but also in those of the same sex, and not only in single births, but even in the case of twins. One may flourish and grow while the other remains puny. The average that is ordinarily expected is that a child should measure about 2 ft by the end of the first year, and should weigh about 20 lb, with proportionate increase from birth upwards.

The following table 9.6 gives the average monthly weights of children during the first year of life. It can be seen that during the first year the gain in weight each month is approximately 1 lb.

Table 9.6

	lb	oz		lb	oz
At birth	6	8	7 months	13	4
1 month	7	4	8 months	14	4
2 months	8	4	9 months	15	8
3 months	9	6	10 months	16	8
4 months	10	8	11 months	17	8
5 months	11	8	12 months	18	8
6 months	12	4			

Age from one year to puberty

When the teeth commence to erupt they form (*vide* p. 197) the most reliable means for the estimation of the age of a child from about the age of six months to puberty, whether the child be living or dead; it is possible by X-ray examination to corroborate such evidence from the ossification of the bones, for which purpose Table 9.7 is here inserted showing the principal points in such ossification. The figures must not be taken too rigidly, but only as implying an average. For a review of the subject see Boyd[20] or Noback.[21]

The female is usually a year or so ahead of the male in fusion dates.

If all the epiphyses are found united, the indi-

Table 9.7A Appearance of other points of ossification[22]

	Foot	Hand
5th–6th month, intra-uterine	Calcaneous (body)	Whole hand cartilaginous during intrauterine life
7th month, intra-uterine	Talus	
9th month, intra-uterine	Cuboid	
1st year, extra-uterine	External cuneiform	Capitate and hamate
2nd year, extra-uterine	(1–2)	First four metacarpal heads
3rd year, extra-uterine	Internal cuneiform, tarsal navicular	Triquetral (2–3)
4th year, extra-uterine	Midcuneiform	Lunate (4–5)
5th year, extra-uterine	Scaphoid (4–5)	Trapezium (5–6), carpal navicular
6th year, extra-uterine		Scaphoid (6–7)
8th year, extra-uterine		Trapezoid
10th year, extra-uterine	Calcaneous (epiphysis) (9–10)	Pisiform (f, 9–10; m, 10–11)

Table 9.7B Appearance of other points of ossification

1st year	Heads of humerus, femur and tibia
2nd year	Lower ends of radius, tibia and fibula
3rd year	Patella
4th year	Upper end of fibula, great trochanter of femur (4–5)
5th year	Lower end of fibula, greater tubercle of humerus
6th year	Head of radius, lower end of ulna
8th–9th years	Rami of ischium and pubis, olecranon
10th–11th years	Trochlea of humerus, lesser trochanter of femur
12th–14th years	External condyle of humerus
14th–16th years	Acromion, iliac crest, lesser trochanter
17th–19th years	Tuber ischii (17 in female, 19 in male), inner clavicle (20–21)

Table 9.7C Union of bones and epiphyses

By 1½ years	The anterior fontanelles should be closed
By 4–5 years	The greater tubercle fuses with head of humerus
By 9 years	The ilium, pubes and ischium should meet in the acetabulum: rami of ischium and pubis fuse
By 13 years	These three should be united but still separable on maceration
By 15 years	The coracoid should be united to the scapula
By 16 years	The olecranon should be united to the ulna
By 16–17 years	The head of the radius and the lower end of the humerus should be joined to their respective shafts
By 17–18 years	The internal epicondyle should be united to the humerus
By 18–20 years	The head of the femur should have joined the diaphysis
By 18–20 years	The epiphyses of the long bones of hand and foot should have united to the diaphyses
By 20 years	The epiphyses of the fibula should be united to the diaphysis. Distal radius unites
By 22 years	The inner (secondary) epiphysis of the clavicle fuses
By 25 years	The crest of the ilium and the articular facets of the ribs should be united

vidual is almost certainly over 25 years of age, and if the three parts of the sternum are united by bone, almost certainly 35 or over.

As stated above, these points can be investigated with almost the same accuracy in the living as in the dead by means of X-rays.

There is a tendency for the epiphyseal centres to appear earlier and for the union of epiphyses to the shafts to take place earlier in the female.

It has also been shown by many observers that in tropical climates ossification takes place earlier than in temperate zones. In Ceylon, for example, Webster & de Saram[23] have shown that ossific centres appear and epiphyseal union takes place at least two years earlier in males and three and a half years earlier in females as compared with standards recognised in temperate climates. Hepworth[24] and Pillai[25] have come to the same conclusion about ossification in India.

Height and weight

These are too variable to be of much use, but the foregoing Table and graph shows the averages with which a given individual may be compared.

Sex changes

The gradual growth of hair on the pubes, commencing with a soft downy growth at about 10 to 13, is a little more reliable, showing at least an approach to puberty. The development of the breasts in girls is variable. In boys the voice undergoes a marked change as puberty comes on, losing its shrill infantile treble and taking on a deeper note, tenor or bass—'the breaking of the voice' in common speech. It must be stated that tastes, habits and inclinations usually vary somewhat with age in children (comparing only members of the same sex), but some boys of 15 are almost men in these respects, and others still children; and the same may be said of girls, some of whom are married at 16, while others at the same age are still schoolgirls.

Precocity

Cases of extraordinary precocity, although not frequent, are by no means rare: many cases of menstruation in girls from six years of age are reported, with excessive development of the breasts and pubic hair.

Kerr[26] records the case of a girl aged six years ten months who began to menstruate at the age of three-and-a-half years. She had well developed breasts and a prominent mons veneris on which there was fine dark hair. The uterus was almost of adult size.

Tumours or excessive development of the suprarenal cortex or of the pituitary gland will, of course, result in anomalies of sex development for the age.

Age in adults

After the age of 25 the estimation of age becomes more uncertain, whether in the living or the dead. It is true that common knowledge comes more or less to our aid, enabling us to make a fair approximation to the decade within which a person may be, but any closer approximation must be made with considerable reservation. Premature ageing may easily be produced by illness, malnutrition, suffering, anxiety or worry; white hair often comes on in quite young people from grief or shock, and often for no reason that can be estimated; calcified arteries and arcus senilis (in the eye) are rarely seen before 40, but after that age they are of little value in estimating the age.

It is difficult to achieve an accuracy of even five years in estimating the age after the full permanent dentition and fusion of all centres of ossification have become established—that is, at about 23 to 25 years. The ossification of cartilage in the hyoid, larynx and ribs, the fusion of the greater horns of the hyoid to the body, and of the manubrium and xyphisternum with the body of the sternum, changes in the appearance of the cartilage lining, the joints and lipping of the bones, all of which occur somewhere between 40 and 60, may be suggestive of advancing age but give no precise evidence. The gradual loss of teeth and changing shape of the lower jaw as it becomes edentulous equally offer no data of precision. Other sources of information on adult age, such as that suggested by Gustafson[27] (*vide* p. 200), may give further evidence on this important matter.

It is manifest that not one of the observations can be relied upon to give a precise age but a careful consideration of all factors may enable us to give an approximation.

Age in skeletal remains

The value of the teeth in estimating the age of skeletal remains has been dealt with in chapter 10. This section will concern itself with the remainder of the skeleton.

The skeleton is largely developed from cartilage through a series of 'centres of ossification' from which bone is laid down in the cartilage. It is estimated that some 800 centres are present by the 11th week of gestation. These centres coalesce and disappear and other ones are formed. At birth there are some 450 centres of ossification present. From birth until 25 years the age may be estimated from the state of development and incorporation of these centres.

The appearance and disappearance of these centres of ossification varies between the sexes, appearing as a general rule earlier in young females. Tables giving their order of appearance and disappearance have been compiled by several workers in this field. There is no place in this text for these details which should be gathered from the original papers.[28-30] Mckern & Stewart[28] developed a point system based upon the state of union of nine epiphyses. By referring this total point count to a table the predicted age and age range can be read off. As the points scale increases so the age range becomes greater.

Over the age of 25, and especially between the ages of 25 and 40, the estimation of age becomes more difficult. For many years the closure of the skull sutures was considered the most accurate method. Recent work has shown that there is too much variation in closure times to merit the use of this method in forensic work. The most accurate of the more recent investigations is that of Todd & Lyon,[31] who studied the closure of the endocranial suture line in white and black males (the closure of the endocranial suture line is more constant than the ectocranial suture line). They eliminated any skulls which showed abnormal suture closure or retardation of closure. These abnormalities in closure, unless very gross, are unlikely to be recognised by anyone other than a skilled anatomist. This, therefore, places a limit upon the value of their

observations to the inexperienced anthropologist.

For many years anthropologists have studied regression changes in long bones. The earlier investigations provided no advance upon the accepted methods of age determination from skeletal remains. More recently, however, advances have been made in this field[32-34] and this method may receive more attention in future from forensic pathologists.

The changes occurring on the articular surface of the symphysis pubis are now considered the best index for ageing male skeletons. In female skeletons, parturition has a modifying effect upon the order of change. When the changes in the symphysis pubis are correlated with other skeletal criteria, Krogman[7] ventures an accuracy of ± two years.

The importance of the symphysis pubis in skeletal age determination was first recognised by Todd [35, 36]. Todd's original work was reviewed and expanded by Brooks[37]. McKern & Stewart[30] developed an alternative system based upon their examination of 349 symphyses of young American males killed during the Korean war. McKern and Stewart's cases are taken mainly from the pre-30 age group, whereas Todd's cases (over 300), were largely from the post-30 age group. Both the Todd and the McKern and Stewart systems are fully described by Stewart[9] in his recent monograph. A system for estimating the age of females from their pubic symphyses has been evolved by Gilbert & McKern[38]. The deviation is greater than with the male symphyses on account of parturition trauma which may be difficult to assess.

HANDEDNESS AND RECONSTRUCTION OF FEATURES

Handedness

Whether the deceased was right or left handed may sometimes be ascertained in the recently dead from greater muscular development in the dominant limb and certain occupational markings. In recent years some work has been done on determining the handedness of skeletal material. These investigations have not proceeded as far as might be anticipated, as there are rarely records of a person's handedness available to the researcher. However, occasionally changes between the upper limbs may be such as to enable a confident opinion to be given. In general terms the dominant limb is longer, the glenoid cavity may show specific changes and arthritic changes are more pronounced in later life. The present state of research may be found in Stewart's monograph.[9]

Reconstruction of the features from the skull

Attempts to reproduce the features of an individual upon a skull have been attempted over many years in both criminal and historical cases without any uniform success. The final reproduction depends much upon the ingenuity of the artist after the anthropologist has presented him with all the information (e.g., sex, stature, age, etc.) amassed from the skeletal remains.

DACTYLOGRAPHY (Fingerprint system)

As long ago as the seventh century finger-tip imprints in ink were in use in the Far East as evidence of good faith in the sealing of bonds or the issue of documents. The British Museum has a MS dated A D 782 bearing such impressions 'Being [marked] in the presence of each other'.[39] Such marks were, however, not comparable with the ball prints used for modern identification, consisting merely of blobs of ink made by the finger-tips; they lacked ridge patterns and cannot, therefore, have been of much use in identifying their signatures.

The first recorded instance of a fingerprint having been used to prove the identity of a murderer was in the Argentine in 1892 (the case of Francesca Rojas). In Great Britain the first case was *R. v. Stratton* and there was another in 1905 although in 1902 fingerprint evidence was used to convict a burglar.

The modern system of dactylography depends upon the development by the time of birth of a fine pattern of ridges on the skin of the balls of the fingers and thumbs, parts of the palms and the soles of the feet. These patterns have a major design which enables them to be placed in groups for primary classification, and a considerable amount of finer detail—of branching and coalescence of ridges, of island, core and delta arrangements permitting subgrouping, and an unlimited quantity of extremely fine pore details along individual ridges. The Henry, Conlay Fleck or Battley 'single-print' systems refer to police methods of classifying such records in such a way as to make them easy to refer to for the purpose of comparison.

Classification

These details enable fingerprints to be classified primarily as loops (about 67%) of which all but some 5% are 'ulnar', i.e., open out towards the ulnar border of the arm, whorls (about 25%) and arches (6 to 7%) or more composite forms comprising the remaining 1 to 2%. Line tracing and counting enables these main groups to be broken down into sub-groups, and final identification is effected by a study of ridge pattern.

In practice 16 to 20 points of fine comparison are accepted as proof of identify, but, of course, an unlimited amount of detail is available in any small area—even a small part of a single print. Details of these can be accurately teleprinted for comparison in modern crime-file departments, so that a search of the records, a comparison and a reply need take only a few hours. The details that are present at birth remain for the rest of the individual's life, unalterable, capable of defacement only at the expense of a series of new identity data—the scars left when the defacing injuries heal.

Palm and footprints may also provide similar material for comparison.

In April 1942, an old pawnbroker was found suffering from head injuries near a rifled safe in the basement of his shop at Shoreditch, London: he died several days later. A single palmprint on the safe door led to the conviction of two men who had planned a raid of this calibre—though possibly never intending murder (*R. v. Dashwood and Silverosa*, C. C. C. 1942).

A safe robbery occurred in Lanarkshire in 1952 and examination of the premises revealed some bare footprints in a film of flour on a hard floor. On the safe two further prints were found, and one of these showed clear ridge details of a great toe. About a month later a well-known safe blower was arrested on enclosed premises, and taken into custody. He was cautioned and charged with the safe blowing robbery: prints of his bare feet gave an exact comparison (from the left big toe) with the print found on the safe at the scene: 22 points of similarity were noted. A conviction followed[40].

Footprints are also used in American maternity hospitals as a means of identifying the babies of maternity cases which might be inadvertently mixed.

The individuality of the fingerprint

The credit of introducing the fingerprint to crime records undoubtedly lies with two Englishmen, Dr Henry Faulds, who first published an account of the method in a letter to *Nature* on 28 October 1880, and to Sir William Herschel. Faulds was undoubtedly aware of the importance not only of the 10 finger records for identification but also of the possibility of recognising chance impressions or identifying mutilated remains in this way; unfortunately, Herschel claimed a precedence for using the method of some 20 years, and had, it would appear, submitted a report in 1877 asking that the method be used as a means of identifying prisoners. An acrimonious dispute over priority achieved no decision, but it appears that Faulds should be given priority. It remained for Sir Francis Galton to prove the individuality and permanence of the fingerprint and to devise a classification for criminal records which was later simplified by Sir Edward Henry of New Scotland Yard.

No doubt can possibly be entertained, as experience has increased, but that the finger ridge patterns emphasised by Locard as being so individual are in fact so—and permanently so.

Galton estimated the chances of similar prints from different fingers as being something like 1 in 64 thousand million: it was a speculation. It is more significant to remark that never yet in the world's crime records have two identical fingerprints been seen, unless from the same finger.

Techniques of fingerprinting

Dactylography is a progressing science and new methods for the recording, lifting and developing of prints under different field conditions, including those on a decomposed body, appear regularly. The technical details are too involved for inclusion in this volume and detailed information should be sought in the various specialist publications upon the subject.

DETERMINATION OF RACE FROM SKELETAL REMAINS

The determination of race from skeletal remains is hazardous as marked facial differences seen in life are not reproduced in the skull except in the stereotypes. In the United States the blacks have tended to lose the pronounced traits of their African forebears and their skulls now closely resemble those of white Americans. Interbreeding between races has made identification very difficult or impossible. Even between skulls of the same race there will be a considerable overlap of features with those of another race. The identity of the race of skeletal remains occasionally arises in forensic cases. These cases should always be referred to an anthropologist.

HAIR AS A FACTOR OF CRIMINAL EVIDENCE

In this connection hair may assume a position of outstanding importance. It is frequently found at the scene of a crime, or upon the victim or suspect, as contact or trace evidence. Not only may a few strands of head hair be found on clothing but some may be found in the hands of a victim of an assault, and in rape pubic hair may be transferred from the assailant to the victim and vice versa. In hit-and-run car accidents, some of the victim's hair may be found upon the vehicle involved in the accident.

In view of its importance as trace evidence much research has been carried out in an attempt to positively identify hair as having come from one individual. In fact, it was hoped at one time that hair would have the specificity of fingerprints. This is not so, but nevertheless the examination of hairs has advanced sufficiently in recent years for the forensic scientist to provide a great deal of information from his examination.

Samples of hair are taken as a routine exhibit from all homicide victims, hit-and-run victims and usually from persons who have been assaulted. Usually samples of head and pubic hair are taken but sometimes eyebrows, moustache or beard and body hair are also removed.

A sample suspected to be hair must be differentiated from a natural or synthetic fibre and it must be decided whether it is of human or animal origin. Human head hair differs in microscopic appearance from animal hair and natural or synthetic fibres have an entirely different appearance from animal or human hair. Hair from different parts of the body, e.g., head, pubic, eyebrows, can be differentiated and there are also characteristic differences between some ethnic groups. Sexing and identification of the owner's blood group may be possible. Variations in head hair of one individual are such that it is not possible to age an adult from its examination. The identity of the origin of hairs becomes more specific the greater the number available for examination.

The questions that the scientist must attempt to answer are:
1. Is the material hair or some other fibre?
2. If a fibre, what is it?
3. If hair, is it human or animal?
4. If human, from what part of the body did it originate?
5. If human, is it male or female?
6. If human, what is the blood group?
7. Are the hairs identical with those of the victim or suspect?
8. Are there any special features?
   a. ethnic,
   b. how and when cut,
   c. presence of dyes, etc.,
   d. any adherent foreign material.

ANTHROPOMETRY (Bertillon's system)

In 1882 Alphonse Bertillon proposed a system of elaborating the general descriptive data circulated for a wanted or missing man by supplying exact measurements of various parts of the body. This system was soon adopted by the French Government, but has now been replaced by the more exact system of dactylography.

IDENTIFICATION OF FRAGMENTARY REMAINS

Not infrequently bones or fragments of soft tissues are found disposed of in the open, in ditches or rubbish dumps, etc., and this material is brought to the forensic pathologist for examination. Many of the procedures and techniques employed have already been discussed and the reader is referred to these sections.

The first problem which confronts the examiner is whether the material is animal or vegetable and, if animal, whether it is of human origin. The variety of objects brought for examination is unending and includes unusual fungi, animal entrails, butcher's bones, animal remains and human remains, including uncrushed cremated remains.

The majority of the objects produced can be identified with little trouble. Thoracic viscera of animals, for example, can be separated from those of human origin by the length of the trachea. Most animal bones can be readily identified as non-human by reference to standard textbooks on anatomy. When one is confronted by small portions of soft tissue, the human precipitin reaction may be employed.

A bear's paw is occasionally confused with a human hand. This problem is well recognised in the United States,[41] and on at least one occasion a bear's paw, which was first mistakenly identified as human, led to extensive police investigations in Great Britain.

Fragments of bone may constitute a difficult problem and the services of a skilled comparative anatomist are required, this investigation being beyond the competence of the medico-legal pathologist.

Where one is in possession of one or more complete bones, the age, height and sex of the individual may be estimated with some degree of accuracy.

HOW LONG HAVE THE REMAINS BEEN INTERRED?

In these days of urban development skeletal remains are often uncovered by workmen and mechanical diggers. The question which must be answered is: are these bones of recent origin or are they ancient remains? Reference to the local archives may be of assistance. It is often found that the development is taking place over the site of an old manor house or near an old church or monastery. In London several uncharted plague pits have been exposed during rebuilding.

Holes and cracks in such bones are more than likely to be due to the inadvertent or frankly careless use of digging or trenching tools. The freshness and lack of healing along fracture edges will indicate their newness.

When all of the soft tissues have disappeared an estimation of the length of interment must be based not only on the appearance of the skeletal remains by also upon all the local information available. It must be understood that merely from the examination of the bones no exact time can be given. One can estimate that the skeleton has lain there in spans of 50 or 100 years and one's opinion should be based upon knowledge derived from the examination of skeletal remains of the same order where the duration of interment is known. Disintegration of bones varies from locality to locality according to the soil and its water content. Bones tend to absorb iron salts, pigments and fine sand from the percolation of water and may become heavily impregnated, so that after many years they are dark in colour and weigh more than the original dry bone. All that is expected of the examiner for medico-legal purposes is an opinion that the bones are of recent or long interment. Police are naturally not interested in interments of over 70 years.

In 1954, suspicion long felt that the famous Piltdown jaw was anthropoid and did not belong to the skull which was alleged to have been found in the same area was confirmed by the finding that it had been artificially coated with mineral pigment, that its fluorine content differed considerably from that of the skull and that the grinding surfaces of the teeth had been artificially filed[42]

SKELETAL REMAINS

Cause of death

Indication of violent death may be obtained long after the disappearance of all soft parts. These consist entirely of vital bony injury, and care must be taken when examining these injuries to exclude any post-mortem damage which may have been caused by a shovel or excavator during disinterment.

If the skeletal remains are found above ground or only lightly covered the bony parts may be attacked by rodents, foxes and dogs. Foxes and dogs may even move individual bones some distance from the main skeleton.

In 1923, during reconstruction of a factory in Egypt, a collection of human bones forming a complete skeleton was found at the foot of a well. A bullet hole of entry lay in the top of the skull but there was no exit, and careful search of the remaining bones with the help of X-ray revealed the spent bullet lying buried in the manubrium of the sternum. It seemed likely that the victim had been shot whilst lying down, possibly during sleep, and then disposed of down the well. A suspect confessed to the crime which had, in fact, been effected in this way.[43]

After World War II, on the instigation of the War Crimes Commission, a number of murders of service personnel by shooting, usually through the neck or back of the head, were established by exhumation of the remains.[44].

The case of Eugene Aram also furnishes an instance of the necessity for closely examining skeletons when it is suspected that the individuals have died from murderous violence. This man conspired with another to murder a person named Clarke who suddenly disappeared in February 1745. In 1758— i.e., 13 years after his disappearance—some bones were accidentally discovered in a cave near the town where he lived. Aram's accomplice was arrested on suspicion; and, losing his presence of mind when charged with the murder, he denied that those were the bones, but mentioned the spot where the bones of Clarke were buried. A skeleton was found there, and a fracture with indentation of the temporal bone was plainly perceptible. The manner in which the murder was committed by the accomplice agreed with the medical evidence. Aram, who was a man of some ability, argued in his defence that it was impossible to identify a skeleton after a lapse of 13 years; that the fracture of the skull and the piece of bone beaten inwards proved nothing; that it might have lain long in the cave where it was found, which had been a hermitage, and therefore a likely place of sepulture in ancient times; and that the violence to the skull might have been produced in times of disorder, when in searching for treasure the graves and coffins of the dead were violated. In spite of the ingenuity of this defence, the facts were too strong against him, and he was convicted and executed.

Aram's defence gives an indication of the questions which are apt to arise when evidence is given from the examination of exhumed bones. Proof of identity is essential, and most careful examination of any fracture so as to enable a medical witness to determine whether it was recent or old, and whether it was likely to have been caused in life or during the exhumation must never be neglected.

In *R. v. Dougal*, what was known as the 'Moat Farm mystery' excited very great interest. The facts were as follows: Dougal, who was a married man, persuaded a Miss Holland to live with him at the Moat Farm. It was proved in evidence by a servant that Miss Holland left the house with the prisoner one day in August 1899, and was never again seen alive. Various excuses were made by the prisoner to account for her non-appearance. Meanwhile the prisoner proceeded to dispose of her property, and was arrested for forging the dead woman's name to a paltry cheque of a few pounds.

Inquiry led the police to believe that Miss Holland had been murdered by the prisoner, and her body disposed of by burial somewhere near the farmhouse. After prolonged search the remains of a human body were found buried in the bank of a ditch which the prisoner had caused to be filled in, and upon the site of which he had had trees planted. Little was found but the bones, a few fragments of personal attire, a pair of boots and traces of internal organs, but there was enough to convict the prisoner, who was hanged. The main items of proof of identity and of the mode of death were the following:

1. portions of a skirt: this was identified by the deceased's dressmaker, who was able to swear to a peculiar mended portion of it, the witness having herself mended the skirt;
2. a comb or hair fastener of a pattern which Miss Holland's maid was able to identify;
3. remains of boots of a peculiarly small size, precisely corresponding to the size which the deceased was known to have worn: they were of French make, and were distinctly identifiable;
4. the skeleton was that (a) of a woman, (b) of a

person about the height of Miss Holland;
5. behind the position of the right ear was found a jagged fracture of the bone, with fragments carried inwards; the brain was sufficiently preserved for Professor Pepper, who performed the autopsy, to trace a wound through it from behind forwards and to the left, at the anterior end of which wound was found a bullet.

With regard to proving that the bullet was one which might have been fired by the prisoner, there was some little difficulty so long after the event, but there could be no doubt whatever that the person whose remains were found had been killed by a bullet fired from behind, and the circumstantial evidence was sufficient to prove

1. that the body was that of Miss Holland,
2. that the prisoner was the only person who could have fired the shot, and
3. that he had opportunity and motive for doing so.

In reference to injuries found in skeletons, it is of great importance to attempt to determine whether the injury had occurred during life or during the exhumation, and if during life, whether it was recent or of old standing. This is difficult in cases in which the injury took place shortly before death, but if any attempt at healing has taken place this will still remain and will prove definitely that the fracture was of some standing.

In this connection it must be remembered that in the skull small portions of bone not infrequently ossify from irregular independent centres and remain for variable periods of time as small bones separable by maceration and disarticulation and known as ossa triquetra. The aperture left by the separation of one of these bones may be mistaken for a fracture produced by a weapon, but the difference is usually well marked. If, on the one hand, the bone has not yet united with the others, the edges of the opening will be found quite thin, and as it were, bevelled off, and possibly membrane may be found on the edge. If, on the other hand, it has united, the then serrate suture or line of junction with the other bones can hardly be mistaken for the appearance of a fracture.

The dead body of a newborn child, wrapped in brown paper and a towel, was found in a pond. The head was much decomposed, and the scalp was extensively lacerated and destroyed over the parietal bones, which readily separated. The brain was fluid. Two apertures were present on one parietal bone; they were small and rounded, and it was at first doubtful whether they had not been wilfully produced by some perforating instrument. Over one aperture the scalp was entire and uninjured, but the other was situated under the lacerated portion of the scalp. No violence had been used in the removal of the body from the water. The bone was macerated, and carefully examined by the aid of a lens. The apertures were quite regular at the edges, which were remarkably thin, evidently merging into a membranous condition. This examination left no doubt that the holes in the bone were not due to any mechanical violence but to deficient ossification. The spaces had been membranous, and the membrane destroyed by decomposition.

Careful search should be made for the hyoid and thyroid bones, for these structures are often fractured in strangulation and seldom by anything else.

In *R. v. Dobkin*[45] (The Baptist Church Cellar Murder) the only evidence that death was due to foul play was a fracture of the right superior cornu of the thyroid cartilage. The medical evidence for the Crown (that this gave the strongest presumptive evidence of manual strangulation) was cross-examined without success. Some dry blood clot in the immediate vicinity showed it to have occurred in life—if only immediately before death.

During decomposition the hyoid and thyroid bones may separate through the anatomical sites of fusion, especially in young persons, and therefore unless actual ante-mortem fractures can be demonstrated the value is limited.

In *R. v. Willis* (Reading C. C. 1978), the body of a young teenage girl was found in a small stream. She had been missing for some months and the soft tissues of the head and neck had largely disappeared. The head was attached to the trunk by a strip of skin. None of the soft tissues of the neck, including the larynx, remained. The head was detached by the pathologist in situ. On examination in the laboratory it was found that a bony process which is connected to the larynx by a ligament was fractured at the base of the skull. The process on the other side was exceptionally long. This suggested that the neck had been manually compressed beneath the angle of the jaw. When the suspect was seen by the police and it was put to him that these were signs of strangulation he immediately confessed that he had strangled the girl and concealed her in the stream.

REFERENCES

1. Mant, A. K. (1962) Med. Sci. Law, **2**, 134.
2. Mant, A. K. (1970) In: Stewart, T. D., ed. Personal Identification in Mass Disasters. Washington, D C: Smithsonian Institute, p. 11.
3. Forbes, G. (1946) Police J., **19**, 266.
4. Sue, J. J. (1755) Mem. Math. Phys. ad. Sci. Paris, **2**, 572.
5. Rollet, E. (1899) De la Mensuration des Os Long des Membres daus ses Rapports avec Anthropologie. La Chirurgie et la Medecine Judiciare. Lyon: Storvi.
6. Pearson, K. (1899) Phil. Trans. R. Soc. A., **192**, 69.
7. Krogman, W. M. (1962) The Human Skeleton in Forensic Medicine. Springfield, Ill.: Charles C. Thomas.
8. Trotter, M. & Gleser, G. C. (1958) Am. J. Phys. Anthrop. N.S., **16**, 79.
9. Stewart, T. D. (1979) Essentials of Forensic Anthropology, ch. 9. Springfield, Ill.: Charles, C. Thomas.
10. Harrison, R. J. (1953) In: Camps, F. E., ed. Medical and Scientific Investigations in the Christie Case. London: Medical Publications Ltd.
11. Dupertuis & Hadden (1951) A.J.P.A. 9(1)–15
12. Davidson, W. H. (1960) Br. Med. J., **ii**, 1901.
13. Barr, X. & Bertram, X. (1949) Nature, Lond., **163**, 676.
14. Giles, E. (1970) In: Stewart, T. D., ed. Personal Identification in Mass Disasters. Washington, D C: Smithsonian Institute, p. 99.
15. Iordanidis, P. (1961–62) Ann. Med. Leg., **41 & 42**.
16. Iordanidis, P. (1962) Ann. Med. Leg., **42**, 231.
17. Eliakis, X. & Iordanidis, P. (1963) Ann. Méd Lég 43: 326
18. Gray's Anatomy (1973) 35th edn. Harlow, Essex: Longman.
19. Hesse.
20. Boyd, J. D. (1953) In: Simpson, C. K., ed. Modern Trends in Forensic Medicine. London: Butterworth.
21. Noback, C. (1944) Anat. Rec., **88**, 91.
22. Flecker, H. (1933) J. Anat., **67**, 118.
23. Webster, G. & de Saram, G. S. M. (1954) J. Crim. Law. Criminal. Police Sci., p. 45.
24. Hepworth, S. M. (1929) Indian Med. Gaz., **64**, 128.
25. Pillai, M. J. S. (1936) Indian J. Med. Res. **23**, 1015.
26. Kerr, W. L. (1937) Br. Med. J., **ii**, 620.
27. Gustafson, G. (1950) J. Am. Dent. Assoc., **41**, 45.
28. Francis, C. C. (1940) Am. J. Phys. Anthrop., **1**, 127.
29. Flecker, H. (1942) Am. J. Roentgen., **47**, 97.
30. McKern, T. W. & Stewart, T. D., (1957) Mass. Tech. Ref.,EP 45. US Army Natick.
31. Todd, T. W. & Lyon, D. W. (1924–25) Am. J. Phys. Anthrop., **7**, 325 & **8**, 23.
32. Am. J. Phys. Anthrop., **23**, 249.

33. Thompson, D. D. (1979) J. For. Sci., **24**, 902.
34. Thompson, D. D. (1981) J. For. Sci., **26**, 470.
35. Todd, T. W. (1920) Am. J. Phys. Anthrop.. **3**, 285.
36. Todd, T. W. (1921) Am. J. Phys. Anthrop., **4**, 1 & 333.
37. Brooks, S. T. (1955) Am. J. Phys. Anthrop., **13**, 567.
38. Gilbert, B. M. & McKern, T. W. (1973) Am. J. Phys. Anthrop., **38**, 31.
39. Giles, L. (1937) Bull. Sch. Orient. Studies, Lond. Univ. **9**.

40. Scott, P. (1953) Police J. **2**, 107.
41. Stewart T. D. (1959) F.B.I. Law Enfor. Bull., **28**, 11, 18.
42. Weiner, J. S. (1955) The Piltdown Forgery. London: Oxford University Press.
43. Smith, S. (1940) Police J., **13**, 23.
44. Mant, A. K. (1962) J. For. Sci. Soc., **1**, 88.
45. Simpson, C. K. (1943) Police J., **16**, 270.

10

Forensic odontology

INTRODUCTION

It is a commonly held view that forensic odontology is a new arrival to scientific investigations in the field of criminal activity but there are numerous references in the literature to case examples in which dental information or data have provided positive evidence of identification where other methods would have proved unsuccessful. Forensic odontology, forensic dentistry and forensic odonto-stomatology are terms used for that branch of forensic medicine which, in the interests of justice, deals with the proper handling and examination of dental evidence and with the proper evaluation and presentation of that evidence.[1] The field of forensic odontology is considered to be a dental speciality since it requires the services of a dental expert to handle and examine the dental evidence with the degree of accuracy that the Courts of law and the legal profession expect. To pursue routinely forensic dental work requires additional training to the accepted and conventional dental education and in which the further forensic knowledge and experience serves to qualify the dental expert as a valued member of an investigating team. Many authorities have found an historical interest in reporting earlier examples of forensic dentistry. Furness[2] in 1973 refers to a form of dental identification in 2500 BC. Two molar teeth linked together by gold wire were found in a tomb at Giza, and this is perhaps the earliest case cited. Harvey[3] cites an interesting case occurring much later in AD 66. Lollia Paulina, the rich divorcee, constituted a threat to the security of Sabina—Nero's mistress and Agrippina, his mother. Agrippina's soldiers were sent to kill Lollia Paulina with instructions to bring back her head when the assassination was com-

pleted. Agrippina was unable at first to recognise the distorted features of her victim, but when she parted the lips of the severed head she saw the discoloured front tooth of Lollia Paulina and paid the requisite assassination fee.

The disfigured body of Charles the Bold was identified after the Battle of Nancy, 1477, by teeth missing from his jaws resulting from an accident with a horse that had occurred some time previously.[4]

Paul Revere was a skilled coppersmith, silversmith and engraver, and he had been taught the art of dentistry by an English surgeon–dentist John Baker. He practised as a dental surgeon from 1768–78. Early in 1775, the same year as his famous ride, he constructed a silver wire and hippopotamus ivory bridge for a close friend Dr Joseph Warren. This latter gentleman had participated with Paul Revere in the incident of the Boston Tea Party as a member of 'The Sons of Liberty' and was one of the leaders in the outbreak of the American Revolution. On the outbreak of war he was elected to the rank of Major-General in the Massachusetts Militia, having first refused an appointment as Surgeon-in-Chief to the Colonial Army. During the Battle of Bunker Hill he was killed by a bullet in the head and buried in an unmarked grave (a common practice to prevent plunder of teeth of victims of battlefields, as a source of teeth for dentures). However Joseph Warren was dug up the following day by the British and exhibited publicly. Ten months after Warren's death in 1776 his brothers and friends, including Paul Revere, disinterred the body to confirm the presence of the silver wire and ivory bridge replacing the upper left canine and first premolar tooth and positively identified Joseph Warren. The body was reburied five times before being left in peace in the family plot in Forest Hills Cemetery.[5]

One of the first crimes to attract the attention of the American Nation was the Webster–Parkman case in 1849. Dr J.W. Webster was Harvard Professor of Chemistry and Mineralogy and although said to be placid at home was sometimes ill tempered and unable to live on a salary of $1200 a year. He borrowed frequently from Dr George Parkman who now practised real estate more often than medicine. Professor Webster had to mortgage his home and goods together with his valuable mineral collection to provide security for the loan. Dr Parkman became more than annoyed when he found out by accident that the professor had not only borrowed further money on the mineral collection elsewhere but had already sold it elsewhere. Naturally Dr Parkman pressed for the recovery of his loan and began to make a nuisance at the professor's lectures, making personal insults and disparaging remarks. Dr Parkman visited the professor's laboratory demanding return of the money and caused a heated argument during which Dr Parkman was either struck on the head or stabbed. Professor Webster then dismembered the body putting the head and some organs into the furnace, retaining other parts after washing the blood carefully away, and disposing of these parts in the furnace over a period of time. The college janitor on receiving a gift of a thanksgiving turkey had his suspicions aroused. When he found a pelvis and two pieces of leg in the dissecting vault he immediately informed the college authorities. Professor Webster denied that any of the remains belonged to Dr Parkman, but the recovered portions of charred teeth fused to gold were identified by Dr Nathan Cooley who had constructed the Parkman denture and by Dr Lester Noble who testified that the study models of Dr Parkman's teeth had been marked by him with the date 'Oct., 1846', and fitted the recovered portion of porcelain denture accurately on the marked model of Dr Parkman's lower jaw. Defence sought to discredit the evidence but the jury were convinced that the dental evidence positively established the identity of the victim and Professor Webster having been found guilty of murder was hanged on 30 August 1850.[5]

The tragic fire at the Bazaar de la Charité in Paris occurred in 1897 and claimed 126 lives. The Bazaar was held annually by the wealthy women of Paris to raise funds for the poor. The bodies were badly burned and mutilated and visual identification was difficult but some identifications were made on clothing and personal effects. Thirty victims remained unidentified until the Paraguayan Consul made a suggestion that the dentists of the known missing persons be requested to chart the teeth of these victims and compare the post-mortem findings with their records of dentistry. Later that year 'The role of the dentists in the identification of the victims of the catastrophe of the Bazaar de la Charité, "4 May 1897" ', was presented by Dr Oscar Amöedo (Professor of the Paris Dental School) in which was recorded the procedures and observations of the dentists engaged in the identification work and pointing out the necessity for the adoption of an international uniform system of charting. Subsequently he enlarged his ideas of dental identification in the text of *L'Art Dentaire en Medecine Legale* published in 1898 in French and in 1899 in German.[6]

In 1942 a workman lifted a stone slab set into the cellar floor under the vestry of a bombed Baptist Church and found a skeleton which he assumed was just another victim of the Blitz. When the police arrived the remains were wrapped in a paper parcel and taken to Southwark Public Mortuary and examined the next day by a young pathologist named Dr Keith Simpson. The neat burial under the slab and absence of bone damage precluded a blitz victim, and neither was it the site an old cemetery. The skeleton could have been on site from 12 to 18 months and it was known that the church had been blitzed two years previously. The head had been severed as were both arms at the elbow and both legs at the knee. Some portions of the limbs were missing. The yellowish deposit on the head and on the earth around it proved to be slaked lime. The calculated height of the victim was 5 ft $\frac{1}{2}$ inch making allowance for the missing parts and soft tissues, and an age estimation on cranial suture closure revealed an age between 40 and 50 years. The enlarged womb revealed no foetal bones of pregnancy. Although the lower jaw was missing the upper jaw presented extensive dental treatment including fillings and marks of denture clasps. Missing persons revealed that a Mrs Rachel Dobkin, the wife of a fire-watcher at the church, had been reported missing 15 months earlier. She was similar in height and had sought advice concerning fibroid growths of the uterus. A dental surgeon, Mr Barnett Kopkin, had kept precise records of Mrs Dobkin's treatment from 1934 to 1940 and was able to sketch a picture of the lady's upper jaw. The further investigation resulted in the arrest and subsequent trial of Harry Dobkin, her husband, who paid the final penalty for murder.[7]

In 1953 a tenant of No. 10 Rillington Place, London, while stripping wallpaper found a cupboard which contained the bodies of three women. Other bodies were found under the floorboards and the remains of skeletons in the garden until six women victims were represented. Two bodies had been discovered in 1949 on the same premises, being those of Mrs Beryl Evans and baby Geraldine and at that time Timothy Evans, husband and father, was thought to be responsible. He stood trial and was found guilty and hanged. Forensic teamwork completed identification of all the victims, but the identification of dental interest was that of Ruth Fuerst. Reconstruction of the burned fragments of skull was carried out and the upper jaw contained a molar tooth with a white metal full crown. Analysis of the crown metal proved it to be made up of alloys frequently used in Central Europe. This information finally positively identified the Austrian girl. The former tenant, John Reginald Halliday Christie, was tried for the murder of his wife—one of the bodies under the floorboards. His defence of insanity was rejected by the jury and he was sentenced to death and executed on 15 July 1953.[8]

One of the most fascinating quests in modern times to achieve positive dental identification has been that of Professor Reidar F. Sognnaes for more than 10 years. His object of research has been to identify post-mortem the party leaders of the Nazi dictatorship, since even today 36 years after 13 bodies were recovered from the bunker at the Chancellery, the Soviet authorities have not released details or statements concerning their autopsies. Professor Sognnaes has established the identities of Hitler and Bormann, the latter's remains being found elsewhere, and eliminated dentally the female remains in the bunker as being those of Eva Braun. Her fate remains unknown but for how long?[9,10,11]

DENTAL IDENTIFICATION

The justification for the identification of dead bodies, especially those resulting from mass disasters, has been constantly argued in the past, with opinion varying from such identifications being a public duty to the reference to Article 6 of the United Nations' Universal Declaration of Human Rights adopted by the United Nations General Assembly in 1948. The article states that 'everyone has the right to recognition everywhere as a person before the law'. The interpretation of one authority is that it is held to imply that a citizen of a United Nation member state has a right 'to possess his personal identity unquestioned', even after death, and the said article considered as an international law prescribes that the identification of the dead must be carried out whenever possible.[12,13]

In general terms the question of justification may be considered under the legal, social and forensic aspects. The legal aspect presumes that it is part of the law of most countries that a dead body must be identified prior to its disposal. Without a valid identity one must consider the ensuing legal problems of death certification, the disposal of the deceased's estate, and the considerable period of time before relatives can claim the accrued money on insurance policies or make claim for compensation where negligence may be involved in transportation accidents. In air disasters evidence is sought relating to the laws concerning simultaneous death or commorientes. If the evidence is unascertainable whether a wife survived a husband in such an accident then it is presumed that the younger survived the elder according to United Kingdom Law (section 184 of the Law of Property Act 1925). The estate may then be disposed of on the basis of presumed survival provided that both husband and wife are testate. If one or both die intestate then section 184 is modified by section 1(4) of the Intestate Estates Act 1952. However, if there is evidence of survivorship, then the Courts will judge the case on its merits and may render the rules inapplicable.[14]

The social aspect of dental identification is concerned with the prevention of unreliable visual identifications being made by distressed and shocked relatives; that the deceased may be accorded the appropriate marks of respect in relation to religion, tradition, or custom; and that the period of natural grief suffered by the relatives may be considerably lessened.

It is claimed that the majority of identifications are made by visual means but it has been found even in normal circumstances that relatives are sometimes unable to identify loved-ones when their facial features are in repose in sleep. In the circumstances of grief and distress relatives often make mistakes in viewing an intact body quite apart from the unpleasant task of trying to recognised a loved-one who has been subjected to the trauma of mutilation, fire or immersion. The advantage of dental identification is that the calcified dental tissues and the jaws appear to withstand a great deal more insult or trauma than the rest of the body can and comparisons are made on specific ante-mortem dental data which obviate the necessity of relatives having to view a mutilated or fragmented body. When the body is correctly identified then the relatives are assured that the deceased is accorded the appropriate funeral rites demanded by religion, custom or tradition, or even superstititon.[15] The relatives reaction to grief may be prolonged if identity is not established and related to the period of time that the loved-one is 'missing' in the belief that one day he or she will return home or the disbelief that the loved-one is buried in a mass grave of unknowns. The psychological effects of prolonged grief are well reported[16] and often it is the dental identification that convinces relatives and averts the possibility of the tendency to identify an unknown body however poor the resemblance.[17–19]

The forensic aspect of dental identification includes homicide in which an early identification of the victim will lead to a prompt discovery of the associates of the victim. It is commonly stated that the majority of homicides are domiciliary and once the identity of the victim is established criminal charges may be brought in good time on apprehension of the perpetrator. In transportation accidents the positive identification can establish who is in charge of the vehicle or aircraft and where the passengers are seated whose injuries may provide evidence as to the cause of the incident.[20] Furthermore dental identification plays an important role in bite mark investigation in cases of homicide, sexual assault and rape, non-accidental injury to children, burglary and housebreaking, and other incidents in which teeth marks are left at the scenes of crime. This particular field of study is described in the last section of this chapter (see p. 202).

Any identification procedure demands the accurate recording of the physical attributes of the unknown body or individual, together with the acquisition and details of the personal effects associated with the unknown individual. From this evidence a full physical description of the unknown individual can be achieved with regard to the sex, race, age, anatomical abnormalities and pathological conditions, occupational and personal habits. It must be remembered, however, that clothing, documents, jewellery and other personal effects, although associated with a particular body, may be misleading in some circumstances especially in major incidents and mass disasters. The most distinctive features of the physical attributes are the personal characteristics of fingerprints and teeth and by these features alone a positive identification can be made.[21]

The techniques of identification, therefore, can be divided into two groups—that of the reconstructive group and that of the comparative group.[22]

Reconstructive group

When an unknown body is found a full and accurate external examination takes place to elicit all the details of the physical attributes of the individual as aforementioned. The description will include details of height, weight, build or degree of obesity, colour of eyes and hair. In addition particulars of the presence or absence of moustache and beard will be noted, as will peculiarities of the fingernails and toenails (bitten or varnished) and whether the ears are pierced or not. Further particulars concerning scars (trauma or operation), tattoos, moles and circumcision will be recorded as reference will be made to the files of missing persons whose descriptions will be compared which may result in a tentative identification if similarities are found. The assessment of these details may be relatively easy if the human remains are recent and intact but in those cases involving decomposition, fire victims, or skeletal remains the important characteristics to be determined are sex, race and age.

The accuracy of sex determination depends on the completeness of the skeletal remains and whether the remains are adult or immature. It is stated that the expert anatomist or forensic anthropologist will achieve an accuracy of 98% if the skeleton is complete, an accuracy of 95% on the pelvic bones alone, and an accuracy of 90% on the skull alone. Recovery of the long bones will result in 80% accuracy in sexing.[23] In conjunction with sex determination is the evaluation of racial characteristics and there is copious information concerning the measurements, proportions and traits of Europiform, Negroid, Mongoloid, Indian, Eskimo groups, etc. Individual skeletal characteristics such as congenital and acquired abnormalities including acromegaly, achondroplasia, cranio–cleido dysostosis and rickets may be present in the bones as may the presentation of healed fractures or 'spontaneous' fractures due to hyperparathyroidism or osteomyelitis which may aid in the identification of the skeletal remains. This is the particular field of study of the expert anatomist and the forensic anthropologist the role of the latter as a member of the investigating team being somewhat neglected at present in the United Kingdom, although being well recognised in the United States.[24] The duties of such an expert extend from the decision that bones recovered from a site may have no forensic significance but may relate to remains from archeological sites which have come to light in forensic investigations, to the evaluation of sex and race when immature remains are recovered.[25] There have been frequent occasions when art has been applied to science in the attempt to reconstruct facial soft tissues from the underlying bone in order to establish a visual means of identification. Various methods have been evolved over the years using the tables of soft tissue thickness of numerous authorities to establish the soft tissue reconstruction. An experiment often referred to is that of Krogman[26], in association with a sculptress, used modelling clay to mould facial features on a dried skull. It is not established how well the appearance of the model compared with the features of the known person in life but such a procedure was considered futile in predicting facial form from skeletal remains by one authority.[27] However, with recent experience in the United States of a demonstration of similar methods being applied to homicide cases with some success, it would appear to provide a procedure to be considered when other

methods of identification have failed.[28]

It has been found in practice that the chronology of dental development is less variable than bone development and that the methods applied to particular periods of life provide more accurate indications of age. The three periods referred to are related to the dental development 'in utero' until just after birth, secondly up to the age of 14 years, which includes the deciduous and permanent dentitions and the replacement of the former by the latter, and thirdly from 14 years until the loss of all teeth and old age to the death of an individual.[29] The assessment of age is inter-related with the sex and the race of the individual, and on comparison of dental development[30] with osseous development of the hand[31] it has been found that if the dental and osseous ages were similar then the individual was male, and if the osseous age was in advance of the dental age then the individual was most likely female. Skeletal development in the female can be in advance of the male up to one year while dental development may differ only from one to four months. By reason of the prime importance of dental age assessment in identification the various means of determination in the three periods of life are discussed subsequently in a separate section in this chapter (see p. 197).

Comparative group

Having established the prime characteristics of sex, race and age and the full physical description of the recently dead unknown body, or as much as skeletal remains will allow, the next phase of the procedure is to apply this information for comparison with ante-mortem data retrieved from various sources. In the circumstances of an air disaster the passenger list will provide a provisional schedule of identification from which relatives and concerned persons can give full descriptions and personal details of their loved-ones to the relevant authorities. In the case of the single unknown body resulting from crime, reference may be made to the Missing Persons Bureau of the police authority in whose jurisdiction the body is found. It may be necessary, therefore, to refer to other Missing Persons Bureaux as part of normal police procedure of the other separate police authorities in the United Kingdom, and through Interpol.

At the locus

It is part of the normal police procedure that the entire scene is recorded photographically to relate the position of the body or bodies to particular locations and to each other. A plan or survey will be drawn which will indicate the relationship and distances of the bodies to other objects at the scene especially if those objects are of forensic interest such as weapons, articles of jewellery, clothing, utensils, displaced dentures, or fragments of natural teeth. Each can be placed in suitable plastic bags and labelled and their position marked on the plan. This part of the procedure is usually under the direction of the senior police officer who is advised by the forensic pathologist. When the forensic pathologist has carried out his preliminary examination it may be possible for the forensic dentist to complete a dental charting prior to removal of the remains to the mortuary and evaluate the significance of any displaced dental evidence associated with the remains. Occasionally, portable X-ray units may be available which will have the dual purpose of locating metal objects in the body if death by firearms or explosive devices is suspected, and the acquisition of standard radiographic views of the teeth and jaws, which in conjunction with the charting may lead to an early identification. Frequently the dental examination may have to be delayed until the body arrives at the mortuary where conditions are more suitable and radiographic examination takes place subsequently in the laboratory or department where a fixed X-ray unit is available. The human remains are removed from the scene in a sealed plastic body bag in a special container so that any evidence associated with the body is not lost in transit to the mortuary. In the past it has been found that bodies recovered in water are not easily introduced into a body bag and should be wrapped and then sealed in plastic sheeting. When bodies are removed from earth sites or shallow graves an attempt is made to introduce a large wooden board to a depth of 6 inches under the body so that it remains relatively undisturbed on its earth surface in transit to the mortuary and after the autopsy the earth can be sifted and examined for teeth, bone fragments and detached restorations. The site from which the body is recovered is carefully examined and sieved for similar evidence that may have become detached from the body. The recovery of evidence from a scene is a highly specialised task and is usually the responsibility of a particular police officer who has considerable experience and training but who relies on the advice of the forensic pathologist, the forensic dentist, and other forensic experts who may have been called by the investigating officer.[32] When bodies have been immersed for a considerable period of time the single rooted front teeth are lost irretrievably, unlike bodies from hard or earth sites where missing teeth may be recovered on careful search after removal of the body. Bodies which have been subjected to intense heat present charring of the facial bones and jaws, which may present a progression of damage from loss of enamel from the labial surfaces of the front teeth which are embedded in the substance of the tongue to extreme damage in which the entire anterior portion of the jaws is burnt away depending on the degree of intensity of heat. In some fire victims it is not always possible to dissect the facial tissues to expose the teeth to a normal dental inspection as manipulation will fragment the brittle or calcined bone and examination of this material is best left to radiographic investigation. At this stage of the investigation, if provisional identities of the human remains are known, the preliminary dental charting may confirm the identities from recent information concerning previous dental treatment submitted by relatives or friends during police enquiries. If a provisional identity is suspected it is relatively easy to establish either a positive identification or eliminate a possible identity. On some occasions the elimination of suspected identities is as useful as achieving a positive identification. With the completely unknown body it may take a number of years to retrieve the relevant information to establish a positive identification. In mass disasters exclusion processes are helpful in separating the known features of victims and therefore lessening the number of other bodies to be identified and on a few occasions have established positive identifications by the presence of physical peculiarities.

Another method that has been frequently used in the past is that of superimposition. One of the earliest successful identifications by this method was that of Mrs Ruxton and Mary in the Ruxton Murder case. Photographs of the two ladies were enlarged to life size for comparison with photographs of the skull. The superimposition revealed similarities which determined the identity of each individual.[33] However it is not always possible to recover suitable photographs of individuals to compare with skulls or radiographs of unknown bodies and it is difficult to relate accurately anatomical landmarks to such photographs of the living. It has been found more appropriate recently to superimpose the irregularities of anterior teeth as presented in photographs with the anterior standing teeth of an unknown skull (Fig. 10.1).[34]

The value of dental means of identification has become fully recognised since the end of the second world war and in the experience of many authorities has provided the most consistent and accurate single means of identification.[21, 35–37] The classic example in which dental identification played an important role was the systematic identification of 118 bodies recovered from the fire on board the S S Noronic in Toronto Harbour in 1949.[38] The routine procedure described has been found to be suitable for the investigation of single individuals and multiple victims and has probably formed the basis of the procedures adopted by disaster victim identification teams throughout the world since that time. The Scandinavian countries, and most notably Denmark, advocated the standing unit of the police officer, the forensic pathologist and the forensic dentist to be readily available at the very beginning of the investigation, having already adopted a system whereby the medical and dental records of missing persons were collected after a specified period of time and retained at a central agency as precautionary registration of comparative data in the event of unknown bodies being recovered during routine investigations.[39] More recently in the United Kingdom the Metropolitan police have introduced a system in which a copy of a missing person's dental chart only is obtained from that person's last known dental practitioner and submitted to the Missing Persons Bureau at New Scotland Yard. The copy of the dental chart is obtained after a specified period of time and only if that person is presumed missing in suspicious circumstances. When unknown bodies are found in routine police investigations, a dental examination is carried out and the charting is compared with those on record at the Missing Persons Bureau at New Scotland Yard. In the process of comparison a number of chartings may present similarities to that of the unknown body and then requests will be made to the various dental practitioners to provide their original dental records in order to obtain a positive identification of the unknown body at best, or eliminate a number of suspected identities at worst. Obviously there is some concern within the professions regarding the confidentiality of medical and dental records when used for identification purposes. When practitioners are confronted with requests to provide original records of patient's treatment they seek guidance from their professional associations and protection societies, who will generally advise that if the records are to be used solely for identification purposes and no

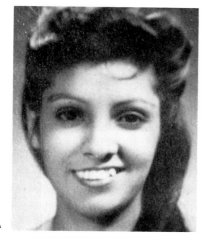

A

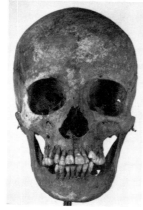

B

Fig. 10.1 Comparison of the photograph of a known person (A) with the skull (B), demonstrating the concordance of the features of the front teeth.

other, then the practitioner's duty to society outweighs a refusal to comply with the request on the grounds of confidentiality.

The routine procedure of the dental examination does not differ greatly from that carried out in normal dental practice other than the location in which the forensic examination takes place. It requires a meticulous attention to detail and the observations and findings must be reproduced in a form that is comprehensible to the police authorities, forensic colleagues and subsequently to Courts of law in the United Kingdom and abroad. The forensic dentist may be requested to carry out the examination at the locus or scene in some circumstances but most often in the mortuary facility and subsequently in the laboratory if specialised techniques are required.

In order to carry out a dental examination for all situations that may be anticipated in forensic investigations it is necessary to provide oneself with a portable diagnostic set to be kept in readiness. The requirements of such sets have been described by a number of experts based on their personal requirements in the field.[40] The basic set of instruments and equipment should be easily transportable by hand and weight should be kept to a minimum as some scenes may be inaccessible to all other means of travel other than on foot. Additional instruments and equipment may be readily available in the armamentarium of the mortuary if saws, knives and skull T-bar chisel are required, or may be borrowed from the forensic pathologist's set of instruments or that of the scenes-of-crime officer or his equivalent if resection of the jaws is contemplated. The simplest collection of diagnostic instruments and materials required for all forensic examinations include:

Normal diagnostic instruments, viz., mirrors, probes and small forceps. In the past dental mirrors with a screw-in mirror face have proved useful since the mirror face can be mounted on the obtuse angle side of the mirror head for normal inspection of the oral cavity and on the acute angle side of the mirror head when the buccal surfaces of the upper molars are to be examined and access is limited by rigor mortis or 'heat stiffening' of burnt facial tissues.[41] Another useful type of mirror is that supplied as part of a patient's oral hygiene kit (Prevdent pa-

tients' mouth mirror). It provides a relatively large surface area and is cheap to buy and is disposable.

A diagnostic torch or illuminated mouth mirror. Conventional diagnostic torches are difficult to sterilise after use in forensic investigations and are relatively expensive to replace. There are diagnostic torches available at the present time which incorporate a miniature bulb on a flexible extension from a sealed battery container (Hoyt flexible examination light). This torch provides an adequate source of light in difficult areas of access without obstruction of vision. Sterilisation is no problem as this torch is disposable and inexpensive to replace. Similarly disposable illuminated mouth mirrors are available as part of patient's oral hygiene kits. However, it has been found that the latter are of limited use as the mirror fitment slides too easily over the barrel of the torch.

Printed work cards. It is necessary to keep a reasonable supply of 6 × 4 inch cards commercially printed with the standard dental grid for use as work cards in the conditions which prevail at the locus or scene and in the mortuary. It is not always possible to have a colleague fill in the details at one's dictation and therefore keep the card unsullied. During the course of the examination the single operator will transfer blood, fat and other noxious material and will therefore contaminate the card as he fills in the dental data. However the relevant dental data can subsequently be transcribed on a fair copy which in the United Kingdom might be that designated for use at the Missing Persons Bureau at New Scotland Yard or any other type of odontogram in use in other countries. It is also recommended to have a rubber stamp with the grid format and an ink pad for the preparation of the Court report, or if printed cards are not available.

Polythene specimen bags and labels. The polythene bags should be of suitable size for individual teeth, bone fragments, dental impressions, and preferably self-sealing. In criminal cases and on some occasions in mass disasters labels will be supplied by police authorities but it is useful to maintain a personal supply of adhesive and tie-on labels.

Disposable impression trays and silicone or rubber base impression materials. Disposable trays weigh considerably less than conventional metal trays and the use of impression materials incorporating a setting catalyst are preferable to the use of alginate which requires the availability of water. In addition the setting time of alginate impression material is considerably prolonged in a cold cadaver.

Modelling wax, wax knife and spirit lamp. Modelling wax can sometimes be adequately softened by warming it in the hands and this material is most commonly used in obtaining wax bite registrations in bite mark cases.

A polished metal tongue depressor. This instrument can be used as a wedge to gently ease open jaws in rigor, or reflect light into the oral cavity, or be used as a spatula to mix the impression materials.

A plastic ruler. Graduated in inches and centimetres and of approved standard measurement and graduated 'Scotch tape' for photographic scales.

Protective clothing, viz., gown, disposable gloves and disposable plastic over-shoes. Ideally the self-contained operator should include a single lens reflex camera with flashlight and capable of close-up focussing, a small battery operated tape recorder, a battery operated ultraviolet lamp for bite mark investigation, and a portable X-ray unit, mains and battery operated (Bendix-Ray model 105).[23] Polaroid land film and other types of self-processing radiographic film can be used with the aforementioned apparatus on site. Access to an automatic developer,[42] or the use of dental radiographic film incorporating a filter dye allowing development in subdued light, are variations of processing which will produce speedy results.

In the mortuary

When the human remains have been removed to the post-mortem room the body or bodies are carefully removed from their sealed recovery bags in order to begin the external examination. In investigations in which there is only a single body to examine this procedure and the subsequent autopsy will take place in an established facility of a public mortuary or a hospital mortuary. In major incidents and mass disasters the facility may only be a temporary one comprising of premises which have been commandeered for the purposes of coping with multiple bodies in an emergency. The premises may include church or school halls, air-craft hangars, warehouses, military and Red Cross tents, and even ice skating rinks. Such premises therefore may not be able to provide all the apparatus one would expect in a well-equipped mortuary and provision must be made to remove material and specimens for radiological and other investigations to more convenient places of study in forensic departments and laboratories. In a mass disaster investigation all the bodies must be retained in the one place until all the comparison procedures have been completed and the coroner or his equivalent has given permission for disposal.

The routine dental examination can take place at any time that is convenient during the course of the external examination providing that it does not impede the requirements of the forensic pathologist or the investigating officer. A dental charting may be obtained at the time the documents and clothing are removed prior to photography, radiography, or after autopsy, when specimens of the teeth and jaws may be removed for laboratory investigations. On numerous occasions the dental procedure can take place in body reception or in the laying out facility well away from the scene of other activity so that a detailed examination can take place by the operator and colleagues in undisturbed circumstances. The principal of making a dental identification is to record all the details of dental treatment, morphology and pathology, and oral characteristics, for comparison with the dental records of missing persons and reconstructive data from information from relatives if dental records are unavailable. The dental examination must take into account the following factors and oral characteristics:

Conservation and restorative dental work. Conservative dental work or fillings provides one of the most reliable means of identification and includes fillings of various materials, root fillings, inlays and crown and bridgework. These restorations are relatively permanent fixtures in the teeth and are generally well recorded on chartings and by radiographs. However, it is well to remember that in the United Kingdom the regulations of the National Health Service do not require the dental practitioner to chart fully the whole mouth when a patient is first seen. He is obliged only to chart teeth present, teeth missing, and the teeth he intends to treat. In England and Wales the dental data is charted on the grid system already described but in Scotland the system requires written details to be recorded. Other countries have adopted charting systems specific to their requirements and it has been estimated that there are more than 200 different methods of charting throughout the world,[13] a figure which appears to have doubled since the survey carried out in 1937. Nearly 100 years ago the necessity and advantages of adopting an international uniform system of charting was described[6] but even the endeavours of the Federation Dentaire Internationale Subcommittee on Forensic odontology have failed to convince many nations of the world of the advantages of the two-digit system of Dr Viohl. This system was rejected by the United Kingdom and the United States and other countries but adopted by Interpol, who incorporated it in the odontogram of their disaster victim identification form. However, over the last 10 years the odontogram itself has proved too cumbersome to complete in mass disasters and the recent air disaster on Mount Erebus confirmed its disadvantages (Churton M.C. 1980, personal communication). As a result of a series of meetings of disaster victim identification teams a number of recommendations have been put forward to modify the format of the DVI form and incorporate a simpler form of charting grid (1st International Multi disciplinary Symposium Disaster Victim Identification' Apeldoorn, Netherlands).

When dental records of missing persons are retrieved it is hoped that they will include dental radiographs which will complete the details missing from the attenuated form of dental charting or provide visual additional information to unfamiliar forms of charting from other countries. It is generally found that the most useful radiographic evidence either in quality or quantity accompanies the dental records of patients who have received more complicated types of dental treatment. A single radiograph may present significant features which will positively identify an individual (Fig. 10.2) even though it has been recommended that a minimum of 12 concordant features be found on comparisons before a firm positive identification is accepted.[13] A further example can be cited in which a radiograph presented root fillings in three roots of a single tooth which could be matched to the treatment of a known individual and the positive identity established.[21] The success rate of comparative methods of identification depends upon the existence and retrieval of the ante-mortem dental records. In the United Kingdom the period of time a dental surgeon is obliged to keep his records varies from four years in Scotland to less than two years in England and Wales. In Sweden a dental surgeon must retain dental records for at least 10 years.[43] Dental records are retained considerably longer in private practice, the dental schools of teaching hospitals, and the armed forces, but less

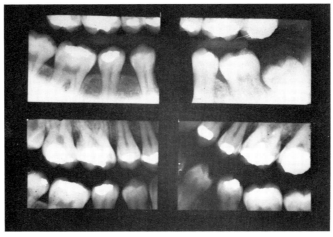

Fig. 10.2 Bite-wing radiograph of the known individual (A) compared to the post-mortem bite-wing radiograph of the unknown body.

than 18 months in the Dental Estimates Board of the National Health Service in England, due mainly to the almost astronomical numbers of records the authority has to deal with in each year. If provisional identities are suspected it is a relatively simple process to retrieve records according to name, address, date of birth, National Health Service number (if relevant), from the Dental Estimates Board. Even if this process results in the recovery of the attenuated form of charting the name of the dental surgeon providing treatment will be included to whom application can be made to provide his practice records, which may provide considerably more information. If the body or bodies are completely unknown the police investigation will commence by interviewing dental practitioners in the local area in which the remains were found and then extending their search by collaboration with other police authorities in this country and abroad. The International Criminal Police Organization complies with constant requests for dental information concerning missing persons throughout the world and communicates the appropriate dental data using the FDI two-digit system. Other methods whereby dental information is requested are by the publication of the physical and dental features of unknown bodies in international dental journals and other professional publications and by the use of television media.

Long periods of time, even years, may elapse before answers are received to these methods of enquiry. In a recent dental publication the Metropolitan police seek help in the identification of a female who was recovered from the river Thames in September 1979 and yet remains unknown despite extensive enquiries in this country and abroad. A remarkable aspect of this case is the presence of five porcelain jacket crowns on the maxillary anterior teeth which one would expect to be a valuable identifiable feature.[44]

In civil aircraft accidents there is the necessity of rapid transmission of acquired dental data to the disaster site. In air disasters involving British aircraft abroad, the Royal Air Force and the Air Accident Identification and Repatriation team adopted a telex code system in 1969 which had been developed several years previously.[18] The code substitutes certain letters of the alphabet for the numerical designation for teeth in the Palmer Notation which is described in the chapter on mass disaster identification.[23] Recently considerable interest has been expressed in the use of the standard telecopier and telephoto equipment for the rapid transmission of a wide variety of ante-mortem data.[45,46] Many legal authorities will accept the ante-mortem data acquired by these methods for the purpose of identification and repatriation of the victims to their countries of origin but may require the Court presentation of original records subsequently.

Partial dentures. Partial dentures are specifically designed to fit and augment a particular individual natural dentition. The denture teeth replace the known missing teeth (by extraction) as presented on the charting and records of a particular person. In common with full dentures the construction of the partial denture can be described with regard to the material used for the base, either metal or acrylic plastic, and the material used for the teeth, either porcelain or acrylic plastic and of particular mould shape and shade. The metals used in the construction of partial dentures of skeletal design are chrome/cobalt alloys, gold alloys, and now less commonly dental plates of stainless steel, and will include the valuable identifying features of occlusal rests clasps and with modern technique, precision attachments. These latter features can be specifically related to individual teeth even if the partial denture is found separate from an intact unknown body or separate from a fragmented jaw in the circumstances of an air disaster. The plastic material used in the construction of a denture base and gumwork may be colourless, pink or stippled. Therefore the description of the partial denture taken in conjunction with the dental charting of the restorative work provides an important means of establishing the identity of an individual.

Full dentures. The provision of a full denture implies the artificial replacement of teeth in an edentulous jaw but does not obviate the possibility of the presence of buried roots or unerupted teeth in that jaw which may only be suspected during the radiographic investigation. Individuals can present combinations of full dentures opposed by natural teeth, or full dentures opposed by partial dentures and natural teeth, total full dentures, or no dentures at all. Full dentures are constructed with the same metal and plastic materials already described, and the possibility of being faced with a vulcanite plate with porcelain teeth in the mortuary nowadays is quite remote. Other identifying features will include the presence of gumwork or its absence anteriorly if the denture was an immediate insertion on extraction of anterior teeth, and the presence of relief areas on the palatal fitting surface of the upper denture.[18] In contrast with partial dentures a degree of suspicion must be reserved when full dentures are found separate from the unknown body. In the edentulous person the alveolar processes are being constantly resorbed during life and therefore the original fit of a full denture deteriorates. The period of time that elapses before the denture apparently becomes loose and ill fitting to the wearer varies with each individual and in fact the effective life of a full denture is considerably less than the patient supposes. The living person tends to cope with the increasing looseness quite automatically and unconciously until the patient is fully aware of the looseness and seeks provision of a new denture. When the separate full denture is placed in the mouth of the unknown body it may appear to have no relationship in the first instance and it is advisable at this juncture to take impressions of the jaw in order to produce a dental stone study model. By this method the morphology of the alveolar process of the jaw can be compared with the fitting surface of the denture to evaluate a favourable or unfavourable match. In the experience of many dental practitioners it is not a rare situation to be told by a patient that they are wearing another person's denture, or that some unfortunate patients have been fitted with the wrong dentures without apparent ill-effects. To prevent the latter occurence it has become establised procedure in busy dental laboratories to inscribe a work number or some indication of the patient's name on the stone production model which is then transferred in processing to the plastic material of the denture. This mark therefore provides a valid identifying feature if found on the denture of an unknown person but many dentures have had the mark erased due to irritation to the wearer when placed on an unsuitable fitting surface. The possibility of marking all dentures for the purpose of identification has been fully discussed over many years. The materials recommended vary from metal tape (originally dental matrix band) on which the identifying mark can be typed on a typewriter set on stencil cutting,[47] to absorbable tapes of linen, nylon or paper which become incorporated in the denture during processing. Metal tape has the disadvantage of having to be inserted into the finished denture and, apart from causing mechanical weakness, the process of insertion may be unacceptable to the patient. A full survey into the materials and techniques was carried out a number of years ago[3] but denture marking has not become generally accepted in the United Kingdom at the present time although the armed forces have carried out the method for a considerable period of time as a means of precautionary registration of dental data.[40] The West German Air Force recommended engraving on metal denture plates using jewellery engraving equipment and recently in Sweden all dentures have to carry an identification mark by law. The British Dental Association has advised dental surgeons to obtain consent from patients before marking a denture as it may imply an intrusion into a patient's privacy. Similar methods of permanent marking or temporary marking is carried out in geriatric hospitals, old folks homes, and similar institutions to prevent the mixing up of dentures and quite apart from the forensic implications of marking dentures it would be of great help in identifying unconscious persons or those suffering from amnesia.

The marking of teeth has now extended into the field of conservation and restorative techniques. One method describes the insertion of a personal dental identifier or information carrier composed of alumina substrate approximately 1.27 mm^2 in dimension with the data recorded in a microminiature mode. The carrier is placed in the prepared tooth cavity prior to the insertion of the filling and its presence can be indicated to the investigator subsequently by a radiographic disclosure pin placed elsewhere in the tooth. The disclosure pin must be suitably modified to prevent its confusion with normal restorative pin techniques. It is claimed that the disclosure pin is easily recognisable during the radiographic investigations in mass disasters and eliminates the lengthy procedures of conventional examination and antemortem and post-mortem comparisons.[49] Another method describes the placement of an encoded information chip sealed within the tooth enamel by a fire resistant filling of red composite material. The information chip consists of a small gold disc approximately 2 mm in diameter on which alphanumeric characters are engraved by an electromechanical engraver using the memory facility of a microprocessing unit. The coloured composite and fire-resistant filling visually indicates the presence of the gold disc to the forensic expert during oral examination of the unknown body.[60]

All of these methods of marking dentures and natural teeth are potentially useful especially when intact and untraumatised bodies are recovered but in the conditions which prevail in high-speed transportation accidents most bodies present extreme trauma to the facial tissues and facial skeleton and sometimes only single teeth and portions of dentures are recovered. The possibility of recovery of the specimens carrying the identifying marker on all occasions and on all bodies is extremely remote and therefore the basic method of full dental examination and comparison of post-mortem findings with ante-mortem data is still the most reliable method of dental identification.

Sex. Until recently the sexing of teeth has had to be assessed in relationship to the bones of the jaw in which they are attached but various techniques are now utilised in sexing individual teeth remote from the jaws. It has been reported that the mandibular canine tooth exhibits the greatest sex difference by reason of its overall greater dimensions in the male when compared to the female. By assessment of the width alone measurement permitted a 74% accuracy of sex determination.[51] Attempts have been made to determine sex by the histological examination of the neonatal line in group sections of the permanent first molar teeth, and by chromosome staining methods in order to identify the male F body in the Y chromosome of pulp cell nuclei even months after extraction.[52] The dental pulp findings can be supplemented by cellular material recovered from saliva since F bodies are consistently shown in a high percentage of trapped male cells in contrast with few cellular remnants recovered from female saliva.[53]

Race. A general knowledge of the florid racial characteristics of teeth are an asset to the forensic dental expert but it is in reality the specific field of the forensic anthropologist. Probably the most distinctive racial characteristic is the 'shovel-shaped'

incisor. This feature occurs in 95% of American Indians, 91% of Chinese, and approximately 50% of the Palestinian Arab population. The Mongoloids present enamel pearls on the occlusal surfaces of premolar teeth, while Prima Indians present paramolar protostylid cusps. Australoid and South African populations exhibit a high proportion of tall pulpal chambers or taurodontism. Mandibular exostoses are present in a high proportion of Aleuts and maxillary exostoses are present in high percentages of Icelanders and Eskimos.[54]

Age. The importance of the role of age assessment in dental identification is well recognised and is a specific field of study that is best left to laboratory techniques and methods which are described in the next section of this chapter. (see p. 197). However, during the course of the dental examination at the scene or locus or in the mortuary, a provisional age assessment can be made based on the clinical experience of the dental expert in relating attrition and level of gingival attachment and other factors in patients of known age.

Morphology. There are normal variations in the shape of teeth which have to be appreciated during the dental examination of separate individual teeth. In most circumstances it is relatively easy to identify a particular tooth and conclude whether it is mandibular or maxillary and from which side of the jaw. On examination of the natural teeth in situ some teeth may be missing as a result of a condition termed as partial anodontia in which certain tooth groups, viz., upper lateral incisors, lower second premolars, and third molars, may be congenitally missing. Other missing teeth may usually be accounted for by a history of previous extraction or not erupted. On many occasions the cuspal pattern of molars can be misleading if some molars are missing or not present in sequence. It is advisable to request a dental colleague to express his opinion on the identification of first, second and third molars as minor discrepancies are often encountered on comparison of the post-mortem charting with the ante-mortem records submitted by dental surgeons. The presence of unerupted or impacted third molars can be determined by the radiographic investigation. Other congenital defects encountered are those produced by osteogenesis imperfecta and the related amelogenesis imperfecta and dentinogenesis imperfecta. Upper lateral incisors are often peg-shaped, and congenital syphilis presents defects in the upper central incisors which are broader at the cervix at gum level than at the incisal edge, and which usually exhibit an elliptical notch (Hutchinson's incisors) and multicuspal molars (Moon's molars). On some upper first molars there is an accessory cusp on the palatal surface which is termed the Cusp of Carabelli and is an identifying feature of the upper first permanent molar.

Acquired defects may be accounted for by habits and occupation of the individual. Notched incisors can be attributed to hairdressers opening hairpins with their teeth or seamstresses biting thread, and formerly cobblers and carpenters constantly gripping nails or tacks between their teeth. Pipe smokers produce marked attrition on opposing teeth on the side of the mouth where they prefer to grip the pipestem for maximum comfort.[55]

Pathology. Individuals who persistently hold boiled sweets or peppermints in the buccal sulcus adjacent to the upper molar teeth present marked cervical decay whilst workers in sugar refining factories present marked cervical decay on the labial cervical surfaces of the upper front teeth. Drug addicts are reported to exhibit marked decay on all teeth as a result of craving for sweet things on removal of the source of their addiction and similar marked decay is attributed to over indulgence of highly sweetened cordials and soft drinks as well as ice lollies or Popsicles. The acid erosion of teeth is encountered as a presenting symptom of hiatus hernia,[56] as well as that caused to the teeth of workers in chemical factories where acid concentrates are produced.[57] Systemic disturbances following infection by measles or mumps in childhood often affect the normal development of the permanent teeth and hypoplastic pits in pairs of teeth or opposing teeth.

Colour Teeth have a natural coloration that appears to darken with age which may be intensified by poor oral hygiene, tobacco staining and tartar. However intrinsic and extrinsic factors are responsible for producing a wide variation of colours. Of the intrinsic factors the presence of pink teeth is worthy of note. It was first recorded by Bell[58] and its significance was not fully appreciated until 1953 when a murder victim presented this sign and a relationship was suspected with carbon

monoxide poisoning. The question was not resolved at that time and the cause of the pinkness of teeth in the cervical region was thought to be a post-mortem break down of red blood corpuscles within the pulp chamber and the altered blood diffusing through the dentinal tubules to appear on the surface of the tooth.[8] Pink teeth have been attributed to asphyxial causes of death but it has been observed on many occasions in the post mortem room with no significance attached to the cause of death. It is also observed in bodies removed from moist conditions[59] and recent research has been in progress to identify specific substances causing the pink colour.[60]

In areas of the country where natural fluoride is in high proportion in the water supply endemic fluorosis produces brown stains in the teeth.

A yellow discoloration is sometimes observed on the anterior teeth of children and can be related to tetracycline treatment at the time of development of the crown of the tooth. Purple or blue-stained teeth have been reported in cases of leprosy.[61]

Extrinsic factors include poor oral hygiene with the build-up of dental plaque and subsequent formation of stained tartar which incorporates numerous substances. Tobacco, tea and coffee contribute to dark staining and mercury poisoning is reported to produce a green stain below gum level due to the presence of sulpho-methalmoglobin.

Palatal rugae; rugoscopy. The pattern of the palatal rugae was at one time considered to be of great importance in identification, especially if study models or photographs were taken of the pattern as precautionary registration of data. This procedure was carried out in a number of South American countries and the details of the rugae entered on the odontogram of an individual's criminal records.[62]

Lips; cheiloscopy. The fissures and grooves on the lips are claimed to be characteristic of the individual and a number of experts believe that lip prints can be of value in identification.[63–65] However in a recent murder investigation in Essex, lip prints were found on a door frame at a murder scene. In spite of exhaustive studies by photography, rubber base impressions of the lips of the suspect, and further lip prints of the suspect, no similarities could be demonstrated in the fissures

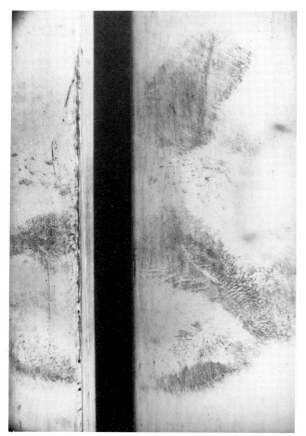

A

and grooves but only in the general outline and dimensions of the lips of the suspect (Fig. 10.3).[66]

AGE DETERMINATION

When human remains are found and prior to the retrieval of ante-mortem data the age of the individual is of prime importance. The approximate age may be determined at the locus and may be of the greatest help in establishing identity but the assessment has to be determined accurately when the body or remains have been removed to a more convenient place of examination. There are suitable methods which will apply according to the type of human remains recovered, and will take into consideration dental development and bone development if skeletal remains are present, or the general physical development if the remains are of recent origin.

If fetal material or children's remains are found a full radiographic examination is completed before the autopsy procedure; in this way the small to minute structures of dental development are located, dissected out of the jaws and subjected to histological study.

The chronology of tooth development would appear to have been studied extensively over the

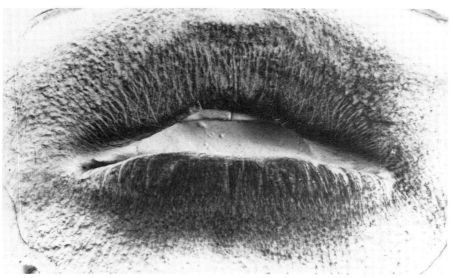

B

Fig. 10.3 Photograph of lip prints on a door frame (A) compared to an impression of the lips of the accused person (B).

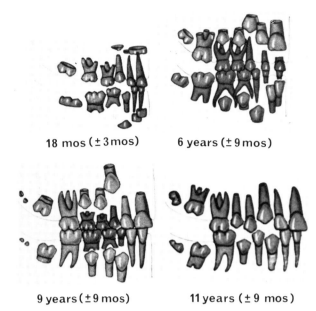

18 mos (± 3 mos)   6 years (± 9 mos)

9 years (± 9 mos)   11 years (± 9 mos)

Fig. 10.4 The development of the dentition, illustrated at four selected ages. Taken from Schour, I. and Massler, M. (1941) published by the American Dental Association.

years by reason of the number of tables published. They present the extent of calcification and eruption of the deciduous and permanent teeth at given ages of children and young persons. Probably that most commonly used even at the present time is the table produced by Schour & Massler[67] (Fig. 10.4). Many investigators find this table to be the most convenient in its pictorial presentation of dental development and eruption although it has been found that the data are of limited value having been derived from the study of a relatively small number of individuals representing one race alone. Moorrees, Fanning & Hunt[68, 69,] (Fig. 10.5) published charts based on a radiographic survey of the details of deciduous and permanent teeth in a large number of American school children. The progress of tooth formation was divided into a series of radiographic landmarks on the chart. The stage of formation of a tooth could then be compared with the chart to obtain the average for attaining a landmark and also the standard deviations either side of the age. Unfortunately this method does not extend to radiographic comparisons of certain posterior teeth as the radiographic appearance of bone structure in the posterior region of the upper jaw masks tooth formation.

Johanson[29] cites a chart published by Gustafson and Koch which covers a period of tooth development from eight months prior to birth up to the age of 16 years. The data collected to produce this chart are derived from 19 sources over a period of approximately 60 years. Four landmarks in tooth development are recorded, the beginning of mineralisation, the completion of crown formation, the completion of tooth eruption and the end of root formation. Each landmark is represented as a small triangle, the apex presenting the average age of attaining a landmark and the angles at the base indicating the earliest and latest ages for the landmarks.

Each of the methods described therefore have drawbacks which the experienced investigator can appreciate when making a choice of which method would be the most suitable in particular circumstances, or whether a combination of methods would be advantageous in determining the identity of an unknown individual by an age assessment.

Age has been determined in a number of young individuals by examination of the structural features of the dentine and enamel tissues of forming teeth. Although it was found that dentine also presented similarities in daily growth when compared to enamel the latter tissue provided clear demarcations that could be readily counted.[70] Microscopic 'cross-striations' of the enamel are generally accepted to be daily increments of growth. The method consists of counting the number of cross-striations formed from birth, indicated in the tissue by an accentuated incremental line called the 'neonatal line', until the point is reached where formation of the enamel tissue has ceased at the time of death of the individual. The method is limited therefore to those cases in which it can be assumed that dentine or enamel was still forming at the time of death of the young individual. The counting procedure of the cross-striations in the enamel is tedious and requires the use of a projection microscope after sectioning the material in its undecalcified state. This procedure, therefore, necessitates the use of facilities of a well-equipped laboratory in the dental school of a teaching hospital. However this is a method of choice when a most accurate estimate of age is to be obtained, and particularly from a few months after birth to three or four years of age, when the age of the individual can be given in

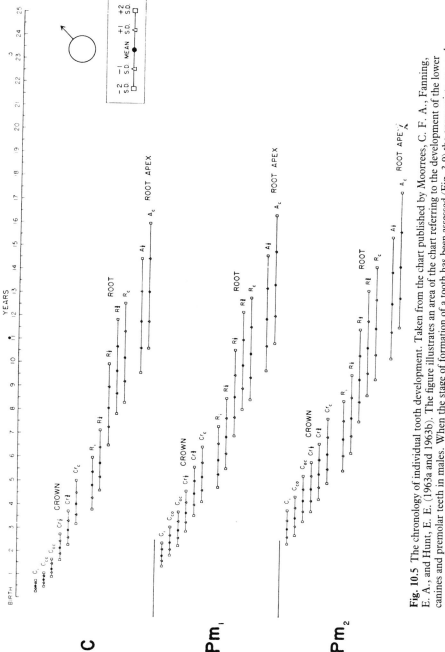

Fig. 10.5 The chronology of individual tooth development. Taken from the chart published by Moorrees, C. F. A., Fanning, E. A., and Hunt, E. E. (1963a and 1963b). The figure illustrates an area of the chart referring to the development of the lower canines and premolar teeth in males. When the stage of formation of a tooth has been assessed (Fig. 3.9) the appropriate age and the ± two standard deviations are obtained by entry in the chart.

days with an experimental error calculated as 20 days either side of the true age.

If tetracycline antibiotic is given to a patient during the period of tooth formation, some of the drug is incorporated in the dentine forming at that time. If subsequently the teeth are sectioned and viewed with ultraviolet light, the areas of dentine marked by the tetracycline fluoresce with a yellow colour. These fluorescent lines represent the dentine forming at the times of the administration of the drug.

Dentine is also laid down in a regular incremental manner, and by measurement of the distances between adjacent fluorescent lines an estimate of the time intervals between successive treatments can be obtained.

In the examination of an unidentified body medical records of missing persons may be available. If the sequence of estimated time intervals between fluorescent lines in the dentine corresponds to the periods between tetracycline treatments recorded in the medical records, some evidence towards the identification of the body will have been obtained.

If medical records are not available it may be possible to measure from the neonatal line (signi-fying the position of the dentine layer forming at birth) to the fluorescent lines. From these measurements estimations of the various ages at which tetracycline treatments were given and the final age of the body may be obtained. (This method was applied to a murder investigation involving the identification of a young girl whose dental records and medical records were incomplete.[71]

An alternative method of some value in which the age of infants is related to the heights and weights of developing teeth has been described but has been infrequently used in the past.[72] The teeth were dissected from the jaws of children of known age and weight and a regression line of weight against age was produced. When the weight of teeth recovered from a human infant of unknown age is compared against the regression line an estimate of age is obtained. This method would only be found to be applicable in the examination of foetal and new born material.

The progressive age changes that occur in the permanent teeth of an adult individual has been frequently used in a method devised more than 30 years ago.[73] This method requires the examination

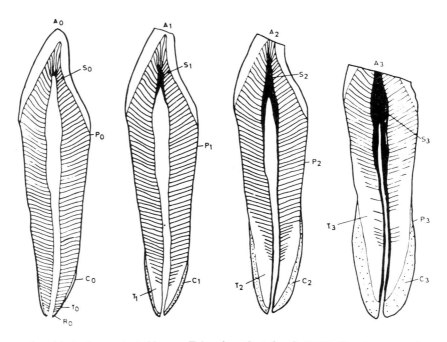

Fig. 10.6 Six changes found in teeth accentuated by age. Taken from Gustafso, G. (1950). The changes are A = attrition, S = secondary dentine deposition, P = apical migration of the periodontal membrane attachment, T = root translucency and R = root resorption (not indicated in the illustration).

of six criteria which includes the attrition of the tooth, the deposition of secondary dentine, the level of the gingival attachment, the deposition of cementum, the translucency of the root, and the resorption of the root. These criteria are assessed both by naked eye examination and in section of the undecalcified specimen and each is given a point value from 0–3 according to the degree of departure from the normal newly erupted tooth which does not exhibit any of the features of senile change or wear (Fig. 10.6). When the total point value has been estimated for a particular tooth this value is then compared with the point values of a tooth series of accurately known age. The comparison is usually carried out on a prepared graph on which is marked the regression line determined from a statistical basis indicating the relation of the total point values of teeth against their known age (Fig. 10.7). In order to achieve an accurate estimation it is necessary to obtain the full point values of all the features of the criteria of the tooth of the unknown individual having first prepared a 'personal' graph with a 'personal' regression line by the collection and assessment of a series of teeth of known age. This method is subjective and it is not entirely satisfactory for another investigator to apply the point values he obtains for each of the criteria against the regression line of Gustafson.

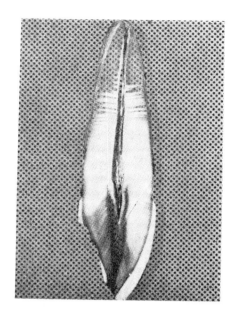

Fig. 10.8

Even with this precaution it is well known that pathological conditions can alter each of the features separately and extensively and extreme care has to be taken in assessing the point values of each of the factors. The average error claimed for this technique is ±3.6 years but Johanson[29] in his critical evaluation of age determinations after 14 years of age concludes that the 95% confidence limit is approximately ±14 years.

However, of the six criteria used by Gustafson, the assessment of root translucent has proved to be the single most reliable age change (Fig. 10.8).[74, 75] This method of age assessment has the advantage that the area of root translucent can be directly measured by use of the microscope, and can be considered to be a true age change, and therefore minimises the subjective error in estimation. In a similar manner to Gustafson's method a regression line is produced on a graph relating length of root translucent against known age of a tooth series and when a tooth from an unknown individual is compared to the graph an error of ±3.6 years is claimed for this method.

In summary, therefore, there are a number of methods of age assessment which may be applied for the periods extending from foetal and neonatal development, through the stages of development

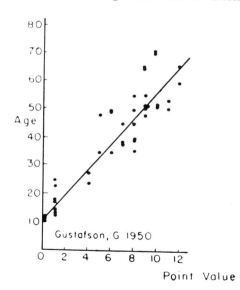

Fig. 10.7 Regression line of point values awarded to individual teeth compared with knowledge. Taken from Gustafson, G. (1950).

and eruption of the deciduous teeth, the mixed period when the deciduous teeth are being replaced by the permanent teeth, and the completion and eruption of the permanent teeth in the early teens. In the latter part of the teens the eruption and development of the third molar or wisdom tooth is the only method that presents information about age. Subsequently when adult dentition is complete, reliance is placed on the senile changes a tooth undergoes to provide an age assessment which may be termed reasonable in accuracy when compared to other methods used in forensic medicine with regard to ossification centres and skeletal development and general physical development. It is well to remember that the chronological or true age is not synonymous with the age presented by dental development, skeletal development or physical development. Until recently the Home Office regarded the skeletal development of the hand and wrist as an accurate means of assessing the age of immigrants to this country when some discrepancy was found in the date of birth on a passport. It was found that any radiographic dental data could provide a more accurate means of age assessment in such cases in spite of the fact that racial, environmental and pathological factors could induce wide variations to the normally accepted values of growth and development tables of a different racial group.[15] At present the charts used in age assessment represent material obtained from few population surveys and it is a field of research that merits greater interest to incorporate many more racial groups.

BITE MARKS

More than 100 years have past since the publication of the first bite-mark case was recorded in the literature.[77] Over the period of time up to the present day the number of reported cases has become more frequent with an increasing variety of types of cases which include bite-mark injuries to the living and the dead, teeth marks in foodstuffs, and damage to inert materials by teeth. Up to 15 years ago it was stated with some authority that in spite of the apparent increase in bite-mark frequency many forensic odontologists had examined few such cases by reason of scarcity.[37] This apparent contradiction

may be explained in the first instance by the fact that although the dental evidence was obvious to the investigating police officer he had no knowledge of the existence of a dental expert who could advise him and even today there are many members of law enforcement and the legal profession who are unaware of trained dental experts who are able to interpret and assess and susequently testify concerning dental evidence in Court. Secondly, the dental expert or forensic odontologist has examined many more cases than he has numerically contributed to the literature. However, bite-mark injuries and damage by teeth are now more frequently recognised by investigating officers. There is an increasing incidence of bite-mark injuries in murder, sexual assaults, affrays, non-accidental injury to children and attacks by animals. In addition there are numerous reports of bite marks in foodstuffs at the scene of a burglary or housebreaking and teeth marks left in inert materials such as wood, plastic cloth and even metal. Therefore the field of study is wide ranging and a simple classification can divide the subject into agents producing bite marks or tooth marks and the substances presenting such marks rather than the very limited classification of bite marks on humans encountered in the Kama Sutra of Vatsyayana. This ancient treatise describes accurately seven types of bite marks on particular sites of the body which are easily recognisable in current bite mark cases.[78]

Agents producing bite marks

Human

Adults. Unlawful killings, sexual assaults, affrays and assault and battery present a high incidence of bite-mark injuries. In numerous cases the victim presents bite-mark injuries as part of the assault or the victim in defence inflicts bite-mark wounds on the assailant. In cases of non-accidental injury to children bite marks feature prominently and it has been found to be distributed approximately equally between father and mother as perpetrators. In addition it has been found an interesting observation that the parent on some occasions who confesses to producing the injury is not necessarily the actual perpetrator.

Children. In some cases of suspected non-accidental injury to children both parents can be eliminated as perpetrators when the size and shape of the bite-mark injuries are consistent with the teeth and arch form of another child in the family, perhaps by reason of jealousy of the new addition to the family, or simple curiosity of the effect that biting has on the new member. However, it is a reasonable precaution to remember that sometimes a child will imitate the example of a 'battering' parent and produce bite marks on an abused child. There are other circumstances in which children bite each other. In nurseries or school where boisterous play and aggressive tendencies are not curbed or under full time supervision.

Animals

The list of members of the animal kingdom which can inflict bite injuries providing they have the correct dental apparatus is almost endless. Injuries can be produced by wild or domestic animals (both farm and pet) and may be either provoked or unprovoked attacks. Wild and domestic animals are sometimes naturally aggressive or will defend their young if they regard the human as a threat. There are numerous reports of adults and children being bitten by dogs, usually domestic pets, but in some circumstances by guard dogs on unsupervised premises often with tragic results. Sometimes bodies of elderly people are found in the open or at home who appear to have suffered a dreadful attack but on examination the wounds are found to be post-mortem and are the result of either wild animals in search of food or even the family pet, cat or dog, who regard the master or mistress as a source of food in order to survive when they are imprisoned in the room in which the human has died.

Fortunately in the temperate climate of the United Kingdom the number of attacks by reptiles or predatory fish are of little importance. The common viper or adder is the only reptile of note and reports of its attacks on humans are infrequent as naturalists observe that the creature is naturally shy and will only bite when disturbed or stepped on. In warmer climates bites of of non-poisonous and poisonous snakes are distinguishable and with the latter the identification of the snake can be ascertained and the appropriate treatment given to the victim. Similarly the bite marks of many fish can be identified especially sharks and a great deal of research has been undertaken in this subject related to survivorship of victims in marine and air disasters in tropical seas.[79] Bodies recovered from water after lengthy immersion exhibit extensive post-mortem injuries as a result of crustacea, fish and mammal mutilation. Hence criminal disposal of bodies at sea could prevent an autopsy establishing the cause of death. An interesting medico-legal case was reported in Australia many years ago in which a newly caught shark when transferred to a public Aquarium disgorged a human arm. The arm was identified as having belonged to a particular individual who had been missing for some time and a murder investigation was immediately instituted. No further remains were ever found and this case has found its place in the literature as the 'Shark-arm' Case.[80]

Mechanical

It was deemed appropriate to include full and partial dentures in this section as the mechanical means of inflicting bite injuries. For many years there had been no reports of edentulous individuals using full dentures to produce bite marks but the situation had been anticipated by Clémençon.[81] Twenty years later the author had experience of a rape and buggery case in which the victim was subjected to bite marks on her breasts and buttocks, whilst in an unconscious state, by the perpetrator who possessed a full upper denture and a few lower natural front teeth. The upper full denture was old and presented wear in relation to the few lower standing teeth. (Fig. 10.9) The differentiation of the marks on the body of the victim could be correlated to both the artificial teeth and to the natural teeth and the assailant stood trial at Nottingham Crown Court. Although the defence strongly contested the evidence the jury was convinced that the man on trial was responsible for the injuries and he was found guilty (R. v. Bowley, Nottingham 1977).

In cases involving partial dentures it is natural to assume that the natural standing teeth are more likely to produce bite marks, but it has been found that artificial teeth in the front of the mouth can produce recognisable marks. Rötzscher[82] presented

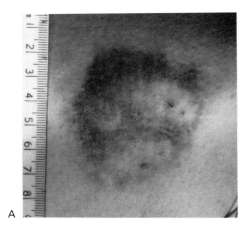

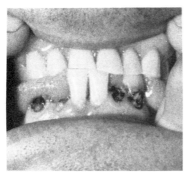

Fig. 10.9 Multiple bite mark on a body. B. Upper full denture and the few lower standing teeth responsible for the bite-mark injury.

a case which clearly illustrated the differentiation a bite makes in relation to the teeth of a partial denture wearer. It is interesting to note that edentulous persons may use their full dentures in biting as an erotic function or concealed masochism.[83]

'Teeth marks' can be produced by true mechanical means if one considers the teeth of a saw. A young girl was found murdered in the Channel Islands and apart from the stab wounds there were minute abrasions of the fingers of the hands which were first thought to be rodent or insect bites. However examination revealed a regularity consistent with the edge of a hacksaw blade which related in evidence to the fact that the murderer was employed in a butcher's shop (*R.* v. *Norton,* Jersey 1966). Sharpened teeth on combs and bicycle-wheel sprockets have been used in football march violence and in a number of murder cases and non-accidental injury to children, even dining

forks have been used to inflict injury (*R.* v. *Taylor,* Hereford 1979).

Substances and materials presenting bite marks

Skin and body tissues

One is unaware at the present time of bite marks on living animals produced by humans but one may anticipate, as in all forensic work, the possibility that it can happen or that it has occurred and has not been reported. Bite marks may occur on any part of the human body but in the adult there appear to be definite sites of election which may be related to the type of offence involved. In the course of an affray fingers and ears are sites of easy access to the assailant or may be the victim's choice of self-defence in rape. Even the genitalia are subject to injury in adults and more especially so in non-accidental injury to children. Such marks may be ill-defined arising from haste compared to the slow deliberate biting that is often seen after sexual crimes of rape and homosexual attack. In sexual crimes the bite marks may be numerous and well defined and are usually found on the neck and breasts, abdomen and thighs of females in rape cases but may be found on the back and buttocks in buggery or homosexual attack in males.[84] However, the presence of such marks does not exclude the possibility of erotic biting on previous occasions of lovemaking when the victim was willing to receive them and should be eliminated and not confused with the injuries of the current attack. The term erotic bite supercedes the previous description of 'love-bite' on the assumption that a painful injury produced is not a true token of love.[85] The true love-bite presents as two ill-defined margins representing the pattern of the upper and lower front teeth containing a diffuse central area of redness and incorporating petechial haemorrhages due to tongue pressure and sucking, and these signs are sometimes seen together with the most severe bite marks. Consequently considerable research has been undertaken in the past and continues in order to elucidate the mechanics and pressures of biting.[86]

Foodstuffs

It would appear that the choice of food bitten into

at scenes of murder, burglary and house breaking must entirely depend on what is available in the household and the personal taste of the intruder. The common factor in each situation is that the food is never entirely eaten but a large portion remains exhibiting the bite almost as if the intruder has deliberately left a 'calling card'. The list of foodstuffs include sandwiches, meat pies, apples, cheese, butter, each of which has its own particular properties of shrinkage and distortion, quite apart from the quality of definition of the bite that the food will exhibit.[87] Considerable thought has been given to preservation of whatever foodstuff is found as evidence at the scene but by far the best procedure is the recording of details by photography which requires the inclusion of a linear scale for subsequent comparisons with suspect teeth, and the use of modern impression materials suitable for the type of food material involved. Preservative substances and refrigeration have been found to be of limited value in the past and the production of a study model in dental stone at the earliest opportunity from the impression materials provides a stable and permanent court exhibit.[88]

Other materials and substances

It is not difficult to assume that this section would be mainly concerned with plastic or softer materials, soap or of plasticene whose physical and chemical properties are such that they are capable of recording a dental imprint. Chewing gum is included in this category since it is a latex substance after the sugars and flavourings are dissolved in the mouth and although it will retain tooth impressions they are subject to considerable distortion but it is a much better source for the recovery of saliva (Fig. 10.10). In a number of cases serological analysis has established the common ABO groups from the secretor status of the individual who chewed the gum.

Pipestems and pencils are common enough to exhibit teeth marks but definition of the marks is not easily comparable to the teeth which may have produced them.[89] Surprisingly it is the harder and more rigid materials that seem to provide most useful information in establishing the identity of the biter. The literature refers to an unusual case of housebreaking in which the thief was disturbed

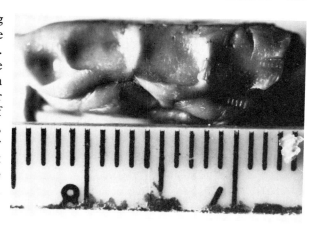

Fig. 10.10 Teeth impression in chewing gum.

by the owner of the household and during the escape through an open window the thief slipped on the window sill and embedded the tips of his upper front teeth in the top of a wooden cabinet. Subsequently an individual was detained whose fractured incisors mechanically fitted the tips of the teeth embedded in the woodwork.[90] An unusual case of suicide has been quoted in which the victim bit through a 'live' electric cable to electrocute himself.[91]

Several years ago a man stood trial at Norwich Crown Court for the murder of his wife. He maintained that her death was caused by the accidental discharge of his shotgun during an argument but it was hard to reconcile the fact that shot entered through the back at the level of the left shoulder blade when the incident was supposed to have taken place as a face to face confrontation. Injuries to the face of the wife were consistent with her having been hit in the mouth with the butt of the shotgun. On examination of the butt of the weapon there were two small linear marks which could be related to the position and angulation of the lower central incisors of the victim. The husband was found guilty of murder and sentenced to life imprisonment (*R. v. Straker*, Norwich 1978) (Fig. 10.11).

More recently a youth alleged that he had been forcibly propelled against a car by a police officer and his face had come in contact with the metal surface of the roof just above the gutter over the door on the driver's side. The upper central incisors and the lower lateral incisors were fractured

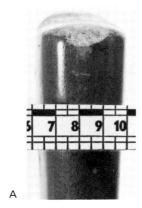

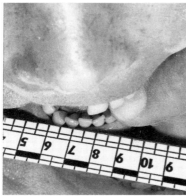

Fig. 10.11 Two marks on the butt of a shot-gun (A) which correspond to the arrangement of the lower central incisors (B).

and there were indentations consistent with the upper teeth on the site described. However, the allegation of the complainant was not consistent with the mode, force and direction of his head to produce the marks on the car from his injuries and the complaint against the police officer was dismissed by the magistrates. This is possibly the first case recorded of teeth marks on the roof of a Ford Escort police panda car (*R. v. Tabel*, Salisbury 1982).

The general methods of recording bite marks

The principle of a routine procedure for the examination of bite marks holds true for whatever material is involved and it is generally accepted by most medico-legalists and law enforcement officers that the forensic odontologist should be called in to the investigation at the earliest opportunity. In cases involving bite marks in human tissues, tooth

indentations and redness and bruising have a tendency to disappear very quickly in the cadaver, and foodstuffs distort by loss of moisture or volatile contents in inappropriate temperatures. If there is a delay in recording the dental characteristics of a bite then evidence may be lost irretrievably. In the living subject bruising changes over a period of days and again there is the possibility that the definition of the marks lessens until it becomes incomparable to the dentition of a number of suspects. It is not always possible to appreciate that there is a bite mark on a human body at the locus if the mark is hidden by clothing and sometimes the injury is not found until autopsy. But in those situations when the mark is evident then the preliminary procedure can be established, either by the police surgeon or the forensic pathologist if in the absence of the forensic odontologist at that time. The presence of the forensic odontologist should ensure that the correct procedures of recording are carried out prior to removal of the body from the scene or prior to the autopsy. However there have been occasions when a distorted bite mark has been examined at the scene and this has given an indication of the posture of the body when it received the injury. The first step in the procedure is to examine the marks on the human body either living or dead with an ultra violet lamp.[92]

In the first instance the illumination may elicit the faint fluorescence associated with saliva which can be collected by swab from the skin surface for subsequent serological analysis. It has been advocated that teased fibres from an old freshly laundered laboratory white coat moistened in distilled water are used, provided the skin surface is not damaged or contaminated from material from clothing or blood from elsewhere which may give false reactions. The saliva may give the ABO blood grouping of the assailant if there is a secretor status of the individual and if not its presence will confirm the mark being examined as a bite mark. Saliva has even been collected using cigarette paper moistened in tap water but serological laboratories are not enthusiastic in analysing material obtained in this manner. After collection swabs should be stored in a deep freeze.[93] However, saliva samples should be taken whatever the circumstances to avoid criticism subsequently that such a procedure was neglected in the investigation.

Secondly, the ultraviolet illumination may elicit other marks on the body which are not visible to the naked eye. Melanocytes or pigment cells have a tendency to migrate to the site of injury and they absorb the ultraviolet radiation and therefore demonstrate the margins of previous wounds as definite dark areas. This method has demonstrated injuries given even months previously and has been found to be extremely useful in eliciting marks on the darker skin of other racial groups, the sites of previous erotic bites in rape victims, and the previous history of injury in non-accidental injury to children.[94] This method has also served to provide a better differentiation of faint marks in photography when standard black and white and colour prints have failed to present an image suitable for comparison purposes.

The two main methods of recording bite marks are by the use of photography and the use of impression materials for the provision of subsequent study models cast in dental stone. Over the years various authorities have refined their methods in order to present the dental evidence in the most appropriate manner for Court presentation. A clear and simple demonstration of comparisons of bitten material with suspect dentitions and a straightforward explanation of the facts are the prerequisite on which a jury may deliberate.

At the locus or in the mortuary the forensic odontologist can direct the photographer to take the exposures at the angles which he feels will best provide the features for comparison. A scale is routinely included so that subsequent enlargements can be reproduced life-size or larger providing the magnification is always noted (Fig. 10.12). Many authorities prefer life-size comparisons while others require magnifications three times life-size or more

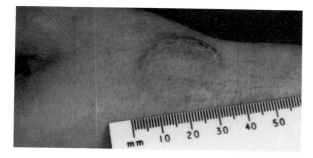

Fig. 10.12 Bite mark on wrist acquired in affray.

before making comparisons.[59] As a photograph only provides a flat representation of marks on curved skin surfaces it is necessary to take successive exposures over the surface with the long axis of the camera lens at right angles to the object plane. In this manner the object plane will always be parallel to the film plane and the centre of the negatives taken and the subsequent prints produced will present an accurate and undistorted view of the particular part of the bite mark under examination. The greater the curvature of the surface on which the mark presents, the greater the number of successive exposures have to be taken to present a series of undistorted portions of the whole mark. If the mark presents on a relatively flat surface then a single view only is necessary or a maximum of three to present the line of the upper teeth, the centre and the lower teeth represented in the mark. Some argument has been generated concerning the type of scale to be included, since some authorities maintain that the use of sticky tape scales provide inaccurate and distorted features for subsequent measurement from photographs and rigid linear scales placed vertically and horizontally near to the mark but not masking any details of the mark are requisite for scientific accuracy. The scale can be in inches or centimetres providing the units of length depicted on the scale conform to approved accuracy standards. In presenting the features of a bite mark on a photograph the normal technical rules in photography are followed. The use of colour or black and white film may depend on the personal choice of the forensic odontologist or the advice of the photographer according to the features to be presented, but the lighting (either normal daylight or artificial from photographic lamps or flashlight) will depend on the skill of the photographer. Angulation of the lighting may enhance the shadowing of indentations in the skin, or the use of filters to bring out shades of coloration, but bitemark photography is concerned with the production of a sharp negative and a clear permanent record of the mark in the finished print.

It has been noted frequently in the past that indentations in the skin both living and dead disappear within a matter of minutes in the living and within 12 h in the dead.[95] If photography and impressions of such marks is delayed then this is another situation in which prime evidence is lost. When the mark appears as a diffuse redness or bruising it is often necessary to rephotograph the injury at 24-h intervals. In the living person bruising is a vital reaction to tissue damage and the bruise develops over a period of time which is specific to the particular individual. In this manner a photograph can be obtained with a better differentiation of the marks due to the natural sequence of events in the living skin. Although bruises do not develop after death it has been noted that post-mortem changes occur in the differentiation of bite-mark bruises, produced, it is thought, by the changes of temperature the body undergoes on removal from the refrigerator at 4°C (39.2°F) to the ambient temperature of the post-mortem room. Re-examination of the marks and photography at the stated intervals sometimes presents a better definition of the marks compared to their presentation at the scene or at the time of autopsy. It is not considered to be good practice to remove the portion of tissue containing the bite mark since tissue specimens shrink considerably on loss of moisture even when kept in a deep freeze and in addition shrink when placed in preservative solutions e.g., formal – saline. However, although bite marks are best preserved in situ on the body there is one specific method of examination of bite-marks for comparison purposes which requires trans-illumination of skin tissues. Other areas of research now include video tape analysis and computerised electronic image enhancement. Great precaution is taken that the excised skin portion and the contained mark retain the same dimensions after removal as before removal from the body.[96]

Other methods have been used in the past which involve infra-red photography and the use of stereoscopic photography to provide greater detail. Each method has inherent problems in demonstration but each method is chosen for those circumstances in which details would not be evident in normal photography.[89, 97] Development of modern impression materials has considerably improved the acquisition of impressions of specimens which were hitherto considered impossible. Water mixed plasters, damaged material containing water-soluble substances and surfaces with fine definition were disrupted by these substances leaching out of the specimen. In addition the physical properties of the impression material in setting could also destroy detail by heat and unsuitable support. The rubber base and silicone base impression compounds have been found to be the most suitable for nearly all the circumstances in which impressions are required. There are numerous proprietary preparations of these compounds with properties suitable for whatever purpose the dental surgeon requires in practice. A material capable of reproducing accurately the dimensions and detail of crown and bridge preparations is eminently suitable for forensic dental purposes. As the choice of impression compound is personal to the practising dental surgeon so is the choice of impression compound to the forensic odontologist for his particular requirements at the locus or in the mortuary. In the existing conditions of ambient temperature at the locus or in the mortuary the setting times of all types of impression compounds are extended beyond proprietary data but the rubber base and silicone base materials which incorporate a setting accelerator catalyst are under the control of the operator. They are less damaging to the specimens under examination and have greater flexible properties compared to plaster of paris and alginate impression compounds. Subsequent study models can be cast in dental plaster or dental stone whose surfaces can be treated with a hardener to provide a permanent study model or models can be produced in acrylic plastic or simulated body tissues in flexible plastic or latex materials.

The next phase of the procedure is to obtain dental impressions of the individual or individuals who are suspected of having made the bite marks. If the suspect is available then the choice of impression compound is the same as that for taking impressions of the bite mark in situ on a victim, or in the foodstuff or other substance, and in addition dependent on the facilities of the medical examination room in a police station or cells. However before the impressions of teeth of the suspect are taken the written consent of that individual must be obtained since an alleged verbal consent can be retracted later by the suspect at a Court appearance and the forensic odontologist could be held guilty of an assault. In the event of refusal by the suspect to be examined or have impressions taken then the refusal can be formally noted and witnessed as should be the consent. There has been only one occasion reported in the United Kingdom on which the authorities have applied for a warrant to force the suspect to comply with undergoing the examination and impression taking, although in the United States a number of suspects have had to comply with a search warrant to provide dental impressions.[5] If consent has been obtained then a routine dental inspection is carried out and noted on a formal dental chart with special reference to abnormalities of tooth or arch form, missing teeth, attrition and types of dental restorations and prostheses. Impressions of the upper and lower teeth of the suspect are taken with the impression compounds of the operator's choice and wax bite registrations. Wax bite registrations are useful as a record of the normal relationship of the upper teeth to the lower teeth in occlusion and in protusive and lateral movements of the jaws. In some circumstances when the movements of the jaw have to be studied in bite analysis the wax bite registrations allow the models of the teeth to be mounted on a dental articulator which can be used to demonstrate normal movements of the jaws of the suspect in the biting process. Having taken the impressions from which study models are subsequently cast it is advisable to produce duplicate study models which can be used as working models while the former can remain as original Court exhibits.

The last phase in the procedure is the comparison of the photographic record and/or study models of the bite marks with the study models of the upper and lower teeth of the suspect or suspects. Various methods have been adopted to demonstrate the similarities or dissimilarities of the teeth of suspects with the bite marks. Some methods have applied a direct comparison of the models of the suspect's teeth with the bite marks in situ on the body which, if held in contact, could produce other marks which could invalidate this evidence in Court. Other methods introduce the phantom model or study model of the part involved but a direct comparison in this manner does not always demonstrate details clearly in Court presentation. A method that has been found to be satisfactory in a number of cases in the past is to accentuate the biting surfaces of the upper and lower front teeth with Indian ink, and the cusps of the premolar

and molar teeth if the bite is considered to involve the latter and photograph the study models including a linear scale. A photographic transparency can then be reproduced life-size from which unwanted detail has been eliminated during photographic development leaving only the pattern of the biting surfaces of the teeth of the suspect. The transparency is laterally inverted and placed over the photograph of the bite marks on a victim or material bitten and a 1:1 comparison made. The comparison will reveal similarities, dissimilarities or even concordance of the teeth of the suspect with the bite marks which will identify or eliminate the suspect as perpetrator. In the absence of photography a sheet of transparent acetate can be prepared by placing the sheet over the study models and marking the underlying arrangement of the biting edges on the transparency with a non-etching draughtsman's ink. In the photographic procedure any number of copies of the transparency can be reproduced by reason of the inclusion of the linear scale whilst in the latter procedure a photostat copy of the master transparency can be used to reproduce unlimited transparencies from the standard copier that produces transparencies for an overhead projector in lecture theatres. There are inherent problems in both methods in obtaining the transparencies, as by the photographic method the transparency may not be particularly clear or not correctly enlarged depending on the skill of the photographer, and by the second method there might be some distortion according to the skill of the dental expert in the free-hand drawing of the details if the sheet of acetate is not firmly fixed above the models of the teeth.[98]

However, when the forensic odontologist has satisfied himself that his personal method is as accurate as he can make it there are further problems associated with the interpretation and assessment of the number of points of similarity which are required to assert that the suspect is the perpetrator of a particular bite mark. Some authorities would consider a minimum number of points of similarity or concordance to be demonstrated before the suspect could be identified as the perpetrator in a similar manner for the requirements of personal identification.[13] Other authorities have set a much lower requirement of a minimum of four to five points of similarity for positive identification, and even fewer

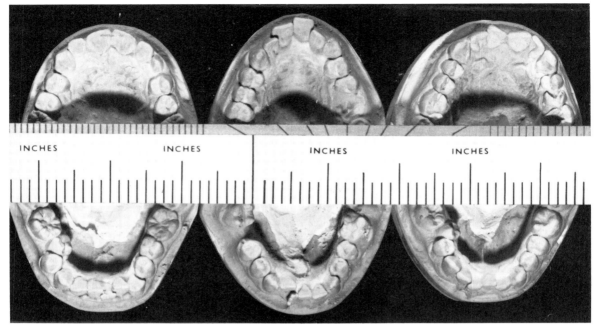

Fig. 10.13 Study models of three individuals, one of whom is the perpetrator of the bite marks on the abdomen and breast of a young female.

points of similarity have provided reliable evidence in the past[90, 99, 100] (Figs 10.13 and 10.14). It was stated by one authority that the evidence in bitemark cases would better serve to eliminate a number of suspects than positively identify the perpetrator.[101] However, it is interesting to note that in the same paper the author describes an experiment in which he is able to positively identify the perpetrator of a bite mark and eliminate two individuals with similar dentitions. Another authority maintains that the interpretation of bite-mark evidence should result in a complete identification or a complete elimination of the suspect, a qualified positive statement in terms of probability based on a degree of similarity not being acceptable.[102] As human tissues, foodstuffs and other materials do not reproduce exactly the character of the teeth biting into them it is not surprising to find so much diversity of opinion based on the cases reported by many contributors to the literature. By reason of the dimensional changes of bitten material it is not always possible to relate tooth measurements to bite marks with the accuracy that scientific experiment requires but the comparison of patterns of marks with the arrangement

of teeth within a dental arch has provided a valid and simple method of demonstrating points of similarity and dissimilarity to the Court and members of a jury. In many circumstances there have been abnormalities in tooth position or arrangement within the dental arch of a suspect that has confirmed him or her as perpetrator of a bite mark and many other times when the comparison of the abnormalities have resulted in complete elimination. A great deal of research has been carried out in the year since the references quoted in the foregoing text on bite marks.

The presentation of bite-mark evidence in Court has probably been considered rare or novel but with the increasing recognition of bite-mark injuries occurring in cases of rape, homosexual assault and non-accidental injury to children such evidence is not only becoming commonplace but becoming the prime evidence and not supporting evidence as before. Perhaps the first reported presentation of such evidence in Court in the United Kingdom to capture professional and public interest was in the Gorringe case in 1948. Almost 20 years later the Biggar Murder Case stimulated even more interest as it was the first occasion that the dental evidence

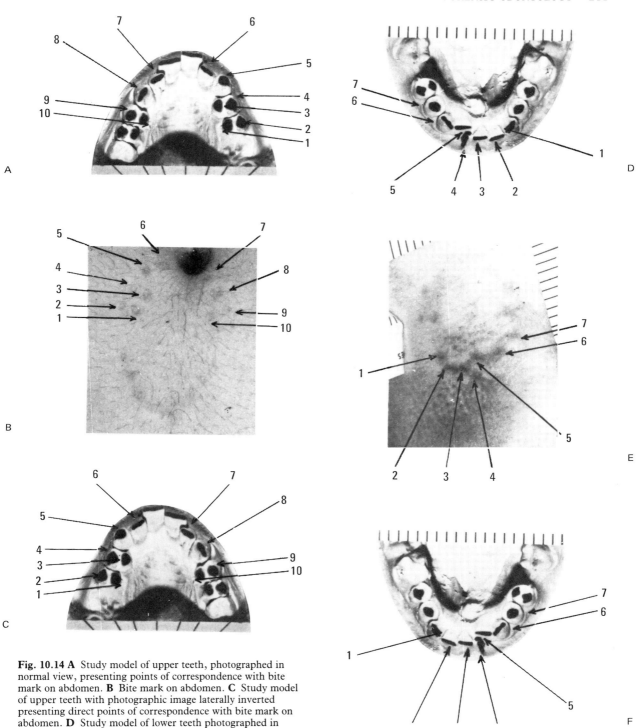

Fig. 10.14 A Study model of upper teeth, photographed in normal view, presenting points of correspondence with bite mark on abdomen. **B** Bite mark on abdomen. **C** Study model of upper teeth with photographic image laterally inverted presenting direct points of correspondence with bite mark on abdomen. **D** Study model of lower teeth photographed in normal view presenting units of correspondence with bite mark on breast. **E** Bite mark on breast. **F** Study model of lower teeth with photographic image laterally inverted presenting direct points of correspondence with bite mark on breast.

was the main evidence in the case and not supportive. Unfortunately there was a great deal of speculation on the part of some authorities concerning the scientific accuracy of the evidence but in view of the fact that the teeth of the perpetrator presented developmental abnormalities which could be matched with specific marks on the breast of the victim and only after careful examination of the upper and lower teeth of 29 suspects, one could conclude that the evidence was entirely correct in the first place. This was yet another occasion when the advice of Professor Keith Simpson was sought, whose experience in this field of study is second to none.[7,103]

In the past few years the interest in the study of bite-mark investigation particularly, and the subject of forensic odontology generally, continues to flourish and the reader is advised to read as widely as possibly the literature on the subject, gain experience in the investigation of forensic dental cases, and seek advice and training in the subject when the opportunity to attend symposia and attachment to departments of forensic medicine arise. Even a cursory perusal of the literature of the subject will acquaint the reader with past authorities and those throughout the world now who continue to extend their research into the wider aspects of the subject by the use of modern techniques and share their knowledge with those who wish to follow.

REFERENCES

1. Keiser-Nielsen, S. (1970) In: Wecht. C. H., ed. Legal Medicine Annual, ch. 2. New York: Appleton–Century Crofts.
2. Furness, J. (1973) Int J. for Dent., 1, 2.
3. Harvey, W. (1966) Br. Dent. J., 121, 344. (Full paper in Int. Police Crime. Rev. 199, 166).
4. Humble BH (1933) Brit. Dent. J., 54, 528
5. Luntz, L. & Luntz, P. (1973) Handbook for Dental Identification. Philadelphia: Lippincott.
6. Amöedo, O. (1897) Dent. Cosmos, 39, 905.
7. Simpson, C. K. (1978) Forty Years of Murder. London: Harrap.
8. Camps, F. E. (1953) Medical and Scientific Investigation in the Christie Case. Tiptree, Essex: Anchor Press.
9. Sognnaes, R. F. (1980) American J. for Med. & Path., 1, 105.
10. Jeffries BMA News Review, 7, 11. (1981)
11. Stevens & Tarlton (1966) Brit. Dent. J., 120, 263.
12. Keiser-Nielsen, S. (1968) Int. Dent J., 18, 668.
13. Keiser-Nielsen, S. (1980) Person Identification by Means of the Teeth. Bristol: John Wright & Sons.
14. Martin, P. & Mason, J. K. (1969) New Law J. 119., 325
15. Radford E, Radford, M.A., Holec. (1978) Superstitions of Death & The Supernatural London: Arrow Books.
16. Smith, J. T. (1982): 34th Annual Meeting of American Academy of Forensic Sciences February 1982 Orlando Florida
17. Knott, N. J. (1967) Br. Dent. J., 122, 144.
18. Haines, D. H. (1967) Br. Dent. J., 123, 336.
19. Ashley, K. F. (1970) Br. Dent. J., 129, 167
20. Mason, J. K. Tarlton, S.W. (1969) Lancet, 1, 431
21. Stevens, P. J. (1970) Fatal Civil Aircraft Disasters: their Medical and Pathological Investigation. Bristol: John Wright & Sons Ltd.
22. Sassouni, V. (1963) J. Dent. Res., 42, 274.
23. Cameron J. & Sims B. G. (1974) Forensic Dentistry Edinburgh: Churchill Livingstone.
24. Snow C. C. (1980) Personal Communication.
25. Hinkes M. J., Brooks, S. T., Brues, A. M., Hoffman J. M., Rhine J. S., Suchey J. M. (1982) 34th Meeting AAFS Feb 82 Orlando Fla.
26. Krogman, W. M. (1946) F. B. I. Law Enf. Bull., 8, 3.
27. Montague, M. F. A. (1947) Technology Rev., 49, 345.
28. Gatliff B. P. & Snow C. C. (1979) Journal of Biocommunication 6, 27
29. Johanson, A. (1971) Odontologisk Revy., 22, supplement 21.
30. Schouri, Massler M. (1941) J. Am Dent Assoc 28, 1153.
31. Greulich, W. W. & Pyle, S. I. (1950) Radiographic Atlas of Skeletal Development of the Hand and Wrist. Stanford, Calif.: Stanford University Press.
32. Venezis P., Sims, B. G. & Grant, J. H. (1978). Med, Sci. Law 18, 209
33. Glaister, J. & Brash, J. C. (1937) Medico-legal Aspects of the Ruxton Case. Edinburgh: Churchill Livingstone
34. Sims, B. G. (1980) Medico-Legal Journal 48, 25
35. Strøm (1946) Norske Tannlaegeforen. Tid 56.153
36. Keiser-Nielsen, S. (1963) J. Dent. Res. 42.303
37. Gustafson, G. (1966) Forensic Odontology. London: Staples Press.
38. Grant, E. A., Prendergast, W. K. & White, E. A. (1952) J. Can. Dent. Assoc., 18, 3.
39. Rigspolitichefen Danmark (1963) Kundgorelse IV, no. 12, 30 January, H G. N R. 1961–84–194.
40. Ford, M. A. (1971) Br. Dent. J., 130, 166.
41. Gradwohl's Legal Medicine, 2nd edn. (1968) Camps, F. E., ed. Bristol: John Wright & Sons Ltd.
42. Petersen K. B. & Kogon S. L. (1971) J Canad Dent. Assoc. 37–275.
43. Frykholm K. O. (1956) Acta. Odont. Scand. 14.11
44. Dental Practice (1982) April 15th Publication Epsom Surrey
45. Vermylen, Y. (1980) Med. Sci. Law. 20, 89
46. Churton, M. C. (1982) Med. Sci. Law 22, 79
47. Kruger-Monsen, A. (1963) 3rd Int. Meeting in For. Immunol. Med. Pathol. Toxicol. Plenary Session IIA, London.
48. Golditz (1967) F. D. I. Commission on Armed Forces

Dental Services. Paris Report III
49. Samis (1978)
50. Muhlemann, H. R., Steiner, E. & Brandestini, M. (1979) J. Forensic Sci. 7, 173
51. Anderson, D. L. & Thompson, G. W. (1973) J. Dent Res. 52, 431
52. Seno, M. & Ishizu, H. (1973) J. Forensic Dent. 1.8
53. Ishizu, H., Ando, K., Seno, M., et al (1973) Japan J. Legmed 27, 239
54. Haines, D. H. (1973) Med. Sci. Law, 12, 131.
55. Harvey (1967) Dental Identification & Forensic Odontology London Kimpton
56. Howden (1971) Brit. Dent. J. 131, 455
57. Furahata, T. & Yamamoto, K. (1967) Forensic Odontology. Springfield, Ill.: Charles C. Thomas.
58. Bell, T. (1829) Anatomy, Physiology and Diseases of the Teeth London, Highley
59. Andrews, E. (1982) Personal Communication
60. Clark, D. & Law, M. (1982) IADR Britain 30th Meeting March 1982 Edinburgh
61. Stanley, H. R. (1972) Oral Surg. 33, 606.
62. Sassouni, V. (1957) J. For. Sci., 2, 428
63. Locard, E. (1932) Rev. Int. Crim. 4, 284
64. Santos, C. M. (1963) Int. Dent. J. 13, 527
65. Suzuki, K. & Tsuchihashi, Y. (1970) J. Forensic Med 17, 52
66. Blythe, P. A. (1981) Police Journal Liv. 300
67. Schour, I. & Massler, M. (1941) J. Am. Dent. Assoc., 28, 1153.
68. Moorrees, C. F. A., Fanning, E. A. & Hunt, E. E. (1963) J. Dent. Res., 42, 1490.
69. Moorrees, C. F. A., Fanning, E. A. & Hunt, E. E. (1963) Am. J. Phys. Anthrop., 21, 205.
70. Boyde, A. (1963) 3rd Int. Meeting in For. Immunol. Med. Toxicol., ch. 7. London.
71. Sullivan (1971) The Ass For Dental Research Int British Division 19th Meeting April Glasgow
72. Stack M. V. (1960) J. Forens Sci Soc 1, 49
73. Gustafson, G. (1950) J. Am. Dent. Assoc., 41, 45.
74. Miles, A. E. W. (1963) J. Dent. Res., 42, 255.
75. Miles, A. E. W. (1963) In: Brothwell, D. R., ed. Dental Anthropology. Oxford: Pergamon.
76. Modi N. J. 1972 Medical Jurisprudence & Toxicology. Bombay: Tripathi
77. Skrzeczkas, A. B., (1974) Vijschr. Gerichtl. Med., 21.
78. Burton, R. & Arbuthnot, F. F. (1963) The Kama Sutra of Vatsyayana. London: Allen and Unwin (translation).
79. Halstead, B. W. (1959) Dangerous Marine Animals. Cambridge, Maryland: Cornell Maritime Press.
80. Davies D. H. J. Royal Naval Medical Service 48, 110.
81. Clémencon (1957) Uber die Aufgabe des Zahnartes bei der Abklärung von Verbrechen und bei der Identifizerung Von Leichen Inaugural Dissertation, 1–31
82. Rötzscher, K. (1972) Deutsch. Stomat., 22, 390.
83. Siegrist H. O. (1970) Kriminalistik 24, 493
84. Furness, J. (1968) Br. Dent. J., 124, 261.

85. Holt (1981)
86. Harvey (1976) Dental Identification & Forensic Odontology London Kimpton
87. Simon, A., Jordan, H. & Pforte, K. (1974) Int. J. Forensic Dent. 2, 17
88. Stoddart, T. J. (1973) Br. Dent. J., 135, 285.
89. Jonason, C. O., Frykholm, K. O. & krykholm, A. Int. J. Foren Dent 2, 70
90. Dedersen P. O., Kerser-Nielson (1961) Retsodontologi Tandlaegebladet 65, 585
91. Scheuer & Petscher (1971) Kriminalistik, 25, 457.
92. Ruddick R. F. (1974) Medical & Biological Illustration 24, 128
93. Dodd (1973) Personal Communication
94. Cameron, J. M., Grant, J. H. & Ruddick, R. (1973) J. Forens. Photog., 1.
95. Sebata, M. (1963) Bull. Tokyo. Dent. Coll 4, 83
96. Beckstead J. W. Rawson R. D., Giles W. S. (1979) J. Amer. Dent. Ass. 99, 69.
97. Frykholm, K. O., Wictorin, L. Torlegard, K. (1970) Sven Tandlak Tidskr 63, 205.
98. Sims, Grant & Cameron (1973) Med., Sci., Law, 13, 207.
99. Berg & Schaidt (1954) Kriminalistik 8, 128
100. Simpson C. K. S. (1969) Personal Communication
101. Fearnhead, R. W. (1961) Med. Sci. Law, 2, 273.
102. Strøm, F. (1963) J. Dent. Res. 42, 312
103. Harvey, W., Butler, O. H., Furness, J. & Laird, R. (1969) J. For. Sci. Soc., 8, 4.

FURTHER READING

Cottone J. A., Standism, S. M. "Outline of Forensic Dentistry" Year Book Medical PuB Inc. Chicago.

Furuhata, T., Yamamoto, K. Forensic Odontology. Springfield, Ill: Charles C. Thomas.

Gladfelter, I. A. Dental Evidence. Handbook for Police. Springfield III: Charles C. Thomas, 1975.

Gustafson, G. Forensic Odontology. London: Staples Press, 1966.

Harvey, W. Dental Identification and Forensic Odontology. London: Henry Kimpton, 1976.

Lunzt, L. L., Luntz, P. Handbook for Dental Identification Techniques in Forensic Dentistry. Philadelphia: J.B.: Lippincott, 1973.

Sopher, I. M. Forensic Dentistry. Springfield, III.: Charles C. Thomas, 1976.

Svadkovsky, B. S. Teaching Aid in Legal Medical Stomatology. (in Russian), Moscow: Medicina Publishers, 1974.

Keiser-Nielsen, K. Person Identification by means of teeth, Bristol: J. Wright & Sons 1980

Vermylen Y, Tormans E, De Valck E, Vanherle G. Gerechtelijke Tandheelkunde. Offset Acco Leuven Copyright Vermyleny Address, Vosweg, 23, 2980 Boortmeerbeek, Belgium.

11

Wounds and their interpretation

The frequency of the various indictable offences that involve injury to the person, which comprise the substance of the following sections, is reflected by the criminal statistics of England and Wales.

Table 11.1 Offences against the person 1980

Total serious offences of violence against the person recorded by police	5968
Homicide	620
Attempted murder	155
Threat or conspiracy to murder	528
Wounding or other act endangering life	4390
Other serious offences	273
Total violence against the person including less serious offences	97 246
Total serious sexual offences recorded by the police	21 107
Including: Buggery	637
Indecent assault on a male	2288
Indecent between males	1421
Rape	1225
Indecent assault on a female	11 498
Unlawful intercourse, girl under 13	254
Unlawful intercourse, girl under 16	3109

The special character of certain of these offences, e.g., infanticide and abortion, rape and other sex crimes, will be considered in detail under the appropriate headings. The sections which follow below are concerned with the nature and interpretation of injuries in general and with the medico-legal complications of wounds of all kinds.

Offences of such a widely differing nature may be inflicted with widely different instruments in an infinity of ways, and demand a consideration of certain general principles before the examination of each in detail.

The characters of an injury caused by some mechanical force are dependent upon:
1. the nature and shape of the weapon;
2. the amount of energy in the weapon or instrument when it strikes the body;
3. whether it is inflicted upon a moving or a fixed body;
4. the nature of the tissues involved.

The consequences of an injury for some mechanical force depend largely on its mass and velocity, the length of time it operates and the tissues injured. The destructive energy liberated when a moving body is suddenly brought to rest is expressed by the formula $MV^2/2$ where M = mass and V = velocity of the object. The mechanics of impact is explored in later sections, but it must be clear from this formula that the velocity is much more important than the weight of the weapon used.

Table 11.2 England and Wales. Deaths from accidents and violence 1978

Total	21 360
Road transport	6772
Poisoning	775
Fire	650
Suicide	4022
Homicide	612
*Undetermined injuries	1485

* This figures refers to cases where a coroner has brought in an open verdict—there being insufficient evidence to determine whether the death was homicidal, suicidal or accidental.

Reference to the table detailing the Registrar General's statistics of injury by cause (in accident and suicide) shows, further, the variety of 'instrument' and other causes for injury—adding more than mere mechanical factors to their potential for harm and indicating a wide field of enquiry and study which we must now discuss at length.

LEGAL CONSIDERATIONS

Wounds and personal injuries may have to be considered both in connection with criminal offences and civil claims to damages. In the criminal law three classes of crime may be distinguished from this point of view, namely homicide, assaults on the person, and certain special offences in which the term 'wound' forms part of the legal definition of the offence.

Homicide

This is not itself the name of a crime in English law but is a general term which includes several distinct crimes. Homicide means the death of one human being as the result of the conduct of another. It may be lawful, as killing in self-defence in certain circumstances, or causing death by sheer misadventure. Unlawful homicide is divided into
1. murder,
2. manslaughter,
3. infanticide, and
4. child destruction.

The scope of the two last-mentioned offences is described in chapter 15. The expression 'culpable homicide' is used in Scots law where it is the equivalent of manslaughter.

For the purposes of homicide the death may be caused either by an act or by an omission but in either case the death must be proved to be the consequence of the alleged killer's conduct. Difficult questions may arise as to the cause of death in the legal sense. In the case of *R. v. Holland* (1841, 2 Mood & R. 351) it was held that it made no difference whether a wound was in its own nature instantly mortal, or whether it became the cause of death by reason of the deceased not having adopted the best mode of treatment; the real question is whether in the end the wound is the cause of death. But if death occurs at too remote a date from the original act or omission it will not be unlawful homicide, for there is an old rule of common law that

to support a charge of murder or manslaughter the death must occur within a year and a day after the receipt of the original injury. The extra day is to make it quite clear that the period of liability is a full 365 days.

Murder

Unlawful homicide implies both the fact of death and an accompanying state of mind on the part of the killer. Certain states of mind make the homicide murder and other states of mind make it manslaughter only. The state of mind necessary in murder is indicated by the highly technical term 'malice aforethought'. A murderer is one who kills another with malice aforethought, expressed or implied. The term is a verbal formula which is liable to mislead, for malice in the usual sense of spite or ill-will is not required, nor is any premeditation or planning in advance. Killing on the spur of the moment may be murder. It will be murder if there is a positive intention to kill some person, whether it be the person actually killed or not, if there is an intention to cause grievous bodily harm to any person and the death of someone in fact results, or even if the intention is merely to do an unlawful voluntary act of such a kind that grievous bodily harm (at the least) is the natural and probable result though not positively intended by the accused. Before 1957 the law was stricter, for where a person killed another in the course or furtherance of any kind of felony it amounted to murder, whatever the intention; this rule of 'constructive malice', as it was called, was abrogated by the Homicide Act of that year.

Manslaughter

The scope of the crime of manslaughter is very wide, ranging from something little short of murder to something which is a technically unlawful homicide for which a nominal penalty is appropriate. The maximum penalty is life imprisonment.

The most serious form of manslaughter occurs when the accused has intentionally attacked the deceased without the necessary intention ('malice aforethought') which is essential to murder. But manslaughter often arises from acts which are not intentional at all, such as the doing of a lawful act recklessly, for instance, driving a car in this way. And it may be committed without any positive act, as in the culpable omission to perform a duty recognised by the criminal law, such as the failure to carry out a safety precaution on a railway. If a homicide would normally amount to murder the offence is reduced to manslaughter if the jury is satisfied that the accused was provoked (whether by things done or by things said or by both together) to lose his self-control. The provocation must be gross, and sufficient to lead to loss of self-control on the part of the normal, reasonable man, and the mode of resentment must bear a reasonable relationship to the provocation.

A person suffering from 'diminished responsibility' who would otherwise be convicted of murder will be convicted of manslaughter instead. This rule was introduced into English law by the Homicide Act 1957, on the lines of Scots law, which takes into account, on charges of murder, lesser forms of mental abnormality than insanity. This special statutory form of diminished responsibility exists if the accused was 'suffering from such abnormality of mind [whether arising from a condition of arrested or retarded development of mind or any inherent causes or induced by disease or injury] as substantially impaired his mental responsibility for his act and omissions in doing, or being a party to, the killing' [section 2 (1)].

Suicide

Suicide and attempted suicide were crimes until the Suicide Act of 1961 abrogated them. For legal purposes other than criminal convictions it may still be necessary to know whether or not a death was suicidal. And it is still a crime to be an accessory before the fact to another person's suicide or attempted suicide, as by persuading him to die (Suicide Act 1961, S.2). It is manslaughter and not murder for a person acting in pursuance of a suicide pact between himself and another to kill the other or be a party to the other being killed by a third party (Homicide Act 1957, S.4). A 'suicide pact' is defined as 'a common agreement between two or more persons having for its object the death of all of them, whether or not each is to take his own life, but nothing done by a person who enters into a suicide pact shall be treated as done by him in pursuance of the pact unless it is done while he has the settled intention of dying in pursuance of the pact'.

In *R. v. Lyons and Reid* (C.C.C. 1981) the accused, both members of Exit, a voluntary euthenasia society, were charged with offences under the Suicide Act 1961 relating to aiding, abetting, counselling and procuring suicide and conspiring together to aid and abet suicide.

Assaults and bodily harm

Assaults vary greatly in legal gravity from an assault with an intent to murder to a 'common' assault. A common assault is contrasted with an 'aggravated' assault where actual bodily harm is caused, or where there are attendant aggravating circumstances, such as an intention to commit a felony or to maim, disfigure or disable any person. The description 'assault and battery' is not tautologous, for the two words indicate distinct offences which may or may not be committed by reason of the same physical act. An assault is an offer or threat or attempt to apply force to the body of another in a hostile manner. A battery is the actual application of force to the body: it is the assault brought to completion.

Inflicting 'grievous bodily harm' is one of the various aggravated assaults included in the Offences Against the Person Act 1861. 'Bodily harm' is not defined by statute for the purpose of this and certain other offences in the definition of which the same phrase is used. It may mean internal as well as external injuries and it need not be permanent or dangerous. It is not grievous unless it seriously interferes with health or comfort. Shooting at a person with intent 'to maim, disfigure or disable any person, or to do some other grievous bodily harm' is a separate offence. In law a maim, or mayhem, is traditionally a bodily hurt whereby a man is rendered less able in fighting to defend himself or to annoy his adversary. Thus it has been held that cutting off, disabling or weakening a man's hand or finger, or striking out his eye or foretooth, are maims but not (at common law) the cutting off of his ear, or nose or the like, because they do not weaken a man but only disfigure him. 'Disfigure', as used in the Act of 1861 seems to mean an external injury which may detract from personal appearance. The word 'disable' in an earlier Act was held to mean permanently and not temporarily disable, but this may be regarded as too strict an interpretation should the point come before the Courts again.

The word 'wound' occurs in the definition of several crimes included in the Offences Against the Person Act 1861. 'Whosoever shall by any means whatsoever wound .... any person with intent to commit murder' is guilty of felony (S. 11), as is anyone who 'shall unlawfully and maliciously by any means whatsoever wound' any person with intent to do grievous bodily harm (S. 18). 'Whatsoever shall unlawfully and maliciously wound .... any other person either with or without any weapon or instrument' is guilty of a misdemeanour (S. 20).

An 'offensive weapon' has been defined by section 1 (4) of the Prevention of Crime Act 1953, as 'any article made or adapted for use for causing injury to the person or intended by the person having it with him for such use by him'. In R. v. *Edmonds and others* (1963, AUE.R.828) three men toured betting shops in London with, it appeared, the intention to rob. When stopped and searched, the car which they were using was found to contain a shotgun and some cartridges. One of the accused had an unloaded starting pistol in his pocket, another had a piece of lead piping and the third a hammer shaft. It was not denied that these could be regarded as 'offensive weapons'.

Grievous bodily harm

The term is to be interpreted literally. Bodily harm includes electric shocks insufficient to damage the skin, tight ligatures placed around the neck, around limbs, or around the penis, foreign bodies inserted into the rectum or vagina, and burns from the throwing of liquids which need not be corrosive, merely staining or irritating the skin. The intent with which hurt is inflicted is of more importance in law than the injury itself.

In R. v. *Davis*[22] a man was charged with wounding with intent to do grievous bodily harm. It appeared from the evidence that the prisoner, half drunk, and during a quarrel, suddenly stabbed the prosecutor, inflicting a serious wound, from the effects of which he was in danger for a fortnight. It was contended that there was no intent to produce grievous bodily harm, but the judge said that the jury might satisfy themselves on that point by considering the circumstances of the case. Could a man inflict such a wound without having an intension to inflict grievous bodily injury? The prisoner was not so drunk as not to know what he was doing, and all the circumstances showed premeditation and intention, namely the nature of the wound, the weapon used, and the part of the body struck, where an injury was likely to be dangerous. The prisoner was found guilty of the intent.

Whilst a man was being forcibly held down, the nozzle of a pressure pump was thrust through a hole in the victim's trousers and into his anus, allowing air to rush into the intestine. On admission the abdomen was highly distended with gas. The lower outlet of the bowel was dilated, and the bowel bulged into it. He died very soon after. A post-mortem examination showed ruptures of the gut. The gut was gangrenous and there was peritonitis, due to the rupture of the gut. There were no marks or bruises on the body of the deceased. Whether the nozzle had been put up the anus was a matter for simple inference.

Several cases of a similar nature, occurring in works where compressed air is used, have since been reported. The force of the issuing stream of air is so great that it is not necessary to thrust a nozzle into the body for 'grievous bodily harm' to ensue.

In 1959 a 12-year-old boy died after an apprentice at a garage had released compressed air from a tyre inflator into his rectum. The transverse colon had ruptured and a fatal peritonitis ensued. It was estimated that as much as 1400 ml of air would be released in one second from the pump nozzle.[1]

Wounds

A wound may be defined as damage to living tissue. The injury may be visible externally but this is not essential as serious and fatal internal injuries may be inflicted in the absence of any external mark of violence.

When a doctor is called upon to give an opinion concerning a wound or wounds he must consider the nature of the wound, i.e., blunt impact, incised or penetrating, whether it appears to be accidental, homicidal or self-inflicted, what sort of instrument (in its widest sense) could have produced the injury, and the amount of force used to inflict such a wound.

The clinician will normally examine the wounds in the living and the pathologist in the dead.

The clinical examination is dealt with in chapter 5 and this chapter will deal with the pathological examination.

In any case of violent death the pathologist must:
1. record the nature and distribution of the injuries;
2. determine the cause of death;
3. assess the contribution, if any, of natural or congenital disease to the death;
4. record the presence of all natural or congenital disease processes which may affect the expectation of life;
5. determine whether there is a novus actus interveniens in addition to his cataloguing and interpretation of the injuries present.
He must determine whether the injuries are due to homicide, suicide or accident.

The manner in which fatal injuries are inflicted, i.e., whether self-inflicted, inflicted by another person or persons, or by accident, is a problem which faces the pathologist, the police and the coroner. Some cases cannot be resolved by mere study of the pattern of injuries and resolution may be difficult or impossible in a small number of cases even after examination of the scene of the death and all other available evidence.

To take a simple example: a person is found dead at the foot of a tall building. The injuries may be the same whether he was pushed, fell, or deliberately jumped. Thus, beyond establishing the cause of death, the autopsy can rarely go further—except sometimes where natural disease, alcohol or drugs may have contributed to a fall. The manner of death in such cases must therefore be elucidated from all the other evidence.

In a number of cases of violent death, especially those involving the use of cutting or penetrating instruments or firearms, the pattern of the injuries points directly to the manner of death. In any form of violent death it is of paramount importance that the pattern of injuries should be fully recorded. Injuries which fall outside the pattern

to be expected from a set of circumstances may indicate homicide.

Dr Barrowcliff[2] records a case of a woman who was attacked with a car jack and the car then driven into a tree to simulate an accident. Three medical practitioners who saw the deceased accepted that the injuries were due to a road traffic accident. Post-mortem examination, however, revealed a pattern and severity of injury not consistent with the minor damage to the vehicle.

Accidental injuries are usually clearly accounted for by examination of the scene. It is the separation of self-inflicted injuries from those inflicted deliberately by another person which provides the greatest difficulty.

Suicidal wounds are deliberate wounds and tend to follow certain well defined patterns, and it is often only a break in a particular pattern which indicates that the case is one of homicide or accident.

When considering the question of self-inflicted wounds the following criteria must be applied:
1. The site of the injury must be accessible to the deceased. The site itself may be characteristic of the type of injury and is then referred to as a site of election vide infra gunshot wounds.
2. Repetitive wounds may be grouped together either at the site of the fatal wound or removed from it. The number of these wounds depends upon their severity.
3. The site of the fatal injury is bare or unclothed, except in the case of firearm wounds.
4. The injuries may be inflicted in front of a mirror.
5. Self-inflicted injuries do not involve the features.
6. They may be grouped in the midline in some of the more bizarre forms of injury.

The severity of the injuries does not preclude self-infliction provided the above criteria are fulfilled.

Difficulty in interpretation may arise where some of the above criteria are fulfilled but the injury is outside the classical site of election.

Suicidal injuries resulting from specific weapons will be described under the relevant sections.

Broadly speaking injuries may be classified into the following groups:
1. blunt injuries;

2. incised wounds;
3. penetrating wounds.
Identification of these classes of wounds is essential for the interpretation of the injuries as a whole.

Blunt impact injuries—external appearances

Blunt impact injuries are caused when some solid object comes in contact with the body. The nature of the wound will depend to a great extent upon the part of the body which receives the impact. For example, a heavy blow with the fist may cause no visible injury if applied to the abdomen but may inflict a laceration if directed against the eyebrow.

Blunt injuries are divided into three groups:
1. abrasions or scratches;
2. contusions or bruises;
3. lacerations.

Abrasions. Abrasions are injuries to the superficial layer of skin—the epidermis—and a true abrasion will heal without leaving a scar. Many injuries classified as abrasions, however, have some deeper areas of subepidermal damage which may result in superficial scarring.

For an abrasion to occur there must be movement between the 'instrument' and the skin. If the movement is horizontal or near horizontal to the skin the epidermis will be heaped up according to the roughness of the surface in contact with the skin. The pattern of the heaping up will indicate the direction of movement of the instrument against the skin.

These 'sliding abrasions' are most commonly seen by the pathologist in road traffic accidents where a pedestrian has been struck and slides over the hard road surface. The presence of clothing will modify the appearance of abrasions.

If the movement of the instrument is around 90° to the skin a pressure type of abrasion occurs. This may be seen in manual strangulation (fingernail abrasions) and in hanging, where the weave of the rope or other ligature may be reproduced. This type of abrasion is usually accompanied by some degree of bruising.

Abrasions, *per se*, by definition are not dangerous to life and, as such, are not usually of medical or surgical significance. However, they are of great forensic importance because they occur at the

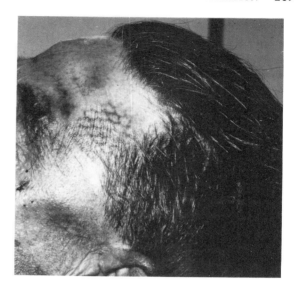

Fig. 11.1 Patterned abrasion on the left forehead due to falling upon a shoe mat.

actual point of contact of the instrument with the body, and they may—if the force is applied at right angles to the skin—reproduce faithfully the pattern of the striking surface of a weapon used to inflict the injury (Fig. 11.1).

Abrasions may be found on any area of the body and may be the only external visible signs of a severe and fatal internal injury.

The appearances of abrasions may be rapidly altered during the post-mortem interval. The abraded area is first moist and this may dry, leaving a tough red-brown or yellow parchment-like area, depending upon the degree or absence of vital reaction to the injury or, if the environment is moist—in summer particularly—the area may be rapidly attacked by insects and fly larvae.

The dried abrasion often appears to be a much more extensive injury than it was at the time of death. This is of particular significance in young children who have some superficial excoriation by urine in the napkin area. At death little may be observed beyond some reddening; some hours later, however, these areas will have dried, leaving depressed yellow or reddish-yellow areas which suggest serious neglect to those not aware of this phenomenon.

Post-mortem abrasions are not infrequently caused by undertakers during their removal of a body. These abrasions may also leave hard yellow areas which can be mistaken for ante-mortem injury.

Contusions or bruises. A contusion is the result of the subcutaneous rupture of blood vessels and the resulting escape of blood into the tissues. There may or may not be some overlying abrasion.

The time interval between the infliction of the blow and the naked eye appearance of the bruise will be influenced by the site of the impact and its force. Bruises become rapidly visible in soft, lax tissue, such as the eyelids, and the 'black eye' is perhaps the most well known of the rapidly forming contusions.

A deep bruise, especially that due to the crushing of tissue against the bony skeleton, may not only take a long time to become visible but may not appear below the actual point of impact. Blood escaping from the damaged vessels will track along the fascial planes (or between muscle layers) which form the least resistance, and may make their appearance some days after the impact where the tissue layers become superficial. For example, a blow to the upper thigh may produce a deep bruise which will appear some days later above the knee.

Bruises inflicted at or about the time of death may not be visible, without dissection, for several days, although their appearance is hastened by an autopsy examination. The reasons for their appearance after a time lapse are:
1. at autopsy blood drains from the blood vessels so that the deep bruises may show up against the white areas as the blood in the contusion will not drain;
2. post-mortem autolytic changes in the blood in the bruise itself, which cause some spreading.

It is always desirable in a case of fatal criminal assaults for the pathologist to re-examine the body some 48 h after his original autopsy to see if further bruises have appeared. It is also highly desirable that the victim of a non-fatal assault be re-examined some 24–48 h after the initial examination.

Artefactual bruising. Bruising may be inflicted post-mortem within a short time of death and this may be indistinguishable from a bruise inflicted immediately before death. In certain organs, however, apparent vital reaction may occur even in an organ contused after its removal from the body. Carscadden[3] illustrates apparent vital changes in a liver contused half an hour after the cessation of heart beat. Moritz[4] states that occasionally it is difficult to distinguish between ante and post-mortem bruising even after the tissue has been examined microscopically.

The type of artefactual bruising which must be carefully avoided by the pathologist is that to the neck in cases of suspected manual strangulation. Autopsies upon suspected crime victims are usually performed shortly after the body is discovered and when the post-mortem interval is short and hypostasis is not fully developed. This provides the ideal circumstances for the production of artefactual bruising. When the neck structures are dissected blood is still in the small vessels of the neck and as the structures are moved the vessels become torn and blood escapes in between the tissues or muscle planes.

To avoid artefactual bruising the area must be drained of blood before it is actually dissected. This is achieved by removing the brain and the internal viscera, cutting the great vessels of the neck and the other tissues level with the thoracic inlet and allowing blood to drain through the cut vessels in the base of the skull and at the base of the neck. The escape of blood can be accelerated by gently lifting and lowering the head. The neck structures are then exposed by making lateral vertical incisions in the skin of the neck and reflecting this skin before removing the soft structures *in toto*.

A further problem relating to the identification of bruising is when it is present in areas where it may be masked by hypostasis. If bruises occur in the pressure areas their presence is obvious but in the hypostatic areas their presence may only be suggested by slight swelling of the area or the presence of an abrasion. Any suspected area should be incised. In an area of hypostatic staining blood will simply run out of the dilated incised vessels, whereas in bruising the blood remains fixed in the tissues.

Disappearance of a contusion. The time taken for a bruise to disappear will depend upon its size and the age of the person. In old people deep bruising may be recognisable many months after its occurrence. The more common superficial bruise, however, resolves and disappears after a succession of visible changes in the bruise itself, due to break down of the haemoglobin or blood pigment.

A fresh bruise is red or dark red. If it involves only the superficial tissues it may not be more than 24 h old. If the bruise is large and deep seated this dark red colour may persist for several days. Around a week later the bruise will develop a greenish tinge which will yellow before it finally disappears. Bruises resolve more rapidly in the young and some animal work suggests that bruises may resolve more rapidly in persons subjected to repeated bruising.

Lacerations. A laceration is the splitting or tearing of the skin by blunt impact and occurs most commonly over bony prominences where the skin is crushed and split against the bone. Thus it is commonly seen over the bony areas of the skull. Lacerations may occur on the limbs and in other regions not only by direct impact but also by tearing, such as may occur in running-over injuries.

The edges of a laceration are usually abraded or irregular to a varying extent depending upon the nature of the instrument and the direction of force. The tissues which may be seen in the depth of the open wound are torn across, but certain structures, nerve cords and tendons may be intact and seen crossing in the depth of the wound. Frequently there is deep bruising around the wound, although this may not be apparent at the time of death.

Haemorrhage will occur from the wound and the depth of the wound will contain blood or blood clot. If, however, the body is immersed in water shortly after death or the injuries occur in water, the blood will become lysed, that is to say the red cells are disintegrated by the water. When the body is removed the wound may be bloodless or blood may still be escaping through cut vessels as it has not clotted due to the presence of water.

Abrasions, contusions and lacerations are the external visible evidence of a blunt impact injury and may give little or no indication of deeper and sometimes fatal injury to the deeper lying structures. Bones may be fractured and vital organs such as the heart or aorta ruptured with the minimum of external signs of impact.

Blunt injuries to specific regions of the body will now be described in more detail and later they will be described in relationship to certain specific forms of blunt impact injury.

Blunt injuries to the head

These are the most common, serious and fatal injuries encountered in practice. The external appearances of the impact, if present, will depend upon the instrument, the point of impact, and whether the point of impact was protected by headgear or hair.

Impacts to the face may result in lacerations over the bony prominences or to the lips from impact with the teeth. Bruises may develop around the eye not only as a result of direct impact but also from anterior basal fractures of the skull. If the impact has occurred over the scalp, the hair may prevent any external laceration, although the inner layers of scalp may be found lacerated upon dissection. This absence of an external laceration is not infrequent even where severe fractures of the skull occur if the instrument is padded or has a broad striking edge.

The cranium is a rigid structure and cannot (except in children) be deformed without fracture.

The skull may be divided for descriptive purposes into the following: the cranium—consisting of vault and base—which contains the brain and the upper and lower jaws and nasal bones. The vault, calvaria or skull cap, is the rounded upper part of the skull which normally has smooth outer and inner surfaces; the base, however, is made up of six paired fossae—the anterior, middle and posterior. The floor of the anterior fossae overlies the eyes, and the middle fossae, which incorporate the ears, are rough, whereas the posterior fossae are relatively smooth. In the posterior fossae there is the foramen magnum—a large opening through which the brain stem passes into the spinal canal.

Fractures of the skull may be:
1. depressed;
2. comminuted;
3. linear or fissured;
4. compound.

Depressed fractures are invariably comminuted and result from a blow of such violence that the bone is fractured and depressed inwards. This may result from a localised impact, such as a hammer head, or from a diffuse impact, such as one sees in road traffic accidents, where a large area of skull may be involved. Linear or fissured fractures may radiate out from depressed fractures. Fissure fractures may be quite simple and single fractures may be seen, for instance, after a fall on to the back of the head. Linear fractures radiating from the point of impact follow the direction of the force.

Violent impacts to the top of the head or transmitted to the base via the spinal column may result in a 'ring fracture' of the base of the skull. This fracture is due to the cervical spine being forced through the skull base.

The immediate principal danger of a closed head injury is the result of the pressure building up inside the rigid skull as a result of haemorrhage or brain swelling (oedema) or usually a combination of the two. As the pressure builds up the brain is forced downwards on to the tough membrane which separates the cerebral hemispheres from the remainder of the brain, and the mid and hind parts of the brain are forced into the foramen magnum at the base of the skull and may cause fatal haemorrhage into the brain stem. If pressure is not relieved permanent brain damage may result in non-fatal cases.

When the head receives an impact, and is free to move as a result of the blow, the brain, which is bathed in cerebrospinal fluid, lags behind the skull in movement with the result that its undersurface is dragged over the irregular base of the skull, small blood vessels between the brain and its coverings become torn and, if the skull is also rotated by the impact, linear damage occurs within the substance of the brain itself.

Owing to the physical forces which cause brain trauma in a closed head injury the most severe damage occurs at a point opposite to the point of impact and direction of force. This is known as the contre-coup injury. The actual damage to the brain and its coverings below the impact point may be local and superficial although the contre-coup injury is most extensive.

Contre-coup injury does not occur when the head is fixed and unable to move. This is of importance when interpreting the cause of the head injury.

Haemorrhage over the brain arising from the injured area is described according to its relationship to the membranes covering the brain, i.e., subarachnoid, subdural and extradural. Although all three may be present following an injury involving a skull fracture it is more satisfactory to deal with each separately.

Subarachnoid haemorrhage. This is haemorrhage which occurs beneath the fine membrane which is actually in contact with the surface of the brain. The potential space between the arachnoid and the brain is known as the subarachnoid space. The arteries which supply the brain run in this space. Traumatic subarachnoid haemorrhage following head injury is the result of the rupture of veins or other small vessels. It occurs anywhere over the brain, depending upon the direction of the force.

Subarachnoid haemorrhage may be due to causes other than direct trauma to the head. These other causes may be natural or traumatic. The most common cause of a natural subarachnoid haemorrhage is the rupture of a congenital aneurysm (sometimes known as a berry aneurysm) on the cerebral circulation. These aneurysms may be very small and develop at the point where the arteries divide. Trauma to the head may cause an existing aneurysm to rupture. Other types of aneurysm may occur naturally in the cerebral circulation but these are rare.

Disorders of the blood which interfere with the normal clotting mechanism may also result in spontaneous subarachnoid haemorrhage. If, however, such a disorder is present, minimal trauma may precipitate haemorrhage.

Subarachnoid haemorrhage due to rupture of a developmental aneurysm is essentially basal and massive, whereas traumatic haemorrhage is relatively less in volume and is common over the cerebral hemispheres rather than beneath them.

A massive, rapidly fatal, traumatic, basal subarachnoid haemorrhage may result from a blow to the side of the upper neck which results in the rupture of the vertebral artery at the base of the skull or in its passage through the first cervical vertebra (*vide infra*).

Subdural haemorrhage. Subdural haemorrhage is one which takes place between the arachnoid and the tough membrane which lines the inner surface of the skull—the dura mater. Haemorrhages in this situation are usually traumatic in origin and due to the rupture of small veins which cross the subdural space. They may accumulate rapidly but not infrequently, especially in the aged, develop slowly into a chronic subdural haematoma. The original haemorrhage gets rapidly sealed off and, as the original clot becomes absorbed, chemical changes occurring in the original clot may cause a further haemorrhage to occur spontaneously without additional trauma, although further trauma often triggers off another haemorrhage. This second haemorrhage then becomes sealed off and may in time be followed by successive haemorrhages until finally the accumulated fresh and old blood reaches such a volume as to cause loss of consciousness or death. This type of chronic haemorrhage, sometimes known as pachymeningitis haemorrhagica (and originally believed to be a manifestation of late syphilis), is usually found in old people. In old age the brain atrophies and there is correspondingly more space in the cranium for blood to accumulate. Very minor impacts to the head may initiate such a haemorrhage and the fatal outcome may not occur for months or even years after the original injury. The original traumatic episode may have been forgotten or may have been so slight as to pass unnoticed. It may be difficult or impossible to give an accurate estimate of the date of the original injury. When a final assessment is made all available clinical data must be considered. It is not infrequent for some acute mental and physical deterioration to occur following a minor head injury. As the deterioration is often relatively minor it may be interpreted at the time to be an acceleration of the natural degenerative processes and it is only in retrospect after death and autopsy examination that the true significance of the deterioration is appreciated.

Subdural haemorrhage is also seen in some cases of child abuse. It may occur if the child is violently shaken. In these cases there may be no external marks of violence upon the child (see ch. 15). Subdural haemorrhage is rarely unassociated with trauma but may occur spontaneously in blood dyscrasias or infection.

Extradural haemorrhage. An extradural haemorrhage is one which takes place between the dura and the skull. It is usually associated with a fracture of the skull which crosses a branch or branches of the middle meningeal artery which runs in grooves in the inner table of the skull. They occur most frequently on the lateral aspects of the brain or in the middle fossae.

An extradural haemorrhage often has a distinct symptomatology owing to the relatively slow accumulation of blood as the bleeding is retarded by the dura which is adherent to the inner table of the skull. The person receiving the head impact will often lose consciousness temporarily but upon recovery will not appear seriously injured. The short loss of consciousness is often diagnosed as a mild concussion. Not infrequently the person will go home and seem quite rational, only to be found unconscious or dead in the morning. It is often considered to be a form of head injury which will respond dramatically to surgical intervention (i.e., removal of the clot and ligation of the blood vessel). Experience has shown, however, that even when the diagnosis is made early the prognosis is not good.

Extradural haemorrhage may occur artefactually in fires where the head is exposed to heat. Heat may also cause post-mortem fractures of the skull. This phenomenon has given rise to suspicion of foul play especially when the death is advantageous to someone about the deceased.

Intracerebral haemorrhage. Intracerebral haemorrhage is usually the result of natural disease processes but may be the direct result of trauma and, should a patient be suffering from natural disease predisposing to intracerebral haemorrhage, minor trauma may cause fatal haemorrhage.

Where there has been violent movement of the head, shearing stresses occur in the brain with resulting haemorrhages along the line of force. These may be small but on occasions initiate larger haemorrhages, and when these occur in the basal nuclei they may be thought to be of natural origin. With severe movement, numerous small or punctate haemorrhages appear throughout the brain, 'commotio cerebri'.

Contusion of the brain may lead to local infarction and although these infarcts are more commonly situated in and beneath the cortex they may be deep in the brain substance and may be complicated by secondary haemorrhage.

The natural causes of intracranial haemorrhage are numerous. The presence of many of these disease processes may be responsible for a fatal haemorrhage following minor blunt injury to the head. The commencement of a natural cerebral haemorrhage may result in the patient falling about and sustaining head injuries which could be diagnosed as the actual cause of the haemorrhage.

The natural disease processes which could cause a spontaneous intracerebral haemorrhage include:
1. hypertension;
2. cerebral atheroma;
3. cerebral thrombosis or embolus—including fat embolus;
4. blood dyscrasias;
5. neoplasms—primary and secondary;
6. congenital malformation of cerebral vessels (angioma);
7. cerebral abcess.

Disease plus injury

These cases may be of great medico-legal interest and require fuller consideration. In one extreme a person may die from a threat of violence which causes a sudden rise in blood pressure and cerebral haemorrhage where there is no trauma to the head, or he may suffer severe head injury which could cause fatal intracerebral haemorrhage even in the absence of existing natural disease. In the former case natural disease is clearly significant but not in the latter.

In *R. v. Woodward and others* (Liverpool C.C. 1974), a number of men broke into a public house after closing time and tied up the manager and locked him in a toilet. He was released the next morning and the following morning was found to have suffered a natural cerebral haemorrhage from which he died. The prosecution case was that the haemorrhage had been precipitated by his treatment at the hands of the accused. The accused was found guilty of manslaughter and sentenced to 15 years' imprisonment.

In the case of *R. v. Harris* (Maidstone C.C. 1974), the accused pleaded guilty to the manslaughter of a man who died from a coronary thrombosis following an assault. He received a sentence of seven years' imprisonment.

Sudden death due to existing heart disease following assaults or even threats have resulted in successful prosecutions for manslaughter although the defendant is usually charged with murder in the first instant. In *R. v. Harris* (Maidstone C.C. 1974), a plea of manslaughter was accepted. The circumstances were similar to those in *R. v. Wood-*

ward except that death was due to a sudden fatal heart attack. Davis[5] has recently written a review of the position in the United States.

Some persons have abnormally thin skulls and a blow which would be insufficient to cause more than a minor injury to a normal person may result in a fatal fracture.

A hydrocephalic, an inmate of a mental hospital, was struck on the jaw by another patient. The base of the skull was so thin that the back of the lower jaw was driven into the skull, killing him.

In general, if a person suffering from some congenital or acquired disease of his skull is assaulted, death is due to homicide although, depending upon the circumstances surrounding the assault, it may be used in mitigation to reduce the verdict from murder to manslaughter.

In old age not only may the skeleton, including the skull, become softened but, owing to the atrophy or shrinkage of the brain, subdural haemorrhage, with or without fracture to the skull, may result from a relatively minor blow to the head.

Having described the effects of blunt impact injuries to the head it is necessary to describe how these injuries arise in practice, the instruments which cause them and the manner of their infliction.

Blunt impact injuries are the most common injuries seen in the living and the most common cause of violent death – the majority resulting from falls or road traffic accidents. The ones of particular interest to the medico-legalist are those deliberately inflicted with a 'blunt instrument'. A blunt instrument in this context is often one that can be wielded by hand and their variety is legion. Some of the more common ones are: hammers; iron bars; axes and cleavers; wooden staves and pick-axe handles; articles of furniture, i.e. chairs; pistol or gun butts; shod feet; fists; pokers; coshes.

Suicide by means of a blunt impact injury inflicted with an easily manipulated weapon is very rare but some cases are recorded. In these cases the pattern of injuries, the presence of the weapon at the scene, the fingerprints of the deceased upon the weapon and the exclusion of any other person from the scene at the relevant time will indicate a deliberate act on the part of the deceased.

In suicidal or self-inflicted blunt impact injuries the injuries are midline and directed to the top of the head and in the very few cases of suicide recorded the injuries are grouped, close to the midline.

In the case of *R. v. Kent* (C.C.C. 1978), the accused phoned the police and informed them that her common law husband had committed suicide by striking his head with a hammer which was still in his grasp. When the police arrived the deceased was found lying face downwards, his right arm lay across his chest and a hammer lay loosely in his grasp. There were numerous circular or semicircular lacerations and abrasions not only to the left side of the back of the head but to the back of the shoulder. There were the most extensive fractures to the back of the skull, resulting from numerous blows, and very extensive brain damage. When confronted with the forensic interpretation of these injuries the accused admitted that she had hit her common law husband as he lay asleep.

In cases of homicide by a blunt instrument the weapon itself is frequently absent from the scene, except in domestic cases, and the pathologist must try to ascertain from his examination the nature of the weapon. As these vary considerably from case to case only general principles will be discussed.

Weapons with a circular leading edge, e.g., a hammer

Both the external wound to the skin or scalp and that of any to the underlying bone will depend upon the angle at which the leading edges strikes the body. The external wound will mark the point of impact; it may faithfully reproduce the whole or part of the leading surface of the instrument. Its site will give an indication of the position of the deceased in relation to the assailant.

The injury to the skull may be a semicircular or circular depressed fracture, depending upon the force used and the actual surface of the striking edge which hits the head. Linear fractures may radiate from the depressed fracture, indicating the direction of force.

The injury to the brain, its covering membranes and blood vessels, will also vary according to the site of impact and the force. Splinters of bone may be driven into the brain substance, lacerating it immediately below the fracture. Contre-coup

injury may be found on the opposite side of the brain if the head is free to move.

Extradural haemorrhage may arise from the middle meningeal artery or its branches which run in grooves in the skull. Haemorrhage may arise from injury to the large venous sinuses or from the smaller veins which pass across the subdural space.

As the skull may be described as a rigid box the first injury will weaken the structure and subsequent blows may cause a degree of damage out of proportion to the force used. A second blow, for instance on an area of skull already fractured, may cause widespread collapse of the skull in that area and the bone fragments and the weapon itself may be driven far into the brain.

If the scalp is lacerated by the first blow, blood will be driven out of the vessels as they are compressed by the instrument away from the point of impact, and although the torn vessels may subsequently bleed considerably the blood will not be projected around the scene. With further blows, however, blood will be projected about the scene under considerable pressure from the already lacerated vessels, and at the same time blood and tissue may adhere to the weapon and be thrown in the direction of the uplift of the weapon. For instance, if this should be vertical, blood will be splattered over the ceiling should the assault take place indoors. With repeated blows blood will be splattered over the assailant and examination of the clothing may not only reveal the stance of the assailant in relation to the deceased whilst the blows were delivered but may also show whether they were delivered with the right or left hand.

An old lady was found dead with severe head wounds in the hallway of her house. The tin box where the old lady kept her money had been rifled. Blood was splattered in all directions around the hallway, the direction of the blood splatters radiating out from where her head lay on the floor. Later, a blood-stained, round-headed poker was found concealed in the vegetation growing in the small garden. After several days investigation suspicion was centred upon a granddaughter, who raised the alarm after returning from school. Examination of the clothing she wore on that day revealed numerous blood spots of such a distribution that she must have been bending over the old lady when the blows were struck, and blood spots on both the outer and inner surface of her right sleeve indicated that the blows had been struck with the right hand. The skull had numerous fractures, including a depressed fracture which fitted the head of the poker, and circular wounds due to the sharp end of the poker having been used as a stabbing instrument.

Blows with cylindrical instruments

The scalp lacerations will be longitudinal and the damage to both the scalp, skull and brain may be extensive if numerous blows are struck with a heavy instrument.

A householder was beaten over the head numerous times with a heavy cylindrical metal bar. A number of lacerations of the scalp and extensive fractures of the skull were inflicted. Brain tissue was found as far as 5 ft from the head of the deceased.

If only one blow is struck, or if the skull is not disintegrated by successive blows, the outline of the weapon may be delineated by the skull fracture, even when the blow was cushioned by headgear.

An elderly man collecting some wages was struck with a pick-axe handle. He was wearing a cap and the only external wound was a pressure abrasion in which was reproduced the weave of his cap. The underlying skull exhibited an almost rectangular depressed fracture with linear fractures radiating directly backwards over the vault of the skull. This fracture not only reproduced the shape of the weapon but also confirmed that the deceased had been facing his assailant when the blow was struck.

When the head has been struck many times with a heavy instrument, a reconstruction following defleshing of the bones may provide valuable information and permit the alleged instrument to be accurately matched with the bony injuries. In *R.* v. *Critchley* (C.C.C. 1981), the defendant had struck his victim a number of blows with one or more blunt instruments. Fragments of skull, brain tissue and blood were widely scattered around the scene. Reconstruction of the skull indicated that the blood-stained hammer at the scene could have inflicted some of the injuries. In this case over 200 fragments of bone from the skull were too small to be used in the reconstruction.

Blows with axes and cleavers

The scalp lacerations will be longitudinal and, if the weapon is sharp, may appear as incised wounds. Owing to the narrow leading or cutting edge the skull may be penetrated to a considerable depth. Blood and brain tissue may be widely dispersed at the scene, depending upon the number of blows.

Fractures to the vault of the skull which have been inflicted with a heavy blunt instrument often extend downwards and across the base of the skull. If the blow is directed to the forehead or above the ears the adjacent base of the skull is often comminuted.

Blows with the fist

Blows with the fist are rarely fatal in themselves but death may ensue because the victim has been knocked unconscious and has been left on his back with blood pouring into his airway from an injured nose or when the victim has fallen backwards as a result of a blow and sustained a head injury.

In one case a husband was unexpectedly at home when his wife's lover knocked at the door. The husband attacked the lover and delivered numerous blows to his face, breaking his nose and knocking him unconscious. He left him lying on his back outside the house, where he was later found dead with his airway filled with blood.

In another case a man had an argument with a doorkeeper. He struck him one blow on the side of the mouth. The doorkeeper fell backwards, striking his head on the pavement, sustaining a fracture of his skull and brain injury, from which he died some 8 h later.

The injuries inflicted with the fist are, with the exception of the broken nose and lost teeth, mainly soft tissue—unless the assailant has a particularly heavy punch when the jaw may be fractured. The soft tissue injuries are bruises around the eyes (black eyes), lacerations over the bony prominences, such as the eyebrows, and lacerations of the inner surfaces of the lips against the teeth.

A variation of a blow to the face with a fist is an upward blow beneath the nose with the side of the palm, the head having been held steady or forced forwards from behind: a technique developed in unarmed combat. The force is transmitted upwards through the nasal septum causing a fracture of the ethmoid bone in the base of the skull above the nose. Fractures may radiate from this centre into the thin supra-orbital plates. Loss of consciousness or even death are immediate. There may be no visible external marks of injury although blood will be issuing from the nostrils.

Kicks with the shod foot

The shod foot is a lethal weapon and can be rendered more lethal with steel or pointed toecaps. Kicks to the head may result in extensive fractures of the skull. As they are often directed against someone lying on the ground, accompanying basal fractures are frequent. The upper and lower jaws are also frequently fractured. The lacerations and surrounding abrasion inflicted with the toe of a shoe or boot may be characteristic.

Kicks to the trunk may result in fatal damage to internal organs, especially the spleen. In elderly persons rib fractures not infrequently lead to fatal pneumonia.

Blunt injuries to the neck

The cervical spine. Injuries to the cervical spine involving the spinal cord may be rapidly fatal or may paralyse the victim in all four limbs.

In practice most cervical spine injuries are sustained in motor vehicle accidents. Few are due to direct impact. Most occur when the head is thrown forwards and then jerked backwards after an impact, causing a dislocation of the spine with the articular surfaces of two vertebrae overlying each other (whiplash injury).

Whiplash injury. This injury is sometimes overlooked in hospital casualty departments and such an oversight may result in prolonged or permanent disability. The most serious injury is a dislocation of the atlanto-occipital joint—the joint between the base of the skull and the first cervical vertebra. This is frequently immediately fatal as the brain stem is crushed by the dislocation. Degrees of this injury are frequently present in fatal road traffic accidents along with other lethal injuries sustained at the same time.

Traumatic subarachnoid haemorrhage due to cervi-

cal spine injury. The mechanism of fatal traumatic subarachnoid haemorrhage due to blows to the upper cervical spine has only been recognised during the last two decades. It is of especial medicolegal significance as it may follow a comparatively light blow. Until fairly recently subarachnoid haemorrhage following minor trauma was considered to be due to the rupture of a small aneurysm on the cerebral circulation, although the actual aneurysm was never located. It is a recognised fact that even with a diligent search the defect in the vessel wall may be so small that it escapes detection. In traumatic subarachnoid haemorrhage a vertebral artery, which supplies part of the cerebral blood flow, is ruptured in the neck, usually where it passes through the foramen in the first cervical vertebra, or between the foramen and where it enters the skull through the foramen magnum.

The actual blow is directed to the side of the neck below the ear—an area of the body not dissected in routine autopsy examination. Usually a small external mark may be found if looked for; as in the supine body it is frequently concealed by the normal skin folds. The transverse process of the first cervical vertebra through which the vertebral artery courses may be fractured and the vessel torn. Blood then tracks along the vessel into the base of the skull, causing death within a few minutes. The vessel may be ruptured without fracture of the transverse process. These blows are usually delivered with the fist, the side of the hand or the shod foot (Fig. 11.2).

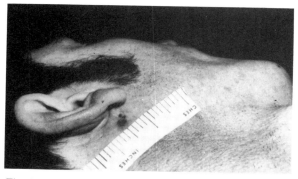

Fig. 11.2 Fatal traumatic subarachnoid haemorrhage. Abrasion below right ear following a kick with the shod foot. The transverse process of the 1st cervical vertebra was fractured and the vertebral artery injured. Death occurred within a few minutes.

In the majority of cases, and especially those where the blow is with the fist, the victim is inebriated. Alcohol not only dilates vessels, rendering them more liable to injury, but also slows the normal defence reactions to a blow. The technique for demonstrating the lesion and a number of illustrative cases are described by Cameron & Mant[6] and Mant[7]. A typical example of such a case is illustrated in *R. v. Rooney* (Reading C.C. 1976). The deceased was attacked and kicked on the side of the neck by Rooney. He collapsed and died shortly afterwards. At autopsy the lace eyelets of Rooney's shoes were reproduced on the side of the deceased's neck. The deceased's blood alcohol was 184 mg/100 ml. Rooney was sentenced to two years' imprisonment for manslaughter.

The larynx and soft tissues of the neck. The structures of the neck, where injury by blunt force may result in death, are the great vessels and the larynx or voicebox. Asphyxial deaths due to compression of the neck are described elsewhere (Ch. 13) and this section will concern itself with injuries other than those due to compression of the neck.

The larynx is a cartilaginous structure which becomes provessively calcified with age. It is generously supplied with sensitive nerve endings, and excessive stimulation of some of the vagal nerve endings may result in sudden cardiac arrest from 'vagal inhibition'.

Blows to the front of the neck may cause instant death when directed against the larynx. Special units during hostilities are trained to strike enemy personnel across the larynx with the side of their hand, causing instant and silent death. Crush injuries of the larynx are occasionally seen in road traffic accidents.

In two cases seen recently husbands killed their wives by blows to the larynx. In one case the wife, whilst lying on the ground, was struck across the throat with a marble-topped occasional table, crushing the larynx against the cervical spine. In the second case the lady was punched twice on her larynx, causing widespread fractures to both the hyoid and thyroid bones. In this case air entered the circulation through torn thyroid veins and was present in the superior vena cava.

Blunt impact to the side of the neck may damage the internal lining of the carotid artery, leading to thrombosis which may be fatal or lead to cerebral infarction by directly cutting off part of the cerebral circulation or by an embolus arising from the injured artery.

Blunt injury to the thorax

The thorax or chest is a bony cage which consists of the thoracic or dorsal spine, the ribs and the breastbone. It contains the heart and the main blood vessels of the body, the aorta, vena cava, the pulmonary artery and veins, and the respiratory passages and lungs. Between each rib lie the intercostal arteries.

The chest cage protects the vital organs it contains and, in an adult, rib fractures usually occur, i.e., the cage collapses before damage is inflicted upon the heart or lungs. In children and young adults, however, the chest wall is very mobile as the calcification is incomplete, and fatal injuries may be inflicted upon the heart, lungs and great vessels, without any fractures of the rib cage or breastbone.

In practice the majority of the fatal blunt impact injuries to the chest are seen in road traffic accidents and falls from a height. More rarely they occur from falling objects or from blows with a heavy blunt instrument, or as the result of having been kicked or having been jumped upon.

The injuries which may be sustained to the chest as a result of blunt impact will be influenced not only by the force and direction of the impact but also by the surface area of the chest involved.

Bony injuries. These may be to the dorsal or thoracic spine, the ribs or the breastbone.

The thoracic spine, excluding the projecting processes, is usually only fractured as the result of great violence such as one sees in air crashes, road traffic accidents and falls from a height. The fracture is then merely an incidental finding amongst a number of fatal injuries. If the spine is diseased and softenend by neoplastic (cancerous) involvement, or other tumours such as myelomatosis, by decalcification (the commonest cause of this is senility) or has become rigid as a result of an arthritic process, fractures may occur readily and, in extreme cases of neoplastic involvement, almost spontaneously.

Fractures may also be caused by direct localised violence such as kicking, and compression fractures as a result of falling heavily on the buttocks —although these latter fractures are more common in the lumbar spine.

Fractures of the thoracic spine may result in permanent deformity if treatment is not satisfactory, and by complete paralysis of the lower limbs if the spinal cord is injured.

A type of compression fracture or collapse of a body of one or more adjacent vertebrae which occurs spontaneously, but is rarely seen today because of treatment, is due to a tuberculous process involving the vertebrae.

Fractures of the ribs and breastbone. These are the commonest chest injuries and are not only seen in those types of violence which result in fracture of the thoracic spine but also as the result of parental or foster violence (e.g., battered babies, ch. 15) and as a result of external cardiac massage where attempts are made to resuscitate a patient after cardiac arrest.

The majority of the fractures seen in practice are those due to frontal violence. The breastbone is depressed into the chest and usually fractured at the manubriosternal junction or below. Ribs on one or both sides are fractured anteriorly but there may be multiple fractures if the force of the impact is severe. The fractured ends of the ribs may become separated and lacerate through the pleura lining the inner chest wall and directly injure the lungs, heart or great vessels. This is more frequently seen when the violence is directed principally to one side of the chest or the other.

When there is a compound fracture of a rib or ribs into the chest cavity the intercostal artery may be torn, and these bleeding arteries may cause death from haemorrhage, if not recognised, even in the absence of injury to the lungs or heart.

Localised rib fractures involving one or more ribs are not uncommon in the aged and infirm who fall around. These fractures are usually to the back or side of the chest. Rarely is the force from such a fall sufficient to cause significant displacement of the ribs. The breathing, however, may be restricted both by the fractures and accompanying pain. This may result in a fatal pneumonia.

A violent, localised impact to the side of the chest, such as may occur with a fall on to an unyeilding narrow projection, or impact with the end of the handlebars in a motor cycle accident,

may cause one or two ribs to penetrate the chest to a great depth.

Fat embolism (*vide infra*) is a possible complication of rib fractures, especially in the very old.

Injuries to the lungs. The healthy lungs are free to move in the chest cavity, their surfaces being lubricated by pleural fluid. The surfaces of both the lungs (visceral) and the inner chest wall (parietal) are lined by a continuous membrane—the pleura. There is a potential space between the visceral and parietal pleura which may become separated by a variety of natural or unnatural phenomena. When lungs or pleura become diseased as a result of infection or neoplasm, or injured in any way—including open chest surgery—they may become adherent.

Following trauma to the lungs, air, blood, or blood and air, may escape into the pleural cavities and these processes are known as pneumothorax, haemothorax or haemopneumothorax. Pus collecting in the cavity is an empyema of chest or pyothorax, and a collection of fluid—usually part of a disease process—is known as a pleural effusion.

Injuries to the lungs or respiratory passages are due to compression or crushing, to sudden diminution of the size of the thoracic cage, to decompression, when the force is released and the chest wall springs back to its normal or near normal size, and to lacerations due to the penetration of ribs.

Compression injuries consist of bruising and laceration of the lungs, with or without loss of continuity of the pleura. In extreme cases the lungs may be torn into several fragments. As the lungs are mobile, and the respiratory passages relatively fixed, the lungs get torn at their attachment to the bronchi and peribronchial and peribronchiolar haemorrhages are seen. If the pleura is torn pneumothorax or haemopneumothorax may result.

In decompression a negative pressure is produced in the pleural cavity and traumatic emphysematous bullae appear on the surface of the lungs. These bullae are air blisters caused by the visceral pleura being pulled from the surface of the lung. They are very thin walled, usually multiple and small, but if large may be filled with blood. Owing to the thinness of their walls they may rupture, leading to a pneumothorax.

If the victim of a chest impact is suffering from

bullous emphysema, a bulla may rupture following relatively minor trauma, leading to a pneumothorax. Emphysematous bullae may rupture spontaneously causing a 'spontaneous pneumothorax'.

Laceration due to penetration of ribs may merely involve the surface of the lungs or a lobe may become transfixed and when the rib springs back the lobe may be torn from its main bronchus.

In one case a mental patient struck another across his back with a rounded stake. There were no bony injuries and yet a lobe of lung had been completely torn from the bronchus. The only external mark was an oblique rectangular contusion upon the back.

When air, blood, pus or fluid collect in a pleural cavity it displaces the lung, causing its partial collapse. Collapse of the lung lowers its efficiency by reducing the area available for oxygenation of the blood. If the collection of fluid or air in the pleural cavity becomes large, the central chest structure, the mediastinum, will be displaced towards the other side of the chest—'mediastinal shift'. The presence of air or fluid in the chest may be the result of natural disease. Pneumothorax may occur suddenly from rupture of bullae on the surface of the lung associated with tuberculous or chronic emphysema. Haemothorax may be due to diseased blood vessels and fluid may collect as the result of heart disease, cancer or pneumonia.

Any chest injury involving the bony thorax or lungs may develop complications which prove fatal. Amongst the more common of these are:
1. pneumonia, especially in the aged;
2. pulmonary embolism due to enforced immobility;
3. accumulation of sufficient air and or fluid in the pleural cavities to impede respiration fatally;
4. haemorrhage from intercostal arteries, major blood vessels in the chest, lung injury;
5. infection of the pleural cavity (emphysema), lung (pneumonia, lung abcess) and infection of bone (osteomyelitis).

Injuries to the heart and great blood vessels. Injuries to the heart and its great vessels—the aorta, the vena cavae and the pulmonary vessels—may occur in the absence of bony injury if the thoracic cage is mobile as in children and young adults. The heart and vessels, however, may escape injury even after heavy impacts to the chest because of their relative mobility inside the thorax.

The aorta. The most common and rapidly fatal injury is a traumatic rupture of the aorta. Although the rupture may occur anywhere along its course it most frequently occurs after it has arched in front of the upper spine, the rupture occurring in the distal arch. In this position it is immobile and a violent impact to the front of the chest will shear it on the left side of the spine, sometimes so cleanly that it might have been cut with a knife. This is clearly the most dramatic rupture and death is virtually instantaneous. Various degrees of rupture may occur, however, so that the blood loss may be slow, especially if the blood pressure has been much reduced by shock. In these cases blood escapes into the central chest structures and accumulates there until it bursts into the chest cavity. If this leak into the mediastinum is recognised it may be successfully treated by surgery. The time interval between injury to the aorta and fatal rupture into the chest cavity may be rarely as long as several days.

The relatively small intercostal arteries may be damaged as they arise from the aorta, but this type of injury is more commonly associated with blast injuries.

If the aorta wall is injured but not ruptured a traumatic aneurysm or swelling may develop. This aneurysm may rupture spontaneously at any time.

The aorta is subject to disease processes which cause it to dilate. Some of these are acquired, i.e., syphilis, some are due to degenerative changes such as atherosclerosis, and others are transmitted genetically, as in 'Marfan's syndrome'. If a person has a diseased aorta this will be more liable to rupture than a healthy one after blunt chest injury.

The aorta may be lacerated directly by the penetration of fractured ribs into the chest cavity.

The heart. The heart may be pierced by fractured bone or crushed against the spine. In the former case any part of the heart may be damaged but in pure crushing injuries it is the right auricle which is most frequently ruptured. The heart may be bruised without rupture, or partially ruptured by blunt impact.

How long may the recipient of a fatal wound remain conscious and perform volitional movements after infliction of the injury?

This is a question which may be raised by both the prosecution and defence in cases of homicide and by the police in cases of suicide where more than one fatal injury has been inflicted. The majority of the questions arise following injuries to the heart. In penetrating wounds of the heart, the heart will normally continue beating until it is prevented from doing so by blood escaping into the tough pericardial sac and building up sufficient pressure to mechanically prevent the heart beating (tamponade)—the blood entering the heart sac more rapidly than it can escape through the perforation made in it by the penetrating instrument. Perforations of the right ventricle bleed more rapidly than those of the left as it is relatively thin walled. Small perforations of the left ventricle may seal themselves and bleeding may be insignificant. If the surgeon can open the chest and pericardial sac before fatal tamponade has developed, the wound in the heart may be sutured and death is unlikely.

Of great interest is the duration of consciousness and volitional activity after the heart has stopped beating either from disease or trauma. After the action of the heart ceases no fresh blood will circulate through the cerebral vessels and consciousness will depend upon the amount of oxygenated blood present in the brain.

Every year drivers of motor vehicles who have died at the wheel of their vehicles are examined and it is only in the most exceptional cases that they have been unable to stop or draw up before they actually collapse. Death in these cases is usually due to a coronary thrombosis[8].

In fatal electrocution in which the heart stops functioning there are several recorded cases of persons walking and talking for some 20 to 30 s before dropping dead.

In stabbed wounds of the right ventricle inflicted with a dagger or kitchen knife it is not unusual for the victim to run some 100 to 200 yards from his assailant before collapsing. Exercise of course shortens the expectation of life in such circumstances.

In suicide by shooting with a pistol through the chest the possibility of homicide is often raised when there have been multiple shots through the heart. Two shots are not uncommon and three shots not rare in suicide and there are several examples of six revolver shots having been fired in indisputable cases of suicide, although in these cases not all the missiles have passed throught the heart. The following two cases are of particular interest as in each case the heart was completely destroyed and yet volitional movement occurred afterwards. In the first case[20] a 17-year-old youth was shot with a 375 magnum pistol whilst standing in a road. He walked around for some 20 to 30 s before collapsing. At autopsy examination it was found that the bullet (a hollow nosed dum dum type) had struck the heart and all four chambers had been destroyed. In the second case[17] a man had been shot through the window with a high velocity rifle whilst sitting in a chair. He got up, walked to a gun rack and removed a gun and started walking towards the window when he collapsed having covered in all some 30 f. At autopsy his heart was completely disintegrated by the missile. In both these cases complete destruction of the heart did not prevent purposeful acts having been carried out for periods of up to about 30 s.

Although these were cases of homicide they illustrate how a suicide may discharge multiple shots into the chest before collapsing.

A recent such suicide[10] was the subject of a Commission of Inquiry. Briefly a police inspector, who never carried a firearm, drew his revolver in the early hours of the morning and a short time later was found shot five times in his chest and abdomen in his locked flat. The wounds were contact and passed from right to left, the fifth wound not entering a body cavity. There was a strong motive for suicide.

Page Hudson[11] reviewed 58 cases of multiple short suicides which occurred in North Carolina during the period 1972–78. He observed that in this series 1.6% of firearm suicides were due to multiple shots. He emphasises the importance of recognising this method of suicide in order to avoid unnecessary homicide investigations. In the majority of the cases in this series the suicide had shot himself through the precordial area—less than 25% through the head, whereas in single shot suicide some 60% shot themselves through the head.

A curious case is recorded by Fatteh et al.[12] A young man shot himself with two guns—one shot to the head and the other to the precordium.

Coronary arteries. The coronary arteries may be injured by bone fragments, which may result in haemorrhage or cause spasm of the vessel, leading to acute myocardial ischaemia.

Direct injury to the coronary arteries, causing death, is unusual. Traumatic coronary thrombosis does occasionally occur when the walls of the artery are injured. The patient may then develop all the signs of myocardial infarction after the vessel becomes occluded. Coronary artery disease is very common from early middle age and sudden death from coronary occlusion may occur in the teens. The assessment of trauma and disease may thus be very difficult, especially if a middle-aged person dies from coronary disease a few months after a chest injury and the occlusion is confined to one small area of artery.

Acute coronary occlusion may be due to a dissecting aneurysm of an atheromatous coronary artery and may follow direct trauma.

Injuries to the more superficial systemic arteries, followed by thrombosis, aneurysm, arteriovenous aneurysm, etc., are well recognised. Coronary arteries, however, occupy a unique position in that direct injury or its sequelae may cause sudden death. Should a patient survive trauma to his coronary arteries their anatomical position renders examination impossible except by special techniques.

Other major vessels. Other major thoracic vessels, the pulmonary arteries and veins and the inferior and superior vena cavae, are rarely injured, except in cases where there have been extensive and fatal injuries to other thoracic organs. In these cases injuries to the pulmonary vessels are more common than to the vena cavae but in both instances are incidental autopsy findings.

Blunt injury to the abdomen

The abdominal cavity is supported by the spine (behind), the pelvis (beneath) and the abdominal muscles (to the front and sides). The abdominal organs are all anchored posteriorly; some have great freedom of movement (e.g., intestines) and others are fixed (kidneys). The diaphragm separates the thoracic and abdominal cavities and during respiration moves up and down—thus the actual position of certain organs alters with respiration (e.g., the liver). Owing to the mobility of the intestines the position of these will also vary according to the stance of the individual.

The anterior abdominal wall consists of three principle layers—skin, fat and muscle—and the inner layer of muscle is separated from the abdominal cavity by peritoneum. By the very nature of its structure the abdominal wall is resilient and may absorb, without visible injury, impacts of such force that if delivered elsewhere might cause lacerations and skeletal damage. Serious injury to the deep lying organs may occur in the absence of any external injury and this will happen more readily should the victim be clothed.

On the posterior wall of the upper abdomen lies a plexus of nerves—the solar plexus. When force is transmitted through the abdomen to this plexus the person may collapse or even die—there being no visible injury. There are recorded cases of boxers dropping dead following a blow to the abdomen during a bout.

In view of the variety of organs present in the abdominal cavity the injuries to each organ or system will be described separately.

Bony injury. The lumbar spine may be fractured, dislocated, or the bodies of the vertebrae may become crushed (crush fracture). As the spinal cord terminates in adults at the level of the second lumbar vertebra the catastrophic sequelae to spinal cord injury as seen in the cervical and, to a lesser extent in the thoracic region, may be absent.

The abdominal aorta passes down in front of the spine and may become injured when the lumbar spine is fractured, especially if the aorta is diseased. Severe atheromatous disease is common in persons over 65 years, and sometimes earlier. However, since the aorta is elastic, complete fractures of the lumbar spine may occur with wide separation of the bony fragments and yet a healthy aorta remains intact.

Blood vessels. Injury to the aorta has already been described. Injury to other vessels, such as the arteries supplying the bowel (the mesenteric arteries), is rare. However, when a branch of such a vessel is traumatised and becomes thrombosed it will lead to gangrene of that part of the bowel it supplies. Unless this is recognised and treated death may occur.

Alimentary tract. The stomach and small bowel are very mobile, whereas the large bowel is relatively fixed. Trauma following blunt impact tends to occur at points where the alimentary tract is fixed by its supporting membrane—the mesentery. In 'battered children' the junction between the duodenum and the jejunum may be ruptured by a blow from the fist, foot or knee. The mesentery may be injured locally from a violent impact delivered over a small area. A golf caddie was struck in the abdomen by a golf ball; he appeared little the worse and spent the evening drinking. The following day he complained of abdominal pain and died. At autopsy it was found that although there was only a small indistinct recent bruise of the anterior abdominal wall an almost circular piece of tissue had been punched out of the mesentery leading to gangrene and ileus. The mesentery of the descending colon may be torn by blunt impact. In children this may be seen after blows or kicks; in adults it is occasionally seen after very violent impacts such as road traffic accidents. Recently there has been recorded a case of strangulation of a bowel herniation through a traumatic tear in the mesentery in an old man, four weeks after a road traffic accident.[15]

Liver. Laceration of the liver is most frequently seen in fatal road traffic accidents but may also be the result of falls from a height, and even from vigorous external cardiac massage. The liver substance is surrounded by a layer of peritoneum and this capsule may not be lacerated by the impact which has injured the deeper parts of the liver. In consequence haemorrhage will be intrahepatic until the pressure inside the liver is sufficient to rupture its capsule. Unless one of the major vessels is injured the liver tends to bleed rather slowly.

The liver is the organ most frequently invaded by carcinoma from some other area of the body. Occasionally these secondary growths may be very large and vascular, in which case the liver will be especially susceptible to blunt injury, and fatal haemorrhage may result from slight trauma or may occur spontaneously.

The liver may be ruptured in 'battered baby' cases where blows have been delivered to the abdomen.

The spleen. The healthy spleen is a relatively small firm organ, lying in the left upper abdomen and largely shielded by the lower ribs. In many conditions the spleen becomes soft and enlarged and, under these circumstances, is very vulnerable to trauma.

In some conditions (certain tropical diseases and chronic leukaemia) the spleen may become very large, occupying much of the upper left and mid-areas of the abdomen. Amongst the more common conditions which cause softening and enlargement of the spleen are infections, malaria and glandular fever or infective mononucleosis. This last condition requires special mention as patients suffering from glandular fever may not feel sufficiently ill to go sick and yet their spleens may be enlarged and very soft. Several deaths occur annually in young adults suffering from glandular fever, whose spleens have ruptured spontaneously or after minimal trauma. Some of these cases are recorded in the literature. One such case appeared recently in the Journal of Forensic Sciences.[9] In athletes, or those following strenuous occupations, the spleen is usually physiologically enlarged.

The normal healthy spleen is infrequently ruptured, except after severe localised trauma such as kicking, or when it is damaged together with other abdominal organs following a violent crushing impact. Although the spleen is a highly vascular organ, haemorrhage from a ruptured healthy spleen is often less brisk than would be anticipated. The ruptured diseased spleen may exsanguinate the patient in a short time.

Kidneys. The kidneys, owing to their depth in the abdominal cavity, are less frequently damaged by frontal impact. Damage may follow blows to the loin and consist of contusions and lacerations. These injuries are seen after kicking over the area of the kidneys or following severe crushing injuries which may occur in road traffic or industrial accidents.

Injury to the kidney may be followed by scarring and a raised blood pressure. Less severe blunt trauma may result in local haemorrhage which may become infected.

Blunt injury to the pelvis. The pelvis is a bony basin consisting of two hip bones which form the front and sides, and the sacrum and coccyx posteriorly. The thigh bones articulate with the hip bone.

The pelvis contains the urinary bladder, the

lower part of the large bowel and, in women, the generative organs and, in men, the prostate.

The pelvis is frequently damaged in road traffic accidents and in elderly persons following falls. The urinary bladder is rarely damaged unless it is distended at the time of the impact. Fracture dislocation of the hip joint may occur in road traffic accidents where the knees of the front seat passenger, or sometimes the driver, strike the fascia when the occupants are thrown forward after frontal impact.

The immediate complications of a fractured pelvis are due to damage inflicted by the fractured bones. The prostatic urethra may be ruptured, the bladder, especially if full, may rupture or be pierced by a bony fragment. This leads to escape of urine between the layers of the abdominal wall, beneath the peritoneal lining of the pelvic cavity or into the pelvic and abdominal cavities. More rarely the rectum may be pierced or even the small bowel if adherent to the pelvis as the result of previous inflammatory disease or malignant adhesions.

One of the more serious complications is laceration of the main arteries and veins (iliac vessels) which cross the pelvic floor to enter the upper thighs. Lacerations lead to massive haemorrhage.

In the female there may be damage to the vagina or to the pregnant uterus. A pregnant uterus may be ruptured causing fatal haemorrhage and extrusion of the foetus into the abdominal cavity. Lesser violence may cause abortion.

Blunt injury to the extremities

Blunt impact to the extremities may result in soft tissue and bony injury.

The force necessary to cause a fracture will depend upon the density of the bone which receives the impact. There are numerous conditions which may cause weakness or fragility of the skeleton, either locally, such as a bone cyst or secondary deposit of carcinoma, or generally due to a variety of pathological states—of which the most frequent encountered is osteoporosis which accompanies old age. If osteoporosis is severe, fractures of the femur may occur with normal weight bearing. Certain congenital skeletal defects must be excluded in alleged 'battered baby' cases.

Although some pathological conditions which are associated with skeletal softening may be present it does not necessarily infer that their presence contributes significantly to the fracture. The fragility of the skeleton can be tested rapidly by a pathologist performing an autopsy examination or, in the living, it can be deduced from radiographs.

Complications of injury

Complications of injury may be directly consequent upon the site of the injury. These have already been discussed under the regional injuries. Alternatively, they may be general, complicating any form of trauma.

Fatal sequelae to injury may result from lack of, or inadequate, treatment, the wrong treatment or abnormal reaction to drugs used to treat the patient. Each such case is often an entity and must be considered in its own context.

There are well recognised fatal complications general to all forms of injury. These complications may arise in spite of rigorous prophylactic therapy and are associated with enforced immobility or bed rest. The old are particularly susceptible to these complications unless they are already bed bound when the trauma occurs.

These decubitus complications are:

Hypostatic pneumonia

Hypostatic pneumonia develops when the usual secretions from the respiratory passages accumulate in the dependent parts of the lungs and then become infected. This is prevented by exercise, preferably under the direction of a trained physiotherapist. It may follow any form of trauma but especially those forms which interfere directly with respiratory movement.

Pulmonary embolism

This complication occurs when blood clots in the veins of the legs and then the clot becomes detached and is carried up in the blood stream to the heart and lungs. It may occur at any age but is especially common in the aged. It is prevented by exercise and by the exhibiton of anti-clotting drugs where this is feasible.

Urinary tract infection

This is more common in the aged, in cases where the trauma has damaged the nerve supply to the bladder and where some interference with the passage of urine exists—e.g., enlarged prostate gland in men and a prolapsed uterus in women.

Trophic ulceration or bed sores

These are classic decubitus lesions and are prone to develop in the aged, in those with poor peripheral blood supplies and those paralysed as a result of trauma or natural disease.

Secondary haemorrhage

This condition follows upon infection of the original injury with break down of the sutures or blood clot resulting in haemorrhage. It is far less common since the introduction of antibiotics.

There are a number of unusual complications which may follow trauma and their possibility should be explored when post-traumatic death occurs unexpectedly and without the development of the more usual general complications listed above.

Patterns of injury

Fatal injuries resulting from blunt impact force will follow a certain pattern, according to the instrument and manner of death.

Blunt impact injuries are usually accidental and are seen in transportation accidents of all types, and in simple falls. Homicidal injuries are usually inflicted with some clubbing weapon, and suicidal injuries are usually inflicted by jumping off tall buildings.

Certain varieties of blunt impact injury merit special description because of their frequency and medico-legal importance. Of all the violent deaths of this type those most commonly examined by pathologists are road traffic accidents.

Road traffic accidents

Injuries to car occupants. Eighty percent of fatal road traffic accidents follow a frontal impact and the injuries are inflicted when the forward motion of the occupants of the car is arrested by internal parts of the cabin or, if thrown out, by contact with the road or some other object.

In a frontal impact the unrestrained occupants are thrown upwards and forwards. If the impact is very violent the injuries to the driver and front seat passenger may be virtually identical although the steering wheel or the hub of the steering wheel may inflict specific injuries upon the driver. Both the driver and front seat passenger will receive injuries from projecting parts of the cabin such as the interior mirror or dash fascia should they come in contact with them.

The cause of death in car occupants following an accident are most commonly related to head, neck or chest injury. In a series of 100 consecutive deaths of car drivers, 42% had fractured skulls, 30% had bony neck injury and 69% had bony chest injury. Fifty-three percent had brain damage, 37% ruptured aortas and 16% traumatic rupture of the heart and 50% had some form of abdominal injury.[18]

A problem which may arise concerns the identity of the driver when all the occupants are thrown out of the vehicle or the occupants have been removed unconscious after the accident and no note made by the rescuers of their positions in the car. The problem is usually resolved by comparison of the patterns of injury upon the casualties with the damage inflicted to the interior of the cabin by the occupants. Pieces of clothing, hairs, skin or blood may be present inside the compartment and the origin of these can be identified by scientific investigation. Methods for the investigation of injuries in road traffic accidents are outlined by Grattan et al.[13]

Contribution of natural disease to road traffic accidents. During the course of a year many persons die whilst in control of a vehicle. The exact figures are not available as such deaths will be classified as natural for the purposes of registration. Mant recorded 100 consecutive cases representing 0.01% of all coroners' autopsies. In only 3% of cases did the vehicle cause serious injury to the driver or some other person. In the majority of cases the driver had either halted his vehicle or had slowed it down to such an extent that minimal or no damage was inflicted to the vehicle or other property.

On the very rare occasions when collapse at the wheel causes the death of other car occupants or pedestrians, the publicity given to the circumstances in the press may convey an impression that persons suffering from coronary artery disease are a menace upon the roads. This is an entirely false assumption. Similar surveys of sudden death at the wheel carried out in the United States and Europe all show a similar lack of injury to a second party or property.[8, 19, 21]

Contribution of alcohol and/or drugs to road traffic accidents. A discussion on the effects of alcohol or drugs upon driving behaviour has no place in this chapter. Alcohol is the most important causative factor in road traffic accidents at certain times of the day. The legal blood alcohol level of 80 mg% in the United Kingdom is *not* a measure of sobriety. The legal limits vary from 0 to 150 mg% in different countries or states. In some countries tests for sobriety are carried out between two statutory blood alcohol levels. If the driver passes these tests he is not charged with an offence. Increasing numbers of drivers stopped by the police after driving erratically or having committed some minor traffic offence are found to be suffering from a degree of drug intoxication. The most common drug found in the blood is valium.

Alcohol will potentiate the action of very many drugs including hypnotics, tranquillisers and antihistamines. Therefore, persons who are taking certain therapeutic preparations may be unfit to drive after a very small alcohol intake.

Seat belts. In many countries and states the wearing of seat belts is mandatory for the driver and front seat passenger and, in some states, for all car occupants. The result of the compulsory use of seat belts has been remarkable in frontal impacts —some states or countries showing a 10–15% drop in the death rate overnight, and eye injuries from broken windscreens showing an even more remarkable reduction. The wearing of seat belts is mandatory in the United Kingdom now. Their lack of use may be taken into consideration when awarding damages after a traffic accident.

Pedestrian injuries. In the United Kingdom the 'hit and run' accident is rare, although it is common in certain countries. The problem, therefore, as to whether or not the injuries were caused by a motor vehicle seldom arises. Occasionally, however, a pedestrian may be struck by one vehicle and then struck or run over by one or more other vehicles.

In an accident where one vehicle and one pedestrian are involved the pattern of injuries upon the pedestrian may result from:
1. primary impact with the vehicle;
2. secondary impact with the roadway, pavement or other object, e.g., bollard, tree, etc.;
3. injuries due to running over or dragging.

The injuries resulting from primary impact will depend upon that part of the car which strikes the pedestrian. In the majority of cases the pedestrian is struck below the knees by the bumper bar, then comes into contact with the bonnet and, possibly, the windscreen. After the primary impact the pedestrian may be thrown into the air, or carried along on the bonnet of the car before falling on to the road, or thrown directly forward.

The sites of the primary impact are important as they reveal the relationship of the pedestrian to the vehicle at the moment of impact. The classical bumper bar injury is a below-knee fracture of one or both lower legs. Examination of the direction of the fracture and the soft tissue injury will usually enable the pathologist to state categorically from which direction the pedestrian has been struck. For example, if a pedestrian was struck on the left side there would be injury to the outer side of the left lower leg and the inner side of the right lower leg.

If the pedestrian is thrown into the air he may be rotated so that the secondary impact injuries are upon the same side as those of the primary impact. Secondary injuries are associated with movement of the body across the roadway and abrasions will accordingly be sustained.

If the victim is dragged by a car there may be severe blunt impact injuries, due to contact with the projecting parts of the engine beneath the level of the chassis, or occasionally burns from contact with the exhaust system. Friction burns may also occur if the victim is dragged along the road. When part of the body is run over by the wheel of a vehicle the skin and the subcutaneous fat may be dragged away from the deeper muscle layers, without any actual break in continuity of the skin. This is known as 'degloving'. The pattern of the tread of the type may be reproduced upon the skin or clothing of the victim.

It is frequently of prime importance to examine the clothing of any victim of a road traffic accident. The clothing may show patterned marks due to contact with some part of the motor vehicle, such as a tyre, radiator or headlamp.

Examination of the shoes of the driver may provide a clue to the cause of the accident when none other is available. One may find exceptionally high heels or sandal-type shoes which catch in the foot controls, or heavy, ill-fitting boots which preclude delicate foot pedal control (Fig. 11.3).

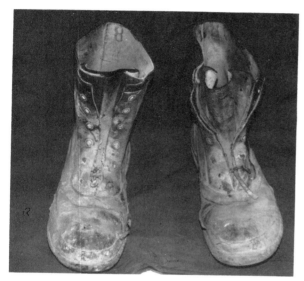

Fig. 11.3 A pair of oversized, unlaced heavy boots worn by a young lorry driver who lost control of his vehicle for no apparent reason.

The laboratory examination of clothing is essential in all 'hit and run' cases as it may reveal contact traces from the vehicle involved, which can lead to its identification. The contact traces most likely to be present are flakes of paint or fragments of glass from headlamps or windscreens.

Hair, blood, pieces of soft tissue or bone fragments may be found on the car involved. In one recent such case when the suspect car was examined a fragment of bone was found beneath the bonnet. The deceased had sustained a comminuted compound fracture of one of her legs. The leg was removed, defleshed and the bones reconstructed.

The fragment of bone recovered from the car had come from the tibia of the deceased.

Incised wounds

An incised wound is a clean cut through the tissues, usually the skin and subcutaneous tissues, including blood vessels. Blood escapes freely through the wound to the surface. Incised wounds have length rather than depth and tend to gape.

Incised wounds are inflicted with sharp cutting instruments such as razors or knives. Their presence indicates an intentional act and, in the United Kingdom, fatal cases are usually suicidal.

The pattern of injury is of great importance in determining whether the wound is self-inflicted or not. Self-inflicted wounds show obvious deliberation and although they are occasionally inflicted in an attempt to achieve publicity, their pattern will be similar to that seen in deliberate attempts at self-destruction. Non-fatal self-inflicted incised wounds are not uncommon in cases where suicide has been achieved by some other means, e.g., by drowning or by ingestion of a poison.

Self-inflicted incised wounds. Cutting one's throat is a form of suicide more common amongst men than women.

The classical fatal self-inflicted incised wound is to the throat, although occasionally the arteries in the wrists, arms or leg are successfully cut. However, before the fatal wounds are inflicted the suicide will almost invariably attack some other part of his or her body with the cutting instrument.

Most commonly the preliminary non-fatal injuries consist of a number of superficial incisions across the front of the wrist but they may appear elsewhere on the body. The characteristic features are that the cut area is bared, the wounds are usually tentative in nature, multiple and parallel, or in parallel groups. The number of wounds inflicted would appear to be directly related to their depth and thus to the pain they have caused. Where the wounds are little more than scratches through the skin there may be 50 or 60 present but where they are deep there may be only two or three. (Fig. 11.4)

The fatal wounds to the throat are preceded by a number of tentative scratches before the deep cut

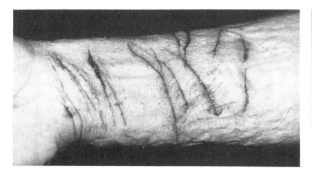

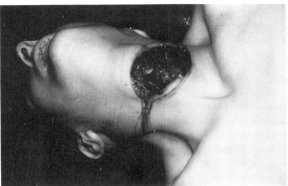

Fig. 11.5 Suicidal cut throat. Numerous tentative wounds are visible to the right of the deep incisions.

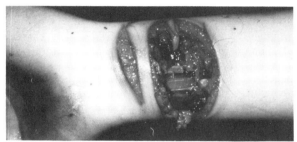

Fig. 11.4 Self inflicted incised wounds of the wrist. The more superficial the cuts, the more numerous they are.

or, more commonly, cuts are made. (Fig. 11.5). In the classic case the suicide throws his head back and the fatal wounds often separate the hyoid and thyroid cartilages and may incise the anterior longitudinal ligament running down the front of the cervical spine. As the head has been thrown back the carotid arteries are pulled behind the transverse processes of the cervical spine and thus are rarely injured. However, as with a number of suicides, the act may be performed in front of a mirror and, if the victim is watching the actual act with his head in the upright or near upright position, the carotids may be incised. Where the carotid arteries are not cut, death is frequently due to blood escaping from the large veins and pouring down the trachea—or to air being sucked into the veins, resulting in fatal air embolism.

An important feature of self-inflicted incised and stabbed wounds is that the clothing is removed from that part of the body which is injured. On many occasions the areas incised are already exposed, e.g., the wrists and neck, but when areas such as the abdomen, breast or forearms are incised the clothing is lifted or removed before the injuries are inflicted. In self-inflicted incised wounds no damage is done to the features.

Homicidal incised wounds. Unless the victim is unconscious, or restrained by some means, the homicidal wounds show none of the deliberation apparent in the suicidal injuries, although in both cases the neck is usually the main target. In homicidal injuries there are slashes usually running obliquely downward on each side of the neck. Slashes to the face or any other part of the body (clothed or unclothed) are common. Injuries from manual compression of the neck or from some blunt instrument may be present.

Defence wounds. Defence wounds are not uncommon upon victims of assaults with sharp penetrating or cutting instruments. They arise when the victim attempts to defend herself or himself and are common on the palmar surfaces of the hand when there has been an attempt to grab the weapon, or upon the arms when the victim has attempted to ward off the weapon. The presence of defensive type injuries indicate an assault by some other person or persons.

If the victim is unconscious the wounds to the throat may appear to be self-inflicted; they are often parallel in nature but differ as they are not as deep, and as the head is not thrown back the carotid artery is commonly incised. The cause of the victim's loss of consciousness may be apparent, e.g., strangulation.

In *R. v. Grimes* (1976) during a family quarrel the accused manually compressed his wife's neck and when she was unconscious he fetched a kitchen knife and cut her throat. The incised wounds bore a superficial resemblance to self-inflicted wounds, in so far as there appeared to be some tentative cuts and there were a number of parallel wounds. The carotid arteries had been severed. Bruising of the neck due to manual pressure and the suffused appearance of the features, due to the petechial haemorrhages which had developed above the line of compression, left no doubt as to the sequence of events.

Although one usually associates fatal incised wounds of the neck with sharp knives or, more frequently in the past, with open (cut-throat) razors, fatal incised wounds inflicted with broken tumblers or bottles are not rare. The broken end of the tumbler or bottle is jabbed at the neck, often with a twisting motion incising the soft tissues and opening one of the large veins resulting in a fatal air embolism.

Modes of dying from incised wounds

Haemorrhage: most fatal incised wounds occur on the neck but major vessels may be incised wherever they run a superficial course. Fatal haemorrhage from incised brachial or radial arteries are sometimes seen in suicide and occasionally a femoral artery is opened. When any major artery is incised death from haemorrhage is the most frequent outcome, although fatal haemorrhage may occur from veins—especially large varicosities in the legs if air embolism (*vide infra*) does not supervene.

Air embolism: when a large vein is opened and the opened vessel lies level with or above the level of the heart, air may enter the cut vessel due to the negative pressure within the vein. The air is then drawn into the right ventricle of the heart and the pulmonary circulation, where it is converted into a froth by the beating of the heart and causes an insurmountable obstruction to the circulation. Some air may enter the general circulation where it may obstruct both the coronary and cerebral arteries.

Respiratory obstruction

This mode of dying applies to incised wounds involving the larynx or trachea. Blood escapes from the cut vessels and enters the trachea or windpipe causing fatal obstruction to respiration.

Delayed deaths

These result from complications associated with the original injury.

Infection local to the wound is rare. Pneumonia, however, may follow inhalation of blood or may occur as a sequel to any serious injury. Fatal pulmonary embolism may arise during the early convalescent period.

Stabbed wounds

Stabbed wounds are by definition those wounds whose depth of penetration is greater than the length of the external wound. Stabbed wounds are usually homicidal although suicidal and accidental wounds are well recognised.

Stabbing instruments include any instrument which is able to produce a wound conforming with the definition given above. Although most stabbed wounds are inflicted by well recognised stabbing instruments such as daggers, sheath knives, kitchen knives or penknives, a very great variety of weapons are occasionally seen in practice including: ice picks (more popular in the United States and the entry wound may easily be mistaken for a bullet wound); pokers; chisels; reamers; bicycle wheel spokes; glass slivers and broken bottle ends; bayonets; screwdrivers; and scissors.

Examination of stabbed wounds. The pathologist examining a fatal case of stabbing has to consider the following:
1. Was death due to the stabbed wound(s)?
2. Is/are the wound(s) homicidal, suicidal or accidental in character?
3. What is/are the nature of the weapon(s) used?
4. What is/are the direction and depth of the wound(s)?
5. What force has been used?

Whether death was directly due to the stabbed wound(s) is usually self evident once the autopsy examination has been conducted and will not be further considered at this stage. The mode of dying from stabbed wounds is described later in this section.

Is/are the wound(s) suicidal, homicidal or accidental in character? Suicidal stabbing is not common and when it occurs follows the general pattern of suicidal wounding. That part of the body injured is

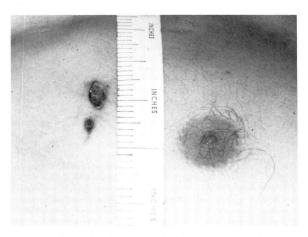

Fig. 11.6 Suicidal stabbed wound of the chest. Note the tentative wound lateral to the main wound.

readily accessible (usually the chest or upper abdomen, rarely the neck). Clothing is removed from the site of the injury (it may be merely lifted or pulled to one side), and tentative 'pricks' are frequently seen around the fatal wound. The stabbing instrument is either in situ or by the body. In suicidal stabbing there is usually, though not invariably, one major wound (Fig. 11.6).

Accidental stabbed wounds may result from falls on to objects such as railings or scissors or knives.

Although homicidal stabbed wounds, like the suicidal wounds, are frequently delivered to the front of the chest or upper abdomen, they differ in that they are often multiple and are delivered through clothing and frequently through sites of difficult or impossible access to the victim, e.g., the back or sides. Defence type injuries are common and may be on the palmar surfaces of the hands,

due to attempts at gripping the instrument, or there may be through and through wounds of arms which were raised in self-defence. Tentative wounds are sometimes present. These occur when the assailant threatens the victim, the victim frequently being held by another assailant. These tentative wounds are usually seen on the face or neck and may be far removed from the fatal injury.

What is/are the nature of the weapon(s) used? In the majority of cases of fatal stabbing only one instrument has been used. Where there has been more than one assailant, each using his own instrument, the pathologist will be asked which instrument caused the fatal wound. In a percentage of cases the police will produce the suspect weapons at the time of the autopsy. The pathological investigation is, however, the same whether or not a weapon is produced.

The most common stabbing instruments are kitchen knives, sheath knives or penknives. A knife blade may be double-edged along its entire length, it may be double-edged for a variable distance or it may have one cutting edge. The external appearance of the skin wound will often depict the type of blade. If the external wound is clean cut at both ends then the knife is either double-edged or the part of the blade which has entered at that point is double-edged. If it is single-edged, one end of the wound will be clean cut whereas the other end may be rounded or square. Exceptions arise when the stabbed wound is not the result of a single in and out thrust but was inflicted with the cutting edge moving forwards as the knife entered the body. Here there may appear to be two cutting edges—the width of the wound, however, will be greater than the width of the knife.

Table 11.3 Comparison of suicidal, accidental and homicidal stabbed wounds

	Suicidal	Homicidal	Accidental
Numbers	Often single	Frequently multiple	Usually single
Tentative wounds	May be present around site of fatal wound	May be present rarely but away from fatal wound	Absent
Clothing	Removed from injured area	Normally not disturbed	Not disturbed
Defence wounds	Absent	Often present	Absent
Site	Accessible pre-cordial area or upper abdomen	May be anywhere	May be anywhere

In a simple thrust and withdrawal the width of the external wound will correspond with the width of the knife blade or may be slightly less owing to the elasticity of the skin. Where there are multiple stabbed wounds it will be found that although there may be a variation in width many will have the identical measurement. The more wounds there are present the more accurate will be the estimation of the width of the blade.

Further characteristics of the weapon are gained from the depth of the individual wounds and the measurements of the wounds, both exit and entry in the internal viscera and especially the heart. These measurements can all be plotted on graph paper and the resulting outline of the dimensions of the knife may be very accurate.

The depth of a wound may not reflect the length of the knife. The knife may not have been inserted to its full length. The depth of the wound may be much greater than the length of the blade. The chest is mobile in young people and may be compressed during the stabbing, and where wounds have been inflicted through the abdominal wall the track may be over twice as long as the blade if an instrument such as a penknife has been used. Many of the internal organs are not fixed but have a variable degree of mobility. This factor must be taken into account when estimating the depth of the wounds.

If the tip of the knife has been turned by striking bone, or was already turned before the wounds were inflicted, it will tend to pull tissue out through the external wound as it is being withdrawn. This may be striking in abdominal injuries where omentum is found protruding through the wound.

The direction of the wound is of particular importance where only one wound has been inflicted. In fatal single stabbed wound homicide cases the most usual defence is that the victim walked on to the knife and that the stabbing was accidental. An upward or downward track is usually quite inconsistent with the defendant's explanation of events.

In these cases where stabbed wounds have been inflicted with an instrument other than the type of knife described above, the entry wound will depend upon the sharpness and shape of the weapon. The blunter the end of the weapon, the more force which will be required to penetrate the

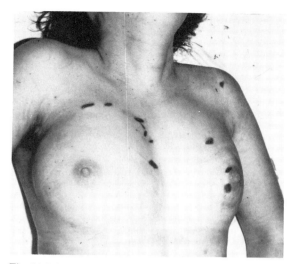

Fig. 11.7 Multiple homicidal stabbed wounds of the chest.

skin, even over an area such as the chest, where the skin is relatively fixed. The more force required, the greater is the extent of the bruising in the surrounding soft tissue. The entry wound will also reflect the shape of the weapon. In the case of an ice pick or sharp chisel the wound may be well defined, but with a poker or scissors it will tend to have lacerated edges and only reflect the general shape of the weapon.

Stabbed wounds are almost invariably inflicted deliberately. Their multiplicity, siting, nature and violence may sometimes give an indication of the state of mind of the assailant.

In homosexual stabbings, and in stabbings committed in unsatisfactory heterosexual relationships, the wounds are generally multiple and many of them, taken singly, could have been lethal. In homosexual stabbings the pattern is often over a very wide area, whereas in the heterosexual group the pattern is closer (Fig. 11.7).

A single fatal stabbed wound which has entered the heart either through the front of the chest or from beneath the ribs suggests deliberation at the time of the act. Some cases occur where a knife is produced and thrust into a person for no apparent reason. These are single wounds and in a number of these cases it appears that there was no intention to kill. The intention of the assailant may have been to frighten his victim or merely to 'show off'.

Once the point of the weapon has passed through the skin it will continue with little thrust until progress is stopped by the haft or the thrusting force ceases unless it strikes bone. The bones most commonly encountered are the ribs, the sternum or breastbone and the spine. A knife often slips between the ribs. It may be deviated by striking them or it may go straight through, severing the bone. The sternum is a firm plate of bone and a knife blade may be gripped by the bone and can only be withdrawn by rocking. The spine also tends to grip the knife.

Where there is a single wound, inflicted with a sharp pointed narrow blade, dagger type or kitchen knife, very little force may have been used to inflict the fatal wound provided the blade has not struck bone. The estimation of force of the thrust may be gauged by bruising around the wound and bony damage.

The causes of death in stabbing. The target in both suicidal and homicidal stabbing is the heart. Wounds of the right ventricle are more rapidly lethal than those of the left owing to the thinness of its wall. In wounds of the heart, assuming there is a solitary penetration, the mode of dying is the rapid filling of the heart sac (pericardial sac) with blood escaping from the ventricle. Blood is pumped out of the heart at a faster rate than it can escape through the perforation of the heart sac so eventually the accumulation of blood in the sac exerts sufficient pressure upon the heart to prevent it beating (tamponade) (*vide supra*). Any increase in heart beat, as from fighting or running after the stabbed wound, will increase the filling of the heart sac and thus hasten tamponade. With wounds of the left ventricle the bleeding is much less owing to the thickness of the muscle. Wounds may close up after the withdrawal of the knife from the left ventricle, the life of the victim thus being preserved. If the victim arrives at hospital alive, his life may often be preserved by rapid surgical intervention to relieve the cardiac tamponade.

Death may be caused by more superficial wounds severing a coronary artery.

Haemorrhage leading to exsanguination follows wounds to the main blood vessels in the chest and abdomen. These vessels include the aorta, the pulmonary arteries and the vena cavae. Haemorrhage is usually massive, blood escaping into the pleural or abdominal cavities. In a few cases a main blood vessel such as the aorta receives only a small perforation and the haemorrhage occurs over a long interval and may not be recognised by the surgeon. Occasionally only the outer layers of the aorta are damaged, leading to a local bulging (traumatic aneurysm) of the wall, which may rupture within hours, days or even months producing a fatal haemorrhage.

Stabbed wounds of the chest involving lung tissue may allow the escape of air or air and blood (pneumothorax or haemopneumothorax) into the chest cavity where pressure builds up and the lungs become compressed so that eventually they cease to function. A pneumothorax is more likely to occur when the victim is suffering from emphysema.

Death may ensue from haemorrhage in the absence of injury to the heart or great vessels or to the lungs if the vessels which run between the ribs (intercostal vessels) are damaged. These vessels are protected by the border of the rib along which they run but when damaged bleed into the chest cavity As haemorrhage is not as brisk as follows injury to a major vessel, the dangerous nature of the wound may not be recognised when the victim is first examined. Death occurs several hours after the wounding in untreated cases.

In stabbed wounds of the neck, death is due to the causes listed under incised wounds. Stabbed wounds inflicted with broken bottles or glass more frequently perforate the jugular vein leading to fatal air embolism.

The causes of death given above are the causes which rapidly follow the initial injury. As with all forms of wounding, death may occur later from complications developing directly from the initial wounding. Traumatic aneurysm has been mentioned above. Other delayed deaths are often associated with secondary infection related to the wound.

Firearm injuries

There are very many varieties of firearms and ammunition, of which only the basic types will be described below. Some knowledge of these basic types is essential in order to interpret and understand the injuries they may inflict.

All firearms have the following features in common. Essentially they consist of a tube (the barrel) which may measure anything from an inch or so to over 3 ft in length. The tube is closed at one end (the breech) and open at the other (the muzzle). The projectile is forced down the barrel by the ignition of the propellant explosive at the breech end. The firing mechanism is operated by a lever (trigger). The firearm is held in the hand or shoulder by the stock. If the weapon carries more than one cartridge or round, these are stored in a box or magazine or in a revolving chamber.

Cartridges either hold a single projectile or bullet or a number of pellets or shot. The latter are intended for sporting purposes, i.e., killing small animals or game.

Firearms fall naturally into two groups: those designed to fire a single projectile and those designed to fire shot.

Firearms designed to fire a single projectile have a spiral groove cut into the inner surface of the barrel (rifling). The diameter or bore of the barrel is smaller than the diameter of the projectile or bullet to ensure an airtight fit when it enters the barrel. The spiral grooves impart a rotational spin to the bullet to ensure that it follows a regular flight.

The raised parts of the barrel lying between the grooves are known as the lands. The bore of a barrel is its maximum diameter and may be measured in millimetres or inches. The number of grooves, the width of the lands and grooves, and the length of the spiral and its direction of twist differ in most makes of firearms, thus enabling a ballistics expert to identify the actual make and type of firearm from which a bullet was fired by examination of the marks left by the rifling upon the surface of the bullet. The interior of each barrel is different from every other and specific scratches on the bullet may enable a gun to be positively identified.

Guns firing single projectiles are divided into two types:

Side arms. These are guns which are held in the hand and are usually called revolvers or pistols. They have short barrels.

Shoulder arms. These are heavy, long-barrelled guns which are fired from the shoulder—one arm supporting the barrel and the other hand holding the stock and operating the trigger mechanism.

Guns are further classified for descriptive purposes by the method used to reload the breech after firing. The non-automatic weapons have to be reloaded by hand or from a magazine by a specific action on the part of the firer. A self-loading or semi-automatic gun (pistols which are semi-automatic are often called automatic) is self-loading after each firing until the magazine is exhausted—the trigger being pressed each time the gun is fired. An automatic gun is one which reloads and fires continuously as long as the trigger is depressed and the magazine is charged.

Light automatic guns are relatively short-barrelled anti-personnel firearms, which are normally fired from the shoulder. The barrel length is intermediate between the hand gun and the conventional shoulder gun.

Modern combat rifles and light automatic guns are designed so that they can fire semi-automatic or full automatic at the control of the firer.

Sporting guns are usually single or double-barrelled shoulder guns and the majority do not carry any form of magazine although 'pump guns', in which extra cartridges are contained in a cylindrical tube beneath the barrel and loaded by a pump action after each firing, are popular in some parts of the world.

Pistols, firing shot cartridges, exist for the shooting of small birds and rodents, but are illegal in Great Britain where a legal shot gun barrel must have a minimum length of 24 inches.

Sporting guns usually have barrel lengths about 28 inches, although for clay bird shooting they may be shorter, and for duck shooting longer.

The bore of a shotgun is measured in inches up to $\frac{1}{2}$ inch diameter e.g., 0.410. Over $\frac{1}{2}$ inch the bore is calculated by the numbers of equal spheres which make up a pound of pure lead which can be placed in the barrel—thus, in a 16 bore there are 16 equal spheres of lead which will fit into the barrel and in a 12 bore, 12 spheres. Therefore the lower the bore number the greater the diameter of the barrel. These guns vary from 20 bore to 4 bore—the latter being used exclusively for duck shooting.

Before discussing gun-shot wounds a brief description of the cartridge or shell is essential for their interpretation. These must be divided into those firing single projectiles and those firing shot. The cartridge for a rifled firearm consists of a brass case in which the bullet or projectile is firmly held and which also contains the propellant charge. At the base of the cartridge case is a cap containing the detonator, a sensitive chemical which explodes upon percussion and ignites the propellant charge. When the propellant charge is ignited it burns rapidly with the production of a large volume of gas, which forces the bullet into the barrel where it is trapped by the rifling and passes up the barrel with increasing speed, reaching it maximum velocity (muzzle velocity) as it leaves the barrel. The pressure of gases inside the barrel varies from about 1 ton/square inch in a revolver to some 25 tons/square inch in the modern rifle.

The enormous pressure generated in the barrel of a gun when it is fired forces the base of the cartridge, and especially the thin copper casing of the detonator, against the firing pin and breech block. A mirror image of any irregularities of the firing pin and breech block is reproduced upon the base of the detonator cap, enabling the ballistics expert to identify the gun from which the cartridge was fired by comparing the marks from the cartridge case at the scene with that fired by the suspect weapon.

Every modern firearm has some means of extracting spent cartridge cases from the breech. This is usually accomplished by a claw which grips the rim of the cartridge, or the groove at the base in the case of automatic weapons, and the case is ejected either by hand or, in automatic weapons, by the employment of some of the gases of the propellant charge. These extractor claws will mark the portion of the base of the cartridge which they grip in a specific manner, leaving marks particular to that gun. These marks will also enable a ballistics expert to match a cartridge case with the gun from which it is fired.

The bullets, other than small calibre bullets used for target shooting, have a lead alloy core, sometimes an aluminium nosepiece—the case and nosepiece being surrounded, except for the base, by a cupronickel casing.

There is a wide variety of ammunition produced for special purposes, such as the duplex or tandem bullet, the partly jacketed bullet 'super vel' and the KTW load—a tungsten cored bullet coated with teflon.

Exploding bullets are staging a revival in the United States and are a hazard not only to the target but also to the surgeon who may have to remove an undetonated explosive bullet from the victim. Ultrasound or microwave diagnostic techniques must be avoided where explosive bullets are present as they can cause the projectiles to detonate.[16]

The muzzle velocity of a bullet or projectile will depend upon the explosive power of the propellant and upon the length of barrel in which the increasing pressure is operative.

The nature of the injury inflicted by a missile is determined not only by the characteristics of the bullet, i.e., lead, partly or fully jacketed, but also by the muzzle velocity. Revolvers have muzzle velocities as low as 680 ft/s, whereas high velocity rifles may exceed 3400 ft/s. As the energy is dependent upon the formula mv^2 it is apparent that there will be an enormous release of energy when a high velocity missile is decelerated as it enters the body.

Velocities are usually classified as low when below the speed of sound, and high when above.

Shot gun cartridges consist of a metal base containing the detonator. The metal base is attached to a cylinder of cardboard which contains the propellant powder, thick plunger wads (which act as a piston behind the shot when the gun is discharged), the shot and a retaining wad or crimp at the end of the cartridge to keep the shot in place.

The propellant powder varies in amount according to the purpose for which the ammunition is designed. The shot also varies in size from fine shot used for shooting small birds, such as snipe, to buckshot used for deer shooting. No. 12 shot is very small, there being roughly 38 000 to the pound, whereas there are only 130 of the larger buckshot to the pound.

The effective range and penetrating power of a shot gun will depend upon the quantity of propellant charge, the size of the shot, the length of the barrel, and whether or not the barrel is narrowed towards the muzzle end (choked). These factors also determine the rate of spread of the shot once it leaves the muzzle.

External characteristics of firearm wounds. When a firearm is discharged the projectile or projectiles leave the muzzle, followed by the gases from the propellant under great pressure, by flame, by unburned powder and by carbon. The gases of the charge also contain carbon monoxide.

The gases, after leaving the muzzle, expand at

once to atmospheric pressure. If the muzzle is in contact with the skin then some of these gases will expand in the tissues immediately below the entry wound. If the gun is held far enough from the skin for the gases to expand without entering the tissues the entry wound will be surrounded by unburnt powder and carbon particles.

Powder tattooing. The size and intensity of the surrounding powder tattooing will depend upon the constituents of the propellant charge, i.e., black powder or smokeless, and the distance between the skin and the muzzle.

Wounds are usually classified by their external appearance as:
1. close contact,
2. near contact,
3. distant.

Close contact. In these wounds, by definition, the muzzle is held in close contact with the skin. The projectile or projectiles, gases of the propellant charge under great pressure, unburned powder and any wads, will all enter the body. If the gun is fired into a body cavity such as the chest or abdomen the cavity will contain the gases, even if there is no exit wound, and the entry wound will be circular. If, however, there is a plate of bone beneath the entry wound (i.e., the forehead) the gases will expand between the skin and the bone and escape through the entry wound, both enlarging, splitting and everting it. The wound, therefore, is stellate, larger than the diameter of the barrel and the skin is blackened on its inner side by powder and carbon.

If the gases are not of sufficient volume, i.e., 0.22 calibre rifle, or the propellant has deteriorated, there may not be sufficient pressure to cause this type of close contact wound and the wound will remain circular although in other respects it follows the criteria for a close contact wound.

Near contact. In these wounds the muzzle is an inch or so away from the skin when fired. The entry wound is circular and the surrounding skin is blackened by smoke and unburned powder. The size of the halo and its intensity will depend upon the distance between the muzzle and the skin and the type and quality of the propellant charge.

Distant wounds. Wounds resulting from guns fired from over 3 ft from the body are divided into:
1. rifled firearms,
2. sporting guns.

Wounds from rifled firearms: the wound is circular unless the missile has riccocheted and will be of slightly smaller diameter than the calibre of the gun. The edges will be narrowly abraded (abrasion collar) due to the inversion and stretching of the skin by the missile as it enters the body. Where a bullet has been greased some grease may be detected in the edges of the wound.

Wounds from sporting guns: at distances further than 3 ft from the end of the muzzle the shot begins to disperse or spread from the cylindrical shape in which they leave the barrel. The rate of spread of shot will depend upon the charge, the size of the pellets, the length of the barrel and whether the barrel is narrowed at the muzzle end (choked) to increase the range of the gun. In order to determine the rate of spread of shot with accuracy it is essential to fire the gun at different distances using the same ammunition. A rough guide, however, may be used for rapid calculation—from a barrel which is a true cylinder the average size of the pattern of spread is 1 inch/yard from the muzzle, less 1 inch. Thus at 5 yards one would expect a pattern of spread of 4 inches.

Internal injuries caused by firearms. The internal injuries due to gunshot wounds vary according to the calibre and velocity of the missile. Once the missile has penetrated the skin, which offers the most resistance to its passage, the missile may pass through the body unless it is slowed or deflected by bone. The character of the internal injury is greatly influenced by the velocity of the missile when it enters the body. When a rapidly travelling object is slowed by passing from a thin to a dense medium, there is a release of kinetic energy which may be so violent as to fracture bones in the immediate vicinity of the track although the bones are not actually struck. Shock waves will also pass through the tissues causing injury remote from the actual wound. For instance, the passage of a high velocity missile through the soft tissues of the thigh may fracture the femur and cause damage to blood vessels in the pelvis as a result of the changes of hydrostatic pressure in the blood vessels.

When a high velocity missile passes through soft tissue it is followed by cavitation as a result of the released energy. This primary cavity then collapses but is followed by lesser secondary cavitation.

When this secondary cavitation occurs a negative pressure is created and debris is sucked into the track and may set up infection, including tetanus. Another feature of a high velocity missile entering a denser medium is that it momentarily tips up on its axis, sometimes even beyond the vertical, and although it corrects itself immediately extensive soft tissue damage will occur at the site of the tipping.

When a high velocity missile strikes a relatively solid internal organ such as the heart, this organ may disintegrate as if an explosive charge has been detonated in its substance.

Internal injuries from shotguns. When the cylinder of shot meets any resistance it breaks up at once—when a gun is discharged through a glass panel the spread may amount to several inches during its passage through the glass. If a hand is held over the muzzle when discharge occurs the pattern may be 3 inches across as it leaves the hand. Thick clothing, such as a leather jacket, will also accelerate dispersal of the shot.

The types of wound depend upon the distance from which the gun is fired, the weight of the charge, the size of the shot and the part of the body struck.

If a standard shotgun (20 bore or greater) with a normal load cartridge is fired at contact range through the head, the skull will often disintegrate, whereas if fired at contact range into the chest no injury other than the entry wound may be visible, the chest cavity containing the expanding gases. In both the skull and the chest cavity the shot is widely dispersed.

When a shot gun is fired from greater distances the penetration of individual pellets will vary. Some may merely penetrate skin. Others will pass deep into the tissues.

The plunger wad will enter the tissues behind the main mass of shot for distances up to several feet and even beyond this may make a circular wound on the skin adjacent to the main entry wound.

If the shot cartridge is loaded with a heavy powder load, or if it contains buckshot, the shot may pass through the chest at close range. Whereas number 6 shot may do little damage to a person at 25 yards, buckshot at this range is lethal if directed against the head or chest.

Exit wounds

Single projectiles: the size, shape and sometimes multiplicity of the exit wound from a single projectile will depend upon the shape and composition of the bullet, its velocity and whether it has rotated, struck bone or altered its shape during its passage through the body.

In other than a close contact entry wound the exit wound is larger than the entry wound. Although the exit wound may be circular it is more commonly elliptical, split or occasionally stellate. With a high velocity missile it may be very many times larger than the entry wound owing to the explosive release of kinetic energy during its passage through the body.

In the majority of cases the difference between the entry and exit wound is easily identifiable. Confusion may arise when the exit wound occurs below some firm resistance, for instance a pocket book against the skin, or where the exit wound is against some resistance such as the back of a wooden chair or bench.

If doubt exists upon external examination the confusion may be resolved by examination of the clothing, by X-rays and by the post-mortem examination.

Shot guns: conventional shot guns with standard loads rarely have an exit wound unless the

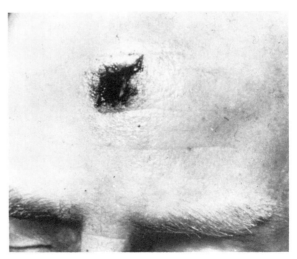

Fig. 11.8 A typical close contact suicidal gunshot wound of the centre forehead (0.455 calibre).

gun is discharged against the head, causing the skull to disintegrate. With heavy charges and a load of large pellets such as B.B. or buckshot exit wounds will occur. As shot rapidly disperses when passing through any resistance the pattern of the exit wounds may be spread over a wide area. The only exception will be with a very heavy load such as buckshot fired from close range. In these cases the dispersal of the shot through the body may be minimal.

Self-inflicted firearm wounds. Self-inflicted gun-shot wounds of the head conform to a pattern that is so exact that any deviation of the entry wound by so much as $\frac{1}{2}$ inch must give rise to suspicion. The wound is contact or near contact and is situated usually with mathematical precision in a 'site of election'. Persons who kill themselves by shooting, even when they are quite unused to firearms, still select these sites. The sites are:

1. centre of the forehead (Fig. 11.8);
2. right or left temple;
3. roof of the mouth;
4. below the chin.

Sites 1, 3 and 4 are in the midline.

Occasionally the site of entry is atypical. When this occurs the suicide has usually used a long barrelled weapon and may have had difficulty in operating the firing mechanism.

Self-inflicted firearm wounds of the chest are not inflicted with such precision and may be found over the front and left side of the chest.

Firearm suicides are not common in the United Kingdom and many police surgeons may never have the opportunity to see more than one or two in a lifetime. Mistakes are not infrequently made between the entry and exit wound when the body is first seen at the scene.

When the scene is examined the relationship of the gun to the deceased must be noted. If the entry wound is in the right temple is the gun in the right hand or close to it? Where a long barrelled gun has been employed measurements of the reach of the deceased and of the distance from the muzzle to the trigger are essential. Suicides may improvise in order to fire the gun, using string tied to the trigger or a twig or piece of wood with a nail driven into it. They may use a toe or even tie a piece of string connected with the trigger to their big toe.

When a gun is fired there is an escape of gases from around the breech and smoke residues will be present on the firer's hand. With old guns this may be very marked. Very often the burned cordite smell is present on the hands of the firer. If any doubt exists, swabs moistened with 5% nitric acid may be rubbed over the suspect area and examined in the laboratory for residues.

With long barrelled guns the suicide may hold the muzzle end against his body, in which case there will be a heavy deposit of powder on his hand, thumb and forefinger.

In any case, where the entry wound is not in one of the sites of election the case should be treated as homicide until proved otherwise.

In homicidal shooting the bullet or projectiles may enter any part of the body. They are rarely situated over one of the sites of election and the range is usually beyond contact.

Investigation of firearm wounds. It is always desirable to X-ray the body in a case of shooting and in a case of homicide or suspected homicide shooting this is essential and especially when a rifled firearm has been used and there is no exit wound. Bullets may be deflected by bone, may break into several fragments or, in the case of frangible bullets, i.e. (iron bullets), completely disintegrate. On rare occasions the bullet may actually enter a major blood vessel and travel in the vessel until it becomes arrested (bullet embolism). Correctly taken X-rays will enable the exact location of the missile to be identified.

The pathologist must recover the missile without causing it further damage for its examination by a ballistics expert. Attempts to locate a bullet blindly are likely to result in its mutilation by instruments.

With shot gun injuries it may be desirable to enumerate all the pellets. This is only feasible by the use of radiographs.

Besides the actual recovery of the missile or missiles the pathologist must ascertain the direction of the missile as it entered the body.

Small calibre guns produce small wounds which may be mistaken for stabbed wounds or missed entirely on external examination of the body.

High explosive injuries

During recent years bomb outrages have occurred

in many countries. It is not intended to discuss the injuries caused by high explosives in warfare but only outline briefly the pathological investigation of a civilian type bombing.

The blast will depend upon the amount and type of explosive used and the effect will be conditioned by its locus—i.e., in the open or indoors.

Pathological problems arising from these cases revolve around identification of the dead, the distribution of injuries, the reconstruction of the positions of those killed in relation to the bomb and the recovery of fragments of the bomb, especially of its firing mechanism.

Identification is dealt with in chapter 9. Recovery of fragments of the bomb and of pieces of the firing mechanism involves good quality radiographs of the bodies and recovery of metallic fragments under direct X-ray control, usually after the soft tissues have been macerated. In one case where five deaths occurred, part of the balance wheel of the watch mechanism was found in the pelvis of one of the victims. This was the only part of the mechanism recovered but nevertheless was sufficient for the make of watch to be identified.

Identification of the type of explosive and the amount used is a problem for the explosive expert and is outside the scope of this book. For those interested in the methods used in the investigation of explosive, *Explosive Investigation* by H. J. Yallop, is to be recommended.[14]

REFERENCES

1. Medico-Legal (1959) Br. Med. J., **2**, 50.
2. Barrowcliff, D. F. (1968) Med. Sci. Law, **8**, 54.
3. Carscadden, W. G. (1927) Arch. Pathol. Lab. Med., **4**, 329.
4. Moritz, A. (1954) Pathology of Trauma, 2nd edn. London: Henry Kimpton.
5. Davis, J. H. (1978) J. For. Sc., **23**, 384.
6. Cameron, J. M. & Mant, A. K. (1972) Med. Sci. Law., **12**, 66.
7. Mant, A. K. (1972) J. For. Sci. Sco., **12**, 567.
8. Mant, A. K (1977) In: Wecht, C., ed. Leg. Med. Annual, ch. 7. New York: Appleton – Century Crofts.
9. Bell, J. S. & Mason, J. M (1980) J. For. Sci., **25**, 20.
10. Report of the Commission of Inquiry into Inspector MacLennan's Case (1981) Government of Hong Kong.
11. Hudson Page (1981) Am. J. For. Med. Pathol., **2**, 239.
12. Fatteh, A., Gore, S. G., Mann, G. T. & Garvin, K. (1980) J. For. Sci., **25**, 883.
13. Grattan, E., Wall, J. G. & Hobbs, J. A. (1973) In: Mant, A. K. Modern Trends in Forensic Medicine, ch. 7, 3rd edn. London: Butterworth.
14. Yallop, H. J. (1980) Explosive Investigation. Harrogate: Forensic Science Society.
15. Brettel, H. L. (1977) Rechtsmedizin, **80**, 167.
16. Knight, B. (1982) Br. Med. J., **I**, 768.
17. Lee, K. A. P. (1980) Personal communication.
18. Mant, A. K. (1978) In: Mason, J. K. Pathology of Violent Injury, ch. 1. London: Edward Arnold.
19. Petersen, B. S. & Petty, C. S. (1962) J. For. Sci., **7**, 274.
20. Thomas, G. (1980) Personal communication.
21. Ysander, L. (1966) Br. J. Ind. Med., **23**, 37.
22. *R.* v. *Davis* 1871 Chelmsford Aut. Assize

12

Deaths from physical and chemical injury, starvation and neglect

HEAT

General effects—hyperpyrexia

The deleterious action of heat upon the body may be the result of its general effects upon the victim as a whole, or the local effects upon particular tissues, such as burns. The general effects, as classified by the Climatic Physiology Committee of the Medical Research Council,[1] included

1. heat stroke;
2. heat hyperpyrexia;
3. heat cramps;
4. anhydrotic heat exhaustion;
5. salt-deficiency heat exhaustion;
6. water-deficiency heat exhaustion.

These conditions are comparatively rarely seen in temperate regions of the world, such as England, and their medico-legal importance in such countries is slight. They normally occur as a result of exposure of the victim to abnormally hot environmental conditions, in tropical areas.

In heat stroke, there is failure of the heat regulating mechanism, with sudden unconsciousness, hence 'stroke'. The condition is likely to prove fatal. Heat hyperpyrexia is due to malfunctioning of the heat regulatory centre, and may lead on to heat stroke. It is defined as a temperature above 106°F (41°C).

The other conditions, due to lack of salt or of water, are of slower onset, and the symptoms are less dramatic, of weakness, muscle pains, faintness, etc.

The occasions on which these conditions will be encountered during medico-legal practice, due purely to climatic conditions, are rare in this country. On the other hand, hyperpyrexia associated with the taking of drugs may occur, and then has considerable medico-legal significance.

Several drugs are liable to be associated with hyperpyrexial reactions, especially in overdosage. Thus atropine has been incriminated as the cause of hyperpyrexia in children.[2] Di-nitro-ortho-cresol and related drugs may also cause high body temperatures, leading to death. Amphetamines may have a similar effect in overdosage, especially if associated with a high environmental temperature.

A youth of 18 took several Durophet tablets, and then attended an all-night dance, during summer, and while there was a heat-wave. The following morning he was seen to be behaving very irrationally, and at midday was found collapsed. On admission to hospital he had a very high temperature, of about 108°F, and died within a few hours in spite of treatment. Autopsy revealed widespread congestion of the organs, with bleeding into the conducting tissue of the heart. Analysis demonstrated small amounts of amphetamine in the body (F.M. 14082A).

Recently an association between anaesthesia and cases of fatal hyperpyrexia has been noted. Such cases were first described in America in 1967, and by 1968 a few had been reported in England.[3] The condition was found to arise rapidly in otherwise healthy persons. A striking feature was the rigidity of voluntary muscles; temperatures rose quickly to 42°C (107.6°F) and in the majority of cases death ensued.

A relationship between the condition and abnormal muscle metabolism was suspected; some of the patients had received suxamethonium as a muscle relaxant as part of the anaesthetic regime. Under experimental conditions pigs which were given suxamethonium during anaesthesia, all developed pyrexia.

Subsequently it was realised that the condition was also liable to occur in association with halothane when this was used as the anaesthetic agent.[4] Enzymes associated with muscle metabolism, creatine phosphokinase and aldolase were found to be raised in persons who had suffered from this condition and had survived, and also in many of their relatives, and this suggested that some form of myopathy was also an integral part of the condition; the anaesthetic agent acted in a triggering capacity. The myopathy would appear to be genetically determined.

Techniques for screening relatives of persons who have suffered malignant hyperpyrexia, to establish whether they too are at risk, have been described recently.[5] The methods include muscle biopsy, neuropharmacological investigation of the contraction of muscle tissue exposed to halothane and suxamethonium, and determination of the serum creatine phosphokinase level. More recently the value of enzyme estimations has been queried.[6,7] The condition has recently formed the basis for legal actions for malpractice in America.[8]

Since the condition of fatal hyperpyrexia, whether during anaesthesia, or from other causes, is rare, the forensic pathologist will see the results of this condition at autopsy very infrequently. However, the pathological findings in cases of heat stroke have been described by Malamud and his colleagues very fully, based on a series of 125 fatal cases in army personnel.[9] They described degenerative changes in the brain which became more pronounced as the length of time between onset of the condition and death increased; neurones became vacuolated, swollen and then pyknotic and disappeared, and there was glial reaction. The changes were most marked in the cerebellum where there was rapid disappearance of Purkinje cells. There were haemorrhages in the meninges, in the walls of the third ventricle, around the aqueduct, and in the floor of the fourth ventricle. There were also haemorrhages into the heart in subepicardial and subendocardial tissues and near the bundle of His, and in the lungs. Later, necrosis of heart muscle, lobar pneumonia, lower nephron nephrosis, centrilobular necrosis of the liver, and degenerative changes in the adrenal cortex occurred. Clinical aspects of the condition are summarised by Kew.[10] A recent study[11] of 10 cases of heat stroke has shown that death was due to disseminated intravascular coagulation.

Local effects—burns and scalds

Just as blunt force may produce a wound so the effect of dry heat on the body may produce an injury, and the intensity of the heat will obviously affect the severity of the injury. However, in the case of heat, the duration of application of the heat will also affect the severity of the burn. Thus if an object at. a relatively low temperature is applied to the body surface for a short period no injury will result, but continued application for a prolonged period will eventually cause a burn. The length of time that heat needs to be applied to the body, at different temperatures, to cause burns was studied by Moritz & Henriques.[12] The minimum temperature capable of causing injury was found to be 44°C. An object at this temperature needed to be applied to the body surface for 5 h before a burn resulted. At 60°C the duration of application of the heat was reduced to 3 s. For full details the work of Moritz and his colleagues should be consulted.[12]

The capacity of objects at relatively low temperatures to produce burns after long periods of contact has practical application. For instance in one case an elderly person fell, became incapacitated by a fractured femur and lay for several hours on a floor which had underfloor heating, the floor temperature being at about 113°F. When found the victim showed first degree burns of those parts of the body which were in contact with the floor.

For purposes of description, burns can be classified according to the depth of involvement of the tissues, and measured by the amount of body surface affected, according to the normal clinical methods.

The classification of Dupytren, in six degrees, allows great precision, but in practice is too detailed.

1st degree = reddening of the skin.
2nd degree = blistering.
3rd degree = skin partly destroyed.
4th degree = skin completely destroyed.
5th degree = subcutaneous tissues burnt.
6th degree = muscle and bone charred.

For normal descriptive purposes, certainly as far as the autopsy is concerned, a classification into three degrees, as originally proposed by Wilson[13] is sufficient:

1st degree = reddening and blistering of the skin only.

2nd degree = charring and destruction of the full thickness of the skin.

3rd degree = charring of the tissues beneath the skin, e.g., fat, muscle and bone.

Since the disability caused by burns is related, to a considerable extent, to the amount of the body surface involved, the clinical method of classification, by the 'Rule-of-Nines', (Fig. 12.1) has value.

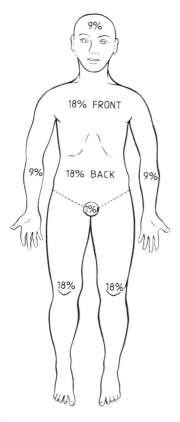

Fig. 12.1 Diagram of 'Rule-of-Nines'.

However, in making an autopsy report an accurate record, by words and diagrams, of the exact distribution, size and depth of each burn is necessary.

This may also become important with regard to the living burnt patient, if the burn has a distinctive shape which may correspond to a particular hot object which was applied to the skin. The agent responsible for the burn may be identified, just as

is the case with abrasions which have distinctive patterns.

In adults such 'patterned burns' are rare, though during the present state of unrest in Northern Ireland examples of burns caused during torture have been described by Professor T. K. Marshall (personal communication).

However, children are always liable to have injuries deliberately inflicted upon them, in the course of the 'battered baby syndrome', and among these injuries may be burns. Thus small rounded burns of about $\frac{1}{4}$ inch diameter may be seen, caused by lighted cigarettes; and Professor Alan Usher has

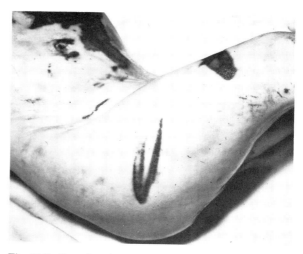

Fig. 12.2. Burn from heated knife blade (on child). Courtesy of Professor Alan Usher.

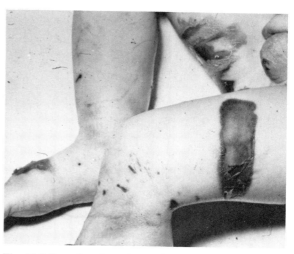

Fig. 12.3 Burn from heated knife blade (on child). Courtesy Professor Alan Usher.

described how a child was injured by its father, who heated a knife blade in the fire and repeatedly pressed it against the child's body, producing characteristically shaped burns (Figs 12.2 and 12.3). In the department at Leeds University an example was seen of a child who had symmetrical burns of both buttocks, caused by being very forcibly sat on top of a hot stove. Circumstances such as these make it imperative that doctors seeing burns on living persons, especially where the injuries have recognisable shapes, should make careful measurements and records, just as with other types of injuries.

Microscopical appearances

At degrees of burning short of actual charring, the effect of the heat on the tissues is to fix them by coagulation of proteins, so that the cell outlines become indistinct and the tissues take up histological stains more intensely.

In the skin, heat causes separation of the epidermis from the dermis, to form blisters, with dilatation of blood vessels in the floor of the blisters. A typical inflammatory reaction with polymorphonuclear leucocyte infiltration occurs in the dermis, within a few hours. Sometimes the epidermis becomes coagulated, thinned and deeply staining. On other occasions, in the process of blister formation, the cells in the deeper layers of the epidermis, adjacent to areas of complete separation of epidermis from dermis, become elongated, with their long axes tending to be orientated more at right angles to the skin surface, closely resembling the 'streaming' of epithelial cells described by Jellinek[14] as a feature of the histology of the electric mark (see below). It seems possible that even in the case of damage caused by electricity, the causative agent is heat.

When epithelial tissues in the interior of the body, notably the lining of the air passages, are exposed to heat, the cells are liable first to become swollen, pale and ballooned (Fig. 12.4). However, they are then relatively rapidly shed into the lumen of the viscus. Thus the smaller peripheral air passages are liable to become choked by a mass of desquamated epithelial cells, mucus and carbon particles (Figs 12.5–12.8). The histological features

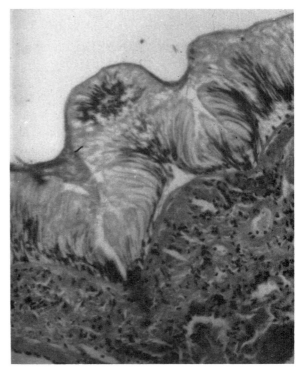

Fig. 12.4 Effect of exposure of bronchial mucosa to hot gases.

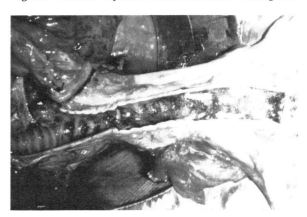

Fig. 12.5 Inhaled soot lining trachea.

of burns have been fully described by Sevitt,[15] and recently reviewed by Pullar.[16]

The age of burns can be determined only in very general terms from a naked eye examination of the injuries. Epithelialisation of the surface takes place in the same way as with other injuries but is liable to be delayed due to infection of the surface, and if the injury extends to the full thickness of the

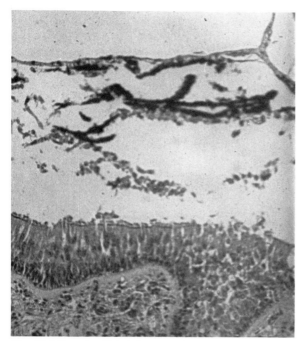

Fig. 12.6 Strands of inhaled soot coating tracheal mucosa.

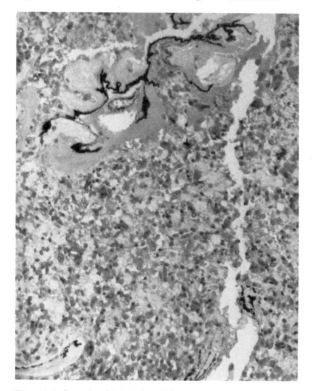

Fig. 12.7 Strands of inhaled soot in air passages.

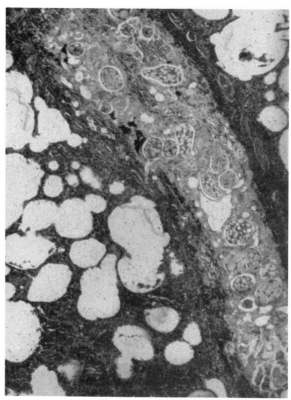

Fig. 12.8 Soot and inhaled stomach contents in air passage of victim of death from inhaling smoke.

skin, or beyond, scarring is liable to be severe. Winter[17] has shown, in pigs, that experimental scalds are completely epithelialised by the 15th day. He comments that tissue regeneration is long delayed. No epithelial regeneration takes place for 8–10 days after infliction of the injury. After this lag phase epidermal cells spread from the edges of the lesion, and the remaining intact hair follicles, to repair the skin loss. After full thickness skin burns scarring is likely; malignant change in the scar may follow.[15]

Ante-mortem and post-mortem burns

It is obvious that the surface of a human body may be burnt, whether or not the person is alive at the time. But determination of whether the burns were sustained before or after death may have considerable medico-legal importance, and it is fortunate that the distinction is usually not difficult, provided that all the skin has not been destroyed. In the intact skin adjacent to a burn, there will normally be a well-marked 'vital reaction', in the form of a reddening of the skin bordering the burn, when the injury was sustained in life. This zone of vital reaction is normally about a ¼ inch in width, although it may be broader where several burns are in close proximity, and, taken in conjunction with the internal findings of the presence of life during the fire, such as soot in the air passages, usually admits of little doubt that the burns were sustained before death.

Blisters of the skin are usually burst and collapsed by the time that the body is examined in the post-mortem room, but if they remain intact, the contained fluid can be examined for the presence of albumen, which is held to be evidence that the blister was caused in life. The 'Albustix' strips supplied by Ames Ltd. make a convenient method of testing. Obviously, for this test to give a positive result there must have been an early inflammatory reaction to the extent of dilatation of blood vessels and exudation of plasma into the tissues. Burns sustained very shortly after death may be indistinguishable, though according to Gonzales et al.[18] any blisters formed will contain no albumen.

Histological methods of distinguishing ante-mortem and post-mortem burns have been described by Mallik[19] using burns inflicted experimentally on guinea pigs, burns of human skin obtained from autopsy examinations, and burns inflicted experimentally on amputated human tissues. The burns were examined by conventional histological and by histochemical techniques. He found that reactions could be detected earlier in the guinea pigs than in humans. In the case of human burns, the earliest histological change in ante-mortem burns was leucocyte infiltration at 6 h after burning. Staining reactions for DNA and RNA, at the margins of the burnt area, increased at the same time, as did the staining reaction for the enzyme alkaline phosphatase. An increase in the reaction for acid phosphatase was detected at 3 h; for leucine aminopeptidase at 2 h and for non-specific esterase at ¾ h.

The histochemical reactions were unaffected by topical surgical dressings, by position on the body, or by a lapse of time between death and post-mortem examination of up to 72 h.

Raekallio[20] has reviewed the application of histo-chemical methods to burns, but states that no reports have been published on any extensive work on human material.

Burns as a cause of death

Death due to burning is a not uncommon event. Thus, in 1971 there were 694 deaths from accidents caused by fires and flames, according to the Registrar General's Statistical Review,[21] 514 deaths being specifically ascribed to burns.

Death may occur at once, or be delayed for days or weeks. The fact that it is a consequence of the burns may be obvious, but the actual cause of death is rarely a direct result of the position and depth of an individual burn, as is the case with other injuries; the cause is more likely to be a remote effect on the body as a whole, and hence it may sometimes be difficult to determine.

The likelihood of a fatal outcome is especially influenced by the age of the victim, the total area of the body affected, and the depth of the burns.

It has been suggested that an index of probable mortality can be obtained by dividing the extent of superficial burns of the body in percentage area by four, and adding the extent of whole thickness skin loss also as a percentage of body surface. Then 35% is taken to be the point where the chances of dying equal those of surviving.[22]

An extensive review of the causes of death after burning has been given by Sevitt.[23] In an analysis of the autopsy findings in 156 persons who died after being burnt, he found that 27 persons died from coincident natural disease. Non-bacterial complications occurred in 91 cases and caused death in 37% of the total. Among such complications he described early shock, respiratory damage (including carbon monoxide poisoning), renal failure, hypokalaemia, pulmonary embolism and acute cardiac failure. The early shock is principally due to loss of fluid from the burned surfaces, resulting in oligaemia and haemoconcentration. There is also often an acute anaemia due to damage to erythrocytes in the burns, to stasis and to internal blood loss.

Among the respiratory effects a characteristic feature may be congestive atalectasis, massive collapse of both lungs resulting in purple airless tissue as seen at autopsy. Sevitt divides his cases of acute renal failure into oliguric and non-oliguric, and says that the determining feature is a gross fall in glomerular filtration rate, rathe. than renal tubular necrosis, although the latter may be present.

Among the bacterial causes of death, which accounted for 63% of his series, were 60 cases of septicaemia and 34 cases of bronchopneumonia. The bacteria were of the same type as those colonising the burns, in most cases. Where infection was by *Pseudomonas pyocyanea*, spread to unburnt skin with ulceration may occur, and internal infection by this organism is especially liable to damage the walls of blood vessels. Gram-negative shock may also occur.

A less common but important complication of burns is the occurrence of duodenal ulcers. Also known as Curling's ulcers. They may occur in association with other conditions, such as brain injuries.[24] Gastric ulcers may also occur, which, it has been suggested, should be called Dupytren's ulcers.[25] These gastric ulcers may occur within a day of burning, but duodenal ulcers never do.[23] There may be bacterial or fungal colonies in the floors of the ulcers, and erosion of large blood vessels, occasionally leading to fatal haemorrhage. Sevitt describes the incidence of duodenal ulceration after burning as being approximately 9%. The manner in which these ulcers are produced by the burns is not known. Various theories, such as local ischaemia, infection, and the effects of stress on adrenocortical function have been suggested.

Circumstances of death from burning

Although the forensic pathologist may on occasion be called upon to make an autopsy examination of the body of a person who has died in hospital several days after sustaining burns, this is only likely if the burns were sustained as a result of some criminal act on the part of another person, or the deceased. More commonly the medico-legal expert will have to examine a body found dead at a scene of conflagration and then his principal duty, apart from establishing identity of the deceased, will be to ascertain whether he was alive in the fire, and died as a result of it, or whether he was already dead when the fire started. In the former case the cause of death will be either immediate shock from the burns, or asphyxiation from the effects of

inhaling fumes. In the latter event, when the deceased's death was not due to the fire, causes of death may range from natural disease, possibly causing a fall and so precipitating the fire, to injuries sustained during a homicidal attack, with attempted subsequent disposal of the body by arson. The pathologist's other duty will be, from the distribution of burns and other features at the scene of conflagration, to reconstruct the circumstances of the death.

The great majority of fatal burnings occur accidentally when the victims are trapped in burning buildings or vehicles. The increase in very large buildings housing many people, either as office workers or occupants of hotels, has resulted, in some other countries, in spectacular fires with heavy loss of life. Even the use of very large aircraft has contributed to the increase in accidental burnings, since a frequent cause of death in major aircraft disasters is burning, when the crashed aircraft catches fire. However, in accidents involving only one person those most often involved are children and the elderly. In an attempt to reduce the incidence of burns to children the Nightdresses (Safety) Regulations 1967,[26] made under the Consumer Protection Act 1961 were introduced, making it illegal to sell children's nightdresses unless they comply with specifications, or are marked as inflammable, though it is still possible for clothing to be prepared from inflammable materials at home of course. Also under the Children and Young Persons Act 1933 and 1952, it is an offence for a person over 16 years to have a child under 12 years in a room with an unguarded fire.

The elderly person is liable to allow clothing to brush against fires, like children, or to drop lighted matches, to fall asleep while smoking a cigarette which drops on to the bed or chair, or to have badly maintained houses with faulty heating appliances or electrical wiring. The vulnerability of these two groups is reflected in the Registrar General's figures for 1971;[21] of 694 deaths due to accidental burning, 250 were under the age of 14, and 364 over the age of 65. Another group of people at risk from accidental burns are drunks, who are, of course, prone to accidents of all kinds.

Suicide by burning is distinctly uncommon, though not unknown, and recently has become rather fashionable as a means of indicating political dissent, for instance in the case of self-immolation of protestors in Hungary and the Far East. In this country it is often achieved by the intended suicide setting alight to himself inside a motor car, after pouring petrol over his clothes. In one such case seen recently by the author the deceased had driven his van down an infrequently used cart track and had evidently then syphoned petrol out of the tank to pour over himself and over the interior of the van. When the scene was examined the pipe used to syphon the petrol had been burnt through, but one end was found in the tank, while the other lay on the ground beneath the filler pipe of the tank (F.M. 17528A).

On another occasion a young man, suffering from schizophrenia, who lived at home with his parents went downstairs in the middle of the night into a bathroom and, after soaking his clothes with paraffin, set fire to himself (F.M. 18302).

Yet another youth soaked himself in petrol and set himself alight in the garden of his house early one morning (F.M. 18574).

Homicidal burning has always been very rare, and scalding is more likely, since boiling liquid is relatively easy to throw at a victim. Recently, however, the practice of setting fire to an enemy's house has increased in some parts of this country, as has the use of petrol bombs. It is not uncommon for people to be burnt to death in the houses thus ignited, and their deaths will then, of course, become the subject of a charge of murder or manslaughter. For instance, the author has recently seen eight such deaths in two households in the course of two years in one town. It seems quite possible that this type of death may become more common.

The examination of the burnt body

External examination

Occasionally a body removed from a burnt building will be completely uninjured by heat, the cause of death then proving to be inhalation of fumes. However, usually the body is burnt, often very extensively so. Sometimes the body has been removed from the room in which it was found, and from the building by the firemen before the pathologist arrives, but if it remains in situ an examination of the scene must be attempted, as with any other scene of suspicious death, note being taken of the position of the body, of any remaining clothing, of any identifiable objects in the room, and so on. For instance, in one case the deceased had been found in his bedsitting room, collapsed over an electric fire, with severe burns. His body had been dragged from the room on to the landing by neighbours who had attempted to rescue him and was first seen in that position by the police and pathologist. However, within the room, burn marks on the carpet indicated that the deceased had probably been seated in an armchair before falling on to the floor and lying against the electric fire. On a table near to the chair was an empty glass which had contained alcohol, and on the floor beneath the chair, and in a drawer of a cabinet in front of the chair were tablets, and bottles containing tablets. The autopsy confirmed that the deceased had consumed an overdose of the tablets and that the burns had only played a relatively minor part in his death (F.M. 17,664A).

The examination of the burns themselves is directed to ascertaining their position and depth, whether they were sustained in life or not, and whether their situation gives any indication of the path taken by the flames, or the position of the body when the fire started. Thus, a man who sat in a car and poured petrol over himself before lighting it was badly burnt over the thighs, front of chest, face and hands, but much less severely damaged elsewhere (F.M. 6893A).

If the body is very severely burnt then all the skin surface may be destroyed, making it impossible from external examination alone to ascertain whether there is any vital reaction to the burns. However, if undamaged skin remains adjacent to the burns, then the appearance of vital reaction should be identifiable as bands of reddening bordering the burns. The appearance of burns caused after death is usually quite distinctive, with an absence of the red margins, and with dried scorching of the skin surface, like burnt paper.

A woman's body was placed in a hospital mortuary overnight after she had died from pneumonia. During the night an intruder broke into the chapel, disarranged the body and set fire to the shroud in which it was wrapped. The resultant burns were superficial, yellowish-black in colour and without any trace of reddening of the skin in relation to them (F.M. 14297A) (Fig. 12.9).

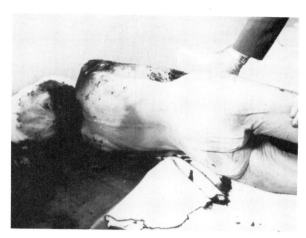

Fig. 12.9 Post-mortem burns—no vital reaction at burn margin.

A body that is badly burnt will almost always assume the appearance known as the 'pugilistic attitude'. This is due to heat stiffening and contraction of the muscles, causing the arms to become flexed at the elbows, and the hands clenched, the head slightly extended and the knees bent. The appearance resembles the position adopted by a person engaged in a fight, and has led on occasion to suspicion that death has occurred during some violent crime. In fact, of course, the body will assume this position whether the deceased was alive when the fire started or not (Fig. 12.10).

In badly burnt parts of the body 'heat ruptures' may be produced. These are splits of the skin, caused by contraction of the heated and coagulated tissues, and the resultant breaches look like lacer-

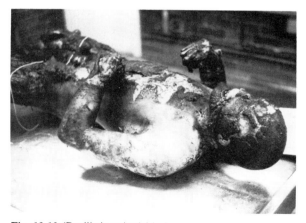

Fig. 12.10 'Pugilistic attitude' in burns.

ated wounds. They are usually only a few inches, but may be up to 1 or 2 ft in length. Normally they lead to no difficulty in interpretation, since they only occur in areas of severe burning, and normally over fleshy areas of the body, like calves and thighs, where lacerations are uncommon. However, when they occur in the scalp they may cause greater difficulties. They can usually be distinguished from wounds inflicted before the body was burnt, by their appearance, position in areas of maximum burning, and on fleshy areas, and by the associated findings on internal examination (Fig. 12.11).

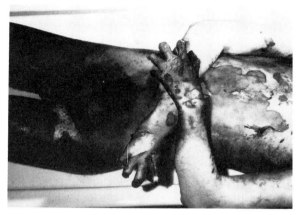

Fig. 12.11 Heat contractures of hands and heat rupture of thigh.

Internal examination

Even when the body appears externally to be very badly burnt, the damage rarely extends beyond the superficial tissues directly beneath the skin. The outermost muscles are coagulated by the heat, and appear rather pallid, though the deeper muscles may have a rich pink hue if the blood contains a high proportion of carboxyhaemoglobin, derived from the fumes. Internal organs, such as the liver and lungs may be coagulated, firm and pallid, and occasionally the body cavities may be opened by partial destruction of their walls, in which hollow organs, like stomach and intestines, may be ruptured. Obviously all these effects may occur, whether the victim was alive or dead during the fire.

The only tissues which yield reliable proof of life of the deceased at the time when the fire commenced, are the air passages and the blood. In most victims of fires in buildings, where there is a considerable production of smoke, the tongue, fauces, larynx and trachea are inflamed, and co-ated by a layer of soot embedded in a film of mucus. If the deceased has inhaled very hot gas or actual flame the mucosa over the tongue and larynx may be blistered or shredded, and the larynx oedematous. Not uncommonly the victim who inhales smoke also vomits and inhales some vomit, presumably due to bouts of coughing, and plugs of regurgitated stomach contents mixed with soot may be found in the smaller bronchi, in the depths of the lungs.

Together with the soot, the smoke which is inhaled usually contains much carbon monoxide, which is absorbed by the blood. The presence of carboxyhaemoglobin is often obvious from the bright pink hue of the blood, the muscles, and even the cut surfaces of the organs. In younger victims of fires, in particular, it may reach high concentrations, even up to 80%, but older persons may only have relatively small amounts present.[27] At all events it is very unwise to rely solely on naked eye impressions of the colour of the tissues from the autopsy; they should be supplemented at least by a spectroscopic examination of the blood by a reversion spectroscope, if not by chemical analysis, such as diffusion into palladium chloride, analysis by the method of Whitehead & Worthington,[28] or by ultraviolet spectroscopy.

Such analyses are important because not only is knowledge of the actual concentration of carboxy-haemoglobin of value in elucidating the circum-stances of the fire, but also because visual impressions at autopsy may be deceptive. The lighting in many mortuaries is liable to give a mis-leading pinkish cast to the tissues when exposed at the autopsy; and some victims of fires, especially of petrol fires, where there is intense heat, may have pulmonary oedema with blood-stained froth of a pronounced pinkish hue exuding from the nos-trils. This gives an impression of a large quantity of carbon monoxide in the fluid, when in fact there is usually none. On occasions death may occur from inhaling hot gases, without any carbon mon-oxide being absorbed into the blood.[29]

Another chemical which may be found in the fumes from a conflagration, especially if substances such as lacquered wood have been burnt, is cya-nide, and it has been shown[30] that fire victims can have quite high levels of cyanide in their blood. In estimating this substance it is important to ensure that the samples analysed are fresh, bearing in mind that cyanide is produced in large quantities in blood stored for some days before analysis, even when refrigerated.[31] Various studies have indicated other toxic products of combustion which can be inhaled.[31–35]

It may be of great assistance, when autopsy reveals internal injuries or haemorrhages, to ascer-tain the quantity of carbon monoxide in the blood composing the haemorrhage or surrounding the injury, and compare that to the circulating blood, in order to elicit the circumstances of the death.

Thus one elderly man was found dead in a badly burnt room, where the source of the fire appeared to be an overturned paraffin heater. Autopsy revealed a massive subarachnoid haemorrhage from a ruptured 'berry' aneurysm. The blood in the general circulation contained 70% carboxyhaemoglobin, while the blood in the subarachnoid haemorrhage contained none. Clearly the sequence of events was spontaneous rupture of the aneurysm, causing collapse, with, in consequence, overturning of the paraffin heater, and a resultant fire.[31]

The estimation of carboxyhaemoglobin in the blood may also be of value in eliciting the circum-stances, when a 'heat haematoma' is revealed by the autopsy. Such a haemorrhage is an artefact, caused by the effect of heat on the skull. It occurs in the extradural space, in cases where the head is exten-sively damaged by fire, and is maximal in amount opposite the site of greatest external damage to the skull. Thus the haemorrhage is often symmetrical and frontal, or occipital, in a position unlike a trau-matic extradural haemorrhage. The blood in the haemorrhage is usually chocolate brown in colour, and the mass contains tiny rounded spaces, like 'Aero' chocolate. The presence of carbon monoxide in the blood serves to confirm the conclusion that the haemorrhage is a heat artefact, and not a fatal injury occurring before the fire. The skull is not usually fractured in relation to the haemorrhage, though the heat may be so great as to burn away part of the bone.

Burning in special circumstances

The development of some new furnishing materials, and some engineering procedures, have recently resulted in unusual hazards of conflagration, which may produce distinctive appearances at the medico-legal autopsy.

Many soft furnishings are nowadays fitted with padding made of expanded polyurethane foam plastic. This material will ignite relatively easily, and then burns very violently indeed. It has been reported[38] that in a fire in a factory in which polyurethane foam was a combustible agent, the fire spread so rapidly and the heat was so intense that many persons were injured. It has been suggested that air preceding the flames may be sufficiently hot to ignite the hair and clothes of fleeing persons.

There have been several tragedies in domestic circumstances, when this material has been involved. In the author's recent experience, three children died in one house, apparently when one of them, while playing, set fire to some furniture. The heat appears to have been so intense that it stripped the plaster from the inside of the room, leaving the brickwork bare, in the space of a few minutes. One child, probably the one causing the fire, appears to have fled to the adjacent kitchen where its grossly burnt body was found crouched in a narrow space between a cooker and the wall. Two other children upstairs died from carbon monoxide poisoning, and the path of hot air could be followed up the stairs, and through the door of their bedroom, exiting through a shattered bedroom window (F.M. 17648 A, B &C).

On another occasion a group of children were playing with a petrol can in an outbuilding containing many fragments of polyurethane foam from discarded furniture. The petrol was ignited, then spilled, and the polyurethane caught fire. The dead child was trapped in the building, and though the fire was extinguished and the body was recovered quickly, it was very badly burnt, with fragments of partly melted plastic foam adhering to the body surface (F.M. 18257A). The principal post-mortem feature is the very intense degree of burning, compared with the period during which the fire was known to be alight. Thus soft tissues are consumed and bone, such as the skull, exposed in a very short time.

The intensity of the fire is such that significant quantities of carbon monoxide are not produced at the seat of the fire, or else the victims do not have

time to inhale any, but die very rapidly from the effects of the heat and lack of oxygen. At all events the bodies of those recovered from the seats of such fires do not seem to have any significant quantities of carbon monoxide in their blood, though other persons dying elsewhere in the building, away from the main seat of the fire, may have inhaled substantial amounts of carbon monoxide. Cyanide may also be detected in the blood, derived from thiocyanates in the plastic.

Another unusual but distinctive variety of rapid intense fire is that occurring in an oxygen enriched atmosphere. The situation was drawn to the world's attention in a dramatic fashion in 1967 when three American astronauts died very rapidly after a fire developed in the space capsule in which they were training. The rapidity of the spread of fire, and of their deaths, was attributed to the oxygen enriched atmosphere within the space craft.

Similar situations occur from time to time in engineering practice when welders are working inside large metal drums, which are almost enclosed, if oxygen is introduced into the drum. On one such occasion a man, welding inside a drum which was almost enclosed save for an entrance hold about 18 inches in diameter, was purging the fumes from the welding operation by using the oxygen line from an oxyacetylene cutting plant. His workmates suddenly noted smoke coming from the drum. When the victim was retrieved, he was dead, suffering from very extensive but superficial burns. The flames had apparently 'flashed over' the surface of his clothing and body. There were extensive 1st degree burns over most of the body surface and his scalp hair was burnt off but body hair was undamaged, presumably being protected by clothing. The appearance suggested that his clothing had become saturated in oxygen and had then become highly inflammable.[39] A closely similar occurrence was noted by Corbett (personal communication 1974) in which another man, also welding inside a metal drum, was fatally burned. Eye-witnesses disagreed as to whether an oxygen line was connected to the tank at the time, but the result makes this appear to be probable. The body was extensively burnt with large heat ruptures of the limbs, but it was notable that there was no formation of a heat haematoma within the skull.

Experiments have been carried out to determine the danger of fires in oxygen enriched atmospheres by Denison and his colleagues.[40, 41] They found that human skin and flesh are almost non-inflammable in air at normal pressure, and in pure oxygen ignite with difficulty, although they may then burn vigorously. However, body hair is highly inflammable in oxygen, and so is the pile of materials such as denim, velvet and brushed nylon, where in atmospheres rich in oxygen the pile propagates the fire, and in very high concentrations of oxygen this has the effect of a very rapid flash fire. They studied the effect on experimental models, and showed that in high concentrations of oxygen a man wearing denims would inevitably suffer 3rd degree burns of at least half his body surface before he could take preventive action. For full details the original articles should be consulted.

'Spontaneous' or 'preternatural' combustion

Compared to many other materials, relatively little is known about the combustibility of human skin and other tissues. Denison found that skin was relatively non-flammable but that human hair was readily flammable in air, as well as oxygen. Sevitt[15] reports studies into heat conduction of skin structures. However no experiments have been conducted recently to discover the relative flammability of the various tissues. In the previous editions of Taylor's *Medical Jurisprudence*, it was stated:

Dry animal solids readily burn, but the soft parts, either in the living or recently dead body, contain as much as 72 per cent of water, which renders them highly incombustible. Until a large proportion of this water is evaporated, the substance does not undergo combustion. In many experiments made on different organs and on different bodies, the author has not observed that different parts of the same body or the parts of different bodies have varied in their degree of combustibility. The bones alone have withstood a greater degree of heat, from the large proportion of earthy matter contained in them. The experiments have led to this result— the flesh and the organs generally are very difficult of combustion and can be completely consumed only in a strong fire and under a powerful arrest of air. Experiments on the bodies of animals have shown that they possess the same property of difficult combustibility. The presence of alcohol in flesh does not render it combustible. The alcohol will burn, but the flesh can only be burned by removing from it the substance which interferes with its combustibility—namely water. Tissues which have undergone extensive fatty degeneration may, nevertheless, become unusually combustible, so as to burn readily on the application of the moderate heat of a spirit lamp.

Against this background of the recognition of the relative non-inflammability of human bodies the occasional case of an apparently very combustible body which has been almost completely consumed in a short space of time, with only a small source of heat and with scarcely any damage to surrounding objects in the room, is particularly striking. Such cases, in the past, were often regarded as manifestations of supernatural intervention, and, within the last century or two, as being associated with alcoholism; presumably the accumulation of alcohol in the tissues was thought to increase their combustibility. Thurston[42] gives an extensive review of the historical features of this condition, and describes a case, and other cases have been reported recently.[39, 43]

The victim is usually an elderly woman, whose body is found lying near a fireplace, grossly incinerated. Often all soft tissues are reduced to ash and most of the bones are calcined. The only part of the body left undamaged, in the author's experience, is likely to be one or both of the lower legs, and between these and the rest of the body there is often a hole in the floor where the floorboards have been burnt through. Usually analysis of the blood remaining in a leg reveals no carbon monoxide, though in one case of the author's a high level was found apparently due to carbon monoxide poisoning prior to the collapse and death, due to a leaking gas poker. The room in which the body is discovered is frequently very hot and the contents, walls, furniture, etc., are heavily soiled by soot, but there is no fire-damage to any of the objects in the room, even to fabrics like tea-towels which may be hanging close to the body.

The overall, bizarre picture is of a body which has been almost totally consumed by fire, in a room, full of inflammable objects which are undamaged. Investigating police officers are often drawn to the initial conclusion that the body has been deliberately destroyed by some person using an accelerant, such as paraffin.

However, experiments have shown that human body fat, when melted, can soak into fabric which will then act as a wick. A temperature of about 250°C is necessary to melt the fat, but once liquid, it will soak into cloth and burn like a wick in a lamp, even when the temperature of the fat has fallen as low as 24°C.

It seems then that the probable course of events in these cases is that the victim collapses, for instance from a heart attack, or from carbon monoxide poisoning, and falls so that part of the body comes into contact with a source of heat, such as a small domestic fire. This part of the body, usually the head, is thus ignited, and adjacent body fat, when melted, soaks into the layers of clothing, which, the victim being an old lady, are likely to be present in abundance. The clothing, acting as a wick, melts the next zone of adjacent fat, and the process is repeated along the length of the body. If floorboards beneath the body are ignited, they will be burnt through, and the sudden increase in draught which results will considerably raise the temperature and incinerate the rest of the body. By the time the lower legs are reached there is less fat, and few if any layers of clothing, so the process ceases. The late Dr Firth, of the Home Office Forensic Science Laboratories, called this the 'candle effect'.

Duration of burning

The forensic pathologist may quite often, as part of a team investigating a fatal burning, be asked for how long a period the burning of the body continued. Thus on one occasion the extent of damage to a room caused forensic science experts to conclude that the fire must have been burning for 1 to 2 h before it was discovered and extinguished. However, those discovering the fire were sure that they heard the occupant of the room cry out only a few minutes before the fire was extinguished and the room entered. The occupant's body was found, near the window, very badly burnt, with features destroyed and abdominal wall burnt away. On this occasion it seemed very unlikely that such extensive damage could have been caused in a short space of time (F.M. 18603A).

However, there is no reliable method of determining the time that has passed during burning, and any opinion given must be very guarded. Obviously the intensity of the fire must be taken into consideration; the more intense the conflagration, as in petrol or polyurethane fires, the more rapidly will the body be consumed. But in a burnt building it is often not possible to determine with any accuracy the intensity of the fire at a particular point for a given length of time. Other factors to be considered may be the amount and type of clothing, obesity of the body, and so on. Even then, an opinion can only be based on the observer's personal experience; there are no universally applicable criteria on which he can base his estimate. Some possible criteria have been suggested by Richards.[44]

The author has no personal experience of a criminal case in which the length of time taken to burn the body was a material point, but in the previous edition of this book such a case was described, in *R. v. Hatto.* Bucks Assize, 1854.

The victim was found dead in her room, her body much burned. She was last known to be living at about a quarter past eight in the evening, and her body was found, still smouldering with fire, on the floor of the room, at about a quarter past eleven. The only persons known to have been in the house were the prisoner and the deceased. The doctor who examined the deceased found that 'both knees were consumed by fire, and the thighs, as well as the private parts, were burnt to a cinder, leaving the shafts of the thigh-bones exposed and charred for several inches. Between the thighs and the feet, the floor underneath had been burnt away, and the leg bones had fallen through the floor, leaving the feet unburnt on the floor'. He expressed an opinion that it would take from two and a half to three hours in order to consume the body to this degree, thus covering the whole interval during which deceased and prisoner were in the house together. The clothing of the deceased was much burned, and beneath the body there was a hempen mat which became highly combustible, owing to the melted human fat with which it was impregnated. Guilt was fortunately established from other circumstances.

It is obvious that an opinion on such a subject must be to some extent conjectural, since the effects depend as much on the intensity as on the duration of the heat. With a more intense flame, the amount of burning met with in R. V. Hatto might have been produced in an hour as in three hours. A confession by the prisoner, made subsequently, showed that the burning must have taken place in $1\frac{1}{2}$ to 2 hours.

Concealment of crime by arson

If a murderer attempts to conceal or destroy the body of his victim, fire is one very convenient agent. It avoids the necessity of removing the body any distance, it can be performed with little preparation, and the subsequent discovery of a dead body at the scene of the fire can be expected to lead to the presumption of death from burning.

It is fortunate then that fire is in fact an inefficient means of removing evidence of a crime. Unless the body is carefully incinerated, a procedure hardly possible if the murderer is to leave the scene of the fire in time to avoid detection, evidence of wounds, fractures, etc., are normally unaffected. The only mode of killing which might be obscured is mechanical asphyxia, such as strangulation.

Two such cases have been seen recently in the department at Leeds.

In one case an old lady's body was found in a fire-damaged room in a house, partially covered by debris. Suspicion was aroused initially by evidence of drawers in other rooms having been ransacked, and the gas meter having been broken into. The post-mortem examination showed multiple head injuries, which proved to have been produced with a poker. There was no soot in the air passages, no carbon monoxide in the blood, and no vital reaction to the burns. The persons responsible were a young couple whom the old lady had befriended and to whom she had lent money on previous occasions (post-mortem by Dr Harbison) (F.M. 13664A).

In another case a middle-aged woman's body was found lying on the floor of her sitting room. Attempts had been made to burn the body by igniting cushions placed against it, but only part of the body was damaged, and evidence of strangulation and of sexual interference remained clearly visible. The assailant was suffering from mental illness (post-mortem by Dr Green) (F.M. 15975A).

The most famous case was that of *R. v. Rouse*, in which the accused apparently stunned his victim, who was seated inside a motor car with blows with a mallet, and then set fire to the vehicle. Sir Bernard Spilsbury found carbon monoxide in the blood, indicating that the deceased had remained alive for a short time after the fire started.

Part of the deceased's clothing in the last case smelt of petrol, and in all such investigations it is important to preserve any fragments of clothing or other material near the body, which could have been contaminated by an accelerant such as petrol or paraffin, for examination by forensic scientists. Gas chromatography may be expected to indicate the nature of the substance.

When injuries are found in a burnt body it is important to differentiate between artefacts caused by heat, such as heat ruptures or heat haematomas described above, and injuries caused in life. Unless the body is severely burnt this should not give rise to much difficulty, but in a badly charred corpse the differentiation may be less easy, and recourse is likely to be needed to microscopical examination, for signs of bleeding or inflammation. The pathologist must beware of accepting evidence of fat embolism as proof that the injuries were produced before the body was burnt, since burns can themselves produce fat embolism. Sevitt[45] says that post-mortem heating of the body and post-mortem burns may liberate droplets of fat into the blood; but these are not crowded and deformed within capillaries like many true pulmonary fat emboli. He points out that slight fat embolism in the lungs is common in patients who die after burns. However if the embolism is more than slight, then it is likely that some other injury preceded death.

Identification of burnt bodies

This problem frequently arises, as the features of burnt bodies are likely to be destroyed. The principles of identification in such cases may be found in chapter 7. The investigator must not overlook portions of clothing or other articles near or on the body. Thus on one occasion a human body was found in a burnt out farm building, and was grossly damaged so as to be unrecognisable. However, a small piece of relatively undamaged shirt was found, wedged in a fold of skin at the back of the neck which had been produced by heat contraction causing extension of the head. The fragment bore a laundry mark by which the body was identified as a boy who had absconded from a special school (F.M. 12678A).

Even on the most badly charred body, fragments of clothing may be found protected in folds of skin or in the flexures of armpits and groins; or traces of jewellery may be found. Unless there is distinctive dental work in the mouth, such extraneous material may be the only means of proving identity, but it can be easily lost or destroyed in careless handling of the body. It is particularly important that relatively protected regions of the body, such as axillae, should be examined, and that any apparent cinders adhering to the body surface, or lying on the mortuary table, should be scrutinised carefully before being discarded.

This is one area of investigation in which the provision of X-ray facilities in the mortuary is especially valuable. In a badly charred body demonstration of old bone deformities, or comparison of X-rays of the corpse with X-rays taken some time previously in hospital, may establish identity, and the presence of foreign bodies, such as bullets, within the body may be demonstrated.

In a body whose face is badly charred by fire, the front teeth, if present, may have partially or completely disintegrated, apparently due to expansion of gas in the pulp spaces. However, those teeth which are situated further back in the jaws, the premolars and molars, will be protected by the soft tissue of the cheeks, and can usually be easily examined, provided that the contracted and coagulated tissue of the cheeks is incised. It is also often necessary to divide the rami of the mandible, so that the mouth can be fully opened, exposing the teeth to visual examination or photography (for further details see ch. 10).

Scalds

As is the case with burns, scalds or injuries caused by hot liquids are usually caused accidentally, and are most likely to affect children and the elderly.

They only affect the superficial layers, of the skin, unless the body is literally 'boiled', and are distinguished from burns by this uniform superficial appearance, with reddening and blistering of the skin, and with an absence of singeing of hairs in the affected areas; also by the shape of the injuries, which may suggest the trickling movement of a liquid. A greater depth of injury can be achieved by such liquids as hot oil or molten metals, which may be many times hotter than boiling water.

It is necessary sometimes to distinguish scalds from skin lesions due to natural disease. Thus toxic epidermal necrolysis, due to disease or drugs, causes blistering and separation of the superficial layers of the skin, leaving a raw weeping surface closely similar, in appearance, to a scald. The variety of this condition known as Lyell's disease, has been specifically cited as a differential diagnosis of scalds.[46]

It is particularly important to bear the distinction in mind when dealing with a possible case of deliberate scalding, as a criminal act. Boiling water, being an easier substance to manipulate than flame, is sometimes used as a weapon; for instance by a jealous wife against her husband. Or a child may be scalded by a parent. Thus, on one occasion, a

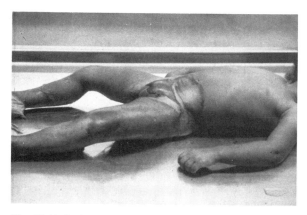

Fig. 12.12 Accidental scalds from bath.

mother, who was a schizophrenic, during an episode of delusion, poured boiling water from a kettle over both her young daughters, aged three years and 18 months, while they were in a bath. They were admitted to hospital as cases of accidental scalding, and it was only after the death of the first from oligaemic shock, that the circumstances became known to the police (F.M. 8634A and B).

In such cases it may be necessary to recognise the pattern of the scalds, distinguishing between an accidental and a homicidal explanation. A child who is placed in a bath of water which is at too high a temperature may be expected to have scalds of the legs and the lower abdomen ending in a line around the waist, or extending up the back (Fig. 12.12). In the case of boiling water poured on to a child cited above (F.M. 8634A) there were scalds, reproducing trickle marks, across the neck and down the arms and trunk, consistent with the water having been poured on to the back of the head. Instead of a uniform scalding of the legs there were many small scalds irregularly distributed, evidently produced as splashes.

Although superficial, scalds can be just as dangerous to life as can burns. Shock, infection, Curling's ulcers, etc., can all occur in the same manner as with burns. However, if survived, scalds are less likely to result in severe scarring.

Chemical burns

Many chemical substances can cause damage to the skin, or even deeper tissues, resembling burns, though in most cases the damage is not caused by heat.

An exception is sulphuric acid, where the combination of the chemical with water from the tissues generates a considerable amount of heat, and the resulting damage is due, in part at least, to this heat.

The other corrosive substances, mineral acids and the caustic alkalis, such as sodium and potassium hydroxide, will also damage the skin, to produce full thickness lesions in many cases. Phenol produces dark brown, leathery lesions, which are painless because of the destruction of nerve endings, and damage to the skin by phenol is especially dangerous, as the chemical is absorbed, affects the central nervous system and can readily cause fatal depression of respiration. In children, other phenol substances, such as cresol, may also damage the skin. Hydrofluoric acid can produce severe burns, and the alkyl halides, in particular methyl bromide, can produce insidious but severe lesions. The latter substance, used in fire extinguishers and in horticulture, is especially dangerous in that it passes through leather, plastics and most materials without hindrance, so that if, for instance, it is poured on to boots, it can penetrate to and burn the feet.[47]

Petrol can cause blistering and reddening of the skin. Other substances which can also cause skin damage include phosphorus, mustard gas and other variants produced for military use, and sodium hypochlorite.

Effects of radiation

Various kinds of radiation can produce tissue damage. The effect of ultraviolet radiation in the form of sunburn is well-known, and in a severe form, as when Europeans visit tropical areas for the first time, can be very disabling, and even dangerous. Damage to the retina can cause blindness.

Atomic explosions generate very great amounts of heat, so that many of the victims of the atomic bombs suffered severe burns. However, atomic radiation, in addition to its other deeper effects, on blood forming organs, etc., can produce penetrating and devitalising skin lesions, resembling deep burns, and there may be malignant change in the damaged area in due course.

In the same way X-rays may also produce skin damage; witness the 'erythema dose' in radiotherapy. Blakely[48] describes the effect of radiation (chiefly beta, gamma or X-rays or neutrons) on the skin as being either epilation, or skin damage, which ranges from erythema, through transepidermal injury with blistering and ulceration, to a severe lesion resembling a 3rd degree burn.

Another recently discovered variety of radiation capable of causing skin and other tissue damage is the laser, or 'Light Amplification by Stimulated Emission of Radiation'. Among people using these radiations the greatest hazard is to the eyes; severe retinal burns can occur very easily. The effect on the skin is to produce charring, the depth depending on the energy of impact of the laser beam. Tissue damage is more severe in pigmented areas.[49]

Part of the effect of lasers, in addition to the production of heat, is due to ultrasonic action. These effects are capable of producing cavitation in tissues. Energy in the form of microwaves may also produce tissue destruction.

COLD

Hypothermia

As is the case with heat, cold may affect the body in two ways, firstly through a general effect caused by lowering of the temperature of the body as a whole or hypothermia. Unlike the effects of heat, this is the most important aspect in medico-legal practice. The less important, local effect of cold is to produce lesions on the extremities, such as frostbite, which is rarely seen in this country of moderate temperatures.

The importance of hypothermia as a cause of illness and death in Britain has only been fully appreciated relatively recently. Series of cases of elderly patients admitted to hospital with very low body temperatures were reported by Duguid, Simpson & Stowers,[50] Prescott, Peard & Wallace[51] and Rosin & Exton Smith[52] among others and there were reports of a Special Committee of the British Medical Association in 1964,[53] and of the Royal College of Physicians in 1966.[54]

The last report finally established the condition as by no means uncommon, especially among elderly people, who constituted 42% of the series. As a result of these reports hypothermia is now defined as the state in which the temperature of the body is below 95°F or 35°C. Mills[55] describes three levels of the condition:

1. From 95° to 90°F, with shivering, attempts at increased exercise and constriction of the skin blood vessels.
2. From 90° to 75°F with failure of shivering, slowing of metabolic process and falling blood pressure.
3. Below 75°F, when heat control fails and the body progressively, and usually irreversibly, cools to the temperature of its surroundings.

Physiology of hypothermia

Only a brief summary is possible here. For more detail the reader should consult standard works on physiology. The subject is well summarised by Cooper,[56] Garry,[57] Keatinge[58] and Kew.[59] The temperature of the peripheral part of the body may vary, according to environmental temperatures and other factors, but the central part of the interior of the body, or core, including the vital organs, is usually kept at a constant temperature. A rectal temperature measurement indicates reasonably accurately the 'core' temperature. There is slight diurnal variation of about 1.5°F.

The internal temperature is regulated by heat production or loss by the body, production being by metabolism, controlled by the thyroid hormone, and muscular activity. Loss is by increasing blood flow through the skin, or by sweating. Modification of such factors as clothing will, of course, also play a part.

The mechanisms for regulating the body temperature are controlled by central receptors, which are presumed to be situated in the hypothalamic region of the brain, and also possibly near the carotid sinus. Peripheral temperature receptors are also known to exist.

In certain natural diseases, infectious fevers or brain lesions, the normal heat-regulating mechanisms are disturbed and abnormalities of temperature occur. Otherwise the body temperature remains relatively constant.

Pugh[60] has shown experimentally with healthy young adults, that when working in conditions of wet clothing and high air currents, provided the work rate was maintained at a sufficiently high level, rectal temperature remained at a constant level, slightly higher than normal, and oxygen consumption was the same as that in warm still conditions. However, at low work rates the oxygen consumption was substantially higher in cold windy conditions, and rectal temperatures fell progressively. The participants described feeling severe discomfort, misery, mental blankness, etc., in the cold, windy conditions.

Circumstances of hypothermia

Hypothermia may be due to exogenous or endogenous causes, or a combination of both factors. Exogenous causes are almost always climatic, a severe cold spell in winter precipitating several cases. Out-of-doors cold, wet and windy conditions may be more dangerous than a very cold, snowy dry spell. Indoors, lack of fuel for heating and the habit of leaving windows open for 'fresh air' during cold spells, lowers room temperatures considerably. Surveys have been made of houses[61] which showed that many old people's homes were below the minimum recommended temperature of 70°F, set by the Department of Health and Social Security. Anderson[62] has commented on the fact that older houses are often so constructed as to be less cold, even if they lack other advantages.

Endogenous factors are disease processes or drugs which modify the normal physiological temperature-regulating mechanism. Obviously brain damage, in so far as it may affect the central heat regulating mechanisms may have this effect.[63] Diseases of endocrine glands, such as hypopituitarism or hypothyroidism, figure in many reported series of cases of hypothermia. Skin lesions, such as exfoliative dermatitis may also have this effect.[55]

Drugs, such as barbiturates, phenothiazine tranquilisers, diazepam, and of course alcohol, have all been described as being associated with hypothermia. Moreover, deliberately induced hypothermia, by means of drugs, has been a well-established technique of anaesthesia since about 1950.[64]

Leaving aside patients undergoing anaesthesia there are three groups of persons who are liable to suffer from accidental hypothermia, i.e., recently born babies, elderly persons and persons engaged in hazardous outdoor activities such as mountaineering, pot-holing and sailing. The features of hypothermia in each of these three groups will be considered separately.

Hypothermia in the elderly

Elderly people are particularly at risk from hypothermia. In the series reported by the Royal College of Physicians,[54] 42% of the patients were over 65 years of age. Such people are especially at risk for several reasons. The temperature of their houses in winter may be unduly low, because they either haven't the money, or the mobility to obtain fuel, and if senile mental deterioration is present, may not realise the need to keep the room temperatures up.

Elderly people are likely to be taking some of the drugs, such as phenothiazines, or barbiturates, which are known to lower body temperature. They are also likely to be suffering from some of the general diseases which are known to predispose to the condition, such as myxoedema, cerebral arteriosclerosis and cardiovascular disease. Also elderly people are prone to accidental falls, with resultant immobility, leading to hypothermia. Another hazard to the elderly is that having once suffered from hypothermia, they appear to be more liable to a recurrence of the condition. Macmillan et al.[65] has shown that a group of survivors from one episode of hypothermia, when exposed to a cold environment under experimental conditions, had low central temperatures which fell progressively; the normal increase of heat production was not evoked.

Such elderly victims of accidental hypothermia are obviously admitted to hospital if found alive, and treated by slow and gentle rewarming, as for instance by means of a warm room, or by immersing a forearm in warm water, or by mediastinal perfusion by warm fluid. Manipulative procedures, such as tracheal intubation or catheterisation are liable to cause sudden death in the hypothermic, by ventricular fibrillation.[66] But of course deaths of such patients in hospital are not likely to be investigated by the forensic pathologist, and he will probably only meet such cases of hypothermia in the elderly when they are found dead at home in suspicious circumstances, and with the cause of death unknown. He is then deprived of one of the most convincing aids to diagnosis, a knowledge of the body temperature in life. Occasionally this

can be assessed, if the time of death is known. Thus in one of the author's cases, an elderly and immobile woman, living in squalor in a badly neglected house, was found partly clothed, lying on the bare floor, in a position which her relatives said she had occupied for several weeks. She was still alive, but died in the arms of a welfare worker at about 8 p.m. When seen by the pathologist at 1.45 a.m. the following morning the rectal temperature of the body was 69 °F. Unless the body had cooled after death at an extremely rapid rate of approximately 6 °F/h, she must otherwise have had a body temperature many degrees below normal when she died (F.M. 18473A).

In the absence of any positive indication by temperature readings, the pathologist must depend for his diagnosis on the features of the scene of death, the rather meagre characteristic post-mortem findings, and the exclusion of other conditions, injuries, etc. Autopsy findings have been reported in some of the published series of cases of hypothermia, notably by Duguid, Simpson & Stowers[50] and the subject has been studied by Mant.[67-69]

Externally there is a tendency to pinkness of areas of hypostasis, instead of the more characteristic purple hue, with patchy erythema of the skin surface, and oedema of the extremities and with a myxoedematous appearance of the facies.

Internally, the most characteristic features described by various workers are the changes of acute pancreatitis. These may consist of gross haemorrhage into the gland, or simply patches of fat necrosis over its surface, with slight irregular congestion of the tissue. Such changes are consistent with the known frequency, in living hypothermic patients, of the finding of a raised serum amylase.

The other common finding is the presence of multiple acute erosions or haemorrhages in the mucosa of the stomach or duodenum. Ulceration of the duodenum, like the Curling's ulcer associated with burns, has been described.[69, 70] However, the more usual appearance is of multiple small blackened areas, up to 5 mm or so in diameter, scattered throughout the mucosa of the stomach.[71]

In Mant's series of 28 cases, 23 showed signs of pancreatitis and 25 exhibited haemorrhages in the gastric mucosa, or acute erosions.

Other features reported in various series include

fatty changes in heart, liver and kidneys, and venous thromboses and microinfarcts, the latter due to 'sludging' of blood in vessels, because of the slowed circulation. Another feature, of practical importance, is the extremely good state of preservation of tissues when examined histologically. This is particularly striking in post-mortem histological material, in which some degree of autolysis is normally almost invariably found.

Other findings, such as bronchopneumonia, cerebral infarct, etc., may be a consequence of hypothermia, but could also have been conditions which preceded and precipitated the condition, and distinction is not likely to be possible. Biochemical investigations may be of some value, bearing in mind the limitations of all post-mortem biochemistry. In the living, blood sugar and urea are often raised, as is the serum amylase and there is often severe ketosis.[72]

One external feature, which the author has come to regard as diagnostic, is the occurrence of large superficial abrasions and areas of reddish-purple discoloration, due to superficial bruises, on the extremities, in those elderly people who suffer injuries and are exposed to cold out of doors.[39] In one such case on Christmas Day an elderly woman, living alone, appeared to have fallen on the concrete yard at the back of her house. She had an exceedingly thin skull, which was fractured, with some extradural haemorrhage, but she had very large purple coloured superficial bruises on the legs and backs of the arms, which had the appearance

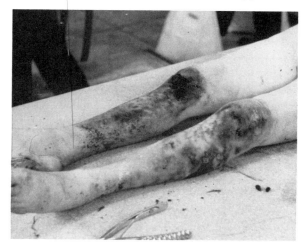

Fig. 12.13 Discolouration of legs in hypothermia.

of being caused by shivering or minor convulsions which had resulted in rubbing of the limbs against the rough concrete (Fig. 12.13). On another occasion, in winter, an elderly woman, suffering from mental illness, wandered off at night, into the grounds of the mental home, and was found the following day, dead, with her legs entangled in some strands of barbed wire. Her body bore multiple scratches and bruises on the legs and arms, with again the widespread reddish-purple discoloration. The impression given by these marks is that they are a response to minor superficial injuries which is modified to produce this unusual appearance by the coldness of superficial parts of the limbs.

Hypothermia in the recently-born

Although the general importance of hypothermia as a cause of death has only recently been established, the danger of cold to newly-born children especially premature infants, has been recognised for a long time. Its forensic significance was discussed by Casper in the nineteenth century:[73]

... drunkards and newborn children die of cold at a temperature of 15° to 20° R = 30°25 to 19°F, a temperature at which the fashionable world in northern cities frolic about on sledges and snow-shoes.

The condition has been fully reviewed by Mant.[68]

That it is a serious cause of infant mortality was shown by Ameil & Kerr.[74] They described a series of 110 babies with hypothermia admitted to three Glasgow hospitals during the winters of 1961–62 and 1962–63. The overall mortality rate was 46%, and even when gross prematurity, congenital abnormalities, etc., were excluded, the mortality rate was 37%.

Physiologically, newborn infants lose heat rapidly soon after birth.[68] If the environment is very cold, then their temperature may fall considerably, and several days may elapse before it returns to normal. The baby, having a large surface area in relation to its weight, is more likely to lose heat by radiation than is an adult, and of course the skin of the newborn is wet, increasing heat lose by evaporation. Normally, chilling causes a metabolic response with increase in heat production, but mild anoxia can depress this response. Heat production in the newborn is particularly connected with the deposits of brown adipose tissue, which are situated on the back and neck and along the spine; nerve impulses from temperature receptor sites stimulate lipolysis, with production of triglycerids, and local heat production.

Ameil & Kerr,[74] distinguished three separate groups in their series: hypothermia on the day of birth, neonatal hypothermia and marasmic hypothermia. In hypothermia at the time of birth, the child, born into a cold environment is lethargic, cyanosed and feels cold.[75] Neonatal cold injury, occurring in the age range of one day to two weeks, includes lethargy, failure to cry, giving the misleading impression of a 'good baby', failure to suck, and redness of the face and limbs. The skin feels cold and there is sclerema, or hardening of the subcutaneous tissues. The abdomen is distended, due to paralytic ileus, with demonstration of fluid levels on X-ray. The condition may terminate in pulmonary haemorrhage.[76] In marasmic infants, who are usually in the age range of two weeks to four months, there is an underlying cause for wasting, and hypothermia becomes insidiously superimposed.

Mant[69] lists some of the conditions predisposing to perinatal hypothermia. Apart from prematurity and neglect, these include asphyxia, birth injuries, congenital heart disease, hypothyroidism, cerebral malformations and acquired sepsis. He reports intrapulmonary haemorrhage as occurring in about one-third of the cases, which he considers is due to inhalation of vomit due to the ileus. Other features of adult hypothermia, such as gastric erosions and/or pancreatitis are rarely seen.

The cases of hypothermia in infants likely to be of especial importance to the forensic pathologist are either in the newly-born, where lack of attention at birth leads to allegations of infanticide, or in the marasmic child, whose wasting may be due to neglect, associated with other forms of cruelty to the child (see ch. 15). In such circumstances in particular, there may be, in addition, evidence of local effects of cold, such as gangrene due to frostbite, or blisters due to cold injury in which there is pallor of the affected epidermis, formation of bullae, and sludging or actual platelet and fibrin thrombi in small blood vessels in the dermis. However hypothermia, as a cause of death, may be easily overlooked in these cases, the attention of the pathologist being distracted by the other, more obtrusive features of the case, such as the wasting, bruises, etc.

Hypothermia in climbers, etc.

It has been realised for a long time that persons exposed to severe, Arctic conditions, such as polar explorers, are at risk of dying from cold. However, it is less well recognised that exposure, in this country, to damp windy conditions, even when the temperature is substantially above freezing, is capable of inducing hypothermia, especially in ill-trained or ill-clad persons. It has only recently been recognised that many people who die from immersion, as in boating accidents, succumb from hypothermia, and not from drowning.[58]

Attention was drawn to the hazards of hypothermia in hill-walkers and climbers by Pugh.[77] He described the features of 23 exposure incidents in various parts of Britain. Eighty-eight people were involved, with 25 deaths. The causes he recognised were bad weather conditions, especially blizzards, being benighted, being wet through, exhaustion, lack of subcutaneous fat (several of the deceased were very thin), sex (women usually surviving conditions which prove fatal for men), and inexperience and lack of training. The sequence of events described was abnormal behaviour, slowing, stumbling, weakness, repeated falling, collapse, stupor, unconsciousness, death. Shivering, present in the early stages, was replaced by muscle rigidity, and some of the unconscious victims had convulsions. Symptoms usually began within 5 or 6 h of setting out and the interval between onset of symptoms and death could be as little as 2 h.

Most of the autopsies reported showed no characteristic abnormalities. A feature commented on was the paucity of subcutaneous fat in several cases. Abrasions and scratches due to falls were noted, and mucopus in the bronchi in one case. In a subsequent paper, Pugh[60] described the results of experiments on volunteers under simulated conditions of exposure. He found that persons exercising at high work rates used equal amounts of oxygen whether they were in warm and dry or cold and wet conditions. However, in the lower work rates oxygen consumption was much higher. Also at the lower work rates, body temperature could not be maintained. In the adverse conditions there was found to be a considerable cooling of the bulk of the muscles and this might contribute to weakness and stumbling noted in the actual victims of hypothermia.

The forensic pathologist may encounter the occasional victim of such circumstances, even in urban areas. In one such case[39] the author examined the body of a woman who, after a quarrel with her husband in a golf club-house, set off alone across the golf course, in light clothing, on an extremely windy and wet night. Her body was found the following day, in a ditch, where she had evidently collapsed and succumbed to hypothermia. The clothing was sodden, but the only striking feature at autopsy was the very bright red colour of the blood, and the fact that a sample was liquid when collected, but coagulated after it had warmed to normal room temperatures. The normal processes of post-mortem thrombosis and fibrolysis appeared to have been inhibited by the cold. On another occasion a boy, who had become accidentally trapped in mud on a quarry edge, succumbed from hypothermia and inhalation of mud. On this occasion also the blood was unusually bright red in colour.

It is now recognised that many people who are found dead floating in water, especially after shipwrecks, have died of hypothermia and not drowning.[58] Although supported by life jackets they lose consciousness from the cold, and may then die from hypothermia or drown when small waves wash over their unprotected faces. Exercise, when the subject is immersed in cold water, is found to increase the rate at which body temperature falls, though clothing and subcutaneous fat have a protective effect. Keatinge[58] reported experiments in which good swimmers were immersed in water at 4–7°C. There was intense stimulation of respiration, and two participants collapsed within a few minutes, and had to be pulled out of the water. It is suggested that this is the reason for some otherwise inexplicable sudden deaths in sailing accidents.

Frost-bite

The condition is well-known in Arctic climates, and graphically described in the annals of explo-

ration. It was studied especially during the Second World War. An important description of the histological features and mechanism was made by Ungley & Blackwood[78] and Ungley.[79] Cold caused dilatation of blood vessels, with loss of plasma into the tissues, and sludging of the red cells left in the blood vessels, with resultant anoxia of the tissues. In seawater the tissues were thought not to freeze, but Keatinge[58] has shown that freezing can occur. The tissues may first become supercooled.

Frost-bitten limbs are at first red, or may appear yellowish or black. After re-heating they become red, swollen and painful. There may be blistering. Residual effects may be vasomotor instability and sensory loss.

ELECTRICITY

Compared to other hazards of our environment, such as burning or drowning, electrocution does not constitute a serious problem, numerically. According to the Registrar General's figures for 1971[21] there were 123 accidental deaths from electrocution. Nevertheless, electricity and electrical appliances are available and are found in the home and workplace of nearly everyone in this country; therefore the possibility of electrocution must be considered when investigating any sudden or suspicious death, especially since the hazard may be totally unsuspected at the scene of death. For instance, on one occasion a vagrant was found collapsed in a yard of some derelict property, near a wall. The probably explanation for the death appeared to be a fatal heart attack, or possibly an assault, but external examination in the mortuary disclosed a black mark on the top of the head, which proved to be an electric mark, with other small electric marks on the hands. Re-examination of the scene revealed a metal conduit on the wall near to the place where the deceased's body had been found, and a mark on the wall nearby, corresponding in shape to the mark on the top of the head. The metal conduit was found to be 'live', due to an electric fault, although it had been thought that all electrical supplies to this property had been disconnected. It appeared that the victim may have entered the building in order to steal metal piping, and so had touched the piece of live conduit (F.M. 11,992, post-mortem by Dr Manock).

Factors concerned in electrocution

Various factors influence the likelihood that electrocution will occur from contact with a source of electricity. Some of these reside in the nature of the electricity supply itself, others in the circumstances of the victim. A knowledge of these factors does not contribute to the diagnosis of electrocution at autopsy, but is valuable subsequently in reconstructing the circumstances of the death.

Recent views of these factors have been made by Wood[80] and Lee.[81,82] The whole subject is very fully reviewed by Polson & Gee.[83] Earlier, classical references are Jex-Blake[84] and Jellinek.[85]

Voltage

The commonest voltage to cause fatal accidents is 240 V. This is probably because the most convenient source, the domestic supply, is at this voltage. Injuries and death can be caused by higher voltages, usually involving high tension cables or pylon lines, when people using vehicles or plant with long upward projections, such as cranes, make contact with the wires, or when people climb pylons with the object of stealing wire, or of committing suicide.

At 240 V any visible damage to the body is limited usually to small electric marks, and death is due to internal derangements of function (see below). At high voltage, however, the body is extensively damaged, with severe and deep burns being a particular feature. The high tension voltages, in the grid distribution system, range from the order of 400 000 to 11 000 000 V in regional systems, and the final supply to domestic use is by the three-phase 415 V network.

Lower voltages than 250 V may prove fatal, though it is unlikely that death will occur at less than 50 V. However, Polson describes a case of fatal electrocution of a man where the source was the batteries of an electric milk float; two 12 V batteries supplied 24 V d.c. The ground was covered by ice and snow. Although tests on the vehicle revealed no abnormality, and the maximum current produced appeared to be about 5 mA, the body of the deceased bore electric marks and no other cause for death was found. (The post-mortem was by Professor C. J. Polson and Dr H. Thompson.)

Current form

Most accidents are from alternating current. The usual supply is 50 cycles/s. The reason for this is evidently, as with voltage, the fact that this is the most readily available source. However, direct current can also prove fatal, as described by Polson & Gee, above.[83]

Amperage

This is probably the most important factor as far as the electricity itself is concerned. The most dangerous level appears to be of the order of 60–180 mA. However, at much smaller currents unpleasant effects may occur. A sensation occurs when a person receives a current of 1 mA, and as the current is increased, contraction of the muscles becomes greater, and more painful. At somewhere between 8 and 20 mA, the person will be unable to let go of the source of the current, and so the victim may be subjected to passage of current for a long time, unless found and released. At much higher currents this factor of 'hold-on' does not occur, and indeed, with high tension accidents the victim is often forcibly thrown clear, a feature which may, of itself, cause injuries. Very high currents, of the order of 4 A, are in fact less dangerous than those of the order of 100 mA.

Resistance

It is well known that the current flowing through a conductor is determined by the voltage and the resistance of the conductor, i.e., $I = V/R$ (where I = current in amperes, V = potential difference in volts and R = resistance in ohms). Therefore the resistance of the body, especially the skin, is an important factor, so that quite high voltages can be withstood if the area of skin making the contact has a high resistance. When a human body forms part of an electric circuit, most of the resistance is located in the skin. The actual amount of resistance can vary from a few hundred to several thousands of ohms, and will depend on the site on the body and the degree of dampness of the skin. Moisture, rain or sweating obviously lowers the resistance. A thick horny skin, as in the palm of the hand, has a greater resistance than thinner, more delicate skin, such as on the trunk or thighs. The tissues within the body offer comparatively little resistance, blood being an especially good conductor.

Earthing

For the current to flow through the human body, it must be connected to the earth. The greater the insulation of the body from earth, the less the risk. This is typified by the industrial accident in which the victim is standing on a wet concrete floor, providing almost no insulation. Dry conditions, rubber shoes and some material such as wood between the body and earth provide much more efficient protection.

Site of contact

This is of importance in two respects. The actual size of the area of contact is significant since a very small area of contact between the skin and the source of electricity will have a higher resistance than will a larger area; for instance, the tip of a finger compared to the palm of a hand. The second factor is the part of the body making contact, and the route of the current through the body. Passage through the region of the heart is the most dangerous, occurring when the path is from hand to hand, or from the left arm to the right leg. Thus in Lee's series,[81] of 118 cases, the route was from arm to arm in 32 cases and from arm to leg in 45.

Other factors

Other factors that have been described as being of importance are general health, constitution and awareness of the victim. The example is quoted in previous editions of Taylor[86] of an engine-driver, who made a habit of catching hold of a 50 V lamp with both hands and letting it go again, as a bet for a glass of beer. He repeated this as often as the beer was forthcoming, until one day he *accidentally* made the same contact and collapsed dead.

Mechanism of death

This subject is dealt with by Lee.[81] Four mechanisms are suggested.

Ventricular fibrillation

This is thought to be the most important form, occurring when current passes through the thorax, from hand-to-hand or hand-to-leg current pathways. The critical level of current appears to be about 100 mA. Lee draws attention to the fact that consciousness need not be lost immediately in these circumstances.

Respiratory muscle spasm

Electric currents passing through the thorax may cause tetanic contractions of the muscles of respiration. Currents of over 30 mA are required. The effects have been shown experimentally by Lee.[81] It is noted that typical signs of mechanical asphyxia are not seen in deaths from electrocution, but it is considered that this is due to the fact that, with the chest wall held rigidly, the lungs are not subjected to negative pressures due to the inspiratory efforts which occur in, for instance, strangulation.

Respiratory failure

This means that the passage of current has caused dysfunction of the respiratory centre in the brain. It is not considered now to be a common mechanism of death, unless the route of passage of the current is directly through the head, which is relatively rare according to published figures.

Late effects

On occasion a victim of electrocution who does not die immediately sustains severe burns, and death may then occur after an interval of a few days, from infection, or from haemorrhage, since damage to blood vessels may be a feature of such injuries.

Neurological sequelae,[87] and damage to the lens of the eye[88] have also been reported.

Signs of electrocution

Electric mark

The point where the electric current enters the body is characterised by the presence of the electric mark, or 'Joule burn'. Although having some features of a small burn, it is easily distinguished from the electric burn which is seen in accidents with high tension currents. It has been studied and described in detail by Jaffe,[89] Jellinek[85] and Polson & Gee.[83]

A typical mark consists of an area of skin, varying in size according to the size of the source with which contact was made, which appears dry and yellow-brown in colour. It may be in the form of a shallow depression, like an ulcer, or slightly raised, so that such a mark has been mistaken for a wart. The shape may also mirror the shape of the contact. The margins are often slightly raised, and in the skin beyond these margins there is usually a narrow reddened border of vital reaction, similar to that seen around a burn caused by heat. Sometimes the skin in the centre of the mark is blackened, at other times it contains some small holes, as though from collapsed blisters. Hairs in the area may be charred.

Professor Polson[83] describes how he and Dr Hainsworth produced electric marks on limbs of dead bodies, and observed the skin blistering and then charring beneath the electrode. They noted on one occasion that a reddened zone appeared surrounding an experimental electric mark, and simulating a vital reaction, even though the tissue had been removed from the dead body and stored in a refrigerator for several days.

Sometimes, if the source of the current is small, and contact made with one hand, the mark may be on the side of one of the fingers, or near a skin crease, and easily overlooked. On other occasions, when contact is with a relatively large source, the mark may be large and obvious, and if the initial contact is with a limb, there may be secondary marks where the limb has come into contact with another part of the body, for instance between the elbow and the side of the trunk, and contraction of the limb may cause the mark to be linear or streaky in appearance.

Histological examination of the mark usually shows coagulation of the dermis, with separation of the epidermis by blister formation in some areas, and in others a pronounced disturbance of the architecture of the epidermis, with the cells becoming elongated and arranged in parallel rows at an acute angle, or almost at right angles to the dermis. The appearance has been ascribed by Jellinek[14] to polarisation of the nuclei by the electric current, but the author has seen a similar appearance of the epidermis in some heat burns. The dermis may become vacuolated, and it is suggested that this is due to the formation of bubbles of steam in the tissues. The comparative appearances of dermal injuries caused by heat and by electricity have been studied.[90, 91]

Exit marks

Sometimes it is possible to find an electric mark at a site on the body which obviously corresponds to the point of exit of the current. In that case the mark resembles the electric mark of entry. It has been suggested that the exit mark would have an everted appearance, but that is not the author's experience.

Electric burns

There may be superficial burns of the body surface, or flash burns due to arcing over of the electric current on to the body. However, exposure to high voltage currents will usually produce very large and deep burns. Soft tissue can be destroyed over a wide area and bone charred or whitened. A limb may be almost severed. On other occasions, electrocution may be associated with almost no external findings, as when it is due to an appliance such as an electric fire falling into a bath of water, or from an electric blanket.

Internal findings

In most cases of electrocution there is a remarkable paucity of evidence to suggest this inside the body. There may be scattered petechial haemorrhages. In one case seen by the author there were haemorrhages on the surface of the interventricular septum of the heart, and congestion of the lungs.

The current is thought to flow along blood vessels, as constituting the routes of least resistance, and damage in the form of disruption of the vessel walls has been described. When contact is directly with the brain, as by a mishap during operation, disruption with gas bubble formation in the brain tissue has been reported.[92]

Metallisation

When an electric current passes from a metallic conductor to the body, some of the metal can be transferred to the skin. For instance, if the conductor contains copper, the electric mark produced can have a bright green colour.

A technique, called the acro-reaction test, has been described by Adjutantis & Skalos[93] which detects traces of metal in suspected electric marks. Small wedges of filter paper are moistened with acid, applied to the mark on the skin, and then removed and tested by drops of reagents which give colour reactions with various metals. Boehm[94] describes the use of scanning electron microscopy in detection of metallic particles in electric marks.

Circumstances of electrocution

The majority of cases of electrocution are accidental. Homicide by this means is exceedingly rare. Most accidents occur at places of employment, due to a multitude of possible varieties of accident involving overhead wires, inspection lamps, power tools, etc. In one major accident in 1973, four workmen were electrocuted during servicing work at Thorpe Marsh power station.

Another major source of accident is the home, where dangers arise from worn electric flex, from amateur and incorrect wiring of houses, or from attempted repair of electrical appliances without removal of the appliance from the source of current.

In one such accident seen at Leeds, a man attempted to wire his own house, but did so incorrectly. His child climbed on to a washing machine, which was plugged into a wall-socket but not switched on, in order to get a drink of water from the kitchen tap. Because of the faulty wiring the

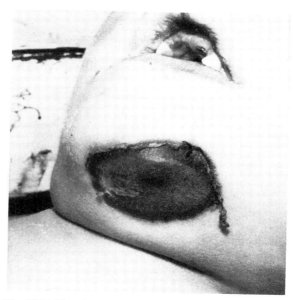

Fig. 12.14 Electric mark, 240 V.

casing of the washing machine was live. When the child turned the tap on, he was connected to earth by the stream of water running down the waste-pipe and died at once. There were large electric marks on the forehead where the child had fallen against the tap, and on the hands and the front of the thighs (F.M. 16, 151) Fig. 12.14.

On another occasion a young child died after touching a fire guard. There was a small electric mark on the hand. The guard had become 'live' due to contact with a flex to a television set; the flex

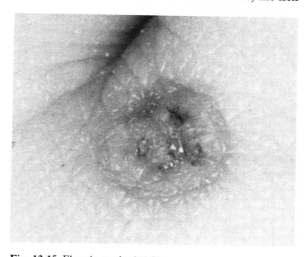

Fig. 12.15 Electric mark, 240 V.

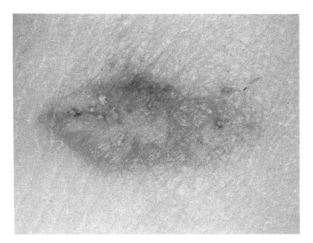

Fig. 12.16 Electric mark, 240 V.

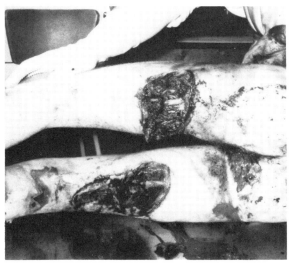

Fig. 12.18 Deep burns from high tension current—grid distribution pylon.

had become worn, with exposure of the wiring. The only signs of electrocution on the child's body were two small rounded electric marks on the forefinger and thumb of one hand (F.M. 13, 642 A) (Figs 12.15 and 12.16).

Electrocution is a relatively infrequent mode of suicide, which is surprising in view of the availability of the means. Whether it will take the place of carbon monoxide, being the most readily available domestic means of suicide, remains to be seen. The victim usually winds wires round the wrists or other parts of the body, connects them to a wall socket and then switches it on. The apparatus is in situ when the body is found, and there are prominent linear electric marks beneath the wires, encircling the limbs (Fig. 12.17). An example is given

of such a suicide in a middle-aged woman by Polson & Gee[83] (F.M. 13, 899). Another example in a teenage boy is given by Randall.[95] In areas where sources of high tension current are accessible, such as on part of the London Underground, suicide may be effected by the victim throwing himself on to the live rail, but other sources, such as pylon lines, are so well protected that only very determined and athletic suicides attempt this (Fig. 12.18)

Attempted homicide by electrocution has been alleged (*R. v. Whybrow*, Chelmsford Assizes 1951) where the husband connected the soap dish in the bathroom used by his wife to a source of electric current. However, such cases are exceedingly rare.

In the United States, in some areas, judicial execution may still be effected by electrocution by the electric chair. Currents of 1700 V are said to be passed through the victim.[18] Paper[96] describes two shocks of 2300 and 550 V, respectively.

Lightning stroke

Although such accidents are comparatively rare (four cases are listed by the Registrar General in 1971[21]), the features which they produce are sufficiently bizarre to require recognition by the forensic pathologist. Unless the accident is witnessed, the fact that the body of the victim is liable to be

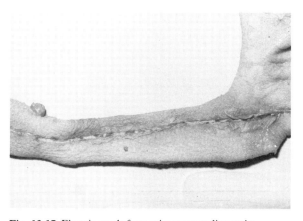

Fig. 12.17 Electric mark from wire surrounding wrist—suicide.

found in an isolated situation with injuries and damage to clothing may arouse suspicion of criminal assault.

The effects of the lightning on the victim are modified from the effects of the ordinary domestic electric supplies by the very high voltage involved, several millions of volts, and by the blast-waves which are associated with the electric discharge.

The victim is usually out-of-doors, during a thunderstorm, and has taken shelter under a tree, or in a solitary building, which attracts the lighting discharge. Occasionally persons inside a house may be affected when lightning strikes a chimney or television aerial and passes down through a living room. It is not uncommon for several people to be injured at the same time, as in the well known incident at Ascot in 1955, when 45 people were affected.[97]

The electric current tends to pass extensively over the surface of the body. As a result there may be found the typical 'arborescent' or 'filigree' burns, a pattern of very superficial burns in the shape of the branches of a tree or the fronds of a fern, usually to be seen radiating over the surface of the chest. Though visible on the corpse, they are not confined to the dead, but can be seen on the body of a living victim for several days after the accident, as shown by Fraenkel & Chassar Moir.[98]

In passing over the body the current tends to produce burns beneath metal objects in contact with the skin, such as wrist watches, bracelets, metal hooks on undergarments, and so on, and the metal in these objects may become magnetised. The effect of metalisation may be to produce a distinctive colouring, for instance browning. This is due to the implantation of metal into the skin. Secondly, associated with the electrical discharge there may be a considerable blast-wave, which of itself may cause extensive damage to the victim. A particularly dramatic example was reported by Skan[99] of an African, inside a hut, who was struck by lightning, with resultant injuries which included tearing away of the left shoulder, a large hole in the left side of the neck, and fractures of the skull and left humerus. The illustration shows injuries resembling those caused by a bomb. Thirdly, the clothing may be extensively damaged, burnt, or more especially, torn. An example is

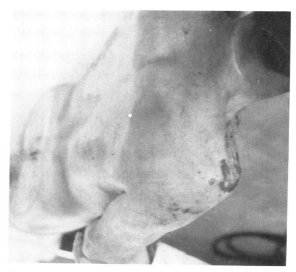

Fig. 12.19 Superficial burn due to lightning stroke.

given by Mant,[100] of a girl, riding a horse, who was killed by lightning which struck the metal stud on top of her riding hat, passed down her body, melting her nylon panties, and tore her jodhpurs. In a case seen in the Department at Leeds, a man, found under a tree near the banks of a river, had apparently been leaning against the tree, since he had a burn on one shoulder (Fig. 12.19), a tear of his anorak and shirt (Fig. 12.20), and a burn beneath a bunch of keys in his pocket; there was a long split in the bark of the tree, directed towards the position where the man had been standing (F.M. 12, 426B, post-mortem by Dr C. H. Manock).

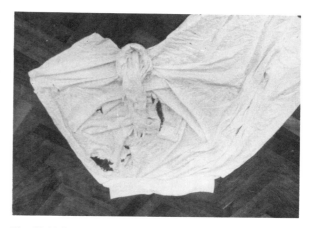

Fig. 12.20 Damage to clothing from lightning stroke.

Other cases have been described in which the clothing was almost totally torn from the body. One example was cited by Polson & Gee.[83]

While lightning stoke is liable to cause death, many victims survive. They are liable to be unconscious or confused for several hours after the event, and may subsequently exhibit neurological signs, such as convulsions, paralyses, deafness or noises in the ears, or visual disturbances. Most of these symptoms and signs resolve within a few days, but persistent headaches or hysterical symptoms may occur, and actual damage to the brain may cause permanent paralysis.[101]

STARVATION AND NEGLECT

Forensic pathologists in Britain are likely to see relatively few cases of death due to starvation, and when these occur they are usually due to complicating factors, such as underlying natural disease or mental abnormality. However, during the Second World War large numbers of people on the continent, especially in concentration and prison camps, suffered starvation from deprivation of food, and the effects were studied by several observers, for instance the relief teams at Belsen.[102] The findings of the observers were reviewed by Keith Simpson in 1953.[103] Extensive famines of recent years in India, Ethiopia, Northern Africa, etc., have made the visual features of starvation a common experience for most people through television.

The minimum food requirement for an adult is about 2000 calories, if that person is not performing any activity. In famine or wartime conditions, food intake may fall well below this level. The effects of such malnutrition were described by Layton[104] and summarised by Keith Simpson[103] as loss of well-being and hunger; apathy and fatigue; loss of flesh; polyuria; pigmentation; cachexia; hypothermia; extreme lethargy, mental retardation and loss of self-respect; hunger oedema; reduced resistance to infection, with development of diarrhoea, and tuberculosis.

The development of oedema is apparently related to a decrease in plasma proteins in starvation. Anaemia, normocytic or macrocytic may also occur. Body weight is lost until a level of about 40% of the original weight is reached, when death is almost inevitable. Specific forms of malnutrition due to lack of certain dietary factors are now well-recognised, such as kwashiorkor, or protein malnutrition, seen especially in African children, and the effects of deprivation of vitamins, such as 'beri-beri', a condition which was rife among prisoners of war in the Far East.

In this country the conditions which may give rise to death from starvation seen by the pathologist are: inability to eat, due to natural disease, such as carcinoma of the oesophagus; voluntary refusal of food as in mental illness, or in 'fasts' for particular reasons, such as political; and accidental entombment, as in colliery disasters. In fact the condition is very infrequently seen.

The post-mortem findings in death from starvation have been well described by Simpson,[103] who lists extreme emaciation; atrophied musculature; demineralisation of the skeleton; deterioration of the skin with loss of elasticity, and increase of pigmentation; atrophy of the coats of the bowel; anaemia, and intercurrent disease.

A typical example of death from starvation, seen by the author, showed the following features. The victim, a woman of 83, had a carcinoma of the stomach. She weighed 63 lb. There was no subcutaneous fat and all the bones were prominent beneath the skin. There was a pressure sore over the right hip. The heart weight 160 g, and the epicardial fat was gelatinous, semi-translucent and brownish in colour. The vessels on the heart surface were tortuous, and the muscle dry and brown in colour. The liver weighed 600 g and was small, firm and greyish in colour. The walls of the bowel appeared thinned, and the gall bladder, filled with dark-green bile, was especially prominent (F.M. 12869) (Fig 12.21).

In any such case it is very difficult to determine, from post-mortem findings alone, the length of time taken for the body to reach the state that it was in when death occurred. In acute starvation, when there is total deprivation of water as well as food, death is likely to occur in about a week to 10 days. However, availability of water can prolong life for many weeks, and of course a diet of sorts, even if well below the minimum required calorific level, will convert the condition to one of slow starvation which may take many weeks or months.

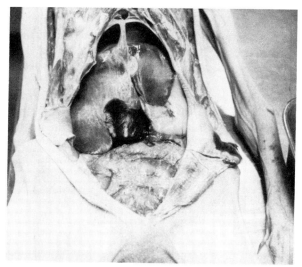

Fig. 12.21 Shrunken liver and dilated gall-bladder due to starvation.

In forensic practice death from starvation may have criminal significance if it appears that food was deliberately denied to the victim. In practice this is very rarely possible these days in the case of an adult, unless the deceased was mentally retarded and unable to fend for himself. However it may be asked, when a person has abstained from food because of mental or physical abnormalities, whether the relatives were negligent in failing to seek medical assistance. In such circumstances it has to be borne in mind that the relatives are themselves frequently mentally subnormal and so less likely to appreciate the gravity of the situation, and that the starvation may have been a slowly progressive condition, less easily noticed by persons seeing the victim every day, than by an outside observer.

The cases which are particularly difficult are those concerning small children. Allegation of deliberate withholding of food must be supported by the evidence of witnesses, for this is not a factor which can be established from the post-mortem examination alone. Wasting and marasmus in children may occur from many different metabolic disorders, some of which have only recently been recognised, and since these are often disorders of metabolic processes, such as deficiencies of single enzymes, their diagnosis may depend on elaborate biochemical studies made in life in a fully equipped

hospital. Exclusion of such conditions can hardly be expected from an autopsy alone. Therefore it is virtually impossible for the pathologist to be completely sure that he has eliminated any question of underlying disease. Such conditions as juvenile diabetes, Fanconi's syndrome, etc., should be considered and searched for. However, the list of possible causes of failure to thrive, or marasmus, in young children is extensive, and for fuller details textbooks of pediatrics should be consulted. It is obviously important that in such children the intestinal contents and samples of blood and urine should be preserved for examination, for evidence of metabolic abnormalities. The possibility of chronic poisoning, e.g., by lead, from flaking paint, etc., should also be considered.

Although the cause of the starvation which caused the child's death may not be capable of proof, the question of neglect on the part of parents or guardians may become the subject of criminal charges, under Section 1 of the Children and Young Persons Act 1933. This section says that a parent shall be deemed to have neglected the child if he has failed to provide medical aid.

Such cases may be gross, and it often seems remarkable that it has been possible for the child's condition to reach the state found at autopsy without comment being aroused in other relatives, or neighbours.

In one case, seen by the author, a child of 10 weeks, whose birth weight was 5 lb, only weighed 4 lb 10 oz when it died. Death was due to bronchopneumonia. There was no body fat, the baby's limbs were shrunken and the bones prominent, the features wizened, like a small monkey, and there was gross ulceration of the perineum, back and legs, due to ammonia dermitis. No underlying cause for the malnutrition was found, but wilful starvation could not be proved. No charges resulted (F.M. 135321).

On another occasion a child aged $3\frac{1}{2}$ years lived with her father, her mother having left them. At death she weighed $19\frac{1}{2}$ lb, was very dirty and had so many head lice that the hair was constantly moving when the body was seen on the autopsy table (FM 16645).

However, the pathologist would be wise to defer expressing an opinion on the culpability of relatives until all the family background is known. Thus one child died, aged only a few months, with a weight well below normal and bronchopneumonia, apparently grossly neglected; but the parents were very young, the father suffered from epilepsy and was constantly losing his job, the family lived in wretched accommodation at an excessive rent, and although attempts had been made by a health visitor, the local authority had failed, until then, to rehouse or help the family.

In fact these children, although grossly malnourished, rarely show evidence of physical illtreatment or injuries, but obviously the picture may overlap on to the features of child abuse and 'battered babies' (see ch. 15).

Neglect, apart from starvation, may be a factor in adult deaths, as well as those of children. Sometimes this may involve relatives. Thus a woman of 60 died from the effects of progressive, undiagnosed multiple sclerosis. She had not moved from a chair for many months, eating, sleeping and performing all other functions in it. She had gross bedsores, exposing bone. No medical aid had been sought, but the daughter and a lodger in the house were of very low intelligence and no charges were made (F.M. 17743).

More often the neglect is on the part of the victims themselves, whether due to mental illness or old age. In one such case, seen by the author, the deceased had lived as a recluse in a disused van, venturing out only at night to eat the refuse brought from dustbins to the adjacent pig farm. The conditions of the van were incredibly filthy and squalid. Such conditions are often associated with hypothermia, and the features of the death cause early suspicions of foul play.

PULMONARY BAROTRAUMA

Alterations in the air in which the human organisms live either as regards the pressure, or its composition, may be reflected by injuries to the body itself. Thus as increase in air pressure may cause damage especially to the lungs, as may a reduction in air pressure. Alteration in the constituents of the air may produce rapid or long-term damage to the interior of the lungs themselves resulting in failure of lung function.

Definition of barotrauma

The name barotrauma normally relates to changes in atmospheric barometric pressure, and in particular to the effects of the ears. Thus after exposure to large pressure waves such as may result after explosions the ear-drums may be perforated. However, in this sense barotrauma may affect other organs of the body notably the lungs and in this section it is the pathology of the damage to the lungs which will be considered primarily.

Pathology of pulmonary barotrauma

Sudden violent change in pressure

Impact injuries. These are likely to result from any form of violent impact on the chest wall as for instance in motor vehicle accidents. Such impacts will result in bruising and laceration of lung tissue with subpleural emphysematous bullae. Lines of bruising are visible over the surface of the lung which may follow the lines of ribs but are commonly more widely distributed. Associated with the subpleural bruising are lines of fine silvery glistening subpleural emphysematous bullae. These are particularly found along the margins of the lobes of the lung and within the areas of bruising. Bruising may be especially noticeable at the backs of the lungs parallel to the sides of the spine. Occasionally larger emphysematous bullae especially on the apices of the lungs may be found. Lacerations of the pleural surfaces are not infrequent especially in relation to the hyla or the base of the lungs and may of course be associated with fractured ribs. In addition to the obvious surface lacerations there are likely to be areas of internal bruising which may be associated with large cavities caused by disruption of lung tissue, especially in the lower lobes. Microscopical examination reveals areas of emphysema associated with extensive haemorrhage which on occasion may show very rapid polymorph reaction. There is obvious disruption of smaller bronchi and alveolar walls. Apart from the massive areas of haemorrhage there may be multiple small areas of haemorrhage scattered throughout the cut surface of the lung tissue.

Blast injury Basically the damage caused as for

instance from bomb explosions is similar to impacts caused by solid objects. However, there may be the additional effect of blast wave entering the various orifices of the body. In addition since the blast may be fairly uniformly distributed over the body surface there may be associated injuries to other internal organs such as liver, diaphragm, etc., as well as the bowel. Such damage may occur to people exposed to blast waves in the air as in bomb explosions or to people floating in the water as from sailors in war time when depth charges are detonated in their vicinity. Similar appearances may be seen on occasions from forcible artificial respiration especially in children where traumatic emphysematous bullae in the margin of the lobes are not uncommon and may indeed result in rupture of the lungs and tension pneumothorax.

Pulmonary decompression. In its acute form this may be seen in divers surfacing from considerable depths at speed. Expansion of the air is likely to cause increased pressure within the lungs with rupture of alveoli and escape of air into the interstitial tissue of the lungs, with rupture of subpleural emphysematous bullae and pneumothorax, and with escape of air into the circulation causing air embolism.

Abnormalities of constituents of the air. Apart form the obvious changes due to inhalation of noxious gases such as carbon monoxide, nitrogen oxide, etc., it is of course well known that the lung may be damaged by increased quantities of oxygen in the inspired air. This may occur under normal pressure or if the oxygen is supplied under increased pressure. By normal pressure the conditions known as respirator lung syndrome may result. In its initial stages this resembles in many respects the condition of respiratory distress syndrome seen in newly-born children, with congested and rather fleshy lungs which on microscopical examination show oedema with the formation of numerous hyaline membranes within the respiratory bronchioles and alveoli. There may be evidence of damage to alveolar lining cells. In the less common situation in which a person is retained on a respirator for some weeks before death ensues, the lungs may show much more extensive damage. In one case seen by the author, in addition to the normal congestion and oedema, the organs showed extensive consolidation with early fibrosis. The appearances resembled in many respects those described in paraquat poisoning. The condition in this case had ultimately led to rupture of a portion of the lungs with resulting widespread emphysema.

When oxygen is administered under high pressure, if the pressure exceeds four atmospheres oxygen poisoning will result with derangement of the central nervous system and death may occur within a few minutes. At lower pressures but above normal atmospheric pressure a similar appearance to respirator lung may occur but with damage to alveolar lining cells, formation of hyaline membranes, etc., but these changes are likely to occur much more rapidly than is the case with oxygen at normal atmospheric pressure.

REFERENCES

1. Climatic Physiology Committee of the Medical Research Council (1958) Br. Med. J., i, 1533.
2. Purcell, M. J. (1966) Br. Med. J., i, 738.
3. Leading article (1968) Br. Med. J., 3, 69.
4. Leading article (1971) Br. Med. J., 3, 441.
5. Ellis, F. R., Kearney, N. P. & Harriman, D. G. F. (1972) Br. Med. J., iii, 559.
6. Macrae, W. A., Miller, K. M. & Watson, A. A. (1979) Med. Sci. Law, 19, 261.
7. Ellis, F. R. & Halsall, P. J. (1980) Br. J. Hosp. Med., 24, 318.
8. Mazzia, V. D. B. & Simon, A. (1978) In: Wecht, C., ed. Leg. Med. Annual. New York: Appleton–Century Crofts, p. 165.
9. Malamud, N., Haymaker, W. & Custer, R. P. (1946) Mil. Surg., 9, 397.
10. Kew, M. C. (1976) Br. J. Hosp. Med., 16, 502.
11. Chao, T. C., Sinniah, R. & Pakiam, J. E. (1981) Pathology, 13, 145.
12. Moritz, A. R. & Henriques, F. C. (1947) Am. J. Pathol., 23, 695.
13. Wilson J. V. (1946) The Pathology of Traumatic Injury. Edinburgh: Livingstone.
14. Jellinek, S. (1957) Triangle, 3, 104.
15. Sevitt, S. (1957) Burns, Pathology and Therapeutic Applications. London: Butterworths.
16. Pullar, P. (1973) In: Mant, A. K., ed. Modern Trends in Forensic Medicine, 3rd edn. London: Butterworths.
17. Winter, G. D. (1972) In: Maibach, H. I. & Rovee, D. T., eds. Epidermal Wound Healing. Chicago: Year Book Medical Publishers Inc.

18. Gonzales, T. A., Vance, M., Helpern, M. & Umberger, C. J. (1954) Legal Medicine, Pathology and Toxicology, 2nd edn. New York: Appleton–Century Crofts.
19. Mallik, M. O. A. (1970) J. For. Sci., 5, 489.
20. Raekallio, J. (1973) Z. Rechtsmed., 73, 83.
21. Registrar General's Statistical Review (1971) London: Her Majesty's Stationery Office.
22. Muir, I. F. K. & Barclay, T. L. (1962) Burns and their Treatment. London: Lloyd-Luke Ltd.
23. Sevitt, S. (1966) Med. Sci. Law, 6, 36.
24. Dalgaard, J. B. (1957) J. For. Med., 4, 110.
25. Leading article (1971) Br. Med. J., 7, 122.
26. Night dress (Safety) Regulations (1967) London: Her Majesty's Stationery Office, No. 839.
27. Tiege, B., Lundeval, J. & Fleischer, E. (1977) Z. Rechtsmed., 80, 17.
28. Whitehead, T. P. & Worthington, S. (1960) Clin. Chim. Acta, 6, 356.
29. Schwerd, W. & Schulz, E. (1978) For. Sci. Int., 12, 233.
30. Wetherall, H. R. (1966) J. For. Sci., 11, 167.
31. Curry, A. S., Price, D. E. & Rutter, E. R. (1967) Acta Pharmacol. Toxicol., 25, 339.
32. Yamamoto, K. (1975) Z. Rechtsmed., 76, 11.
33. Yamamoto, K. (1976) Z. Rechtsmed., 78, 303.
34. Yamamoto, K. & Yamamoto, Y. (1978) Z. Rechtsmed., 81, 173.
35. Napier, D. H. (1977) Med. Sci. Law, 17, 83.
36. Bowes, P. C. (1976) Med. Sci. Law, 16, 104.
37. Gee, D. J. & Dalley, R. A. (1967) Med. Sci. Law, 7, 56.
38. Accidents (1972) London: Her Majesty's Stationery Office, 93.
39. Gee, D. J. (1974) Police Surg., 5, 63.
40. Denison, D. M. (1966) In: Wallace, A. B. & Wilkinson, A. W., eds. Research in Burns. Edinburgh and London: E & S Livingstone.
41. Denison, D. M., Emsting, J., Tonkins, W. T. & Cresswell, A. W. (1968) Nature, 218, 1110.
42. Thurston, G. (1961) Med.-Leg. J., 29, 100.
43. Gee, D. J. (1965) Med. Sci. Law, 5, 37.
44. Richards, N. F. (1977) Med. Sci. Law, 17, 79.
45. Sevitt, S. (1962) Fat Embolism. London: Butterworths.
46. Catto, J. V. F. (1959) Br. med. J., 2, 544.
47. Polson, C. J. & Tattersall, R. N. (1969) Clinical Toxicology. London: Pitman.
48. Blakely, J. (1968) The care of Radiation Casualties. London: Heinemann.
49. Goldman, L. (1967) Biomedical Aspects of the Laser. Bristol: John Wright & Sons.
50. Duguid, H., Simpson, R. G. & Stowers, J. M. (1961) Lancet, ii 1213.
51. Prescott, L. F., Peard, M. C. & Wallace, I. R. (1962) Br. Med. J., ii, 1367.
52. Rosin, A. J. & Exton Smith, A. N. (1964) Br. Med. J., i, 16.
53. British Medical Associate Special Comittee (1964) Br. Med. J., ii, 1255.
54. Report of Committee on Accidental Hypothermia (1966) London: Royal College of Physicians.
55. Mills, G. L. (1973) Br.J. Hosp. Med., 10, 6961.
56. Cooper, K. E. (1969) Br. J. Hosp. Med., 2, 1064.
57. Garry, R. C. (1969) Med. Sci. Law, 9 242.
58. Keatinge, W. R. (1969) Survival in Cold Water. Oxford and Edinburgh: Blackwell.
59. Kew, M. C. (1976) Br. J. Hosp. Med., 16, 502.
60. Pugh, L. G. C. E. (1967) Br. Med. J., i, 333.
61. Fox, R. H., Woodward, P. M., Exton Smith, A. N., Green, M. F., Dennison, D. V. & Wicks, M. H. (1973) Br. Med. J., i, 200.
62. Anderson, W. F. (1969) Med. Sci. Law, 9, 228.
63. Fox, R. H., Davies, T. W., March, F. P. & Urick, H. (1970) Lancet, ii, 185.
64. Forrester, A. C. (1969) Med. Sci. Law, 9, 233.
65. Macmillan, A. L., Corbett, J. L., Johnson, R. H., Smith, A. C., Spalding, J. M. K. & Woolner, L. (1967) Lancet, ii, 165.
66. Hockaday, T. D. R. (1969) Br. J. Hosp. Med., 2, 1083.
67. Mant, A. K. (1964) Med. Sci. Law, 4, 44.
68. Mant, A. K. (1967) Modern Trends in Forensic Medicine. London: Butterworth.
69. Mant, A. K. (1969) Br. J. Hosp. Med., 2, 1095.
70. Dalgaard, J. B. (1958) J. For. Med., 5, 16.
71. Hirvonen, J. & Elfring, R. (1974) Z. Rechtsmed., 74, 273.
72. Muir, A. L. (1967) In: Davies, C. N. et al, eds. The Effects of Abnormal Physical Conditions at Work. Edinburgh: E. & S. Livingstone.
73. Casper, J. L. (1861) A Handbook of the Practice of Forensic Medicine. London: The Sydenham Society.
74. Ameil, G. C. & Kerr, M. M. (1963) Lancet, ii, 756.
75. Hutchinson, J. H. (1969) Med. Sci. Law, 9, 224.
76. Aherne, W. A. (1964) In: Dyke, S. C., ed. Recent Advances in Clinical Pathology, series IV. London: J. & A. Churchill.
77. Pugh, L. G. C. E. (1966) Br. Med. J., i, 123.
78. Ungley, C. C. & Blackwood, W. (1942) Lancet, ii, 447.
79. Ungley, C. C., Channell, G. D. & Richards R. L. (1945) Br. J. Surg., 33, 17.
80. Wood, J. L. (1965) Med. Sci. Law, 5 192.
81. Lee, W. R. (1965) Med. Sci. Law, 5, 23.
82. Lee, W. R. (1965) Br. Med. J., 2, 616.
83. Polson. C. J. & Gee, D. J. (1973) Essentials of Forensic Medicine, 3rd edn. Oxford: Pergamon.
84. Jex-Blake, A. J. (1913) Br. Med. J., i, 425. 492, 548, 601.
85. Jellinek, S. (1932) Die Elekrisden Verletzunder. Leipsig: Barth.
86. Taylor, A. S. (1965) Principles and Practice of Forensic Medicine. London: Churchill.
87. Critchley, M. (1934) Lancet, i, 68.
88. Lee, W. R. (1961) Br. J. Ind. Med., 18, 260.
89. Jaffe, R. H. (1928) Arch. Pathol., 59, 837.
90. Danielsen, L., Thomsen, H. K., Nielsen, O., Aalund, O., Nielsen, K. G., Karlsmark, T. & Genefke, I. K. (1978) For. Sci. Int., 12, 211.
91. Thomsen, H. K., Danielsen, L., Nielsen, O., Aalund, O., Nielsen, K. G., Karlsmark, T. & Genefke, I. K. (1981) For. Sci. Int., 17, 133.
92. Dickson, W. C. (1947) J. Path. Bact., 59, 359.
93. Adjutantis, G. & Skalos, G. (1962) J. For. Med., 9, 101.
94. Boehm, E. (1975) Proc. 8th Ann. Meeting, ITT Res. Inst., Chicago, p. 563.
95. Randall, K. J. (1966) Med. Sci. Law, 6, 45.
96. Perper, J. A. (1976) Leg. Med. Annu., 135.
97. Arden, G. P., Harrison, S. H., Lister, J. H. (1956) Br. Med. J., i, 1450.
98. Fraenkel, G. J. & Chassar Moir, J. (1963) Br. Med. J., i, 1329.
99. Skan, D. A. (1949) Br. Med. J. i, 666.

100. Mant, A. K. (1968) In: Gradwohl's Legal Medicine, 2nd edn. Bristol: John Wright.
101. Leading article (1946) Lancet, **i**, 35.
102. Mollison, P. L. (1946) Br. Med. J., **i**, 5.
103. Simpson, K. (1953) Modern Trends in Forensic Medicine. London; Butterworths.
104. Layton, G. B. (1946) Lancet, **ii**, 73.

FURTHER READING

Armstrong, J. A., Fryer, D. I., Stewart. W. K. & Whittingham, H. E. (1955) Lancet, **i** 1135.
Children and Young Persons Act 1933, s.11.
Children and Young Persons (Amendment) Act 1952, s.8.

Ernsting, J. (1963) Guy's Hosp. Gaz., 367.
Hitchcock, F. A. (1964) In: Handbook of Physiology, Section 4, 835. American Physiological Society.
Lambertsen, C. J. (1965) In: Handbook of Physiology. Washington, D. C.: American Physiological Society, p. 1027.
Leading Article (1971) Br. Med. J., **iv**, 66.
Mason, J. K. (1962) Aviation Accident Pathology. London: Butterworths.
Mason, J. K. (1962) Aviation Accident Pathology. London: Chicago: College of American Pathologists Foundation.
Moritz, A. R. (1947) Am. J. Pathol., **23**, 915.
Respirator Lung Syndrome (Dr Parkinson's collection of reprints).
Waterworth, T. A. (1975) Injury. **1**, 89.

13

Mechanical asphyxia

Asphyxia may be defined as a state in which the body lacks oxygen because of some mechanical interference with the process of breathing. As pointed out by Taylor[1] in the first edition of this work under the term *asphyxia* are included those forms of violent death in which the act of respiration is primarily arrested. He noted that the literal translation from the Greek was 'pulselessness'. He suggested that since the state was induced by any cause which arrested the function of respiration the term *apnoea* (Greek 'respire') was more appropriate. In subsequent editions and elsewhere objections to the use of the term have been raised mainly on etymological grounds. Without indulging in semantics it may be recalled that similar objections can be applied to the various other terms which have been offered as substitutes. It is also a term which is well established in medico-legal affairs. Its continued use, therefore, seems appropriate within well defined limits.

The purpose of breathing is to convey oxygen from the atmosphere into the lungs and remove carbon dioxide from the lungs to the atmosphere. When the process is impeded there will be interference with the passage of both of these substances. Thus, in a standard text on the physiology of respiration[2] the definition of asphyxia is extended to a state in which two elements are combined.

1. *Hypoxia*, being a condition in which there is an inadequate supply of oxygen to the tissues, and

2. *Hypercapnoea*, being an increase in the carbon dioxide tension in the blood and tissues.

The normal levels of oxygen in arterial blood (Po_2) with a 95% saturation of haemoglobin range in value from 90 to 100 mmHg (12 to 13.5 kPa) at the age of 30 years to 65 to 80 mmHg (8 to 10 kPa)

at 60 years or more. Reduction to 60 mmHg (8 kPa) results in hypoxia even although the haemoglobin is 90% saturated. Forty mmHg (5 kPa) represents severe hypoxia and death might be expected when the level falls to 20 mmHg (3 kPa).[3]

Hypoxia can arise from a wide range of causes including natural disease. The various classifications are somewhat confusing, some being based on the physiological adaptation of the body to hypoxia, others to its pathological cause. A classification such as that illustrated by McIntyre[4] represents a useful summary. Most classifications of oxygen lack stem from Barcroft[5] who arranged hypoxia under three main headings:

1. *anoxic*—where the oxygen from the atmosphere cannot reach the blood;

2. *stagnant*—where the circulation of the blood is impaired;

3. *anaemic*—where the blood cannot contain enough oxygen.

Histotoxic—where there may be no oxygen lack but the tissues cannot utilise it was added later by Peters & van Slyke[6].

Thus, the forms of hypoxia which are mainly of forensic interest are those in which the process is primarily due to airways obstruction—*anoxic* (sometimes also called arterial) and *stagnant* (also known as hypokinetic) which results from a decreased blood flow.

It is perhaps useful to recall that asphyxia is a term which indicates a mode of dying rather than a cause of death, a factor of which we are reminded in a footnote which appears on the front of the Medical Certificate of Cause of Death at present in use in England.

It is clear that hypoxia can result from a number

of conditions apart from those in which there is mechanical interference with breathing. Some of the features in asphyxial deaths are those which are indicative only of hypoxia. Before they can be interpreted as evidence of mechanical asphyxia other features must be sought. These are:

1. evidence of mechanical interference with breathing such as pressure marks on the face or neck;
2. the local intensification of the hypoxic features indicating that the hypoxia is not general.

GENERAL FEATURES OF HYPOXIA

The general features of hypoxia associated with the hypoxic state are:

1. cyanosis;
2. increased capillary permeability;
3. petechial haemorrhages.

Cyanosis

From the Greek meaning 'dark blue', cyanosis indicates a blue colour of the skin, mucous membranes and of the internal organs, notably spleen, liver and kidneys. It may be general but is usually more marked in some regions than in others. The colour change is more pronounced in the skin, where hypostatic livid stains develop, and in the parts in which there is an abundant capillary and venous circulation, notably lips, ears, cheeks, and internally the lungs, liver, spleen, kidneys and meninges.

It is due to a change in the character of the circulating blood, being apparent when more than 5 g 100 ml of whole blood is in the form of reduced haemoglobin regardless of the total haemoglobin concentration.

The capillary dilatation that accompanies a reduction in oxygen tension promotes stasis and therefore a vicious cycle of suboxygenation of the blood commences. The return of blood to the heart is diminished. The resultant impaired oxygenation leads to further capillary dilatation, further stasis, with deepening cyanosis.

The margin between cyanosis and fatal hypoxia is small.[3]

While the diminished oxygen tension in the blood with a rise in proportion of the reduced hae-moglobin is the essential cause of cyanosis, there are modifying factors which may vary the threshold concentration of reduced haemoglobin in the capillary blood necessary to produce visible cyanosis.

These factors may also considerably change the intensity of cyanosis caused by a given amount of oxygen unsaturation.[7]

The factors are:

1. the thickness of the epidermis (which in itself has no blood vessels);
2. physiological or pathological pigmentation of the skin;
3. variation in the colour of the blood plasma;
4. variation in the concentration of oxidised hae-moglobin in blood;
5. variation in the number, width and length of blood-filled capillaries in a given surface area.

These modifying factors cannot, however, produce cyanosis themselves. They can influence the amount of oxygen unsaturation necessary to give the skin a perceptible blue colour and can modify the shade of colour produced.

Increased capillary permeability

Probably results from a combination of stasis and hypoxia. Fluid exudes into the tissue spaces. This may result in the moistening of tissues in the more affected parts, recognisable with the naked eye in the brain or possibly oedema in the mediastinal tissues and the lungs, and later the development of excess fluid in the pericardial and pleural sacs.

It must be stressed that this is a common finding in deaths due to various forms of natural cause, particularly when the lesions are only recognisable at microscopic level, such as pink coagulum as shown by H & E stains in the air spaces of the lungs.

It has been maintained that the amount of pulmonary oedema can be used to estimate the time interval between injury and death. In practice it is seldom of value as it is common experience that the changes described can develop with great rapidity when a patient dies after choking. It is also frequently found in various forms of rapidly fatal accidents in which there is probably some hypoxic element. Mason[8] has described pulmonary oedema in sudden deaths in aircraft accidents.

Swann[9] concludes from an experimental study

using animals that in various forms of 'sudden asphyxial deaths' pulmonary oedema occurs during the agonal period, which he describes as the time between the cessation of breathing and the cessation of heart action.

Petechial haemorrhages

Petechial haemorrhages occupy a hallowed place in the literature on asphyxial deaths. Although often referred to as 'Tardieu spots' they are not, as suggested by Tardieu[10] pathognomonic of asphyxiation. They are tiny haemorrhages, perhaps about pinpoint in size, often seen in the conjunctivae and the face (Fig. 13.1). They may be difficult to see, their presence being identified with certainty by the use of a hand lens. They may be more numerous, in some instances coalescing. Larger haemorrhages are sometimes seen in the upper chest, sometimes on the back of the body, apparently superimposed on intense post-mortem congestion.

Internally a careful search may reveal their presence in the larynx, air passages, pleurae and epi-

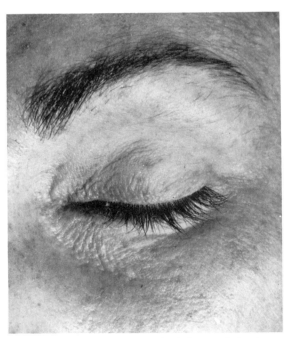

Fig. 13.1 A 31-year-old woman dead of strangulation by ligature. Petechiae are present around the eyes.

cardium. Occasionally they may be found in the bowel.

The criticism of their over-ready acceptance as proof of an asphyxial form of death is well summarised by Shapiro.[11]

As regards internal petechial haemorrhages these have been described by Gordon & Mansfield as developing spontaneously after death in serous membranes, i.e., visceral pericardium and visceral pleura.[12] They offer as an explanation the possibility that the haemorrhages on the ventral side of the heart may result from the trapping of blood in a group of dependent venules causing a rise in hydrostatic pressure followed with rupture of the walls. Serial sections showed that they were probably caused by rupture of the venules.

It appears likely that petechiae indicate stasis and increased capillary permeability which may be associated with hypoxia. There is no doubt that they tend to develop most pronouncedly in parts where the capillary pressure and dilatation are more rapidly developed, for instance in the scalp, eyelids and conjunctivae.

Local venous obstruction is in part responsible for the more rapidly developed capillary turgidity, early oedema and petechial haemorrhages that are a feature of slower deaths from constriction of the neck or compression of the chest.

As pointed out by Simpson[13] the distribution of such changes may often be diagnostic. They are important guides when the hypoxic state is not necessarily a general one but may be due to some local constriction.

Our findings in a large forensic practice are in accord with those of Polson & Gee[14] who note that petechial haemorrhages are not rare in sudden deaths from coronary disease. This does not, however, lead them to the belief that external petechial haemorrhages of the kind and distribution found in death from mechanical asphyxia occur in deaths from natural causes, even coronary disease, unless there is an asphyxial element in the circumstances of the death. Their significance on all occasions must be correlated with the circumstances. Their main value and importance is that they serve as a warning to the observer that he must consider mechanical asphyxia as a possible cause of, or factor in, the death.

SIGNS AND SYMPTOMS OF ASPHYXIA

The cellular response to hypoxia is complex as outlined by Alberti.[15] Equally complex are the various regulatory mechanisms of the cardiopulmonary system[4] which a lack of oxygen sets in motion and whose function is to control optimum gas tensions in the body tissues. They are complex and still not completely understood but well described in a standard physiological textbook such as Best & Taylor.[2] However, the successive phases of asphyxia which depend on this complex interrelationship of oxygen lack and increased levels of carbon dioxide appear to be fairly well established following numerous clinical observations.

The successive phases of asphyxiation are:

1. The respiratory rate is quickened and the depth of excursion increased: cyanosis develops. The pulse rate is accelerated and the blood pressure rises. These are signs of physiological response to the decreasing oxygen saturation of the blood.

2. Cyanosis deepens and respiration becomes more laboured; oedema develops in the lungs and salivation adds to the fluid in the throat and glottis. The pulse becomes more rapid and bounding, the blood pressure rises. The face, eyes and tongue may, when the throat is constricted, become turgid and bulge. Consciousness is clouded.

3. Respiration becomes irregular, punctuated by expiratory gasps; unconsciousness supervenes and convulsive movements may ensue. Minute vessels rupture both in the skin and internally, and blood may tinge the saliva and bronchial fluid. Vomit may regurgitate into the throat, and urine and faeces may be voided. The pulse becomes feebler and irregular, the blood pressure falls and death supervenes.

Asphyxia by violence

The features mentioned above are indicative only of hypoxia. Their presence alerts the pathologist to the possibility that death may be asphyxial in type, i.e., hypoxia associated with some mechanical interference with the process of breathing.

The two features which strengthen this view must then be sought:
1. evidence on the body of some mechanical interference with the process of breathing, and
2. a local intensification of hypoxial features indicating that the hypoxia is not general.

Thus, in some deaths with the features of hypoxia there may be local marks of injury, such as pressure marks on the face and neck, foreign material in the air passages. These give sound evidence as to the cause of the hypoxic process and they will be described in detail in the following pages.

Where hypoxic changes are localised to a certain part of the body, say in the head and neck, and are less pronounced elsewhere it is reasonable to suggest that there has been some local venous constriction as well as the obstruction of respiration, and their presence strongly suggests local violence. In an ideal situation there is intensified local distribution of hypoxic changes which coincide or can be matched with marks of violence.

Asphyxia can usually be distinguished from other forms of hypoxia but the findings are likely to be equivocal when:
1. there are no marks of injury as is often seen in suffocation by some soft object, or
2. the hypoxic changes are slight.

In the absence of marks of injury, the distribution of petechiae may strongly suggest the way in which breathing was obstructed although the pathologist is unable to offer conclusive evidence as to what happened. Thus there may be strong suspicion of mechanical interference with respiration and particularly the absence of any other cause of profound hypoxia must lend weight to this suspicion.

It is, therefore, essential that a forensic postmortem must include the detailed examination of all major organs in the body and microscopic preparations made to exclude thereby any reasonable possibility that there is any other cause for this hypoxic state.

If breathing is interfered with for a sufficient period of time unconsciousness and death will supervene. Pathologists are frequently asked as to how long an interval of time may have elapsed between the significant part of an assault and the loss of consciousness, and also the interval between the onset of unconsciousness and the time of death.

These questions are difficult to answer with any

certanty for the time interval involved must vary with a number of variable factors.

These must surely include:
1. the age of the victim;
2. the presence of natural disease;
3. the action of drugs and/or alcohol;
4. the degree of respiratory obstruction;
5. the way in which the obstruction has been applied.

Conclusions are sometimes based on experiments such as those described by Swann & Brucer[16] in which various animals were subjected to rapid anoxic death. These were conducted under laboratory conditions and how much of their findings can be translated to human affairs is arguable.

Direct unbiased evidence of the time intervals involved in human subjects is very uncommon. Nevertheless the time interval may be of the greatest importance to the proper understanding of the case.

Precise figures may not be possible and if ventured into can be misleading. In general terms it might be reasonable to suggest that evidence of mechanical obstruction in the complete absence of hypoxial features is consistent with death occurring almost immediately, possibly within a few seconds.

In cases where the obstructive process appears to have been less forcibly applied, or possibly intermittent, and the hypoxial features are pronounced, it again might be considered reasonable to suggest that these are more compatible with a longer period of time but unlikely to have exceeded 1 min. Some of the factors involved will be considered in more detail in the section on strangulation.

It appears, however, quite certain that in many instances unconsciousness can occur in several seconds.

The classical case described by Simpson[17] of *R. v. Southam.*

In *R. v. Southam* (Lewes Assizes 1950) an unusual case of deliberate suffocation was witnessed by a nurse. In her presence, the matron of a nursing home was seen to be forcibly restraining an elderly woman who refused to swallow a sleeping draught. The matron pinned her down on to the bed, holding her arms, and drew a pillow across her face by means of her teeth, pressing it there for what the nurse describes as 'several minutes' during which the old lady's struggles gradually ceased. It seems unlikely, however (from other evidence) that as long as 'several minutes' could have elapsed.

This matter will be considered again in the section on strangulation.

CONDITIONS ASSOCIATED WITH MECHANICAL ASPHYXIA

These include:
1. *Suffocation*—where the interference with the process of breathing is at the level of the nose or mouth.

Terms which may also be included in this category are *smothering* when some object, usually soft, is placed against the face, and *gagging* where something is stuffed into the mouth.
2. *Choking*—where foreign bodies block the internal air passages (larynx and bronchi).
3. *Drowning*—where the air passages are occluded by fluid.
4. *Strangulation*—where there is compression of the neck, either by:
a. the human hand (manual strangulation or throttling);
b. a ligature.
5. *Hanging*—when a ligature is applied to the neck and the force necessary for constriction is the weight of the body.
6. *Traumatic asphyxia*—where the respiratory movements are impaired by compression of the chest.

In each of these categories the obstructive process at the various levels will result in the development of the symptoms and signs associated with asphyxia previously described. These must vary with the type of interference, with the process of breathing and the amount of force involved. Their rapidity of onset and results must also vary with the health and general condition of the victim.

However, in each case one can expect to find, albeit in a varying degree, some of the general features of the hypoxic state and some local evidence of the type of mechanical interference, and possibly the amount of force involved. To support a suggestion that death resulted from a process of asphyxia their presence must be demonstrated.

Suffocation

Obstruction at the level of the nose and mouth may

occur when the face is pressed deeply into some yielding substance such as sand, corn, bedding and the like. The circumstances are usually accidental. Suicide or homicide are more likely when the occluding object is applied to the face.

General features

The changes associated with hypoxia are usually present and intense, as the obstruction may be intermittent or incomplete with a struggle to breathe. Less often, and usually in children and the aged, the hypoxic changes may be slight.

The head and face may show intense congestion and cyanosis with numerous petechiae. Blood exudes from the mouth and nose. Blood tinged frothy fluid is present in air passages. Mucus may be found at the back of the mouth and throat and is usually found in considerable quantity when associated with a gag.

Sometimes an area of pallor in an otherwise suffused face delineates a mark which may indicate the agent which caused the respiratory obstruction. Even in those cases where hypoxic changes are slight a careful search will usually reveal the presence of petechiae (Fig. 13.2).

Microscopically the presence of intense conges-

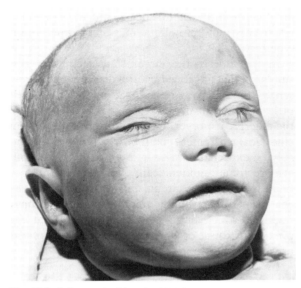

Fig. 13.2 A five-week-old male child found face downwards in carry-cot. Face suffused apart from an area around the nose and mouth. Scanty petechiae in the eyelids and numerous petechiae found internally.

tion in the major organs will be confirmed with sometimes the presence of tiny areas of haemorrhage.

The lungs, which are of particular interest, usually show in addition to congestion of inter-alveolar capillaries, the presence of oedema fluid in the alveoli, areas of haemorrhage and collapse with intervening emphysema.

The air passages often contain eosinophilic fluid with red blood cells and varying amounts of desquamated respiratory type epithelium.

The local evidence of mechanical interference with breathing must vary from the obvious cases in which the causative agent is still with the body, thus the presence of sand, gags and plastic bags are self-evident.

The presence of blood and mucus in the mouth and nose of someone found face downwards in bedding is obvious, but perhaps their precise role in the production of death is more difficult to evaluate.

When the human hand is the local factor there may be very little evidence, particularly if the amount of force applied is not greatly in excess of that required to occlude the air passages.

A careful search with proper mortuary facilities may reveal slight bruising of the inner aspect of the lips and tiny cuts in relation to the teeth against which the lips have been compressed.

The application of a soft object such as a pillow may leave no trace on the victim, especially in the young and the old.

Accident, suicide or murder?

The features mentioned above suggest how difficult it can be to determine how the asphyxial state has been caused and it is possibly more difficult still to demonstrate findings which can support a criminal charge.

The possibility of death related to natural causes must be considered.

Experienced forensic pathologists are well used to incidents where adults are found dead with the general features of hypoxia but no localising signs. Detailed autopsies fail to reveal any evidence of natural organic disease. On further investigation often the only significant finding is a history of epilepsy which has often been concealed from close

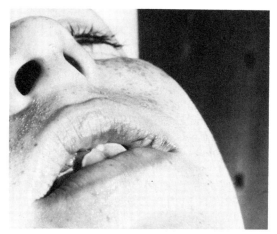

Fig. 13.3 A seven-year-old girl dead of homicidal suffocation. Two tiny cuts on the left upper lip (see illustrative case P. 21873).

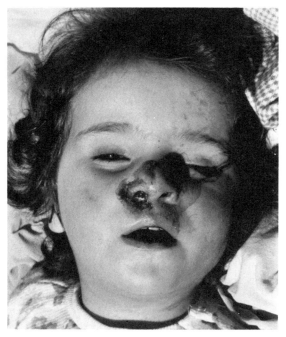

Fig. 13.4 Girl aged two years. Suffocation by hand (see illustrative case P. 24573).

associates. Adult deaths from this category usually occur when the person is already weak or unconscious either from disease or drugs. In these circumstances the involvement of another person and the possibility of homicide must be considered. Similarly with young children and old people little or no resistance might be expected. Evidence, therefore, of injury may be minimal (Fig. 13.3).

There is now widespread recognition that the vast majority of infant deaths previously thought to be due to suffocation or overlaying can rightly be included in the so-called 'Sudden Unexpected Death in Infancy Syndrome',[18] these being deaths which are natural but of undetermined cause. Thus the unfortunate relatives of the children of these 'cot deaths' are spared the anxieties associated with police investigation and possible Court appearances as has happened so often in earlier times.

In our own practice about 50% of 'cot deaths' show no abnormal features either at post-mortem examination or in subsequent laboratory investigations. In many there is evidence only of a generalised hypoxic process.

It must also be agreed that often the precise way in which the infant has died of suffocation is not revealed at autopsy. Thus, it is considered a hazard that there may be the over-ready use of the convenient label of 'cot death' in cases with essentially negative post-mortem findings, particularly those with some hypoxial features which may include some cases of suffocation (Fig. 13.4).

The background to the death and the circumstances in which the body was found are often of help in the absence of localising signs at autopsy.

Also the forensic scientist may help if he can find material from the victim such as mucus, squamous respiratory type epithelium, on suitable smothering type material.[19]

In the elderly the circumstances are not dissimilar in that advanced natural disease may be present. This may be at the stage in which there is little impairment of the restricted daily routine of the elderly. However, unusual physical exertion or emotional excitement, both of which might reasonably be expected to arise in attempted suffocation, can precipitate sudden death, with atypical autopsy findings. Again the circumstances surrounding the death must be considered together with the autopsy findings, which often may only suggest that the proximate cause of death was obstruction of the process of breathing (Fig. 13.5).

In adults the problem is usually more easily solved with well developed hypoxial features and recognisable localising marks, because of the degree of force necessary.

Those deaths in which difficulties can arise in

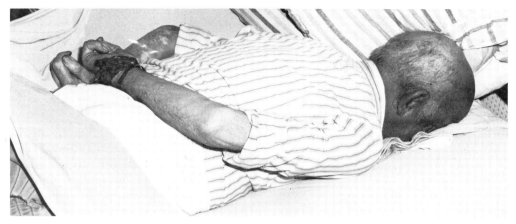

Fig. 13.5 A 64-year-old man found face downwards with his hands tied behind his back. Death was considered to be due to advanced coronary atherosclerosis in the course of an erotic exercise.

practice are usually related to sexual activity.

The first group usually concerns women who are found partially unclothed and dead, face downwards. The mechanical blockage of the nose and mouth by the usual bedding has been aggravated by an apparently rapid accumulation of saliva, mucus and possibly blood, the combination leading to suffocation (Fig. 13.6).

The problem here is how much force was involved and how long it has taken for death to ensue. It may be suggested that death was of the vasovagal type and instantaneous and that the accumulations of secretions were a post-mortem or agonal phenomenon.

An evaluation of the extent of the hypoxic features, the type and nature of marks, together with microscopic examination of the relevant areas usually are of assistance.

In Simpson's classical case:[17]

R. v. Heath (C. C. C. 1946) the first of two victims, Margery Gardner, was found dead, face upwards in bed with her hands tied by the wrists behind her, and her ankles also tied. She was naked, and both bite marks and whipping impressions were visible on the body. Some of these lay across the back, and as the face was turgid and blotchy—and asphyxial petechiae were present in the lungs—it was suspected that, whilst turned face down into the bedding and being whipped she had met her death from suffocation. In fact, enquiry revealed a scarf soiled by saliva in an attaché case left by Heath at Bournemouth railway station, and he subsequently admitted having bound and gagged his victim before assaulting her. There was nothing at autopsy to indicate these details.

Since the widespread publicity on the dangers associated with plastic bags accidental suffocation

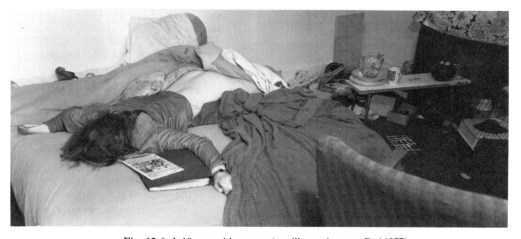

Fig. 13.6 A 19-year-old woman (see illustrative case P. 16377).

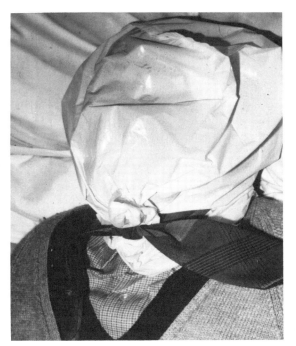

Fig. 13.7 A 65-year-old man found dead in bed. No signs of injury or disease. A suicide note was left.

of children by this means has become rare. They are still, however, the method of choice by some for suicide. The circumstances usually are such that there is little difficulty in establishing this. In our practice the number of cases of suicide with plastic bags is divided equally between the sexes (Fig. 13.7).

When cases of frank suicide are eliminated we are left with a second group of cases in which the plastic bag appears to be associated with sexual activity. These cases in our own practice to date occur only in males.

In such cases the hypoxic features may be slight. Often the head and face enclosed in a plastic bag are pale. There may be a few petechial haemorrhages in the eyelids; frequently these are not detected.

Internally there are subepicardial petechiae of the heart but usually there is little else of note.

In about half our cases some stomach content is present in the upper air passages and this is not usually associated with any great inflammatory response.

Usually the interior of the bag contains abundant droplets of moisture and, as pointed out by Polson

& Gee[20], it is misleading to suggest that this could be the result of breathing inside the bag as we can confirm that the organs and moist inanimate objects also can 'breathe' when enclosed in plastic.

The circumstances in which the body is found usually clearly indicate auto-erotic activity. The scene of death is a secluded place such as a locked room or deserted woodland. It may be naked or dressed in female clothing. If normally dressed the genitalia are often exposed. Erotic literature is often arranged nearby and mirrors may be placed so that the practitioner can view himself.

The process is sometimes combined with the inhalation of 'sniffing substances' such as ether, amyl nitrate or cleaning fluids, and pads soaked with the appropriate solution are found with the bag (Fig. 13.8).

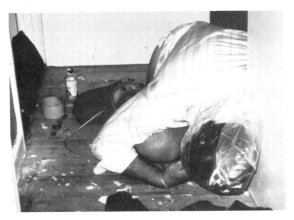

Fig. 13.8 A 29-year-old man. A pad containing cleaning fluid was enclosed in the plastic bag. Pornographic literature was present in his briefcase nearby.

The bag may be secured around the neck by an elastic band or a ligature. This ligature may form part of a system of bondage which also is attached to the genitalia. Bondage can be very elaborate and evidence considerable ingenuity and industry by the deceased. In addition to ropes and string, electric flex, lengths of chain with padlocks are often applied. The bondage is of obvious interest to the investigating police officer. The complexity of the arrangement when examined in detail at autopsy can cause difficulty and sometimes it has to be suggested that the assistance of another person in applying the bondage must be considered. An interesting recent account of a homicide masquerading as sexual asphyxia is that given by Wright & Davis.[21]

Illustrative cases

Accidental suffocation—baby—11 weeks. After feeding the baby the mother left it for some 20 min. On returning she found the two-year-old child sitting on a cushion which was on top of the baby's head. The face was suffused apart from an area of pallor on the brow, nose and upper cheeks. Some mucoid material exuded from the left nostril. Internally there was intense congestion of the lungs with large subpleural haemorrhages, particularly in the lower lobes, subepicardial petechiae at the base of the heart and some large haemorrhages in the thymus. Microscopy showed only intense congestion with haemorrhage throughout all lobes of the lungs (p. 25576).

Homicidal suffocation—boy four years—girl two years. Father admitted killing them by placing his hands over their faces. In the elder child the face was pale apart from the lips which were cyanosed. Tiny petechiae were present in the left eye. No recent marks of injury were detected either on the outside or after detailed internal dissection. The younger child's face was pale. A little white frothy mucus exuded from the right side of the mouth. The front of the nose, the upper lip and the left side of the face were smeared with blood which appeared to have trickled from the left nostril and run across the face. There were no injuries. Hypostasis, which was intense, was confined to the posterior dependent parts of the body apart from the areas of contact flattening. The only petechiae detected were a few in the subepicardium at the base of the heart. Dissection of the head and neck structures showed no obvious injury (P. 24573) (see Fig. 13.4).

Homicidal suffocation—girl—seven years. The body of a seven-year-old girl was found on a canal bank, partially concealed by bushes. The accused man was alleged to have subsequently stated: 'I came over funny and I suffocated her with my coat'. The injuries which were slight included: a $\frac{1}{8}$ inch circular bruise on the front of the nose, barely discernable; a semi-circular scratch on the left brow, $1\frac{1}{4}$ inches in length; a horizontal scratch on the left brow, 1 inch in length; two cuts on the

inside of the left upper lip close to the margin, each $\frac{1}{8}$ inch in length; some blood tinged mucus exuded from the nostrils; petechiae were not found on the face which was suffused. Numerous subepicardial petechiae were present at the base of the heart posteriorly. The genitalia were uninjured although dark pubic type hairs were recovered and a recent $\frac{1}{8}$ inch bruise was present on the upper posterior margin of the anus (P. 21873) (see Fig. 13.3).

Homicidal suffocation—woman—19 years. A 19-year-old woman was found naked from the waist, face downwards on a bed. Hypostasis, which was intense, was confined to the front of the body. The face and upper chest were intensely suffused apart from a white pressure type mark on the left cheek. Numerous petechiae were present in the eyelids. A large strand of hair lay across the face and front of the mouth. Internally a $\frac{1}{8}$ inch cut was present on the inside of the right lower lip. The soft tissues at the back of the mouth and in the neck were congested with numerous petechiae around the epiglottis. Abundant blood tinged froth filled the air passages. The neck showed no mark of injury and no recognisable impression from a fine silver chain and medallion which encircled the neck and was intact. The accused admitted to anal intercourse. A plea of manslaughter was accepted (P 16377) (see Fig. 13.6).

Homicidal suffocation—woman—71 years. A 71-year-old woman was found on the floor of a cupboard, fully dressed. The hands were secured to the front of the lower chest by two ligatures. A gag composed of two strips of towelling type material encircled the face and was tightly applied to the mouth. The face was intensely suffused apart from a pale band which corresponded with the ligature. Petechiae were widespread and particularly numerous in the eyelids. The eyes showed larger areas of bleeding. Seven relatively superficial wounds were present on the top of the head. Internally a lower set of dentures had been displaced backwards by the gag. Numerous petechiae were present in the upper lip, back of the tongue and larynx. It was thought that the head injuries had rendered the deceased unconscious and that she was then carried upstairs and placed in the cupboard when the accumulation of fluid and the gag caused death from suffocation. The post-mortem findings were considered to be consistent with this. One accused was found guilty to murder and the other to manslaughter (P 21476).

Choking

This category as a cause of an asphyxial type of death is closely related to suffocation in its mechanics and effects. It refers to the blockage of the upper air passages (the glottis, larynx, trachea and main bronchi) by some solid substance. It must be distinguished from those conditions in which the stomach content is found in the air passages, as this latter condition represents a reflux to food which has already been swallowed.

Choking as a cause of sudden death has been recognised since the time of Hippocrates and there are numerous records of the process throughout history.[22]

Almost all chokings are accidental; they occur mainly in the very young and the elderly and when they do occur in adults they are largely seen in patients from mental hospitals. These patients are usually described by the clinical staff as 'greedy people who bolt their food'.

Pieces of food, such as lumps of meat, orange, onion and potato, are the commonest agents found. They usually show no evidence of having been chewed.

Most pathologists have a list of other objects which are numerous and varied. Our own cases include socks, draughtsmen, bottle tops, coins and solid faecal material.

In some instances there must be suspicion that the death is homicidal and in these, with the absence of other marks, it is not possible to disprove accident on autopsy findings alone.

Microscopic examination of the lungs are nonspecific in that there is intense interalveolar congestion, haemorrhages of varying size with intraalveolar oedema and collections of desquamated respiratory type epithelium. Occasional fragments of the causal agent are sometimes seen.

In the majority of cases reliable observations are available by trained observers such as nursing staff, and in some, death appears to be a sudden collapse in the course of a meal and the autopsy findings do not indicate a hypoxic type of death. These may be attributed to some vagal inhibitory process.

In others there is a struggle to breathe and

attempts to remove the occluding object are unsuccessful. In these cases hypoxic features are usually well pronounced.

Of forensic interest are those cases of assault in which a person with head or facial injuries is found at autopsy to have a large collection of blood and mucus at the back of the throat and sometimes lower down in the air passages as far as the smaller bronchioles.

It may be suggested that as these victims have a high level of alcohol and a stomach distended by drink, the increased tendency of a drunk to vomit may be the significant factor in the cause of death. It must be agreed that these cases can cause difficulty.

It is perhaps worth recalling that the presence of stomach content in the air passages is by definition not necessarily choking and the significance of finding stomach content in the respiratory tract after death can present some problems.

Most forensic pathologists can readily support the experimental work of Gardner[22]. A reasonable explanation is the lack of normal protective mechanisms of the air passages—being no longer available after death.

Knight[23] in a pilot series found that 25% of deaths from various causes revealed macroscopic evidence of gastric contents in the air passages. In no case did the clinical history suggest regurgitation of stomach content in life. Our own observations would suggest that this is a relatively low figure.

In addition it seems that the regurgitation of stomach contents into the air passages is more likely to occur in an asphyxial type of death from any cause.

Our own experience using routine microscopy in such cases is that it is generally possible, even in sudden deaths, to make a reasonable suggestion that the process occurred at or about the time of death and is not purely a post-mortem phenomenon.

Drowning

The mechanism of death in drowning is complex. It is now widely accepted that the earlier definition of an asphyxial death due to submersion in water is an oversimplification of the matter. The other factors involved will be considered shortly.

It has been suggested[24] that the term 'drowning' should be used to denote the process resulting from submersion in water in which there is loss of consciousness and a threat to life. Drowning occurs when an individual is unable to remain afloat in water.

There are sufficient eye witness reports to outline the sequence of events as it generally happens. The swimmer remains on the surface until he is exhausted and then the sequence of events is apparently similar to that which affects those unable to swim. If the person falls into the water the momentum of the body will cause it to sink further.

A drowning person apparently sinks and rises a number of times in the water, inhaling a little water into the air passages causing violent coughing. He continues to rise and sink with further coughing and choking. Some water is inhaled into the lungs. With the increasing hypoxia consciousness is lost, vomiting may take place and large amounts of water are inhaled. Some water may also enter the stomach. The body then sinks.

The permeability of the alveolar membrane and hydrostatic and osmotic force play an important part in the direction of movement of the inhaled fluid and its solutes.

The ultimate cause of death in drowning has been studied in detail in animals by Swann & Brucer.[16] In general the sequence of events they noted is essentially similar to those mentioned above. Once the water reached the alveoli which, of course, presents an enormous area through which osmotic interchange can take place, the course of events is different, depending on whether the drowning fluid is freshwater or seawater.

When freshwater enters the alveolar spaces it is rapidly taken up by the pulmonary circulation resulting in gross local haemodilution. There is also local haemolysis and free haemoglobin is present in the plasma. The animal's blood streams are inundated with water, usually by the 3rd minute after submergence. Dilution of the blood components after 3 min reaches a disastrous level.

In seawater drowning a reverse osmotic flow occurs due to the higher saline content of the seawater. Water leaves the circulation and enters the alveolar spaces resulting in local haemoconcentration in the pulmonary circulation.

The changes observed in the two types of exper-imental drowning are explained by Swann & Spafford[25] by contrasting tonicity of the drowning medium with that of blood. It is apparent that the pulmonary epithelium is extremely permeable to all ions except sulphate. In seawater drowning salts diffuse in one direction while waters diffuse in the reverse direction. Pulmonary oedema, however, appears to take place simultaneously with the diffusion process in both types of drowning.

Death tends to occur earlier in freshwater drowning, with an abrupt fall in pulse pressure. This is considered due to the onset of ventricular fibrillation which did not occur in dogs drowned in seawater and is believed to be due to the fall in the sodium concentration of the blood reaching the left heart.

The potassium concentration is less reduced—because of haemolysis and the increase in plasma potassium following anoxia. This disturbance of the potassium/sodium ratio is an additional factor in the production of ventricular fibrillation.

While these studies are in keeping with the widely held clinical impression that drowning in freshwater is produced more rapidly, how far the findings can be extrapolated to human cases of drowning is in some doubt. A further difficulty, as pointed out by Crosfill[26] is that these experiments were conducted on animals which were totally immersed.

The biochemical findings in human subjects who have survived drowning are much less definite. In clinical cases[27] it is noted that atrial fibrillation was only seen in one case.

It is also pointed out that in discussing the theory of Swann & Spafford[25] the ventricular fibrillation is thought to be the result of haemolysis of red blood cells with the liberation of potassium, which in the presence of hypoxaemia leads to ventricular fibrillation.

In the dog erythrocyte, however, the main intracellular cation is not potassium but sodium and hence the release of intercellular potassium cannot be the full explanation. It is considered that ventricular fibrillation or any cardiac arrhythmia is rare in near drowning.

It must be recalled that irrespective of the type of water inhaled it will contain significant quantities of particular matter, such as Diatoms and other chemical material, some inert and some reactive. Once this material comes into contact with the alveolar membrane an inflammatory reaction will occur. This situation will interfere with gaseous exchange across the alveolar-capillary membrane.

Giammona[28] commenting on the findings of Swann notes that both Fuller and Modell have emphasised the importance of the hypoxaemia being due to an inadequacy of gas exchange across the lungs because of the presence of fluid in the lungs. Giammona & Modell[29] also stress the importance of changes in pulmonary surfactants in characterising some of the differences between freshwater and seawater drowning. They note that all authors who have reported on drowning studies have emphasised that the volume and electrolyte changes are of lesser importance than hypoxaemia in those victims who are resuscitable and brought to the hospital for further therapy.

As the circulation is usually maintained for a time after the lungs are filled, changes may be expected earlier and are more noticeable in the blood on the left side of the heart.

Gettler in 1921[30] made chloride determination of 22 people who died from causes other than drowning, 19 who drowned in saltwater and three who had drowned in freshwater. He believed that a difference of 25 mg of sodium chloride between the two sides of the heart would indicate death by drowning. In freshwater drowning the chloride of the blood on the left side of the heart was lower than that on the right side and the reverse situation was noted in saltwater drowning. He did, of course, point out that there might be no significant difference if death was caused by the shock of immersion rather than drowning. In drowned or nearly drowned humans evidence of substantial fluid shift was found.

Durlacher, Freimuth & Swann,[31] comparing the biochemical data of the plasma in the right and left atria of drowned human subjects, found no difference between fresh and seawater groups as far as potassium, sodium and chloride was concerned. Five out of 10 control (non-drowning) cases would have been diagnosed as drowning cases.

Fuller[32] in a review of 50 cases of near drowning could find no differences in the electrolyte conditions of the blood in sea or freshwater victims. This is also the view of Rivers, Orr & Lee[27] from laboratory findings of cases of secondary drowning, i.e., cases which survive.

Gettler's test may be considered to be possibly valid when water entered the lungs and the heart subsequently beats a few times.

Modell et al,[33] state that if aspiration in humans has been pronounced and provided that the determinations are done very early in the resuscitative period, definite, although small, differences may be found. They suppose that in the surviving human there is a rapid spontaneous redistribution that masks any fluid shift.

As regards post-mortem cases, in general terms these findings are probably of interest if the examinations are carried out soon after death.

Differences of significance tend to disappear as putrefaction progresses and as, therefore, in forensic work, in which victims of drowning have either been immersed for some time and possibly more important there has been some delay between recovery of the body and autopsy, such findings are of limited value.

Jetter & Moritz[34] found that in both dogs and man there is a progressive loss of plasma chlorides accompanied by an increase in plasma magnesium which is a normal post-mortem phenomenon. The changes do not always occur at the same rate in the two sides of the heart. In freshwater drowning the plasma chloride may be reduced in both sides of the heart to levels below those usually encountered in comparable samples from control subjects and their reduction may be considered greater in the left side than in the right.

In a forensic practice in which both fresh and saltwater drowning cases are not infrequent we have been unable to find any significant differences in an admittedly small number of cases in which some degree of putrefactive change has not been present.

Further experimental work by den Otter[35] on dogs in which one lung was drowned, the other being kept ventilated, suggested that the electrolyte changes were less pronounced than those induced by Swann,[9] thus confirming the important role of reactionary pulmonary oedema 'which is a collateral phenomenon increasing the aqueous inundation' and hence contributing to the fatal outcome.

Therefore, these biochemical findings are of limited value in forensic practice, or rather in solving the practical problems which arise in forensic practice, a view which we share with Timperman[36].

Post-mortem appearances in the drowned

These must vary according to the time during which the body has remained in water and the period which has elapsed before it is examined.

It may be a convenient point to recall that certain factors influencing the process of decomposition are peculiar to immersion. The body may be found in still or running water, polluted or clean water, fresh or saltwater. All of these have their own influence on subsequent decomposition because of their varying bacterial and animal content.

Owing to the more rapid cooling of the body in water and since for the greater part of the year in England the temperature of the water remains below the atmospheric temperature for the whole of the 24 h, decomposition *per se* tends to proceed more slowly than in air. When the water temperature is persistently below 40 to 45°F the body may show no appreciable decomposition after several weeks immersion. At 50 to 70°F it may be expected after—say—three to five days.

It is a common finding that while the lower part of the body may be in reasonably fresh condition the upper part, including the head, shows the colour changes of decomposition. This may be explained by the fact that the head floats lower than the rest of the body and blood gravitates first to the head and neck. On removing the body from water further putrefactive change develops with remarkable rapidity.

External appearances

When a body has been in the water for a matter of hours and the subsequent autopsy performed within a short period of time cyanosis may be present, but the skin is more often pallid and cold. It shows pimpling in the form of cutis anserina (goose skin). This is not uncommon since rigor of the erector pilae muscles can produce a similar reaction in many other forms of death. The skin is generally sodden, particularly the hands and feet, with more prolonged immersion whether life is present or not (Fig. 13.9). The skin is often blotchy from irregularly distributed areas of discoloration because

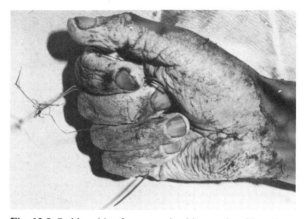

Fig. 13.9 Sodden skin after seven days' immersion. Note the grass firmly clenched in the hand.

movements of the body in the water have prevented the usual development of the livid stains which occur in bodies which have not moved. These may be pink or even bright red if the body is cold, but again in some cases hypostasis is confined to the head, neck and front of the chest as these parts are at a lower level than the rest of the body in a drowned person.

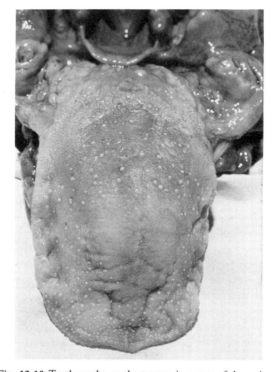

Fig. 13.10 Teeth marks on the tongue in a case of drowning.

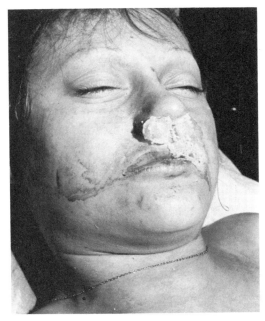

Fig. 13.11 Drowning in the bath. Note fine foam. Nail mark on cheek.

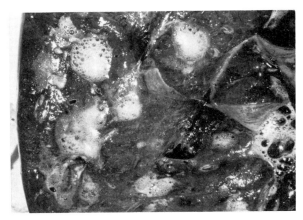

Fig. 13.12 Section of lung showing abundant froth exuding from the cut surface.

The tongue may be thrust between the lips and sometimes has teeth marks (Fig. 13.10). The lips and nostrils may be covered by a fine foam oozing from them (Fig. 13.11). It may be tinged with blood. It can be wiped away but will come back.

The eyes are often congested but petechial haemorrhages are rare. The pupils may be dilated.

Sometimes substances floating in the water or forming the base of the river or sea, such as gravel, mud, sand, weeds, are found in the ears or under the nails.

Internal appearances

In those cases which are examined before putrefaction has developed the main findings are in the lungs which will be distended, completely filling the chest cavity. They are crepitant and do not collapse on sectioning.

In freshwater drowning the tissues contain some foam and little fluid. On sectioning some frothy fluid tinged with blood may escape.

In drowning cases in saltwater, when they are examined sufficiently early, the lungs may be heavier, more markedly waterlogged and on sec-

tioning a much larger quantity of fluid pours out (Fig. 13.12).

In practice the distinction between drowning in the two types of fluid is perhaps less clear cut than one may be led to believe from the literature.

The air passages from the glottis to the smaller bronchi usually contain fine froth, sometimes tinged with blood. Silt, sand and pieces of water weed may also be seen (Fig. 13.13). Sometimes regurgitated stomach content can be found in the air passages. Occasionally some subpleural haemorrhages are seen but this is unusual. They may be present elsewhere, in the subepicardial region of the heart posteriorly. The stomach content may contain water and foreign material, such as sand and weeds, which are sometimes also seen in the lungs.

Microscopy

There is distension of the alveoli, some of the alveolar ducts and sometimes terminal bronchioles. Some of the alveolar walls are ruptured. Reh[37] is quoted by Timperman[36] as describing four stages as revealed by the Gomori silver impregnation method. There is progressive reduction in width of the alveolar walls, later complete intraseptal ruptures. In the terminal stage there are multiple ruptures. The septal stumps are retracted and appear thickened. Similar findings to some extent can be identified with routine H & E stained sections.

In some cases of drowning, usually in deep sea-

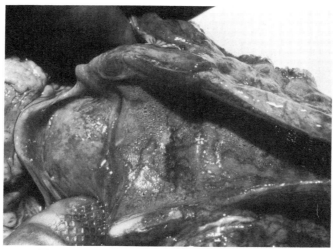

Fig. 13.13 Blood tinged froth in the upper air passages.

water, haemorrhage can be found in the middle ear and mastoid air cells as described by Niles,[38] although it has been recorded in cases from shallow water.

Massive haemorrhage can be recognised in the region of the middle ear at the base of the skull without removing the temporal bones. In less well marked cases the bone must be removed for their demonstration and minor cases can be detected only by microscopic examination.

The pathogenesis of temporal bone haemorrhage is not known but is thought to be that of barotrauma. Thus, the pressure differential between the middle ear and the surrounding water causes the formation of a relative vacuum. This negative pressure within the closed cavity causes inward stretching of the tympanic membrane.

Another possible mechanism is the aspiration of fluid into the eustachian tube with related haemorrhage from either an increase in pressure within the middle ear or from an irritant effect on the vascular mucosa.

Late effects following immersion

In those cases which have survived, delayed death may be accompanied by inflammation of the lung with development of bronchopneumonic consolidation with hyaline membranes in alveoli and alveolar ducts.

Regardless of the drowning medium, the organic and inorganic content of the inhaled fluid produces an inflammatory reaction in the alveolar capillary membrane which quickly leads to an out-pouring of plasma-rich exudate into the alveoli. This is further complicated by the loss of the normal surfactant by the inhaled water which can result in large areas of atelectasis.

In longer survivors granulomatous inflammation can occur with foreign body type reactions. This is presumably due to contamination with toxic substances in the immersion fluid.

Fuller[32] reported a fatal immersion syndrome in which the victims were unconscious but clinically resuscitated. Autopsy demonstrated haemorrhagic desquamative pneumonia. In those surviving more than a few days empyema and multiple abscesses were often found, cerebral oedema with anoxic changes in the frontal and parietal cortex with patchy loss of neurones and spotty necrosis in the hippocampus and thalamus. Focal necrosis of the spleen and renal tubular necrosis were found occasionally. All these findings were attributed to hypoxia and pulmonary oedema secondary to aspiration.

Diatoms

These findings, particularly when decomposition has set in, can be no more than suggestive that death was due to drowning. Other possible causes associated with immersion will be considered later.

A major advance in the diagnosis of death by drowning was made in 1904 by Revenstorf[39] who showed that microscopic particular matter could penetrate the peripheral regions of the lung and be detected there by microscopic examination. The particular matter, generally called plankton (the Greek 'drifting') includes algae, a variety of microscopic debris, and Diatoms.

Diatoms or Bacillariophyceae are a class of microscopic unicellular algae which are found whenever there is water and sufficient light to support photosynthesis.

There are about 15 000 species known to science. Roughly half of them live in freshwater while the remainder live in sea or in brackish water.

The systematic classification of Diatoms is based on the structure of their siliceous valves and is, therefore, somewhat involved.[40]

For forensic purposes their precise classification is of less importance than their distribution, and if in difficulty the help of an expert biologist is usually available.

It is now widely accepted that in cases of drowning in water containing Diatoms a number of these are taken into the lungs (Fig. 13.14).

The extensive literature has been admirably summarised by Timperman.[41]. His own studies with Thomas clarify the somewhat conflicting reports which appear throughout the literature.

Their value depended on the supposition that once Diatoms had reached the lungs only in a live body could they be carried by the blood stream to other parts of the body, such as the brain and marrow. This presupposed that the heart was still beating and pumping blood around the body.

While a Diatom differs little from many other plant cells if it is regarded solely as a physiological unit, in the structure of the cell it is unique in that it secretes a hard siliceous outer box-like skeleton called a frustule and as this is chemically inert and almost indestructible it tends to persist for long periods of time. Thus, when tissue is chopped up and digested in strong acids it is possible to remove the soft tissues and to be left with the acid-resistant Diatoms.

The earlier enthusiasm for their value was dampened by reports such as those of Spitz & Schnei-

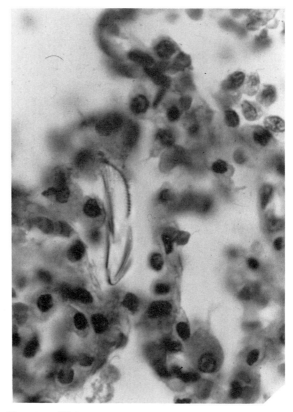

Fig. 13.14 High power photograph of lung showing Diatom in situ.

der[42] and Spitz, Schmidt & Fett[43] who found Diatoms in 96% of non-drowning cases.

Other workers, notably Muller,[44] provided detailed evidence of their absence in carefully controlled conditions.

The detailed studies of Thomas, Van Hecke & Timperman[45] have shown that the method is reliable provided adequate precautions are taken to prevent contamination at each stage in the process.

In our own series of cases we have, but rarely, found Diatoms in the lungs of persons who have not died from drowning. In these cases Diatoms are scanty and a possibility of post-mortem contamination was considered to be likely. For instance, tap water can contain Diatoms and tap water may be filtered through sand or diatomite. Ordinary laboratory filter paper can contain Diatoms.

We have found Diatoms in putrefied lungs from cases in which the submerged body was probably dead before immersion. In these cases Diatoms have not been found in other organs. The organs examined routinely comprise lung, liver, brain and bone marrow.

Rigorous precautions are taken at all stages of collection and preparation. Controlled preparations are prepared to exclude the possibility of contamination from materials. A series of random non-drowning cases, i.e., the first body to be examined on Tuesday mornings, has not shown any Diatoms.

We are, therefore, convinced that in a body in which there is no gross mutilation, their presence in organs other than lung is diagnostic of death due to drowning.

Hendey[46] suggests that the full significance of the method is not apparent until the problem is approached from a totally non-medical point of view, until it is regarded as an exercise in plant ecology and the Diatom is considered as an organism in its own right.

He points out that one must bear in mind that when examining tissues for Diatoms from persons believed to have died from drowning it is most important that every care should be taken to see that if Diatoms are found they belong to the flora inhabiting the water mass at the point where the body was found.

He also reminds us that the pattern of Diatom reproduction is somewhat unusual and the number of Diatoms present in water will vary at different times of the year with a population peak in the spring and another, but less pronounced, in the autumn.

Timperman also reminds us that increasing pollution can have a considerable effect on the number of Diatoms available.

Thus from the biologist's point of view criticisms of the Diatom test can be answered, namely that some known cases of death from drowning have shown no Diatoms. Obviously the details of the season are important, the concentration of the flora and the amount of water inhaled.

As regards the second criticism that Diatoms have been found in the organs of persons who have died from causes other than drowning Hendey[46] points out that:

1. A large number of Diatoms are ingested with unprepared foods eaten raw, such as salads, watercress, which come into contact with the soil Diatoms, and particularly shellfish such as mussels, limpets, winkles, cockles and oysters, which feed exclusively on Diatoms.

2. There is extensive use of diatomaceous earth for industrial purposes. It is used extensively in building, chemical processes and insulating material. It is reasonable, therefore, that people living in the immediate vicinity of such industry will be exposed to Diatoms in the atmosphere.

3. There is contamination by Diatom-containing dusting powder, formerly extensively used by pathologists on rubber gloves.

Hendey[46] considers, however, that their presence from the sources outlined above amply confirm that the Diatom test is only valid if it can be shown that the species recovered from the pathological specimens are all present in the sample from the site of drowning. All species of Diatoms in the pathological specimens other than those represented in the site sample must be ignored.

These conditions place the Diatom test on a firm scientific basis and satisfactorily combat criticisms which have been levelled against this test.

Other causes of death on immersion

There are undoubtedly cases in which signs of drowning are absent altogether or minimal. These constitute in most series some 10 to 15% of deaths associated with immersion. There is a marked lack of water in the lungs at necropsy. It is usual to postulate a sudden acute laryngospasm. In others some form of reflex inhibition of the heart is postulated.

In this connection Keatinge et al,[47] in experimental studies on the effect of cold water on swimming, noted that before rectal temperature fell the swimmer suddenly floundered after developing respiratory distress. Two fatter men in Keatinge's series were able to swim through this period of uncontrolled hyperventilation. Keatinge suggests that their greater buoyancy led to the expenditure of less effort in simply keeping afloat. He postulates that the respiratory distress can be explained by the effect of reflexes from cutaneous cold receptors. He admits that reflexly-induced cardiac arrhythmias may occasionally cause the deaths of healthy young men in water but considers that this is a rare occurrence and that acute respiratory conditions are a far more frequent hazard in life.

Another possible cause occurs sometimes in

trained swimmers who take several deep breaths before submerging to prolong their underwater swimming time. This hyperventilation appears to cause an increase in arterial oxygen content which is negligible. The hyperventilation is also associated with a rapid fall in the level of carbon dioxide. This can result, in addition to the apparently desired lack of stimulus to breathe, in a reduced cerebral blood flow leading to underwater loss of consciousness which usually leads to death.[48]

Submersion deaths in association with alcohol are well known to forensic pathologists and have been considered by Giertsen.[49] A reasonable explanation, he suggests, is that alcohol can produce a cutaneous vasodilation with loss of heat and a fall in body temperature. The skin temperature rises leading to an increased gradient between skin and water temperature. Consequently the stimulus reacting on the cold receptors in the skin on immersion becomes stronger.

The recovery of an immersed body

After drowning has occurred the body usually sinks and then may reappear after a variable period of time. The time interval depends on:
1. the nature of the water—salt or fresh;
2. the specific gravity of the body;
3. the rate of putrefactive change.

It may be recalled that according to the principle of Archimedes a body in water will experience a buoyant force equal to the weight of water it displaces. Also the specific gravity of the body relates the weight and volume of the body to that of the water. The specific gravity of the human body is very close to that of water. Small variations, therefore, have considerable effect on the buoyancy.

In a study in which the specific gravity and buoyancy were calculated related to specific volume of air in the lungs of each subject Donoghue & Minnigerode[50] concluded that all subjects would be capable of floating in either freshwater or seawater at total lung capacity. At functional residual capacity (the approximate lung volume of a dead body), 69% of the subjects would float in seawater whereas only 7% would float in freshwater.

In addition to the amount of air in the lungs, the specific gravity of the human body varies with the size and composition of that body. The weight of the skeleton is balanced against the amount of fat present. Thus women generally have a lower specific gravity than men while infants and young children appear to float more readily than adults.

Clothing will tend to support the body initially with natural buoyancy and later perhaps assist in sinking because of its weight. The addition of weights to the body will also assist the process.

Thus, as a general rule the body with water in the lungs and stomach will sink. It will go down to the bottom because hydrostatic pressure which increases with depth will compress what gas is present and thus increase specific gravity. There it may remain until, if it is free to move, the formation of the gases of putrefaction will decrease the specific gravity. It will then rise to the surface and float.

In any consideration of the rate of putrefaction in water the following features must be considered:
1. The route which has been taken by the body from its entry point to the place where it was found. In the Thames a difference of 9°C has been noted in the temperature of the water at different sides of the river at the same level.
2. The body may have been caught at a deep level where the temperature is lower and the putrefactive process is thus slower.
3. The time between the body being again exposed to air and its recovery—such exposure accelerates the process.

Simpson[13] suggests that in the Thames the time of the year is as good a guide as any. The intervals involved are some two days in June to August, three to five days in April, May, September and October, 10 to 14 days in early winter (November and December), and in January and February, the coldest months, the body may not come up at all as the process of decomposition is at a standstill.

Accident, murder or suicide?

The investigation of drowning by the pathologist can be difficult. His role in determining whether the findings are consistent with accidental death, suicide or homicide, is complicated by the frequency with which drowned bodies show the changes of decomposition. However, in many instances evidence from other sources helps to resolve the matter.

In practice it is helpful to consider the possibilities under two main headings:

1. Bodies in which death can be attributed to drowning with reasonable certainty, that is, those cases in which the post-mortem findings are as described above and routine microscopic examination confirms the presence of Diatoms, again as mentioned above.

These may conveniently be subdivided into:

a. Those which do not have injuries, and

i the deceased entered the water voluntarily, or

ii he entered it involuntarily while under the influence of alcohol or drugs, or

iii natural disease, such as ischaemic heart disease or epilepsy, caused a sudden collapse with subsequent drowning.

b. Cases with injuries:

i the deceased was injured by another person or persons and put into the water while unable to save himself—thereby drowning;

ii the injuries did not involve another person and were caused when the deceased struck some projection while entering or in the water.

2. Those cases in which the signs of drowning are not demonstrable. Again there may be:

(a) Those which do not have injuries. The possibility of death occurring in the course of immersion rather than from classical drowning, place these deaths in the category of some form of inhibitory process. They are commonly seen and, as considered above, are probably related to cold.

(b) Cases with injuries. The person may have fallen into the water after a collapse from natural causes—the injuries being sustained at that time. Alternatively death may be due to violence and the body disposed of by immersion.

It will be clear from this that the pathological investigation of such cases is difficult and it must be agreed that this is an area of forensic practice in which the pathologist is unable to give an opinion which is sufficiently positive as to satisfy the requirements usually demanded in a medico-legal investigation.

Cases which illustrate these various points will follow but certain features appear to be sufficiently common as to warrant special attention.

It emerges that the investigation must be carried out without any preconceived idea that because a body has been found in water drowning is the cause of death. The examinations must, therefore, include a detailed examination of the clothing and the body for marks.

The internal examination, in addition to a search for the findings associated with drowning, must include detailed microscopy to determine the nature, extent and stage of antecedent disease.

In practice most cases fall into one of two main groups:

1. Those in which a person is found dead in a bath. Here often natural disease is found such as cerebrovascular disease or coronary occlusion are at a stage at which a collapse might reasonably be expected.

Examination of these cases must include an analysis for alcohol, drugs and carbon monoxide, as faults associated with water heaters are, in our practice, a common cause of such deaths.

Cases are found in which young people are found drowned in which the possibility of any other person being involved can be excluded with reasonable certainty and with no indication of suicidal intent. Some of these are possibly attributable to some form of epilepsy. Marks on the body in the bath present some difficulty in interpretation and, of course, the classic case of *R. v. Smith* underlines how homicide in the bath can be accompanied by only slight injury.

In the case of *R. v. Smith*, known as 'the brides in the bath case', no less than three women were murdered by drowning in a bath. The murderer in each case had immersed the victim by lifting the legs up and pushing the head under water. In only one of the cases was there any signs of violence—that of Miss Lofty, in which there were three bruises on the arm. Suspicion was only aroused by the chance reading in a newspaper of what seemed a curiously repetitive series of 'accidents' involving the same man.

2. Outdoors in rivers and in the sea additional problems arise because not infrequently the bodies have been extensively damaged and it is sometimes difficult if not impossible to do more than determine by microscopy that these injuries were caused at or about the time of death.[51]

Those injuries which have been sustained after the deceased has been in the water for some time are usually distinctive. Such injuries include tears, fractures, particularly of the skull, but are not usually associated with any damage to the internal organs.

The possibility that some of the marks may be

associated with the body being struck by passing boats must be borne in mind and finally soft tissues particularly can be extensively mutilated by the action of fish and other water creatures. Their investigation and interpretation must follow the guidelines outlined elsewhere in this work.

Illustrative cases

Drowning—man—65 years. A man in poor general health was found in a kneeling position with his face and part of his head submerged in approximately 6 inches of water, in a trough. His nearby caravan was destroyed by fire. The previous evening the deceased had been found by friends having fallen off his moped after leaving a bar. He declined assistance. Internally the findings were consistent with drowning. There were double fractures of ribs on the right side of the chest. Microscopy of the adjacent soft tissues showed effusion of red cells and fibrin with some exudation of polymorphs. Diatoms were not demonstrable in the lung, brain or bone marrow. Enquiries eliminated the possibility of others being involved. The death was considered to be accidental (P. 11777).

Immersion injuries—woman—65 years. A woman prepared lunch for her husband then disappeared. Two days later the body was found on a beach some five miles distant. The only clothing was a pair of stockings, a girdle, bra and vest. The remaining clothing, if any, could not be found. Early putrefactive change affected the face but in addition there was bruising of both orbits, a linear laceration on the top of the head, 1 inch in length, a $\frac{3}{4}$ inch laceration on the back of the head and extensive bruising on the arms. There was some bruising of the undersurface of the scalp but the skull was intact and the brain showed no evidence of injury. There was a complete fracture dislocation of the cervical spine between the 4th and 5th vertebrae, associated with extensive haemorrhage into the muscles and soft tissues around the fracture. The cord was intact but there was slight bleeding into the adjacent meninges. Sand was present in the larynx and throughout the air passages as far as the smaller bronchioles. Microscopic examination of the wounds and bruised areas showed effusion of red cells but no organisation. Diatoms of marine type were present in the lung but not in

the liver, brain or bone marrow. It was suggested that the injuries were sustained with a fall from a height into the sea. The microscopy of the wounds suggested that they were sustained at or about the time of death and the distribution of Diatoms that death occurred almost immediately on immersion if not earlier (P. 25177).

Drowning and homicide—man—55 years. A man was found in the centre of a stream, almost directly underneath the edge of a small bridge, the drop being about 7 ft. The body was fully dressed in normal outdoor type clothing. Some 70 yards away were found numerous blood stains. Various personal articles belonging to the deceased were scattered around this area. There were several and extensive injuries to the head and face which could be arranged in nine separate groups. Internally there were multiple fractures of the bones of the nose. The back of the throat contained a large quantity of partly clotted blood mixed with mud. Microscopy of the lungs showed extensive haemorrhagic collapse with abundant blood and scanty silt like material in the larger air passages of the right

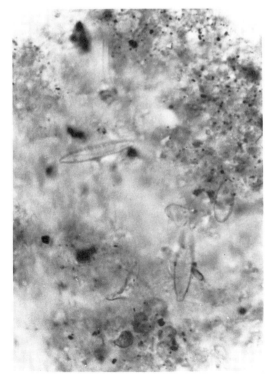

Fig. 13.15 Diatoms.

side and abundant silt like material on the left side. Diatoms were demonstrated in the lungs but not in the brain, liver or marrow. The cause of death was considered to be multiple injuries to the head and face and the microscopic findings suggested that the deceased, if not already dead, died almost immediately on immersion (P. 12676) (see Fig. 13.15).

Possible homicide—woman—56 years. A routine post-mortem examination on the body of a woman found drowned revealed some haemorrhages in the tissues around the top of the shoulders. Further examination revealed a group of three faint bruises on the front of the neck, one on the right side of the neck, one on the right lower shoulder blade and five on the back of the right elbow. The only internal mark of injury was a tiny ($\frac{1}{8}$ inch) bruise in the soft tissues joining the left side of the hyoid bone to the undersurface of the tongue. The findings in the lungs were consistent with death due to drowning. Diatoms were not detected in the body organs or the bath water. The person who found the body committed suicide shortly afterwards. Further enquiries were not helpful (P. 231073).

? Accidental drowning—woman—26 years. A woman was found in the middle of a stream underneath a road bridge. She lay floating on the surface of the water, face upwards, nose and face above the water level, hands and arms folded across the front of the lower chest, legs out-stretched and close together. The face was covered in blood and the possibility of an assault was raised. The internal findings were typically those associated with drowning and showed no evidence of any significant natural disease or injury. Closer examination showed that the bleeding came from multiple superficial erosions of the skin on the front of the brow, eyes, nose, cheeks and front of neck. From many of these blood continued to exude and various forms of pond life were still adherent in some quantity. The deceased had a history of epilepsy (P. 20770) (see Fig. 13.16).

Suicide—man—52 years. A moderately obese man was found in a pond. Early putrefactive changes were evident, the face and neck tissues being swollen with greenish discoloration and some desquamation of the skin. The skin of the hands was also largely desquamated. There was no recognisable external mark of injury. The finger nails

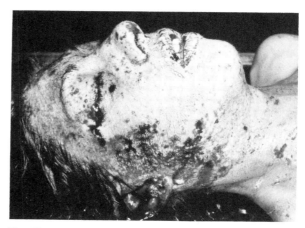

Fig. 13.16 Drowning.

were long, reasonably clean and completely unbroken. The clothing, which was wet, was female in type. In order of removal from the body: a black 'home-made' hood covered the face and head, auburn coloured wig, one pair of green ankle socks, one rubber bootee on the left foot, one pair of black net self-supporting stockings, one black coarse cloth crudely made frock, one blue woollen short-sleeved pullover, one pair of women's type black panties, a black bra the cups of which were filled with foam rubber sponges. The clothing showed no evidence of tearing or other form of injury. A length of two core $\frac{1}{4}$ inch electric flex encircled the middle part of the body: it extended from a slip type loop in the middle of the back, encircled the body once and then bound both elbows to the side of the chest and continued to be wound round the wrists tightly, where it was secured by a series of loops. The testicles were lodged at the level of the internal inguinal ring. Internally the findings were typically those of drowning. Acid digest preparations of brain and lung showed the presence of Diatoms. It was considered that death was due to drowning and that the ligature could have been applied by the deceased without the assistance of any other person (P. 21270) (see Figs 13.17 and 13.18).

Strangulation

The asphyxial state in strangulation may follow compression of the neck either by:
1. the application of a ligature, the ligature not

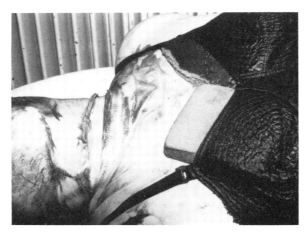

Fig. 13.17 Drowning.

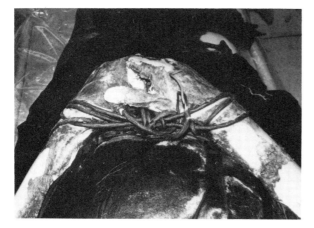

Fig. 13.18 Drowning.

being attached to a suspension point as in hanging, 2. the application by human hand or hands (throttling).

It is not uncommon to find that both methods have been employed in the same case.

Cause of death

Most people can hold their breath for a considerable period without distress. It is, therefore, remarkable that a sudden compression of the windpipe should so often render a person powerless to call for assistance and cause almost immediate insensibility and death. That this can occur is widely recognised in cases of criminal throttling. Death is clearly not a matter of uncomplicated

asphyxiation and some pathologists prefer, in such cases, to give 'compression of the neck' as the cause of death.

The reason is that irrespective of the degree of asphyxia that develops there is an element of cardiac inhibition (vasovagal) operating in many cases of sudden pressure on the neck.

The findings at post-mortem in a case in which sudden death occurs during compression of the neck can be negligible. The diagnosis then must involve the exclusion of other possible causes of sudden death.

The precise mechanisms involved in such a case of death are still not fully understood but they are connected to a reflex inhibition of the heart through the stimulation of the vagus, its branches, notably the superior laryngeal nerves, or the carotid sinus.

The carotid sinus, it may be recalled, is a dilated part of the wall of the carotid artery. It contains numerous nerve endings from the glossopharyngeal nerve and it also communicates with the medullary cardiovascular centre in the brain and the dorsal motor-nucleus of the vagus. It is intimately concerned with the control of blood pressure and heart rate. It is situated in the wall of the carotid artery at its bifurcation which is at the level of the upper border of the thyroid cartilage, a site commonly involved in strangulation. Whatever may be the precise mechanism involved there are well documented cases in the literature since Brouardel[52] drew attention to this concept as a mode of death.

Simpson[53] has analysed a series of 87 such deaths from various causes including six cases of manual strangulation. Such deaths are of considerable medico-legal importance as death may well result from circumstances in which there has been no intent to cause such a death. These circumstances will be considered in detail later.

It is, therefore, important to consider how far the elements of asphyxia and inhibition can be separated.

The amounts of force necessary to compress a blood vessel will depend on the thickness of the wall and the pressure within the vessel. It follows that it is more difficult to block the arterial flow of blood in the neck than that of the veins. When the venous drainage only is impaired blood will accumulate above the level of the constriction with hypoxic features. When the entry of blood into the

Table 13.1

Form	Signs and symptoms	Autopsy features
Vagal inhibition	Sudden loss of consciousness. Arrest of respiration and circulation	None
Slight vagal effect. Some venous obstruction	Muscular weakness, vertigo, clouding of consciousness	Slight congestion, occasional petechiae.
Some respiratory obstruction. Pronounced venous obstruction	Loss of consciousness	Congestion and cyanosis of head and neck. Petechiae and ecchymosis of eyes. (Less pronounced where there is arterial compression)
Extreme respiratory and venous obstruction	Unconsciousness	Intense congestion, deep cyanosis, bulging of eyes and tongue, numerous petechiae in eyelids, eyes, face and scalp. (Again lessened by arterial compression)

neck is also occluded these features may be expected to be less pronounced.

The vast majority of cases would fall into one of four groups shown in Table 13.1.

Post-mortem appearances in strangulation

As will be seen from the above it is possible in strangulation that death can result from slight injury and, therefore, with trivial, if any, marks to indicate the way in which violence was applied and, when death has occurred, few if any post-mortem findings.

In the vast majority of cases, however, the general features associated with an asphyxial type of death are evident, and there is usually some evidence of their localised intensification.

In such cases it is often possible to suggest the way in which the neck has been compressed even when the constricting objects—hands or ligatures—have been removed.

A careful search in suitable mortuary conditions will usually reveal either external or internal evidence of the area where the constriction has occurred. The findings will be considered under the following headings:

1. General appearances—external and internal.
2. Local appearances—external and internal.

General external features. The general external features of asphyxial deaths found in strangled bodies show that the face may be blotchy and swollen, the eyes suffused and bulging with dilated pupils, the tongue protruding, sometimes caught between the teeth. Frothy blood tinged fluid exudes from the nose and mouth. Tardieu's spots are usually seen in the skin of the eyelids, the face, the scalp and sometimes larger haemorrhages are present in the eyes (Fig. 13.19).

As suggested earlier these features are not in themselves pathognomic. Their local distribution in the head and neck is, however, strongly presumptive of strangling. Marks on the neck will confirm this.

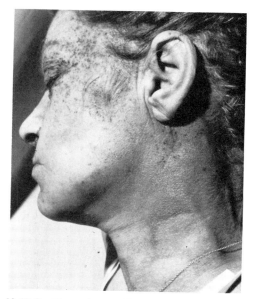

Fig. 13.19 See illustrative case P. 12674.

The voiding of urine and faeces and the omission of seminal fluid are all commonly found in this group but also occur in deaths from many other causes.

General internal appearances. Internally the air passages contain fine froth, often blood stained. The lungs are congested with subpleural petechiae. Microscopically there is usually intense interalveolar congestion with haemorrhages of varying size, fluid in the alveoli, areas of collapse and intervening areas of ruptured alveoli. The air passages often contain large areas of desquamated respiratory type epithelium, red blood cells and fluid. The remaining organs show only congestive changes. Petechiae are usually more common in the brain than elsewhere.

Local features—external. These comprise marks as of a ligature or constricting fingers. It is doubtful whether strangulation ever takes place without some mark being left on the neck but the possibility that death could be caused in this manner without leaving any appreciable trace of violence does exist.

Thus, a ligature, when something soft and yielding, may produce nothing more than a slight depression or flushing of the skin.

These conditions are rare as because of the circumstances the assailants usually employ considerably more force than would appear to be necessary to ensure that death takes place.

In general terms the mark on the neck is usually of the same width as the constricting object and the depth is about half its diameter.

Most often the ligature comprises something which is readily to hand. Wire, electric flex, pieces of bathroom chain, tights, scarves, binder twine and dog leads, are objects commonly used (Fig. 13.20). While it is possible to form a view as to the nature of the ligature from the impressions of the marks left on the neck, it can be difficult and misleading to attempt to read too much into such surface marks.

If the ligature is still present the number of turns and the types of knots require detailed study and are frequently of help in deciding whether it is an accident, suicide or murder. Multiple turns produce a complex mark in which it may be possible to trace the number of turns but again the possi-

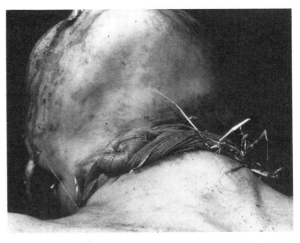

Fig. 13.20 Homicidal strangulation with tights on a golf course. Vegetation is included in ligature.

bility of the single application of a doubled or quadrupled ligature cannot be excluded.

Finger marks

In manual strangulation the marks of bruising will be on the front or sides of the neck, chiefly about the larynx and above it. Marks of pressure of fingers may, however, be slight. These bruising marks of the fingers will, of course, vary. The absence of bruising upon the skin, especially when deep-seated bruising is present, can be accounted for by the maintenance of pressure until death has supervened, since compression of the skin will empty the vessels in it with comparative ease during life and the heart may have ceased to beat before the pressure has been removed.

The distribution of these marks when present will vary with the circumstances, and factors which will affect it include the relative position of the assailant and victim, the manner of gripping the neck, being greater if the grip is shifted or has been reapplied if the victim struggles, and the degree of pressure. Their interpretation is a matter for experience (Fig. 13.21).

Fingernail marks are perhaps less common than bruises in cases of manual strangulation and when present may be self-inflicted by the deceased in a struggle to release the strangling hold. Their relative infrequency compared with finger marks, as

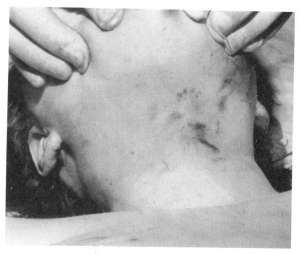

Fig. 13.21 Manual strangulation of child by mother. Multiple bruises and scratches.

pointed out by Polson & Gee,[14] that it is a prerequisite of clear-crescent type nail marks that the assailant has well manicured finger nails but most who embark on throttling are careless with their nails (Fig. 13.22).

Irregular scratch marks are, however, much more common but again these may be reasonably

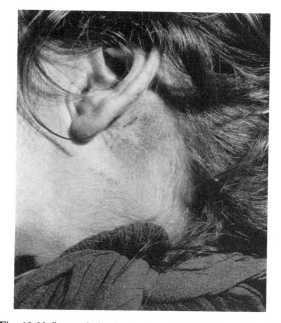

Fig. 13.22 Strangulation by ligature (tights). Clear nail mark behind ear.

suggested to have been caused by the deceased trying to free him or herself.

Local features—internal

These are conveniently considered under two headings, soft tissues and solid tissues. The soft tissues comprise the subcutaneous fat, fascia, muscles, blood vessels and nodes.

It is usual to find bruising in the soft tissues of the neck in cases of strangulation even when there are no external marks on the skin. It must be recalled that bruising does not invariably result from the application of a ligature during life, especially when the ligature has been tightly secured and not removed until after circulation has ceased. If a ligature is involved, the bruising will usually be at the same level. Several areas of bruising at different levels is good evidence of pressure from fingers rather than a ligature.

Injuries to the blood vessels are extremely rare in strangulation and raise the possibility of direct blows.

The solid tissues of the neck are of extreme importance in cases of suspected strangulation. A brief review of the normal anatomy may be helpful.

The solid structures comprise the hyoid bone and the cartilages forming the larynx.

The hyoid bone is 'U' shaped and composed of five parts: the body, two greater and two lesser horns. It is relatively protected, lying at the root of the tongue where the body is difficult to feel. The greater horn, which can be felt more easily, lies behind the front part of the strap muscles (sternomastoid), 3 cm below the angle of the lower jaw and 1.5 cm from the midline. The bone ossifies from six centres, a pair for the body and one for each horn. The greater horns are, in early life, connected to the body by cartilage but after middle life they are usually united by bone. The lesser horns are situated close to the junction of the greater horns in the body. They are connected to the body of the bone by fibrous tissue and occasionally to the greater horns by synovial joints which usually persist throughout life but occasionally become ankylosed.

Our own findings suggest that although the hardening of the bone is related to age there can be considerable variation and elderly people sometimes show only slight ossification.

From the above consideration of the anatomy it will be appreciated that while injuries to the body are unlikely, a grip high up on the neck may readily produce fractures of the greater horns. Sometimes it would appear that the local pressure from the thumb causes a fracture on one side only.

While the amount of force in manual strangulation would often appear to be greatly in excess of that required to cause death, the application of such force, as evidenced by extensive external and soft tissue injuries, make it unusual to find fractures of the hyoid bone in a person under the age of 40 years.

As stated, even in older people in which ossification is incomplete, considerable violence may leave this bone intact. This view is confirmed by Green.[54] He gives interesting figures: in 34 cases of manual strangulation the hyoid was fractured in 12 (35%) as compared with the classic paper of Gonzales[55] who reported four fractures in 24 cases. The figures in strangulation by ligature show that the percentage of hyoid fractures was 13. Our own figures are similar to those of Green.

It would appear that the fracture can be caused in one of two ways: direct lateral compression from the sides of the neck, this being the commonest and to produce it pressure must be applied high up under the angles of the jaw. The second mechanism is indirect violence as described by Camps & Hunt[56] in which the hyoid bone is drawn upwards and immobilised by the numerous muscles which are attached to its upper surface when the neck muscles are contracted, as in an attempt to resist strangulation. Violent downward or lateral movement of the thyroid cartilage will exert traction through the thyrohyoid membrane and ligament and cause a traction.

The larynx occupies the front of the neck. The position differs with age and sex, being opposite the 3rd to 6th cervical vertebrae in the adult male and somewhat higher in adult females and children.

In the midline the laryngeal prominence (Adam's apple) is some 2 to 5 cm below the hyoid bone when the chin is held up as would appear to be usual in strangulation.

It is composed of nine cartilages—thyroid, cri-

coid, epiglottis and the much smaller pairs of cuneiform, corniculate and arytenoids. These small paired structures are not usually involved in injury. In forensic practice the two most important components are the larger thyroid and cricoid.

The thyroid comprises a central shield-shaped body which is angled forwards at some 90° in males and some 120° in females. This is a vulnerable structure as it lies on the front of the neck covered merely by skin and two thin layers of fascia. At the back of the body upper and lower horns are attached on both sides. The superior horn is firmly attached to the hyoid bone. The thyroid consists of hyaline cartilage and tends to become more or less ossified as age advances. Ossification is generally considered to commence about 25 years although this is variable and it is not unusual to find a thyroid still completely cartilaginous in old age.

The cricoid, which is shaped like a signet ring with the signet part at the back, is the only solid structure which completely encircles the neck. It also consists of hyaline cartilage. Ossification appears to occur later than in the thyroid and is frequently incomplete if present at all.

Thyroid fractures are common as might be expected from its position and the mechanism of throttling, particularly manual strangulation, as maximum pressure is likely to be effected at this site. Again as might be inferred from the anatomy when fractures do occur they are more likely to involve the horns (usually the upper) rather than the body. Fractures of the horns comprise 50% of Green's cases in manual strangulation and 34% in strangulation by ligature.[54] They may be unilateral or bilateral. Fractures of the body are much less common and probably seen more often in cases involving direct violence. Green did not find any in strangulation by ligature and in 12% of his cases of throttling.

In our own practice fractures of the body are very infrequent and usually in those cases in which there is direct violence involved. The age of the person concerned is of considerable importance.

The cricoid, being less accessible and very often still cartilagenous, is rarely injured. When it does occur it would appear to be associated with the application of considerable force with anteroposterior compression of it against the spine, either with two hands from the front or a forearm from the back. Again direct violence would appear to be a more likely explanation.

Accident

As a general rule cases of accidental strangulation present little difficulty when the body is found with the constricting agent undisturbed.

Should the body have been removed from the scene of death or the ligature removed, as frequently happens, the pathologist can only establish presumption of accident from the description given or possibly from a study of the photographs, and state whether the post-mortem findings are consistent with death having occurred in the manner suggested.

It is for this reason that whenever possible we prefer to join the investigating officers at the scene.

Usually these cases occur at the extremes of life. Even before birth or during the process of birth some infants are strangled by their own umbilical cord. The old and infirm sometimes fall into a situation from which they cannot escape and compression of the neck results. Otherwise healthy adults can be caught in machinery, compression of the neck following the twisting of loose clothing such as neck ties and scarves. In this age group those under the influence of alcohol or drugs die when the neck is compressed in a position from which they are unable to extricate themselves (see Fig. 13.19).

Suicide or homicide?

Again it is generally very helpful to examine the body at the scene of death if it has not been disturbed or, if it has, a visit to the scene can still be helpful when its position can be reconstructed by those who first had to confirm that life was extinct. In most instances the circumstances at the scene of death together with the findings at autopsy and further investigations in the laboratory usually make it possible to distinguish with reasonable certainty in which of these two categories the death should be placed. It is helpful to review the main points which may help in forming an opinion.

In such cases the features placing the death into the asphyxial group with localising signs are usually well marked. The position is very different in those cases in which death occurs suddenly with few or no post-mortem findings suggesting a vasovagal mechanism and trivial injuries if any at all. The pathologist in these cases can only agree that such a mechanism is a possible explanation and the question as to whether it was accident or design is a matter for a jury.

Examination at the scene of death can be of the greatest assistance. If the body is found to have died with marks on the neck which indicate manual strangulation and this is subsequently confirmed in the mortuary and laboratory the case must be regarded as a killing by another person. It is inconceivable that anyone could die from compression of the neck by his own hand because loss of consciousness would cause relaxation of the constricting fingers. When a ligature is involved the matter is different. If the ligature is found in situ suicide is unusual but a distinct possibility.

As most cases of strangulation involve females and are associated with sexual activity, signs of a struggle must be sought together with any evidence of disturbance or tearing of the clothing of the appropriate parts.

The subsequent investigation falls into three main headings, viz., to distinguish between homicide and suicide it can be helpful when death is associated with compression of the neck to establish:
1. how it was applied;
2. how much force was used, and
3. for how long was the force maintained?

If the constriction was the result of the human hand the case must be regarded as one of homicide.

Self-strangulation involving a ligature may occur in four ways:

1. When the neck is constricted by multiple turns which are sufficient to maintain constriction without a knot or fewer turns secured either by a half or double knot at a point accessible to the person's own hands.

2. More frequently a rod of some sort is either inserted under a knot or included in it, the neck being compressed by twisting in the fashion of a tourniquet. This, in our experience is the commonest method used.

3. A running noose with a weight attached to the free end.

4. A running noose with the free end attached to the hand, the weight of the hand and forearm affecting compression.

The type of ligature involved is seldom helpful in that it is usually something which is readily to hand, although cases have occurred in which the matching of the ligature with material torn from a place associated with the suspect has provided the connection between the two.

The types and positions of the knot are also seldom of assistance.

The position of the marks on the neck, it will be recalled, depends on the relative position of the victim and assailant and the way in which the neck was gripped.

Thus, in addition to examining the neck for finger type bruises and nail marks, the examination must include a careful search at the back of the head and neck for possible bruising indicative of thumb marks. Again, particularly in cases which appear to be associated with sexual activity, it is essential to examine the back of the body over the pressure areas such as the shoulders, buttocks and elbows for marks of pressure or internal bruising.

The examination must also determine that the injuries were caused before death.

It is worth recalling that artefacts can be produced after death and these include, in babies and fat people with short necks, marks due to folding in the skin associated with bending of the neck. The ritual of laying out a body involving the propping up of the sagging lifeless chin with a sandbag not infrequently leads to forensic enquiry.

Clothing or other articles around the neck can produce marks apparently suggestive of a ligature in a body when the tissues are swelling as the result of putrefactive change. This appears to be particularly common after bodies have been immersed in water (see Fig. 13.17).

It is also important for the pathologist to exclude artefacts during the course of the internal examination. It is not unknown for fractures to be produced by the rough handling and unskilled removal of the neck structures. This will not arise when the removal of the body from the scene and its subsequent arrangement in the mortuary is supervised by the pathologist and experienced police officers and skilled mortuary technicians.

Areas of apparent bruising can be produced particularly by rough handling.[57]

These occur usually in fresh bodies in which the neck structures are suffused. This can be minimised by the removal of the brain initially and the drainage of the neck or by incision in the superior vena cava. Division of the neck structures at this stage is considered inadvisable as it can lead to distortion. Further dissection is a matter for personal preference but in general it must be conducted in layers, the areas of bruising recorded and possible fracture sites identified by evidence of bleeding at that site. Removal is then completed as a matter of some delicacy, the neck structures being preserved with fixative then examined by X-ray, and, thereafter, areas of haemorrhage and fractures further dissected with removal of tissues for microscopic examination. It is as well to recall that all marks on the neck are not necessarily evidence of direct violence. Noteworthy are the haemorrhages at the back of the larynx usually at the level of the cricoid cartilage. Most of these, as pointed out by Camps & Hunt[56] are due to over-distension and rupture of a group of thin-walled venous sinuses forming the pharyngo-laryngeal plexus.

Paparo & Siegel[58] noted an incidence of about 1% of such haemorrhages in 1500 medico-legal autopsies. They found evidence of 'asphyxial' petechial haemorrhages in other sites of the body in over 50% of the cases and suggest that in the remainder, where petechiae could not be found, this did not exclude asphyxia as a possible cause of death.

These haemorrhages are usually much larger than one finds in those which are due to direct trauma and we can confirm an incidence of about 1% and again mainly in cases in which intense asphyxial changes from other causes may be evident.

With ligatures the amount of force employed determines the severity of the injuries, but an important factor is the elasticity of the ligature. This will limit the pressure which can be applied to the neck. Stockings and tights (commonly used as ligatures in strangulation) are elastic structures.

Cases which can cause some difficulty are those in which severe internal injuries are accompanied by trivial external marks if any. This must raise the possibility of a stranglehold applied from behind by a firm, broad, smooth object such as the human forearm in cases of mugging.

The length of time for which the force was maintained is a matter to which considerable importance must be attached, as it may be related to whether or not intent to cause death was present. It is also one in which it is impossible for a pathologist to be dogmatic. It is unusual to have any direct evidence of the time involved and even when people give an estimate of that time it is usual that most people considerably overestimate the time involved. Thirty seconds in these circumstances as suggested by Polson & Gee[14] can seem like an eternity.

In general terms the post-mortem findings will range from those which are consistent with an immediate vagal type of death to those in which the local changes associated with an asphyxial process are pronounced. The former might be associated with an immediate and sudden collapse, possibly associated with pre-existing natural disease which, of course, will be revealed at the routine autopsy; in the latter a longer period of time is involved, probably at least half a minute or so.

In an interesting case such a time interval was given by a pathologist who suggested that death had occurred after 30 s continuous pressure on the neck. On appeal a second pathologist agreed that death was due to pressure on the neck but not as to the time involved, it being considered that there was no evidence to support the view of firm continuous pressure for at least 30 s. He considered that the pressure could well have been for a very few seconds only. A verdict of manslaughter was substituted.[59]

Illustrative cases

Strangulation—natural causes—man—55 years. A man had a dispute with a younger man over some money owed for household repairs. The younger man put his right arm around the neck while with his left hand he pushed the head forwards. The deceased's wife tried to separate them. The deceased staggered into another room where he collapsed, became unconscious and died within a few minutes. The only marks on the body were faint bruising of the right orbit, brow and upper cheek.

Some blood exuded from the left nostril. Detailed dissection of the neck and radiological examination showed no evidence of injury. Elsewhere there were the changes of advanced chronic bronchitis with emphysema and advanced pulmonary heart disease with lipid atheroma reducing the coronary arteries to some 70% of normal at several points. Microscopy confirmed the presence of pulmonary hypertension. Compression of the neck was considered to be a minor but contributory cause, the cause being the pulmonary heart disease. No criminal proceedings were initiated (P. 14375).

? Strangulation—accidental—woman—51 years. A woman was found face upwards on a twin bed in her bedroom. Two areas of pallor were noted on the front and left side of the neck. On the front of the neck it was roughly triangular with the base crossing the midline at some 10° to the vertical plane, each limb measuring, some $1\frac{3}{4}$ inch in length and it was centred some $3\frac{1}{2}$ inches below the point of the chin. On the left side of the neck the mark was roughly rectangular. It measured $1\frac{1}{8} \times 1\frac{1}{2}$ inches and was centred $3\frac{1}{2}$ inches below the lobe of the ear and 3 inches to the left of the midline. Blood tinged fluid exuded from the nose. The side of the neck and top of the shoulders were intensely suffused with numerous petechiae. A thin chain with a cross was intact around the neck and not associated with any related pressure marks. The clothing, a bra and pants, was intact and undisturbed. A thin fluted pressed steel radiator was present on the wall close to this bed. Some spots of blood were present on the intervening carpet. When the body was placed with the nose in relation to these blood spots the marks on the neck coincided with the design on the radiator. The liver showed advanced alcoholic type cirrhosis. An analysis showed a blood alcohol level of 417 mg%. On further enquiry it was found that the person finding the body agreed that the reconstruction was how he had found the body initially. It was subsequently placed on the bed by ambulance men (P. 12674) (see Fig. 13.19).

Self-strangulation—woman. The body of an unidentified middle-aged woman was found on a bench at the back of a beach hut. She was dressed in outdoor type clothing. No shoes were present and she did not wear any underwear. A strip of wood lay alongside the back of the head and appeared to be connected to the body by a scarf which encircled the neck in the form of a ligature. The ligature comprised a scarf of silk type material which was deeply embedded in the neck. It was secured at the front by a granny knot. At the back a quarter circle wooden batten had been passed through the ligature and turned through two complete circles. The two straight edges of the batten measured $\frac{7}{8}$ inch each and it had a total length of some $28\frac{1}{2}$ inches. A deep impression was present on the neck underneath the ligature. It had a maximum width of about 1 inch, passed $2\frac{1}{2}$ inches below the lobe of the right ear, $2\frac{1}{2}$ inches below the lobe of the left ear and 3 inches below the point of the chin, with an irregular area, about 1 inch in diameter, which corresponded with the knot. A group of three recent roughly horizontal superficial cuts on the front of the left wrist, each about 2 inch in length, were the only other marks on the body. These were considered to be of the type usually associated with a suicidal gesture. The examination did not disclose any other marks of violence, particularly those of a defensive nature. The site and nature of the ligature on the neck were such that it could have been a deliberate act on the part of the deceased (P. 10974) (see Fig. 13.23).

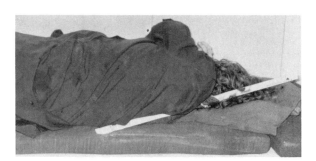

Fig. 13.23 Self strangulation.

Manual strangulation—male child—15 months. A male child of normal physique and showing no evidence of any significant natural disease. Frothy brown fluid exuded from both nostrils. The face was suffused and petechiae were present in the brow and both eyelids. Hypostasis was confined to the posterior dependent parts of the body. Three bruises associated with some abrasion of the skin were present on the left side of the head. These

were considered to be consistent with having been caused by an earlier fall. In addition:
1. An irregular area of faint bruising on the left side of the neck, centred $1\frac{1}{2}$ inches below the lobe of the ear. In the centre of this mark there were six very faint vertical scratches, each about $\frac{1}{4}$ inch in length and $\frac{1}{4}$ inch apart from each other.
2. Two faint scratches on the right side of the neck which ran down and to the right at some 45°, each about $\frac{1}{4}$ inch in length. They were situated $2\frac{1}{2}$ and 3 inches below the point of the chin and $1\frac{1}{2}$ inches to the right of the midline. Tiny areas of bruising, each about $\frac{1}{16}$ inch in diameter, were present throughout the upper part of the strap muscle on the left side of the neck in relation to external injury (1). An $\frac{1}{8}$ inch bruise on the middle of the strap muscle on the right side of the neck. The only other findings were numerous areas of subpleural haemorrhage. The cause of death was considered to be manual strangulation. The mother subsequently admitted causing the death of her child in this way (P. 11672).

Strangulation by ligature—girl—eight years. A girl was found lying outside the back door of a terraced house. She was dressed in normal outdoor clothing apart from the buttocks which were bare and exposed. A pair of turquoise slacks were completely detached from the body but gripped between the thighs. On moving the body a pair of crumpled grey flannel knickers were found underneath the right hip. The perineum and anus were moist and a single dark hair was found to be adherent to the margin of the right side of the anus. Numerous petechiae were present in both eyelids and the face was suffused above a ligature mark, 7 inches in length, which was present on the front of the neck. It passed 2 inches below the point of the chin and ran backwards on the right side of the neck $1\frac{3}{4}$ inches below the lobe of the ear to terminate $1\frac{1}{2}$ inches behind it. On the left side it ran backwards $1\frac{3}{4}$ inches below the lobe of the ear to terminate 1 inch behind it. The mark was fairly deep and irregular with a maximum width of $\frac{1}{2}$ inch. At the outer edge of both sides it bifurcated into single thinner marks. Around the left end of the ligature mark there were multiple irregular scratches, each about $\frac{1}{8}$ inch in diameter. The only other mark was a roughly triangular bruised abrasion on the right side of the neck, centred $1\frac{1}{4}$ inches above the end of the ligature mark. Internally there was extensive bruising of the muscles and soft tissues at the front of the neck at the level of the thyroid cartilage, with some bruising of both lateral lobes of the gland. A youth subsequently admitted placing a dog chain around her neck. He was found guilty of manslaughter (P. 13574).

Strangulation by ligature—woman—17 years. The body of a woman was found naked and face downwards on a mattress. The clothing, which was of the normal outdoor type, was scattered around the room. The head was wrapped in a red piece of cloth which proved to be part of a torn mini-dress, tightly knotted on the right side of the head. The knot included several strands of hair. A pair of brown nylon tights encircled the neck three times, the panty part being tucked underneath a loop in the region of the nape of the neck and including several strands of hair. They then ran under the left armpit, across the back and under the right armpit where the other end, the feet, were tightly tied around the top of the shoulder. The face above the ligature mark was suffused with numerous petechiae in the eyelids. Nine areas of bruising were present on the face and jaw, four of these were considered to be consistent with blows and four with forcible gripping, but an irregular bruise on the right side of the neck, $\frac{3}{4} \times \frac{1}{4}$ inch, centred $3\frac{1}{2}$ inches below the lobe of the ear and $3\frac{1}{2}$ inches to the right of the midline, was considered to be slightly older than the other injuries. This was confirmed by subsequent microscopic examination. In a statement the accused admitted holding her by the neck and pushing her down on to the floor. He then punched her and after undressing her attached the clothing to the head and face as described. He also alleged that she taunted him after he had questioned her about a 'love bite' on her neck. The older injury on the neck was considered to be consistent with this account. He was found guilty of manslaughter (P. 71072).

Hanging

In hanging the body is wholly or partially suspended by the neck so that the constricting force applied to the neck is the weight of the body. It differs from strangulation where the neck is constricted irrespective of any effect caused by the weight of the body. In practice the distinction between the two groups is important because strangulation is usually homicidal and in hanging the vast majority are considered to be suicidal.

The symptoms of hanging

There are a number of cases on record in which survivors of hanging have given an account of their experiences.[14] The accounts of the process in so far as they can be relied upon because of the differing degree of amnesia, stress how rapidly unconsciousness supervenes and it is noteworthy that often, even before unconsciousness supervenes, they are unable to move their hands to save themselves.

Despite the prevalence of partial hanging for autoerotic purposes, remarkably little information appears to be available from this source.

Litman & Swearingen[60] who succeeded in securing the co-operation of nine practitioners record that one who had made a study of the time taken for unconsciousness to ensue noted that a thin rope around the neck will cause unconsciousness in 15 seconds.

The cause of death in hanging

The autopsy findings in cases of hanging are varied and it appears that the actual cause of death depends on which of a number of factors predominates. These factors are:
1. Injury to the spinal cord.
2. Sudden stoppage of the heart due to vasovagal inhibition.
3. a. Blockage of the air passages (producing asphyxia).
   b. Obstruction of the venous drainage in the brain by pressure on the jugular veins.
   c. Obstruction of the arterial blood flow to the brain by pressure on the carotid arteries.

Injuries to the spinal cord. These occur when injury to the neck structures is associated with a drop. It was, of course, found in judicial hanging where a drop of some 6 ft effected fracture dislocations at the level of the 2nd and 3rd or 3rd and 4th vertebrae. Less commonly fractures are found in the 1st and 2nd vertebrae. The cord is usually separated from its junction with the medulla of the brain. This method is rare in cases of suicidal hanging.

Vagal inhibition. The essential features are similar to those considered under strangulation. It must be considered as a possible cause of death when there are no features as of hypoxia, and where death does not appear to have been intended.

Experiments and observations in persons hanged have shown that this is very easily brought about, its occurrence to some extent depending on the position of the ligature and on the degree of force used.

Almost all published series record that in suicidal hanging the ligature is above the level of the larynx in the vast majority of cases. This can be explained when hanging takes place in the vertical position as the ligature will slip up until it is held by the jaw.

The pressure of the ligature compresses the tissues of the neck and forces the base of the tongue against the back of the pharynx.

This does not appear to occur so readily when the ligature is below the level of the thyroid cartilage.

The amount of force required to produce constriction and the amount which can be produced by the weight of the body are generally underestimated.

Blockage of the air passages. Brouardel[52] showed that tension of 33 lb was sufficient to close the trachea. When the air passages are thus blocked asphyxia must naturally be the cause of death and the autopsy findings indicative of a profound general hypoxia.

Obstruction of the venous drainage. When a ligature is tightened around the neck the principal venous trunks forming the main channels for the return of the blood from the brain are compressed and stasis in the venous circulation in the brain is likely to be produced. It is well established that this can cause unconsciousness and may play a major part in the production of death from hanging.

Brouardel[52] showed that the jugular veins were closed by a tension of 4.4 lb.

It is in these conditions that the most pronounced external hypoxic changes become developed and the head and neck become intensely engorged above the level of constriction.

Obstruction of arterial flow. Brouardel[52] records

that 11 lb of tension can close the carotid arteries, this being confirmed by the experiments of Polson & Gee.[14, 20] This, no doubt, contributes to the rapid loss of consciousness commonly observed in hanging.

Post-mortem findings

The general features will depend on the predominance and combination of the above mechanisms. These give pressure:

1. On both the air tubes and the blood vessels, the pressure on the air tubes being only partial. Death will probably result from a combination of obstructive asphyxia and an interference with the cerebral circulation, but primarily from asphyxia.

2. Given pressure in such a way that the airway is more or less protected death may occur from interference with the cerebral circulation and will then be slow. The features of suboxia will not be so pronounced generally.

3. Given complete constriction so that the entrance of air into the lungs is entirely prevented death will result from intense asphyxia and may be extremely rapid but not as sudden as (4).

4. Where sudden local pressure on the vagus or carotid sinus may show no abnormal findings whatsoever.

General external appearances

As indicated above this must depend on the mode of dying.

The face is usually pale although may occasionally be livid and swollen with protruding eyes and tongue, but the swelling of the face often disappears when the body is cut down and is no longer evident by the time it has reached the autopsy room.

Saliva may have dribbled from the mouth but blood stained froth, common in strangulation, is unusual. Occasionally the pupils of the eyes differ in size. Petechial haemorrhages occur as in other asphyxial deaths in the face, forehead and eyes, but are relatively infrequent in hanging.

A state of engorgement or semi-erection of the penis has been frequently noted and there may be some dribbling of seminal fluid.

Post-mortem lividity is most marked in the

dependent parts and ecchymoses may be seen in the skin of the lower arms and legs.

Full suspension is not necessary as long as adequate constriction of the neck can take place. Thus, a victim may kneel, sit, slump back or forward, or lie prone with only the face and chest off the ground. It is in these hangings from a low point of suspension with a lessened constricting force that the congestive changes are more pronounced.

General internal appearances

The general internal appearances are those associated with an asphyxial death.

There is usually intense congestion of the brain, lungs, heart and other major organs. Subpleural petechiae are common. Subarachnoid effusions are not uncommon.

The interpretation of neck marks is usually less difficult than those found in cases of strangling. The width and character depends on the nature of the ligature. It may be deep and patterned and if the ligature is well defined the pattern may be impressed on the mark on the skin, or it may be shallow and difficult to define with a broader fold when some softer agent, such as cloth, has been used (see illustrative case P. 22573).

Ligatures comprise a wide range of articles and are usually chosen from those which are readily available.

The impression left on the skin is deepest around that part of the neck opposite the point of suspension. In the region of the knot the mark follows an upward course to form an inverted 'V', the apex of the 'V' corresponding with the site of the knot. The mark is generally yellowish or yellow/brown and often dried from an exudation of tissue fluid. Often a thin line of congestion will be seen above or below the groove at some point but usually the deepest.

When the ligatures comprise multiple strands of twine or wire there may be multiple congested areas where the skin has been caught between the various strands. The knot marks may or may not be left depending on where the tie lay.

Although as a rule the deepest impression is opposite the suspension point, marks are generally deeper on the front and side of the neck than at the back where the neck structures are firmer and less accommodating to a noose.

When the suspension point is behind the ligature may encircle the neck almost horizontally, particularly when only part of the body is suspended.

When the body is fully suspended its weight will tend to pull the noose to the level above the larynx and this is more likely when the knot is on the front when lifting the chin and tilting the head will facilitate such a rise.

Internal injuries are remarkably infrequent and when present suggest that some violence has occurred such as from a drop. In addition to soft tissue injuries, which are infrequent, fractures may occur in both larynx and hyoid. The frequency with which these occur varies considerably in different series. In our own practice fractures of the superior horn of the thyroid cartilage are approximately equal to fractures of the greater horn of the hyoid. They are considerably less common than is found in strangulation and are, as might reasonably be expected, normally related to the state of ossification of these structures and in general, therefore, to the age of the deceased. The infrequency in our own findings may, therefore, be explained by saying that perhaps two-thirds of our cases of hanging are under the age of 30 years.

Was death due to hanging or was the body hanged after death?

The circumstances in which the body was found may often be of considerable help. As may be surmised the general findings may be non-specific and particularly if there is no evidence of localised asphyxial changes or these do not correspond with the ligature mark difficulties can arise. It is for this reason that a detailed systematic autopsy, supported by adequate laboratory investigations, is essential.

Points which are of assistance include:

1. The presence of any other possible cause of death, with particular reference to marks of violence which cannot be explained by the deceased having attempted other forms of suicide prior to suspension. The possibility of marks sustained when the body is cut down, particularly from a height, must be considered.

2. The distribution of hypostasis which is not in keeping with suspension as in the classic case of

R. v. Emmett-Dunne when, it will be recalled, the victim of an assault had been concealed in the boot of a car and later suspended from a stairway.[61]

The ligature mark itself is not necessarily the deciding factor. If the mark is dried and brown in colour it may have been applied before or after death, and if there is no evidence of any local lividity at the edges it may be impossible to say from the mark alone whether the body was alive or dead when suspended.

A detailed microscopic examination of the mark may confirm the presence of effusion of red cells, possibly with separation of fibrin and cellular elements, but no evidence of tissue reaction. It is then still worth quoting, as in previous editions, the original experiments of Casper:[62]

1. The body of a man, aged 28, was suspended, an hour after death, by a double cord passed round the neck above the larynx. The body was cut down and examined 24 hours afterwards. Between the larynx and hyoid bone there were two parallel depressions, about ¼ inch deep, the skin having a brown colour with a slight tinge of blue, and a leathery consistency: in certain parts it was slightly excoriated. There was no effusion of blood beneath, but the muscles which lay above the compression were of a dark purple colour, and the blood-vessels of the neck were congested. The appearance of the body was such that any person unacquainted with the facts would have supposed, on looking at it, that the hanging had really taken place during life, for there was nothing to indicate that the body had been hanged an hour after death.
2. The body of another young man was hanged an hour after death, and an examination was made the following day. The two depressions produced by the double cord were of a yellowish brown colour, without ecchymoses; the skin 'appeared as if it had been burnt', and felt like parchment.
3. The body of an old man who had died from dropsy, was hung up two hours after death. The impressions presented exactly the same characters as in the preceding case. When the hanging took place at a later period than two hours after death, there was no particular effect produced.

It is clear that the mark which is usually seen on the neck where hanging took place during life may be produced also by a ligature applied within 2 h, or even later after death—consequently, this kind of mark is not conclusive proof that the hanging took place during life.

Accident, suicide or homicide?

When a body is found hanging in the vast majority of cases the death is due to suicide. It is assumed to be unlikely that an adult person can be overcome and hanged unless that person is either old or infirm. A physically healthy person may be hanged while rendered defenceless through the influence of drugs, alcohol or other injury, or when a sufficient number of people are present to overpower any resistance.

Circumstances which suggest that apparent suicides warrant further investigation include:
1. The scene of death where there are signs of violence or disorder of furniture and other objects.
2. Where the clothing of the deceased is torn or disarranged.
3. Where there are any marks on the body, either defensive or offensive. Of particular interest are scratch marks around the neck.

Sometimes people bent on suicide have attempted other methods. Therefore, the body may have cuts and other injuries. The room may be in some disorder and extensively stained with blood.

Other factors which may be considered must include the extent and nature of the injuries in the neck.

Although severe injury to the neck can be met with in suicidal hanging, evidence of violence should ordinarily arouse some suspicion.

In addition to injuries mentioned, which may have been caused intentionally by the deceased himself, there may be others which have been accidental in that the person may have sustained them when throwing himself from a table or chair.

The method of application of the ligature has already been considered as regards vital reaction, or rather the lack of it.

In general terms, as considered above, in suspension when the full weight of the body is applied it is usual to have a ligature above the larynx, whereas in strangulation it is usually below. Difficulties can arise when the noose has been initially placed lower on the neck and has been pulled up later.

Incomplete suspension, as already mentioned, can have a mark which is almost horizontal and does not rise up to a suspension point, particularly if the noose is of the running type.

Accidental death is unusual in adults. It occurs in someone overcome by alcohol and whose head is caught in some constricting situation. Children playing with cords and ribbons occasionally perish in this manner (see illustrative case P. 31075 and Fig. 13.24).

The association with accidental deaths which

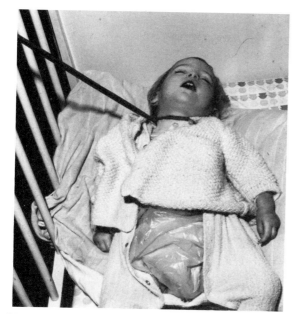

Fig. 13.24 See illustrative case P. 30175.

the case reported by Wright & Davis.[21]

The circumstances appear to result from the seeking of erotic stimulation, apparently resulting from the hypoxic state which can arise from constriction of the neck. This is achieved by self-suspension. This form of suspension is often extremely complex. It is often associated with bondage in which the neck ligatures are connected to either the hands and feet or the genitals. The neck is also often padded to prevent injury.

It is usually done in conditions of secrecy. It is often accompanied by pornographic photographs and occasionally mirrors so that the suspended person can observe what is going on. Sometimes the suspension is complicated by the use of a plastic bag and the inhalation of substances such as ether, cleaning fluids, amyl nitrate.

Difficulties can arise when the relatives who first find the body remove the various pieces of apparatus before investigating officers can examine the scene.

Although it is apparently a solitary exercise, Litman & Swearingen[60] note that the practitioners who co-operated in their study often appreciated the services of a companion for reasons of safety. Evidence of such a person having been present at the scene of death can cause problems for the investigating officer.

occur in the course of auto-erotic exercises, the so-called sexual asphyxias, is now well recognised.

Most psychiatrists agree that there is an element of masochism in these exercises. It would appear, however, that in the vast majority death is not intended. There are numerous reports now of such cases, usually in the young and almost all males.

Henry[63] reports a sex-related case in a 19-year-old woman from accidental hanging. It involved a complicated system of bondage but he specifically notes that mechanical asphyxia, as in males, was not an integral part of this system of loops. He notes that he had been unable to find a single report of such deaths in females in the literature. He found that the death of the female in this reported case was due to the accidental malfunctioning of a part of the victim's costume which resulted in an unintentional hanging.

Sass[64] has reported what appears to be a clearly defined accidental masochistic hanging in the female who had clothes-pegs on her nipples.

The psychiatric background has been considered by Litman & Swearingen.[60] From the forensic point of view these cases can cause some difficulty in that although the findings may seem typical enough it is possible that homicidal hanging can occasionally masquerade as sexual asphyxia as in

Illustrative cases

Hanging—woman—20 years. A married woman was found dead by her husband between the sink and the bath. An interrupted ligature mark was present on the neck. The face was suffused. Petechiae were present in both eyelids. The only internal injury was a $\frac{1}{8} \times 2$ inch bruise in the muscles of the front of the neck between the hyoid bone and the cricoid cartilage. The husband stated that he found the deceased with the chain of the washbasin tightly secured around her neck. The marks on the neck coincided with those on the chain. After initial doubts because of the length of the chain, experiments with it showed that it could have happened in the manner described (P. 22573) (Fig. 13.25).

Hanging—accidental?—female child—13 months. A five-year-old child awakened parents by saying 'baby has a red thing around her neck'.

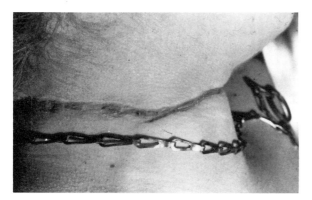

Fig. 13.25 See illustrative case P. 22573.

Numerous petechiae were present on the neck and face above the level of the mark on the neck. This comprised a dried mark as of a ligature, some 6 inches in length, which completely encircled the neck but was least developed at the back of the head on the right side where there was a series of five roughly circular congested areas, each about $\frac{1}{8}$ inch in diameter, separated by areas of pallor. The mark was consistent with having been caused by a red ribbon, some 27 inches in length, attached to the edge of the cot (P. 31075) (Fig. 13.24).

Hanging (sexual)—man—17 years. A young man was found hanging by the neck from a large fir tree, some 10 ft above the ground. The lower chest and abdomen were unclothed with a pair of blue denim jeans at the level of the ankles. The zip was undone and the belt completely unbuckled. A pair of white cotton underpants were present at the same level. Three ligatures were applied to the body:

1. A loosely plaited rope comprising seven strands of $\frac{1}{8}$ inch coarse twine surrounded the neck through a loose slip type knot on the right side. The ligature was separated from the skin by the innermost of three sweaters.

2. Both ankles were firmly secured by a $\frac{3}{8}$ inch coarse rope which encircled them four times and was secured on the front of the right ankle by a firm granny type knot.

3. A $\frac{3}{8}$ inch single strand of rope encircled the lower abdomen. It then ran between the top of the left thigh and the genitalia, around the thigh, crossing the outer aspect of the left hip. One end then ran around the front of the abdomen and the other around the back where they were attached to both wrists, across the midline, by loose slip type knots.

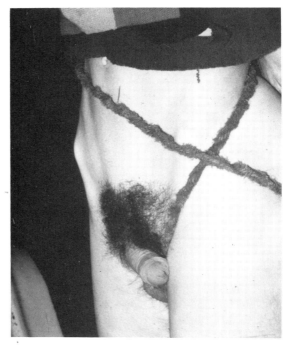

Fig. 13.26 Erotic hanging.

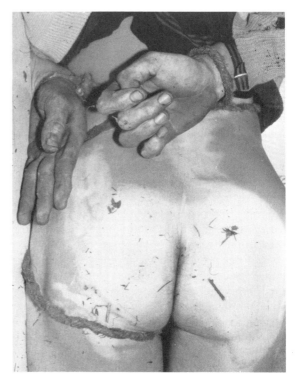

Fig. 13.27 Erotic hanging.

This ligature was only moderately tight.

The examination in the mortuary showed a mark around the neck consistent with an act of self-suspension, the suspension point being to the right of the occiput. The only other mark was a superficial bruised abrasion on the front of the root of the nose $\frac{1}{8}$ inch in diameter. The left side of the face was slightly suffused and the lips and lobes of the ears were cyanotic. Internally there were congestive changes but no marks of injury. It was concluded that the post-mortem findings and the circumstances surrounding the death were consistent with it having occurred in the course of an erotic exercise (P. 14471) (Figs 13.26 and 13.27).

Traumatic asphyxia

The air flow in and out of the lungs occurs as the result of pressure differential between the outer and inner ends of the airways. The supplying of oxygen and removing of carbon dioxide is accomplished by the flow of air in and out of the lungs with each breath. This is a mechanical process for which the muscles of respiration provide the force, i.e., the diaphragm, the inter-costal muscles and accessory muscles. Expiration is the result of the elastic recoil of the lungs and the thoracic cage and the action of gravity when the respiratory muscles relax.

It follows that forcible compression of the chest can rapidly produce the hypoxic state and the obstruction to the flow of venous blood can cause a rapid increase in pressure in the neck, head and shoulders, these being the parts which characteristically become intensely cyanosed.

The external appearances are those of intense cyanosis in the areas mentioned, viz., head, neck and upper chest, and generally fairly sharply demarcated from the lower parts which are considerably less cyanosed or even pale.

Pale marks in the cyanotic areas may show remarkably well delineated patterns which correspond with clothing such as the collar or braces worn by the deceased. Petechiae or frank haemorrhage into the eyes are common.

Microscopic examination of these areas confirms intense dilatation of blood vessels with extensive areas of frank haemorrhage. Sometimes there are fractures of ribs but in the majority of cases which we have examined the lack of fractures was a remarkable feature, considering the amount of force which was applied.

The circumstances can readily be imagined, as when a person is crushed by a mob of persons who find themselves in a situation from which they cannot escape. It would appear that traumatic asphyxia was a major factor in the Black Hole of Calcutta, from the account of Holwell as described by Bayon.[65] He writes:

It might be surmised that many of the one hundred and twenty-three dead were simply stifled by pressure on the ribs paralysing the lung and cardiac action. This would occur among those pushing against the door.

One of the worst examples in modern times was described by Simpson[66] during the Second World War:

During the bombing of London in the second great war an alarm sounded and several hundreds of people, mostly women and children, pressed forward to make their way into the deep shelter at Bethnal Green Tube Station. A woman stumbled and fell on the stairway, and before anyone could intervene people had started piling up over her on a landing: they became inextricably tangled and it was several hours before the pile of victims was cleared. One hundred and seventy-three were dead of suffocation, pinning and crushing of the neck, chest or abdomen, vagal inhibition, regurgitated vomit inhalation, prolonged suboxia, etc.

In addition to such cases where the pinning force is heavy and maintained, cases are seen in which the force moves and rolls over the chest and in some of these the blood appears to be pushed backwards into the smaller veins and capillaries of the head and neck and with such a sudden increase in pressure they burst with the production of numerous petechiae and areas of larger haemorrhage. Cases of this sort are seen in accidents involving various forms of industrial machinery and in road traffic accidents. This appears to be a particular hazard when a person is partially ejected from an overturning open-top sports car.

Sometimes the effect of the local constriction is augmented by other asphyxial producing features. This appears to have been so in the method adopted by William Burke when he killed Margery Campbell. Hare, who gave 'King's evidence', described how Burke got stride-legs on top of the woman on the floor, put one hand under the nose and the other under the chin. This process is now sometimes referred to as 'Burking'.[67]

It is agreed that the degree of force required to produce traumatic asphyxia and the manner of its application is such that a fatality can usually only occur by accident. This would appear to be true in the majority of cases but the position is less clear cut when the complexity of the case is increased by the effects of alcohol and drugs, which are notable adjuvants in this respect.

This occasionally presents problems in sexual offences when the victim is face downwards, and compressed against some firm surface by the weight of the attacker, while the mouth and nose may be partially occluded by bedding.

Illustrative cases

Compression of the chest—male child—2½ years. A child was found dead in a garage near a pushchair. The face was slightly suffused and numerous petechiae were present in both eyelids. Hypostasis, which was faint, was confined to the posterior dependent parts of the body apart from the areas of contact flattening. The only mark of injury was a faint rectangular bruise on the back of the right lower chest, ½ × 1½ inches, centred 8¾ inches below the nape of the neck, 19½ inches above the heel and 1 inch to the right of the midline. Internally the air passages were acutely congested and contained some frothy blood tinged mucus. All lobes of the lungs were intensely congested with areas of recent haemorrhagic collapse. A few subepicardial petechiae were present at the base of the heart posteriorly. It was considered that the cause of death was traumatic asphyxia due to compression of the chest by the pushchair (P. 14774).

Traumatic asphyxia—woman—37 years. A circular mark as of pressure comprising a central area of pallor surrounded by an area of intense congestion on the right side of the face, with two almost horizontal linear similar pressure marks on the right side of the neck, ¼ inch apart, 3 and 2½ inches in length and ¼ inch in maximum width. Marks were also present on both arms. Hypostasis, which was intense and cyanotic, was present on the posterior dependent parts of the body and also on the front of the head and neck, which was intensely suffused with numerous petechiae. Internally there was bruising of the strap muscles of the neck on the left side in the region of the greater horn of the thyroid cartilage. Blood tinged froth was present in the air passages. The daughter of the deceased found her lying face downwards under an overturned gas stove. It appeared that the deceased was trapped by the gas stove which was insecurely fastened and had overturned (P. 14172).

Mechanical asphyxia—man—25 years. A man was found face downwards by the side of a small stream at the foot of a steep embankment. Embedded in the stream was a consolidated pneumatic generator which had two large rubber tyres. This was normally kept at the top of the embankment. The findings were those of intense hypoxia in the head and upper chest. The only marks of injury were semi-circular bruised abrasions on the outer aspect of the left side of the trunk and thigh and a group of semi-circular bruises on the outer aspect of the left side of the chest, arranged in a roughly circular manner. Internally the only findings were intense congestion of the lungs with subpleural haemorrhages and a few subepicardial petechiae at the base of the heart posteriorly. A suggestion that the deceased had been run over while 'fooling about' was supported by tyre and other marks on the embankment (P. 81073).

REFERENCES

1. Taylor, A. S. (1865) Principles and Practice of Medical Jurisprudence. London: Churchill.
2. Best, T. K. & Taylor, M. R. (1973) In: Brobeck, J. R., ed. Physiological Basis of Medical Practice, 9th edn. Baltimore: Williams and Wilkins.
3. Eastham, R. D. (1971) Biochemical Values in Clinical Medicine, 4th edn. Bristol: John Wright & Sons.
4. McIntyre, J. P. (1969) Br. J. Hosp. Med., 2, 1113.
5. Barcroft, J. (1925) The Respiratory Functions of the Blood. London: Cambridge University Press.
6. Peters, J. P. & Van Slyke, D. D. (1931) Quantitive Clinical Chemistry. Baltimore: Williams and Wilkins.
7. Lundsgaard, C. & Van Slyke, D. D. (1923) Medicine, 2, 1.
8. Mason J. K. (1962) Aviation Accident Pathology. London: Butterworths.
9. Swann, H. E. (1964) J. For. Sci., 9, 360.
10. Tardieu, H. (1866) Ann. d'Hyg. Publ. Med. Leg., 2, 357.
11. Shapiro, H. A. (1955) J. For. Med., 2, 1.
12. Gordon, I. & Mansfield, R. A. (1955) J. For. Med., 2, 31.

13. Simpson, K., ed. (1965) Taylor's Principles and Practice of Medical Jurisprudence. London: J. & A. Churchill.
14. Polson, C. J. & Gee, D. J. (1973) The Essentials of Forensic Medicine. Oxford: Pergamon Press.
15. Alberti, K. G. M., M. (1977) J. Clin. Pathol., 30. R. Coll. Pathol., 11, suppl., 14.
16. Swann, H. G. & Brucer, M. (1949) Tex. Rep. Biol. Med., 7, 604.
17. Simpson, K. (1953) Police J., 26, 22.
18. Lyons, M. M. (1973) In: Mant, A. K., ed. Modern Trends in Forensic Medicine, Vol. 3. London: Butterworths, p. 1.
19. Luke, J. L. (1969) J. For. Sci., 14, 398.
20. Polson, C. J. & Gee, D. J. (1972) Z. Rechtsmed., 70, 184.
21. Wright, R. K. & Davis, J. (1976) J. For. Sci., 21, 387.
22. Gardner, A. m. N. (1958) Q. J. Med. N.S., XXVII, no. 106, 227.
23. Knight, B. H. (1975) For. Sci., 6, 229.
24. Miles, S. (1968) Br. Med.J., iii, 597.
25. Swann, H. G. & Spafford, N. R. (1951) Tex. Rep. Biol. Med., 9, 356.
26. Crosfill, J. W. L. (1956) Proc. R. Soc. Med., 49, 1051.
27. Rivers, J. F., Orr, G. & Lee, H. A. (1970) Br. Med. J., ii, 157.
28. Giammona, S. . (1971) Curr. Problems Pediatr., 1, 3.
29. Giammona, S. T. & Modell, J. H. (1967) Am. J. Dis. Child., 114, 612.
30. Gettler, A. O. (1921) J. Am. Med. Assoc., 77, 1650.
31. Durlacher, S. H., Freimuth, H. C. & Swann, H. E. (1953) Arch. Pathol., 56, 454.
32. Fuller, R. H. (1963) Milit. Med., 128, 22.
33. Modell, J. H., Davis, J. H., Giammona, S. T., Moya, F. & Mann, J. B. (1968) J. A. M. A., 203, 99.
34. Jetter, W. W. & Moritz, A. R. (1943) Arch. Pathol., 35, 601.
35. den Otter, G. (1973) For. Sci., 2, 305.
36. Timperman, J. (1972) For. Sci., 1, 397.
37. Reh, H. (1965) Der Ertrinkungstod Med. Mschr., 19, 487.
38. Niles, N. R. (1963) Am. J. Clin. Pathol., 40, 281.
39. Revenstorf, (1904) Vjschr. Gerichtl. Med., 27, 274.
40. Hendey, N. I. (1964) Ministry of Agriculture, Fisheries and Food. Fishery Investigations, series IV, part V. Bacillariophyceae (Diatoms). London: Her Majesty's Stationery Office.
41. Timperman, J. (1969) J. For. Med., 16, 45.
42. Spitz, W. U. & Schneider, V. (1964) J. For. Sci., 9, 11.
43. Spitz, W. U., Schmidt, H. & Fett, W. (1965) Dtsch. Z. Gerichtl. Med., 56, 116.
44. Müller, B. (1952) Dtsch. Z. Gerichtl. Med., 41, 400.
45. Thomas, F., Van Hecke, W. & Timperman, J. (1963) J. For. Sci., 8, 1.
46. Hendey, N. I. (1973) Med. Sci. Law, 13, 23.
47. Keatinge, W. R., Prys-Roberts, C., Cooper, K. E., Honour, A. J. & Haight, J. (1969) Br. Med. J., i, 480.
48. Davis, J. H. (1961) J. For. Sci., 6, 301.
49. Giertsen, J. C. (1970) Med. Sci. Law, 10, 216.
50. Donoghue, E. R. & Minnigerode, S. C. (1977) J. For. Sci., 22, 573.
51. Pullar, P. (1973) In: Mant, A. K. Modern Trends in Forensic Medicine, Vol. 3. London: Butterworth, p. 64.
52. Brouardel, P. (1897) La Pendaison, la Strangulation, la Suffocation, la Submersion. Paris: Bailliere.
53. Simpson, K. (1949) Lancet, i, 558.
54. Green, M. A. (1973) For. Sci., 2, 317.
55. Gonzales, T. A. (1933) Arch. Pathol., 15, 55.
56. Camps, F. E. & Hunt, A. C. (1959) J. For. Med., 6, 116.
57. Prinsloo, I. & Gordon, I. (1951) S. Afr. Med. J., 25, 358.
58. Paparo, G. P. & Siegel, H. (1976) For. Sci., 7, 61.
59. Court of Appeal (Criminal Division) Reports (1969) p. 256.
60. Litman, R. E. & Swearingen, C. (1972) Arch. Gen. Psychiat., 27, 80.
61. Camps, F. E. (1959) Med. Leg. J., 27, 156.
62. Casper, J. L. (1861) A Handbook of the Practice of Forensic Medicine. London: The New Sydenham Society.
63. Henry, R. C. (1971) Med. -Leg. Bull., 24.
64. Sass, F. A. (1975) J. For. Sci., 20, 181.
65. Bayon, H. P. (1944–45) Proc. R. Soc. Med., 83, 15.
66. Simpson, K. (1943) Lancet, ii, 309.
67. Roughead, W. (1948) Notable British Trials, 2nd edn. London: Wm. Hodge.

FURTHER READING

Brouardel, P. (1904) Ann. Hyg. Publ. (Paris), 2, 193.
Fuller, R. H. (1963) Proc. R. Soc. Med., 56, 33.
Swann, H. G. & Brucer, M. (1949) Tex. Rep. Biol. Med., 7, 511.

14

Abortion

Certain clinical and pathological aspects of forensic medicine have remained unchanged over the past decade whilst others, due to the emergence of hitherto uncommon injuries or advances of laboratory investigation, have required considerable reappraisal. In this context the 1967 Abortion Act has been responsible for a dramatic change in the incidence and attitude to therapeutic abortion whilst at the same time fatalities from criminal abortion have continued their downward trend in the practice of forensic pathology. There has been very little change noted in the methods of criminal abortion and therefore virtually no advances in this particular field of forensic medicine under review.

Miscarriage is synonymous, in a legal sense, with the word abortion, the fetus being regarded as a human life to be protected by the criminal law from the moment of fertilisation. Prior to 1806 the unborn child was afforded legal protection only when quickening had occurred, a circumstance which arose from ancient speculation regarding the time of commencement of life.

The procuring of an abortion was an offence under the common law of England before Parliament existed and it was made a statutory offence in the reign of George III with further legislation in 1861 which chiefly concerned the administration of poisons to procure an abortion.

The statutory law relating to abortion is in the Offences Against the Person Act 1861, Section 58 and 59 which deems it unlawful to adminster any poison or other noxious thing or use unlawfully any instrument or other means whatsoever with intent to procure the miscarriage of any woman. In addition, it is an offence in law to procure unlawfully, or supply any poison or noxious thing or instrument for the purposes of procuring the miscarriage

of a woman. The poison or other noxious thing includes any recognised poison, indeed any substance used with intent to procure abortion.

Section 58. Any woman, being with child, who, with intent to procure her own miscarriage, shall unlawfully administer to herself any poison or other noxious thing, or shall unlawfully use any instrument or other means whatsoever with the like intent, and whosoever, with intent to procure the miscarriage of any woman, whether she be or not be with child, shall unlawfully administer to her or cause to be taken by her any poison or other noxious thing, or shall unlawfully use any instrument or other means whatsoever with like intent, shall be guilty of felony and being convicted thereof shall be liable to be imprisoned.

Section 59. Whosoever shall unlawfully supply or procure any poison or other noxious thing, or any instrument or thing whatsoever, knowing that the same is intended to be unlawfully used or employed with intent to procure the miscarriage of any woman, whether she be or not be with child, shall be guilty of a misdemeanour, and being convicted thereof shall be liable to be imprisoned.

It should be noted that the terms felony and misdemeanor were abolished in the Criminal Justice Act 1967 and the word offence was substituted. On conviction under Section 58 a term of imprisonment not less than two years was prescribed, the maximum penalty being life imprisonment and under Section 59 a term of imprisonment not exceeding two years.

There are therefore three categories of persons who may be involved in a criminal act: any woman who being with child attempts to procure her own miscarriage, any person attempting or assisting the woman to procure a miscarriage whether she be or not be pregnant and any person who supplies a drug or instrument knowing it is to be used unlawfully for the above purpose. Although the full penalty on conviction is life imprisonment a shorter term is usually prescribed depending on the type of person involved and the circumstances. It is

322

worth emphasising that it is a criminal offence to attempt to procure a miscarriage; the outcome being irrelevant and this is also true whether or not the woman is pregnant but self-inflicted abortion is criminal only if the woman is pregnant although it should make no difference to a charge of conspiracy. In practice, prosecution in self-inflicted abortions is seldom contemplated let alone carried out. If the victim of an illegal abortion dies, a charge of murder can be preferred only if the accused contemplated that death or grievous bodily harm would result; manslaughter is the usual charge.

The Infant Life Preservation Act 1929 also has some bearing on legal termination of pregnancy as it gives sanction to a practitioner to destroy the fetus but only in order to preserve the life of the mother.

THE INFANT LIFE PRESERVATION ACT 1929

Any person who, with intent to destroy the life of a child capable of being born alive by any wilful act causes the child to die before it has an existence independent of its mother, shall be guilty of child destruction... provided that no person shall be found guilty of an offence under these sections unless it is proved that the act which caused the death of the child was not done in good faith for the purpose only of preserving the life of the mother.

For the purposes of this Act evidence that a woman had at any material time been pregnant for a period of 28 weeks or more shall be prima facie evidence that she was at that time pregnant of a child capable of being born alive. This Act sanctioned destruction of an unborn child provided it had survived 28 weeks gestation and was a legal issue in the case of *R. v. Bourne* (1939, 1K.B. 687).

HISTORICAL DEVELOPMENT OF THE ABORTION ACT

Before the Second World War when mortality from criminal abortion was considerable (432 deaths in the United Kingdom in 1930) interest in legal reform was promoted by the National Council of Women and by the formation of the Abortion Law Reform Association in 1935. Three years later an important test case was heard at the Central Criminal Court. It concerned a 14-year-old girl who had become pregnant following rape. A distinguished gynaecologist, Mr Alec Bourne, after being approached through the School's Care Committee and the Abortion Law Reform Association and after proper consultation, terminated a six week pregnancy on the grounds that continuation of it could endanger the girl's life. The matter was reported to police and subsequently a charge of procuring an unlawful abortion was made. At the Magistrates' Court the word 'unlawful' implicit in the Act of 1861 and omitted in the charge was added at the specific request of counsel for the defence who inferred that its inclusion could imply that there might be a lawful instrumentation to procure a miscarriage. The Crown case was that an operation contrary to the Offences against the Person Act 1861 had been carried out and that it was a grave offence which involved destruction of an unborn child, there being a clear distinction between danger to life and danger to health. The defence view was that the surgeon had acted from the highest motives; he had carried out that which was lawfully right and honest, his view being that the patient's health was endangered by pregnancy. The Judge, Mr McNaghten, directed the jury in his interpretation of the law, drawing attention to the Infant Life Preservation Act 1929, which contained the words 'no person could be found guilty of the offence of child destruction provided it was done in good faith to preserve the life of the mother'. In the judge's view the act referred explicitly to the law with regard to procurement of abortion and that a person should not be convicted unless the act was not done in good faith in preserving the life of the mother, the burden of proof resting on the Crown. The latter maintained that there was a perfectly clear distinction between a danger to life and a danger to health but in Judge McNaghten's view such a distinction was artificial in that impairment of health might reach a stage where there was a danger to life and if a doctor, on reasonable grounds and knowledge, thought that the probable circumstances of pregnancy continuing would render the person concerned a physical or mental wreck then an operation terminating pregnancy could be performed. The surgeon was acquitted and further cases confirmed this view.

In 1966 a United Kingdom Parliamentary Bill was introduced which became Statute Law in April 1968 known as the Abortion Act 1967, being applied to England, Wales and Scotland but not Northern Ireland. It permitted termination of pregnancy by a registered medical practitioner subject to the following conditions:

1. That two registered medical practitioners form, in good faith, the opinion that the continuance of the pregnancy would involve risk to the life of the pregnant woman, greater than if the pregnancy was terminated.

2. That it would involve risk of injury to the physical or mental health of the pregnant woman greater than if the pregnancy were terminated.

3. That it would involve risk of injury to the physical or mental health of any existing child of the pregnant woman's family, greater than if the pregnancy were terminated.

4. That there is a substantial risk that the child born would suffer from some physical or mental abnormality so as to be seriously handicapped.

The following factors should be noted: in determining whether continuance of a pregnancy would involve risk of injury to the physical or mental health of the pregnant woman, the practitioner should consider the pregnant woman's actual or reasonably forseeable environment. Except in the case of termination on an emergency basis, operation must be carried out in a hospital or in other places approved by the Secretary of State. The opinion of two registered medical practitioners is not required for the termination of pregnancy by a doctor acting on his own if he believes that it is necessary to save life or to prevent grave permanent injury.

The procedure of termination should be notified within seven days on a prescribed form (available from the Department of Social Security) to the Chief Medical Officer of the appropriate department of England, Wales or Scotland by the doctor or appropriate authority. This form was redesigned in 1981. The gynaecologist is required not only to identify reasons for termination and establish legality for operation by 'ticking' boxes but also to give specific reasons for termination in order to collate results.

Notification forms include information as to the place of termination, the practitioner's signature, the name, status and occupation of the woman, details of previous pregnancies and births; date of admission and discharge from the hospital or approved place and the grounds for termination; procedures adopted and any complications which might have arisen following the operation.

Such information may only be disclosed at the discretion of the Chief Medical Officer in the following circumstances:

1. To an officer of the ministry authorised by the chief medical officer or to the Registrar General for the purposes of carrying out duties or for the same reasons to the Director of Public Prosecutions or an authorised member of his staff.

2. Similarly to a police officer not below the rank of superintendent in the course of his duties or in pursuing criminal proceedings already commenced.

3. For bona fide research.

4. To a registered medical practitioner provided the written consent of the patient is obtained.

The Office of Population Census and Survey undertakes statistical processing and analysis of notification forms by arrangement with the chief medical officer and annual figures for therapeutic abortion operations are issued as a supplement to the Registrar General's Statistical Review.

The regulations of the Abortion Act govern the form in which registered medical practitioners are to certify their opinion which must be preserved for a minimum of three years either by the operator or a hospital authority, the disclosure of such information being prohibited except to certain persons. Schedule I of the regulations concerns the practitioner's certificate, ordinarily Certificate A being used, the form being signed by two practitioners, one of whom, though not necessarily, will be the practitioner who performs the operation of termination. In emergency cases Certificate B is used. Certificate A must be completed before the operation commences and if an emergency Certificate B is used with insufficient time to complete it before the operation it must be completed within 24 h of termination of pregnancy. Both surgeon and anaesthetist should not act on hearsay evidence of the existence of a certificate but should ensure that it is examined in detail.

Certain provisions of the Act must be given careful consideration. The pregnant woman's actual or reasonably forseeable environment has given rise to the view that a therapeutic abortion may be obtained on 'social' grounds, unjustifiably so, as on many occasions a doctor may have to consider the patient's family background or environment in relation to treatment in the course of any illness. Existing children of a family may include adopted, illegitimate, step children or a subnormal child within the family over the age of 21 years. Section 4 of the Abortion Act relates to a substantial risk that the child, if born alive, might suffer from physical or mental abnormality so as to seriously handicap its life. This risk requires a certain amount of inspired guess work on the part of the practitioner as applied to each individual case although there are well recognized diseases, e.g., rubella, which may carry a substantial risk. Conscientious objection to the Act does not exclude a doctor discharging his responsibility to advise and treat a patient. Should a doctor consider a therapeutic abortion cannot be recommended on grounds of conscientious objection to it, it is his/her duty to recommend the patient to seek advice and possible treatment elsewhere. Conscientious objection does not apply necessarily to religious grounds only. Although a doctor may be required to prove his conscientious objection in law, a statement on oath in Court would suffice. It should also be noted that under the Offences against the Person Act 1861, it remains a criminal offence to perform an abortion illegally, other than under the Abortion Act 1967.

Consent

As in any surgical procedure it is essential for the patient to give her written consent to termination of pregnancy and normally a husband's assent would be implied during the course of conversation or discussion after the practitioner has reviewed the case. However, it is by no means mandatory to obtain his permission in order to terminate a pregnancy. Should he be unwilling for it to take place it is highly unlikely that legal redress could occur.

Between 16 and 18 years of age the Family Law Reform Act 1969 would be applicable. Under 16 years of age the girl's parents should be informed of the girl's pregnancy and given the practitioner's opinion as to its continuation but under the Abortion Act, if the girl's consent is forthcoming, the parent's view to the contrary may be disregarded. Conversely should a parent demand termination of a daughter's pregnancy contrary to the patient's wishes no termination should take place.

At all times, therefore, the patient's wishes, interest and consent are paramount and a reasonable opinion which recommends termination of pregnancy, given in good faith, should be acceptable to any subsequent Court of legal procedure.

ETHICS AND DUTY OF A PRACTITIONER IN ABORTION

In therapeutic abortion a registered medical practitioner may decide whether there are sufficient grounds for termination of pregnancy depending on the regulations of the Abortion Act and also if it is necessary on clinical grounds in the interests of the patient. It is possible that the practitioner might risk criminal proceedings for negligence if he should refuse an emergency termination of pregnancy should it at a later date constitute (in the eyes of the law a reckless act, or should it indicate a failure to take proper care) a case for negligent practice.

With regard to criminal abortion, a doctor's duty was put on record in 1916 when the Royal College of Physicians of London advised practitioners that their duty to the patient superseded their common law duty and that information regarding abortion should only be divulged for the purposes of a criminal investigation. This followed Mr Justice Avory's opinion given two years previously at Birmingham Assize. A woman had died following a criminal abortion and despite the fact that she had informed the doctor of the abortionist's name no action was taken. The judge told the practitioner that he should have communicated with the police and supplied information to assist the administration of justice, his view being that a doctor–patient relationship should be subordinated to the process of common law. In practice, if a practitioner has knowledge of possible criminal interference in pregnancy, particularly to the extent of involving a doctor in treating or admitting a patient to hospital for treatment, informal discussion is advisable with senior police officers. A doctor should always urge a patient to make a statement but even if she refuses to do so there is no legal obligation to take further action except to report a death, should it occur, to the coroner.

In general practice a practitioner may be consulted by a patient in the hope that an abortion might be initiated, or by attempting to mislead a doctor as to the state of a pregnancy, in order that an examination be made which could accelerate a threatened abortion. The practitioner must be most careful to avoid falling into this trap particularly in regard to an examination carried out in his surgery which could form the basis of a criminal charge, an assault or blackmail; apart from taking emergency measures of treatment, arrangements should be made for the patient to be seen at hospital without delay, if necessary asking a colleague's advice on the matter. In effect, therefore, a practitioner should decide whether his duty lies solely with the patient and her pregnancy respecting confidentiality in any matter relating to abortion bearing in mind that evidence may be required to be given in a Court of law at a later date.

THE EFFECT OF THE ABORTION ACT ON THERAPEUTIC ABORTION

The Abortion Act 1967 has been the subject of much discussion and dispute. In particular, objections have been voiced against termination of pregnancies in patients from overseas and in approved places and private clinics. However, the Act does contain powers for the Secretary of State to enforce regulations relating to the licensing of premises for termination operations. The Lane Committee (1974) made recommendations concerning specialist abortion services within the National Health Service which would lessen the need for private treatment and clinics; there should be licensing of medical referral abortion services and breaches of the abortion law should incur criminal penalties; also there should be an upper limit of 24 weeks for termination of pregnancy, and the pregnant woman should be examined by both practitioners

Table 14.1 Therapeutic abortions in England and Wales

1970	86 565
1971	126 777
1972	159 884
1973	167 149
1974	162 940
1975	140 521
1976	127 904
1977	132 999
1978	141 558
1979	146 453
1980	163 126

Source: Office of Population Censuses and Surveys.

signing the certificate. Finally, the chief medical officer should be able to disclose to the General Medical Council matters relating to possible serious professional misconduct. These recommendations were referred to a Select Committee on Abortion, as constituted by Parliament.

Since 1968, the first complete year for annual return for operations performed under the Abortion Act, the number of therapeutic abortions performed has risen steadily (see Table 14.1) to a peak in 1973. Since then there has been a diminution in numbers of terminations reported to the chief medical officer, this fall being due to a decrease in the number of patients entering the country from abroad. Deaths following therapeutic abortion are reported to the coroner as well as being notified to the chief medical officer. They are small in number (see Table 14.2). Prior to the Abortion Act 1967, relatively few therapeutic abortions were performed.

Analysis of deaths over the years 1970–73 indicates that of the total deaths reported (36) only 19 were directly attributed to abortion operations.

Table 14.2 Deaths from therapeutic abortion induced for medical indications. England, Wales and Scotland per 100 000 abortions

1968	3
1969	15
1970	14
1971	10
1972	13
1973	4
1974	5
1975	2
1976	1
1977	8
1979	6

Source: Office of Population Censuses and Surveys.

THERAPEUTIC ABORTION IN OTHER COUNTRIES

Mortality from therapeutic abortion varies according to whether abortion is regarded as being legally acceptable, the mortality being lower in those countries where abortion is permissible. In the United States of America legal abortion has been recognised since 1965 in many states. New York State has a liberal law. Since 1970 abortion is permitted if, in the physician's view, the life of a pregnant woman is in jeopardy regardless of reason or motive. In the first year 139 042 abortions occurred, over 50% on non-residents. In the same year the American Medical Association established that an abortion be performed by a licensed physician in an accredited hospital after consultation with two competent physicians with a clause allowing a physician to withdraw from a case. In 1973 the United States Supreme Court acted to supersede most state restrictive laws on abortion and in 1976 to bypass parental or husband's consent in most cases, an action which has led to law suits being taken out over parental consent.

In East European countries, notably Czechoslovakia and Hungary, some restrictions have been imposed in the hitherto 'free' abortion demand due partly to the increased incidence of cervical scarring following therapeutic abortions and partly on economic grounds.

SPONTANEOUS ABORTION

The incidence of spontaneous abortion in all pregnancies is generally recognised to be about 10% and numerous factors have been held responsible. Any systemic disease, especially hypertensive heart disease or chronic renal failure, may cause abortion; also acute infections including the spirochete of syphilis which, unlike other organisms, can cross the placental barrier. Other conditions include chronic inflammatory pelvic disease and abnormal uterine positions which may play a part but more important are abnormalities of the ovum leading to foetal maldevelopment. Tupper and his colleagues[1] investigated 135 cases of spontaneous abortion; they confirmed lower circulating eostrogen and progesterone levels and found degenerative changes in the chorionic villae with fibrinous necrosis and hyalinasion though it is not clear whether these findings were the cause or result of foetal abnormality. Gray[2] in an extensive study of placental lesions in early abortions reported hyalinasion of villae following the break down of collagen and the formation of fibrinoid necroses. More recently attention has been directed to genetic abnormalities in spontaneous abortion. Carr[3] analysed chromosomal abnormalities in 227 spontaneous abortions and whilst 50 showed abnormality none were seen in chromosome studies of 51 other induced abortions. Genetic abnormality may be more important, especially translocation of chromosomes, as the majority of spontaneous abortions occur in very early pregnancy.[4] Pathological changes in the ground substance of chorionic villae or stromal network is found in most cases of spontaneous abortion.

It is also known that ABO incompatibility may cause abortion and similarly rhesus sensitivity may occur following transplacental haemorrhage.

METHODS OF THERAPEUTIC ABORTION

Methods of termination of pregnancy have advanced considerably in the last decade and complications nowadays arise largely in relation to the advancing age of the pregnant woman and to increasing duration of pregnancy, in common with obstetrical conditions generally. The injection of uterine pastes and the use of laminarial tents have been replaced by other techniques. Recently synthetic prostaglandin compounds in the form of a vaginal suppository in the first few weeks of pregnancy may cause uterine contraction and expulsion of the embryo; similarly in early pregnancy menstrual aspiration is a simple procedure.[5] Vacuum aspiration, first used in China in 1958, is a simple safe procedure with little risk of uterine perforation attended by minimal blood loss.[6] In the second trimester methods involving intra-uterine injections of foreign substances such as urea or glucose, prostaglandins or salt have been widely used.[7] Intra-uterine injection of hypertonic saline was first used in the 1930s[8] and increasingly used in other countries, e.g., Japan and the United States of America.[9] Numerous complications have been reported following these techniques including DIC syndrome (disseminated intravascular coagulation syndrome.[10–12]

In the United Kingdom, Cameron & Dayan[13] reported three cases of intracerebral haemorrhage with cerebral oedema and compression (acute haemorrhagic infarction) following intra-uterine injection of hypertonic saline. Further experimental work on pigs caused salt poisoning but no specific brain changes.[14] Prostoglandins F2D have also been used to induce termination of pregnancy during the second trimester either via amniocentesis or cervix.[15] Johnson, Cushner & Stephens[16] reported cardiac and respiratory changes following hypertonic saline entering the pulmonary circulation but Keranyi, Mandelman & Sherman[17] performed 5000 intra-amniotic injections with no deaths or vascular complications. It is not completely clear how intra-amniotic saline causes abortion but Galen et al,[18] thought that acute salt retention, hypernatrimia and dehydration occurred, the fetus dying from acute sodium poisoning, the alternative view being that placental damage was more significant.

CRIMINAL ABORTION

There has always been considerable difficulty in obtaining an accurate incidence of criminal abortion in the United Kingdom. The Home Office Inter-departmental Committee on Abortion 1939, estimated between 100 000 and 150 000 abortions occurred annually, about 40% following criminal interference. These figures have been questioned by Goodhart[19,20] on the grounds that deaths due to criminal abortion (Table 14.3) should have been

Table 14.3 Deaths from criminal abortion

1942	76
1952	47
1962	29
1972	8
1973	4
1974	3
1975	1
1976	1
1977	1
1978	—
1979	—

Source: Office of Population Censuses and Surveys.

considerably higher than reported if the estimate of annual abortions was correct. There were between 200–400 offences involving abortion known to the police between 1960 and 1963 but these have fallen considerably in recent years, to 14 in 1975. Numerous estimates have been published over the years concerning possible incidence of criminal interference of abortions admitted to hospital. Davis[21] considered spontaneous abortion occurred in only 10% of his series and Teare[22] estimated 28% of fatal abortion cases examined in the London area had been self-induced, the remainder following some form of criminal interference. Cameron[23] reporting a series of 74 fatal cases between 1960 and 1967 concluded that 60% were due to illegal interference with pregnancy.

Methods of abortion are legion and may be considered to be due either to the administration of abortifacient drugs or by mechanical interference with pregnancy, almost always by the intra-uterine injection of fluid or the use of instruments. Accidental or intentional direct abdominal trauma does not disturb the amniotic sac unless injuries are of such severity that they are associated with numerous fractures of the pelvis, etc. There are numerous examples of unsuccessful attempts to produce abortion despite gross trauma by blows or kicks.

Drugs

It is doubtful whether any drug can be affective without endangering the health or life of the pregnant woman, although almost every common drug must have been used at some time in an attempt to produce abortion. In general, pregnant women resort to increasingly dangerous methods of abortion as the time of gestation advances and it is therefore more common for irritant drugs to be used in the early stages of pregnancy before resorting to instrumental interference later. Again, the use of abortifacient drugs depends to some extent on local fashions, custom and availability as well as on faith engendered by advice from well meaning amateur abortionists. The mode of action of all drugs in abortion must be either to destroy the embryo or interfere with the maternal reaction to pregnancy and there is no doubt that should a safe effective pharmaceutical preparation be available for terminating pregnancy it would be widely used in lieu of operative termination.[24] Purgatives are all relatively mild in action and include castor oil, rhubarb, senna, aloes and cascara.[25] More drastic are vegetable products of the jalap or colocynth group which contain resinous glucocides and acids; also included in this group are scammony and podophyllum, the latter being very toxic and having antimitotic, cytotoxic and teratogenic effect on rats.[26]

Essential oils are volatile odoriferous materials derived from plants known chemically as terpines. Volatile oils include a large number of preparations derived from flowers of plants of the order *Labiatae umbelliferae, cruciferae, coniferae* and *aurantiacae*. From this group the oils of savin, juniper, tansy, saffron, apiol (common parsley), arborvitae, pulegone (pennyroyal) are derived. Most of the substances mentioned above are of historical interest only and a part of folk medicine as regards their use and effect on pregnancy nowadays. In general their action is to produce pelvic congestion and possible irritation of the uterine endometrium although generalised toxic symptoms including vomiting and diarrhoea with convulsions and coma may result from the administration of volatile oils.

Any drug or substance capable of contracting the uterine wall during the early months of pregnancy is unlikely to be effective if the os cervix is closed and the drug is not likely to affect the placental circulation to any extent. It is known that ionising radiation[27] and mitotic drugs such as ergocornine and vinblastine may destroy the embryo or placenta, also antimetabolic drugs such as aminopterin.[28] Substances which interfere with the maternal reaction in pregnancy include exogenous steroids, monoamine oxidaze inhibitors[29] and acetylated diphenyl alkalines. Cytotoxic drugs given to pregnant women with leukaemia may also produce abortion.[30]

Other drugs and substances which have a reputation for their use as abortifacients are oxytocin, ergot, posterior pituitary extract and synthetic eostrogens. Ergot[31] either in the form of crude extract or in alkaloid form has a uterine action which increases as pregnancy advances but its toxic circulatory side-effects result in arterial spasm and gangrene of the extremities. Posterior pituitary extract (oxytocin)[32] will only cause uterine contraction near term, effective by intramuscular injection

or as snuff but ineffective orally. Synthetic eostrogens have also been used as abortifacients but as they tend to stimulate production of steroids by the placenta they may protect rather than disturb the foetal sac.

Quinine has largely fallen into disrepute as an abortifacient following stricter control of this drug in the last decade. An alkaloid from the cinchona tree, it may cause toxic symptoms due to idiosyncrasy to the drug, or in larger quantities produce characteristic symptoms of cinchonism, visual impairment and lead to convulsions. It may also produce an acute haemolytic anaemia resulting in skin discoloration not dissimilar to that of *Clostridium welchii* septicaemia.

Potassium permanganate has been widely used as a chemical abortifacient, possibly following its original use as a fluid for vaginal douching.[33] A potassium permanganate tablet in contact with the cervical mucosa will result in a chemical burn and ulceration.[34] The permanganate ulcer has a punched out appearance with raised edges and a granular black base, liable to result in acute severe haemorrhage following erosion of subjacent blood vessels.[35] Its appearance may also simulate a syphilitic ulcer or an antepartum haemorrhage. Brudenell[36] reviewed 650 cases from the literature; only 10% had resulted in abortion. Potassium permanganate breaks down into potassium hydroxide and manganese dioxide and after absorption may produce intravenous haemolysis and methaemoglobinaemia.[37] Outbreaks of permanganate poisoning following its use as an abortifacient have been reported by Cabaniss & Clark,[38] Bobrow & Friedman[39] and Obeng.[40] Other substances which may produce corrosion of the vaginal mucosa include heavy metals such as mercury and copper sulphate and diachlyon plasters containing oleate of lead have also resulted in poisoning when the substance has been consumed orally. In practice, the composition of 'abortifacients' available to the public are legion, disguised when sold under a proprietary name and David[41] found that the most common ingredients were aloes and apiol.

Criminal abortion by instruments

The commonest form of mechanical interference with pregnancy is by a very large number of metallic objects and instruments, including hair pins, hat pins, bobby pins, knitting needles, crochet hooks, umbrella spokes, metal syringe tips as well as surgical bougies; also non-metallic compounds of plastic or celluloid material, including urethral catheters or glycerol urethral bougies, formerly used for dilating urethral strictures. If a foreign intraperitoneal body is suspected following attempted abortion X-ray examination is advisable prior to a laparotomy.[42] Slippery elm bark (*Ulmus fulva*) derived from a tree in Central America has been frequently used in the past, interfering with pregnancy following its insertion into the cervical canal, in portions 1–3 inches long, where it absorbs the moisture causing cervical dilatation in a manner similar to a laminarial tent.[43]

Gross trauma following criminal abortion may produce laceration of the uterine fundus necessitating removal of portions of the small bowel.[44] The instrument most commonly used in former years was the enema syringe, being readily obtainable for many purposes and in the past responsible for more fatalities than any other instrument. It may be used to inject soap or antiseptic solutions such as lysol,[45] turpentine,[46] formaldehyde[47] and ethyl alcohol.[48] The addition of an antiseptic or chemical compound results in corrosion of the uterine mucous membrane and intense shock. The danger of intra-uterine injection of any fluid through the enema syringe is that a mixture of air and fluid may enter the systemic circulation after separating the placental membranes from the uterine wall, spreading along large vascular spaces leading to the entry of soap and air into the large veins, vena cava and eventually the pulmonary arterial circulation and via alveolar capillaries to the coronary and cerebral circulation.[49] The risk of air embolism increases as pregnancy advances and emboli may reach the brain through the placental venous plexus[50] or the abdominal and thoracic veins which anastamose with the vertebral venous plexus. In early pregnancy antiseptic fluid may enter the peritoneal cavity via the fallopian tubes causing shock and chemical peritonitis and it may also cause widespread venous thrombosis and uterine infarction.[51] Mant[52] reported fatal intravascular thrombosis due to polyethylene glycol used as a vehicle base for xylocaine. Maternal aspiration of amniotic fluid is possible following a laceration of the uterine wall and intestinal wall allowing amniotic elements to reach the stomach via reflex peristasis, subsequent vomiting causing amniotic debris to be inhaled.[53].

Utus paste

Intrauterine injection of utus paste is of particular interest as death has followed its use in therapeutic and criminal abortion. First described by Leunbach,[54] it was widely used in Europe in the 1930 era and subsequently in the United States of America by criminal abortionists with numerous fatalities, Dutra[55] recording four deaths following its use. The paste consists of soft soap containing potassium iodide and an aromatic substance injected into the uterus only after closure of the fallopian tubes occurs. Barns[56] used it successfully therapeutically in the United Kingdom and Berthelsen & Ostervaard[57] in 1235 cases of therapeutic abortion in Denmark without fatality but more recently Thomas, Galizia & Wensley[58] reported a case of consumptive coagulopathy and intravenous haemolysis following its use. Similar related substances are Hexol, a pine distillate like turpentine.[59]

CAUSES OF DEATH

Therapeutic abortion (see Fig. 14.2)

Deaths are due in the most part to errors in surgical technique or inexperience and are more likely to occur in circumstances where large numbers of therapeutic abortions are performed without adequate facilities, including transfusions, with a lessening of standards of surgery.

Criminal abortion

Immediate

It is well recognised that vagal inhibition or reflex shock may result in cardiac arrest if the cervix or uterus is manipulated particularly in the unanaesthetised state and if the patient is in a state of apprehension. Severe haemorrhage may occur following vaginal or uterine laceration from instrumental procedures and air embolism is a common complication following the use of an enema syringe. The latter usually causes sudden collapse and death but delayed death from air embolism has been reported. Simpson[60] found that a minimum of 2 h may elapse before death occurs following introduction of air into the uterine cavity. It is therefore unwise to be too dogmatic as to the time interval between criminal interference and death in cases of air embolism, a medico-legal point of considerable importance.

Delayed

The principle delayed causes of death in criminal abortion are sepsis and hepato-renal failure but cardiorespiratory failure can occur following toxic shock. Utian[61] reported 9700 cases of abortion in over 32 000 gynaecological admissions with 0.29% deaths (28 cases), 50% being due to criminal interference; Burnett[62] reported a death rate of 0.09% in 2300 cases of abortion and Perera[63] a 0.06% death rate in 8347 abortions. In the United States of America Schwarz & Emich[64] found 0.20% deaths out of 10 000 abortions. Infection is easily conveyed from an instrument or the perineum into the uterine cavity and any injury to the uterine wall or the presence of irritant products with necrosis of tissue will favour such infection, particularly following criminal interference.[65] Infection may also occur almost immediately, days or weeks later. Bacterial shock resulting from endotoxins or bacterial hypersensitivity may be associated with enterobacillary septicaemia.[66] Septicaemia may result from organisms varying from *Escherichia coli* to staphylococci and non-haemolytic streptococcus and occurs more rapidly from uterine invasion by anaerobic organisms, particularly *Cl. welchii*.[67] The latter produces a classical reddish-brown discoloration of the skin (bronze cyanosis), an infective process which may cause death within 24 h of interference with pregnancy. Infections that may occur later are SABE,[68] osteomyelitis,[69] actinomycosis[70] and systemic moniliasis.[71] Tetanus is also a hazard[72] and haemorrhagic syndromes due to DIC may occur.[73] Renal failure following acute tubular necrosis was a common cause of death prior to methods of dialysis.[74]

POST-MORTEM CHANGES

There have been relatively few deaths in recent years in the United Kingdom following criminal abortion and most pathologists may only very rarely encounter a case but it must always be borne in mind in the investigation of any unexpected death in a female of child bearing age. Prompt action to prevent dispersal of evidence by investigating police officers is also essential.

Autopsy examination will include formal identification of the deceased and careful examination of the clothing which must be retained for contact traces of any foreign substances particularly on the underclothing, e.g., antiseptic solution.

The general characteristics, e.g., height, weight, scars and injuries on the deceased and particularly the areas and distribution and colour of hypostasis and body temperature will be recorded.

As it is essential to confirm or exclude air embolism, the body must not be opened before the pathologist's examination and radiological examination may show translucency of the right ventricle and pulmonary artery as well as pelvic soft tissues and veins.[75] If death occurs more than 18 h before autopsy in a temperate climate the possibility of pseudo-embolism due to gas formation in the systemic vessels should be borne in mind.[76] The vaginal contents should be pipetted and stored in a clean sterile container for possible chemicals, drugs or soap.

Following the initial abdominal incision it is preferable to ascertain and confirm pregnancy by uterine palpation. The preliminary incision, being a small suprapubic one to inspect uterine and adnexal tissues, assessing, if suspected, crepitation due to gas formation in the uterine wall and venous channels and inspecting the inferior vena cava for air or soap embolism bubbles. The external incision may then be extended upwards to the zyphysternal notch without severing large blood vessels and the chest opened in the usual manner after severing the costochondral cartilages, leaving the upper ones intact prior to inspection of the heart. Incision of the pericardial sac will lead to inspection of the coronary vessels for air or gas emboli. The skull vault must then be carefully removed, avoiding puncture of the meninges and vessels over the brain surface which allows air to enter these vessels; a detailed examination of the basal sinuses, veins and arteries is made for the presence of air embolism.

Returning to the thoracic cavity, the right ventricle is opened to elucidate the presence of frothy blood which is often seen in air embolism, within the pulmonary trunk and vessels. It may then be possible to trace bubbles of air, gas or fluid from the uterine vein, via the inferior vena cava into the coronary vessels. Samples of blood from the inferior vena cava and both cardiac ventricles should be collected.

Following removal of the thoracic and abdominal organs in the usual manner, the pelvic organs must be excised *en masse*, following severence of the symphysis pubis and a circular dissection to include vagina, vulva and rectum with adjacent skin, taking care to collect any foreign fluid or material evident.

Further samples of vaginal contents may be collected and the state of the cervix noted, also possible minor abrasions, bruises or lacerations of the lower tract are significant. The vagina and uterus are opened along their anterior surface because injuries are more likely to occur on the posterior vaginal wall following criminal interference. Following incision of the uterus from the cervix upwards any fluid must be collected, the uterine cavity opened without disturbing the amniotic sac. Swabs of the uterine wall should be taken for microbiology and the specimen preserved for fixation and further examination in 10% formal saline.

Fetal maturity may be checked against established tables.[77] Samples of blood, urine and stomach contents should be collected for toxicology, as well as pubic hair, also tissues for histology from all organs. Photographs for the purpose of identification and to show external colouration of the body and to preserve the presence of air embolism in internal organs should be taken.

The post-mortem examination should be performed to answer the following questions:
1. Evidence of recent pregnancy and/or the presence or signs of recent pregnancy?
2. Evidence of abortion and possible criminal interference by drugs or instrument?
3. To relate the cause of death to abortion.
4. To assess any natural disease found.
It must be remembered that there are few other pathological conditions where the pathologist will be required to make an examination at the minimum time after death, not only to demonstrate air embolism but to give the investigating authority an opportunity to apprehend a possible criminal abortionist and instruments or equipment.

It should be borne in mind that any criminal charge must be substantiated not only by positive evidence of interference relating to the deceased's death but also to exclude the possibility of self-induced abortion.

Post-mortem laboratory investigation of abortion death

The investigation of embolism by soap, antiseptic fluid or detergent substances may be elucidated in the laboratory. It is rare for soft soaps to be used nowadays, toilet soaps, detergents or antiseptics being more likely to be used. In soap abortion dispersion occurs rapidly and it is only possible to test for the presence of sodium or potassium iodide, cellulose, optical clarifiers and inorganic components of soap.[78]

Histological changes following soap abortion have revealed necrotic degeneration of the uterine muscle and fatty deposits in the wall of blood vessels with toxic changes in the kidney and liver.

REFERENCES

1. Tupper, C., Moya, F., Stewart, L. C., Weil, R. J. & Gray, J. D. (1957) Am. J. Obstet. Gynecol., **73**, 313.
2. Gray, J. D. (1957) Am. J. Obstet. Gynecol., **74**, 111.
3. Carr, D. H. (1967) Am. J. Obstet. Gynecol., **97**, 283.
4. Roberts, C. J. & Lowe, C. R. (1975) Lancet, **1**, 498.
5. Goldthorpe, W. O. (1977) Br. Med. J., **ii**, 562.
6. Vojta, M. (1967) J. Obstet. Gynaecol. Br. Commonw., **74**, 768.
7. Wood, C., Booth., R. T. & Pinkerton, J. H. M. (1962) Br. Med. J., **2**, 706.
8. Aburel, E. (1939) Rev. Med. Chir. Jassy, **50**, 121.
9. Wagatsuma. T. (1965) Am. J. Obstet. Gynecol., **43**, 743.
10. Beller, F. K., Rosenberg, M., Kolker, M. & Douglas, G. W. (1972) J. Obstet. Gynaecol., **112**, 534.
11. Lemkin, S. R. & Kattlove, A. E. (1973) J. Obstet. Gynaecol., **42**, 233.

12. Weiss, A. E. & Easterling, W. E. Jr. & Odom, M. H. (1972) Am. J. Obstet. Gynecol., 113, 868.
13. Cameron, J. M. & Dayan, A. D. (1966) Br. Med. J., 1, 1010.
14. Cameron, J. M., Morgan, A. G., Robinson, A. E. & Urich, H. (1969) J. Obstet. Gynaecol. Br. Commonw., 76, 168.
15. Roberts, G., Gomershall, R., Adams, M. & Turnbull, A. C. (1972) Br. Med. J., 4, 12.
16. Johnson, J. W. C., Cushner, I. N. & Stephens, N. L. (1966) Am. J. Obstet. Gynecol., 94, 225.
17. Keranyi, D., Mandelman, N. & Sherman, D. H. (1973) Am. J. Obstet. Gynecol., 116, 593.
18. Galen, R. S., Chauhan, P., Wietzner, H. & Navarro, C. (1974) Am. J. Obstet. Gynecol., 1, 47.
19. Goodhart, C. B. (1964) Eugen. Rev., 55, 197.
20. Goodhart, C. B. (1969) J. Biosoc. Sci., 1, 235.
21. Davis, A. (1950) Br. Med. J. 2, 123.
22. Teare, R. D. (1952) Br. Med. J., 1, 915.
23. Cameron, J. M. (1969) Recent Advances in Forensic Pathology. London: J. A. Churchill, p. 89.
24. Potts, D. M. (1970) Br. Med. Bull., 26, 65.
25. Gollman, A. (1965) Pharmacology and Therapeutics, 6th edn. London: H. Kimpton.
26. Chamberlain, M. J., Reynolds, A. L. & Yeoman, W. B. (1972) Br. Med. J., 3, 391.
27. Stern, S. (1928) Am. J. Roent., 19, 133.
28. Emerson, D. J. (1962) Am. J. Obstet. Gynecol., 84, 356.
29. Koren, Z., Pfeifer, Y. & Sulman, F. G. (1966) J. Repro. Fert., 12, 75.
30. Nicholson, H. O. (1968) J. Obstet. Gynaecol. Br. Commonw., 75, 307.
31. Brost, U. (1959) Geburtsh. Frauenheilk., 16, 698.
32. Goodman, S. & Gilman, A. (1956) The Pharmacological Basis of Therapeutics, 3rd edn. New York: Macmillan.
33. Posner, L. B., Waller, R. W. & Posner, A. C. (1960) Harlem Hosp. Bull., 1, 139.
34. Koback, A. J. & Wishnick, S. (1955) Am. J. Obstet. Gynecol., 70, 409.
35. McDonough, J. H. (1945) New. Engl. J. Med. 232, 189.
36. Brudenell, J. M. (1961) J. Obstet. Gynaecol. Br. Commonw., 68, 115.
37. Jetter, W. W. & Hunter, F. T. (1949) New. Engl. J. Med., 240, 794.
38. Cabaniss, C. M. & Clark, J. F. J. (1962) Am. J. Obstet. Gynecol. 83, 13.
39. Bobrow, M. L. & Friedman, S. (1958) Am. J. Surg., 95, 938.
40. Obeng, B. B. (1968) Br. J. Clin. Prac., 22, 465.
41. David, T. J. (1974) Med. Sci. Law, 14, 120.
42. Veprovski, E. C. & Ostreich, L. L. (1954) Am. J. Obstet. Gynecol., 68, 1615.
43. Cook, R. G. (1938) Br. Med. J., 1, 1045.
44. Shenoi, P. M., Smits, B. J. & Davidson, S. (1966) Br. Med. J., 2, 929.
45. Finzer, K. H. (1961) Can. Med. Ass., 84, 549.
46. Martin, I. A. (1957) Obstet. Gynaecol., 9, 523.
47. Jaujoks, H. (1952) Dtsch. Med. Wochenschr., 77, 1381.
48. Marcinkowski, T. (1973) For. Sci., 2, 245.
49. Prag, J. J. (1951) S. Afr. Med. J., 25, 566.
50. Batson, O. V. (1940) Ann. Surg. 112, 138.
51. Elstub, J. (1956) J. Obstet. Gynaecol. Br. Commonw., 63, 748.
52. Mant, A. K. (1975) Acta. Med. Leg. Soc., 24, 326.
53. Adelson, L. (1963) J. For. Sci., 8, 132.
54. Leunbach, H. J. (1931) Monatschr. Gerburtsch. Gynäk., 87, 509.
55. Dutra, F. R., Cleveland, F. P. & Lyle, H. P. (1950) J. Am. Med. Ass., 143, 865.
56. Barns, H. H. F. (1947) Lancet, 2, 825.
57. Berthelsen, H. G. & Ostervaard, E. (1959) Dan. Med. Bull., 6, 105.
58. Thomas, T. A., Galizia, E. G. & Wensley, R. T. (1975) Br. Med. J., 1, 375.
59. Gornel, D. L. & Goldman, R. (1968) J. Am. Med. Assoc., 203, 146.
60. Simpson, C. K. (1958) Med.-Leg. J., 26, 132.
61. Utian, W. H. (1968) J. Obstet. Gynaecol. Br. Commonw., 75, 705.
62. Burnett, C. F. W. (1952) Br. Med. J., 1, 886.
63. Perera, W. S. E. (1961) Br. Med. J., 1, 705.
64. Schwarz, R. H. & Emich, J. P. (1965) Obstet. Gynaecol., 26, 767.
65. Parish, T. N. (1935) J. Obstet. Gynaecol. Br. Commonw., 42, 1107.
66. Deane, R. M. & Russell, K. P. (1960) Am. J. Obstet. Gynecol., 79, 528.
67. Gear, E. J., Paxson, N. F. & Penman, W. R. (1956) Am. J. Obstet. Gynecol., 72, 652.
68. Lein, J. N. & Stander, R. W. (1959) Obstet. Gynaecol., 13, 568.
69. Sherman, M. & Schneider, G. T. (1955) Sth. Med. J., 48, 333.
70. Hauptstein, P. (1960) Munch. Med. Wochenschr., 102, 1778.
71. Janowski, N. A. Weiner, L. & Obwer, W. D. (1963) N.Y. State J. Med., 63, 1463.
72. Adedevoh, B. K. & Akinla, O. (1970) J. Obstet. Gynaecol. Br. Commonw., 77, 1019.
73. Norburn, L. M. (1957) J. Obstet. Gynaecol. Br. Commonw., 64, 220.
74. Bratton, A. B. (1941) Lancet, 1, 345.
75. Ritico, M. & Nikolaides, D. (1962) Am. J. Roentg., 88, 119.
76. Zeldenrust, J., Makkink, B. & Voortman, M. (1963) Med. Sci. Law, 3, 277.
77. Camps, F. E. & Purchase, W. B. (1956) Practical Forensic Medicine. London: Hutchinson & Co., p. 23.
78. Schwerd, W. (1965) In: Curry, A. S., ed. Methods of Forensic Science, vol. 4. London, New York, Sydney: Interscience Publishers.

15

Infant deaths

In fine nothing is said now that has not been said before (Terence, 185–159 BC).

INTRODUCTION

Live births

The number of live births in England and Wales in the calendar leap year 1980 (656 234) was almost 15% higher than that of 1977. The increase in the number of live births in 1980 was mainly a result of it being a leap year and of the increase in the rate of childbearing and only partly due to the greater number of women of childbearing age. The crude birth rate rose from the lowest recorded level of 11.6 live births per 1000 population of all ages in 1977 to 13.3 in 1980, an increase of over 14%. Relating live births to women of childbearing age, the fertility rate in 1980 at 65 (live births per 1000 women aged 15–44 years) was over 10% higher than in 1977.

The difference between 1977 and 1980 in the proportionate changes of numbers of births (Table 15.1), in the crude birth and in the fertility rate reflect changes in population size as well as structure.

Table 15.1 Live births and deaths

Year and quarter	Live birth occurrences Number	Percentage change from preceding year
1977	569.3	−2.6
1978	596.4	+4.8
1979	638.0	+7.0
1980 (leap year)	656.2	+2.9

Since the child has little control of his environment and the infant virtually none, social and environmental factors will play an even greater part in determining well being or ill health in the early years than they do in adult life. Often such factors as disease are inextricably combined, and it may be impossible to determine the relative importance of any of them. All children are susceptible, like adults to natural disease from which they could die. They could also die as a result of congenital abnormalities; but one should seek guidance for these in textbooks on paediatric medicine, surgery and pathology. One must however remember that foul play either by commission or omission must also be considered in medico-legal cases.

Stillbirths and infant mortality

Although the number of live births in 1980 rose by about 15% compared with 1977, there was a continuing fall in the number of stillbirths. The result of stillbirth rate of 7.2 per 1000 total births (live and stillbirths) in 1980 represents an improvement on the previous year of almost treble the average annual reduction over the previous five years. Deaths in the first week of life in 1979 numbered 4307, which, when combined with the stillbirths, gives a perinatal mortality rate of 14.7 per 1000 total births. This substantial reduction from the 1977 rate of 17 is almost as striking as that between 1975 and 1976, which had been the greatest for almost 30 years. The proportional reduction in the perinatal mortality rate between 1975 and 1978 is greater than at any corresponding interval since the rate was introduced 50 years ago. The infant mortality rate for the year 1979 was 13 per 1000 live births. The stillbirth rate has been reduced to 40%

of its level in 1960 (20 per 1000 live and stillbirths). Although the reduction in the rate of first-week deaths in 1979 to 51% of the 1960 level of 13 per 1000 live births is not as great as that for stillbirths, the rate of reduction of the past three years, in proportional terms, is approaching three times that for the period as a whole. In a list of 35 countries with perinatal mortality rates available for 1976 England and Wales were placed 15th. Perinatal rate for Sweden, for example, in 1976 was 10.7 while that for England was 17.26. The causes of stillbirth are of medico-legal importance in relation to infanticide and abortion. Table 15.2 shows the causes of stillbirth (1979) in England and Wales.

Table 15.2 Stillbirths (1979) by cause and sex

Cause	Male	Female	Total
Disease in mother	129	125	254
Toxaemias of pregnancy	232	234	466
Difficulties in labour	64	58	122
Complications of placenta, cord and membranes	1184	897	2081
Birth trauma	11	12	23
Congenital malformation of foetus	377	562	939
Diseases of foetus and ill-defined cases	654	575	1229
Total	2651	2463	5114

From the medico-legal point of view the importance of neonatal deaths can be divided into four groups:

1. The establishment of whether the child has had a separate existence and, if not, the reason.

2. The establishment as to whether the process of birth or mechanical assistance has played a part in the failure to survive, i.e., whether, for example, the pressure of the forceps has played a part, in which case the death becomes accidental; on the other hand, destruction by craniotomy is clearly before birth and no survival could take place.

3. The occurrence of infection of the child before birth, during birth, or after birth demands an investigation as to the source of the infection. Thus, if there have been other cases arising from a common source there may be grounds for civil action.

4. In cases of failure to survive being due to asphyxia, clearly the possibility of some act of omission or commission must be considered.

Neonatal deaths and deaths in infancy may be classified as follows (the list is not intended to be comprehensive):

1. Congenital abnormalities (including treatment),
   a. oesophageal fistula,
   b. cardiac malformations,
   c. transposition of viscera,
   d. rhesus and other incompatibilities.
2. Diseases of unknown aetiology,
   a. fibroelastosis,
   b. cardiomegaly.
3. Infective,
   a. Acute infection of air passages: bronchopneumonia, capillary bronchitis, acute epiglottitis,
   b. acute pyogenic infection as caused by the following organisms: *Meningococcus* (Waterhouse-Friederichsen syndrome), *Pneumococcus, Staphylococcus, Streptococcus*, and others,
   c. diphtheria,
   d. acute viral infection: acute anterior poliomyelitis, vaccinal encephalitis,
   e. protozoal infection: toxoplasmosis.
4. Mechanical: strangulated hernia, intussusception and volvulus.
5. Traumatic (accidental or with intent) including:
   a. suffocation by plastic bags, material (soft pillows and mattresses) or impacted foreign bodies,
   b. strangulation: hanging by toys and furniture,
   c. burns and scalds,
   d. electrocution,
   e. asphyxia due to gases (mainly carbon monoxide) including incomplete combustion (calor or bottled gas), oil stoves and fires,
   f. poisoning from:
   a. (i) household poisons:
      a. acids: scourers and alkalis,
      b. tablets and drugs,
      c. lead toys and paintwork,
   b. (ii) therapeutic drugs: chloramphenicol, penicillin, mercury (grey powder), borax (marking ink), mistletoe etc.

OFFENCES AGAINST CHILDREN

The law

Nothing offends the public conscience more than cruelty to children and animals. It is perhaps a sign of the changes which have taken place in the past 50 years that charitable organisations established in the past days of poverty to care for 'waifs and strays' (the children who were neglected, ill-treated, starved and even deserted) now devote a large part of their money and efforts to caring for the physically handicapped, mentally backward and maladjusted children in the present state of affluence. In addition, they also attempt to improve some of the parents. Yet, in spite of this, cases of cruelty, possibly more overt and with no real excuse, are daily reported in the newspapers alongside acts of aggression by young persons which were never evident at the beginning of the century.

From the point of view of the law, offences of cruelty and neglect of children are covered by the following legislation.

Offences against children may be dealt with on the same basis as if the victim were an adult, for example, murder, manslaughter, or the various types of assault. In English law, however, there are special provisions dealing with certain offences against children.

The Infanticide Act 1938, section 1, provides that:

> Where a woman by any wilful act or omission causes the death of her child, being a child under the age of twelve months, but at the time of the act or omission the balance of her mind was disturbed by reason of her not having fully recovered from the effect of giving birth to the child or by reason of the effect of lactation consequent upon the birth of the child, then, notwithstanding that the circumstances were such that but for this Act the offence would have amounted to murder, she shall be guilty of infanticide.

Her sentence is at the discretion of the court.

Part I of the Children's and Young Persons Act 1933, deals with the prevention of cruelty and exposure to moral and physical danger of children and young persons. In particular, section 1 of the Act provides that:

> If any person who has attained the age of sixteen and has custody, charge or care of any child or young person under that age, wilfully assaults, ill-treats, neglects, abandons, or exposes him, or causes or procures him to be assaulted, ill-treated or abandoned, or exposed in a manner likely to cause him unnecessary suffering or injury to health (including injury to or loss of sight, or hearing, or limb, or organs of the body, and any mental derangement), that person shall be guilty of an offence punishable on indictment with up to two years' imprisonment and/or up to £100 fine.

Part III of the 1933 Act, as amended by the 1963 Act of the same name, includes provision for children and young persons 'in need of care and protection'. A child or young person is deemed in need of care or protection, amongst other things, if it lacks 'such care, protection and guidance as a good parent may reasonably be expected to give to such an extent that this is likely to cause him unnecessary suffering or seriously to affect his health or proper development'. The same applies if certain offences are committed against him.

A juvenile court which is satisfied that any child brought before it by a local authority, constable, or other authorised person is in need of care and protection may, amongst other things, commit him to the care of a fit person willing to undertake the care of him or order his parent or guardian to enter into a recognisance to exercise proper care and guardianship.

Infanticide

The killing of the newborn or young child was a recognised practice in many primitive communities and took place for a variety of reasons in the past. Probably one of the basic motives was survival of the fittest, or safety of the tribe, which was the explanation for the destruction of those suffering from malformations, or of less potential value to the community, such as females, among certain religious groups. Other reasons for such destruction were tribal superstitions which involved the question of 'unlucky' and included twins, the presence of teeth at birth, and even leg presentations. So too there was also involved the age-long desire for strength and fertility which led to destruction of the first-born which if eaten added strength to those who devoured it. In the more civilised communities there can be no doubt that killing of the newborn child, particularly if the mother was unmarried, has been associated with expediency, whether it be from breach of convention, or inconvenience, or inability to support it, and is closely linked with the reason for criminal abortion. It is therefore of interest that in one country at least where the state automatically assumes responsibility for the illegitimate child, the infanticide rate decreased considerably, which in some ways supports the fact that the infant mortality rate of illegitimate children is higher than that of those born in wedlock.

The law in respect of infanticide differs in different countries, but the English law and its evolution are of considerable interest. Until 1922 the killing of a newborn child was murder, no matter by whom it was done. However, by that year public opinion had reached a state when it was embarrassed by a procedure which involved a trial of the mother for murder, whilst if conviction resulted it would involve passing the death sentence on a person who would almost inevitably be reprieved and who was commonly mentally unbalanced at the time of commission of the act. In that year (1922) the Infanticide Act was passed which applies only to England and not to Ireland or Scotland. In Scotland, the crime is known as child murder. This laid down that:

Where a woman by wilful act or omission causes the death of her newly born child in circumstances which but for the Act would have amounted to murder, but at the time of such act or omission, she had not fully recovered from the effects of the birth and by reason thereof the balance of her mind was disturbed, or by reason of the effect of lactation consequent upon the birth of the child. She shall be guilty of infanticide and shall be punishable as for manslaughter.

Whereas the drafting of this Act undoubtedly was clarity itself, the omission of a limitation of age led to difficulties, and in 1926 it was re-enacted to limit the age of the child to 'under 12 months'.

There are certain important points which must be underlined:
1. it is only the mother who can be charged with the offence;
2. the child must be born alive (and, of course, be viable);
3. it must have been killed;
4. there must be evidence to establish that the accused person is suffering from disease of the mind for the reasons mentioned.

The Act clearly says 'the mother': if anyone else is involved the charge must be homicide (murder or manslaughter) and this will apply also to any person who assists the woman. Thus a woman was charged with infanticide and her husband, who assisted her, with murder. In England the definition of stillbirth is 'any child which has issued forth from its mother after the twenty-eighth week

of pregnancy and which did not at any time after being completely expelled from its mother, breathe or show any other signs of life' (Births and Deaths Registration Act 1953, section 41).

Such a definition clearly can lead to some problems. For example, should the mother, whilst one foot of the child is still in the vagina, strangle it or kill it by some other means, even if it has cried since the delivery of the head, she is not guilty of the offence because the child is on this definition a 'stillbirth', having not been completely expelled. Such cases have occurred and the woman has been acquitted. From a practical point of view it is highly unlikely that a woman who does not know the law would invent the story of incomplete expulsion; hence, if she volunteers it in her original statement it will be difficult to refute, whilst another aspect is that in cases in which the child has been found without identification, it may be clearly impossible for the pathologist, even if he finds evidence of breathing, to say that it had a separate existence at any subsequent inquest. Evidence to establish whether the child has had a separate existence is discussed below.

The child must have died from the act

In respect of acts of violence, provided that the pathologist can produce adequate evidence to satisfy the Court that death was due to such violence, this presents little difficulty, but in cases of omission it is usually held that such an omission must be proved to be deliberate. Thus, because a woman has made no provision for the birth and death results from precipitate labour—although this might be held to be due to lack of proper attention at the time—it is unlikely that a charge would be made. Such emergencies can occur (though rarely) even in the best of conditions and circumstances.

The most important point is that the pathologist must be able to prove the cause of death and not allow the circumstances of the case to prejudice such an opinion. Logically, from the wording of the Act, it would be expected that the injuries to the child and the cause of death would be of the nature which might be expected from a mentally unbalanced woman, and not be those which might be associated with premeditation, and in practice this is commonly so, but, as a psychiatric or medical opinion is essential to establish the mental state of the woman at the time of the act, it may well be that such a witness will assist the Court as to what might be expected, i.e., gross violence or otherwise.

It must be noted that it is at the time of the act that the disease of the mind must exist, and it must be due to the effects of the birth or lactation. In practice as it is often difficult to prove the mental condition at the time even from the evidence of any practitioner who sees the woman shortly afterwards, the opinion of an experienced forensic psychiatrist who has had the accused under observation is usually proffered.

The Infant Life (Preservation) Act 1929, although it is rarely used, covers the eventuality that the child was deliberately destroyed before birth. It is an offence 'punishable with imprisonment for life, if any person with intent to destroy the life of a child capable of being born alive, by any wilful act, causes the child to die before it has an existance independent of its mother, subject to the proviso that no person shall be found guilty of the offence, unless it be proved that the act which caused the death of the child was not done in good faith for the purpose only of preserving the life of the child'.

The definition of 'viable' is again in the 1929 Act and means that it is more than 28 weeks' gestation. This will depend upon the various criteria of maturity (see below) and on occasions greater reliability can be placed upon the anatomical findings than upon the clinical opinions of those who have examined the mother before birth.

Maturity and identity

If should be pointed out that a non-viable child from the point of view of gestation period can be born alive and in such cases the opinion to be expressed should be in such terms.

The maturity of a newborn child may be difficult to establish, and in many cases it is always simpler to have radiological examination of the entire body, rather than carry out an extensive dissection of the epiphyses.

The maturity is based upon the following observations, but in special cases the assistance of a specialist anatomist and odontologist should be sought.

Full term. Traditional, but subject to variation of sex, race and individual.
1. Size: usual length 50 cm (18–21 inches) (crown-heel); 30 cm (12 inches) (crown-rump). Usual weight 2270–3630 g (5–8 lb)
2. Lanugo has disappeared; head hair about 2 cm or more long.
3. Male testicles descended and in scrotum; female vulva closed and labia minora covered by fully developed labia majora.
4. Finger and toenails beyond tips of fingers and toes.
5. Lower end of femur may show centre of ossification about $\frac{1}{4}$ inch in diameter.

Viable (28 weeks' gestation).
1. Length 35 cm (CH), 23 cm (CR).
2. Weight 900 g.
3. Other signs: eyelids separated.

Evidence of recent birth.
1. Caput succedaneum: if present this usually disappears within one to two days. It is of value in establishing the presentation and rapidity of birth (in head presentation).
2. The umbilical cord:
   (a) if attached to placenta newborn;
   (b) if clamped or tied—if there is no evidence of reaction it is newborn;
   (c) site of severance and method of severance should both be noted, but whether cut or torn may not always be easy to decide. It is best to remove the cord and examine it in the laboratory;
   (d) length (total), weight of placenta.

Evidence of life

The proof of live birth when taken in connection with complete expulsion is on a par with the proof of time of death, and at the moment is just as much an insoluble problem as an educated guess from experience. There are two traditional methods of establishment, neither of which can overcome the criterion of complete expulsion.

The traditional naked-eye appearances. The aeration of the lungs: this is based upon the expansion of the alveoli by post-natal breathing and is ascertained by evidence of the eye. It does not, however, take into consideration the phenomenon of partial aeration or the fact that the child may cry in utero or breathe after expulsion of the head and before complete expulsion. Clearly the degree of aeration must play a part in the interpretation, whilst the presence of gases of decomposition with concomitant bullae must modify any decision or attempts at 'mouth to mouth' resuscitation, may evoke a false positive, but it is difficult to see why a person who desires the death of the child should endeavour to resuscitate it on the one hand, whilst whoever desires to save it will do so. On the other hand, it is possible that the ultra-criminal mind might do so to avoid arrest.

The hydrostatic test was first noted by early German writers of the seventeenth century. The lungs should be removed at autopsy with the bronchi, trachea and larynx intact. The 'pluck' is placed in water, and if it floats (provided decomposition is absent) the test is positive. Each lung is tested separately, and again, if it floats the test is positive. Finally, each lung is cut into fragments which are again tested, and if they float the test is positive (this should exclude irregular and partial aeration).

Air in the stomach: traditionally a bubble of air in the stomach indicates respiration after birth but nowadays the presence of air at autopsy is no longer regarded as an irreversible fact, and the circumstances must be taken into consideration before deciding that the child has been born alive, for here again artificial respiration must play a part and in any event air can enter the stomach.

Cause of death

As already mentioned, in the majority of cases of infanticide the mind of the mother is unbalanced, and hence the usual pattern is one of gross violence which will conform to the pattern already described under various headings such as 'wounds', 'strangulation', and the like.

1. Multiple Injuries (see also Battered Child Syndrome, p. 346)—these will include head injuries due to deliberate striking of the child's head against some object or swinging it by the legs (grip marks on the legs). The interpretation will be as for other wounds and will depend upon external bruising, fractures, and cerebral haemorrhage and bruising. Usually there will be bruising in other parts of the body. Sometimes the child is struck by some blunt object which may leave a definite pattern or shape. The defence in the case of head injuries may be precipitate labour or accidental dropping of the child. If older it may be alleged to have fallen from its cot or from a table, sometimes accidentally knocking itself against some object such as a doorpost or cot side. Most of such stories should be capable of confirmation or contradiction.

2. Stabbing—this type of killing is usually done with some easily accessible weapon such as a pair of scissors, penknife, domestic knife, or even a tool. Very rarely some very thin weapon is used such as a long needle, and a careful search for punctures should be carried out before making a dissection.

3. Cutting—incised wounds are not very common but cases have occurred when instruments such as razor blades have been used. The distinctive features of this type of injury are that the wounds may be well arranged and parallel, due to the fact that a small child can be immobilised.

4. Strangulation—this presents little difficulty in interpretation when a stocking, pair of nylon tights, or other form of ligature is tied tightly around the neck of a newborn child; the picture is one of ante-mortem compression with petechial haemorrhages and congestion above the level of the ligature. There may be some difficulty when decomposition has taken place, and under such circumstances it is wiser to err on the side of 'cause of death unascertained' than to 'press' on inconclusive evidence which can be challenged.

5. Smothering—this presents the most difficult problem because of the incorrect tradition which has associated petechial haemorrhages in the lungs and pericardium, fluid blood, and cyanosis with asphyxia. Unfortunately the word 'asphyxia' has become synonymous with mechanical asphyxia, whereas it is a feature of many deaths with venous congestion. In order to prove death from smothering it is essential to show evidence of the act itself and this, as in the cases of alleged 'overlying' or 'cot deaths', is by no means easy to demonstrate if associated with a soft surface. Evidence of smothering will include bruising of the lips or gums and sometimes counter-pressure on the back of the neck, whilst obstruction to breathing will cause small pleural areas of emphysema.

Smothering can also take the form of material

such as handkerchiefs, pieces of sheet, and the like being stuffed down the throat. Provided that there is proof of the child being alive at the time this represents little problem of interpretation.

From this it can be seen that, although in the cases in which the cause of death is obvious and post-mortem changes are not marked it is not difficult to offer an opinion provided that there is proper identification, in those in which the cause of death is obscured (usually by decomposition), even when identification is made, it would be impossible to succeed with a prosecution of infanticide where evidence of mental unbalance is available. Such cases are, however, covered by the offence of 'concealment of birth': 'It is an offence for any person (mother or other) by any secret disposal of the body of a newly born child to conceal the fact of the birth, whether it was live birth or still birth'. Such an offence can only be proved if the body is properly concealed, i.e., buried in the garden or hidden in some normally inaccessible spot, or when attempted destruction has taken place, such as partial incineration.

The law in Scotland

At Common Law in Scotland, there is no difference between the murder of a child and the murder of an adult. However, the crime became one of such frequent occurrence and the difficulty of proving it so great, that an Act was passed in 1690 which provided that if certain facts were proved, the jury were entitled to presume that the crime of child murder had been committed. Owing to its severe nature, this enactment was repealed by the Concealment of Pregnancy Act 1809, which reduced the crime to one of culpable homicide.

The Act of 1809 provides that if any woman conceals her being with child during the whole period of her pregnancy and does not call for and make use of help or assistance at the birth, and the child is found dead or amissing, she may be convicted and imprisoned.

Under this Act the onus is on the Crown to prove
1. that the woman was pregnant and that she concealed this fact during the whole period of pregnancy,
2. that she failed to call for or make use of help at the birth, and

3. that the child has been found dead or amissing.

At Common Law, to constitute 'live birth' the child must have been fully extruded from the parts of the mother, and have achieved an independent existence, but it is not necessary that the child should have breathed, or that the cord should have been cut, but the child must have given some active evidence of life.

The legal definition of live birth will be seen to be divergent from the medical definition, as in the latter, evidence of respiratory action of the child whether initiated partly within or wholly without the maternal parts, is indicative of live birth. Frequently, on account of the difficulty in determining by physical appearances of the body whether respiratory function was initiated while a portion of the child was within the maternal parts, or after complete extrusion, the alternative charge to infanticide or child murder, namely a charge of concealment of birth, in England, or of pregnancy, in Scotland, is returned as the verdict of the jury.

The law in Ireland

Registration of births and deaths
Until the Registration of Births and Deaths Act (Ireland) was passed in 1863, there was no civil registration of births or deaths in Ireland. The system of registration established in 1863 has not been altered in any major respect up to the present. It is based on local registrars (who generally have been the district medical officers) under the supervision of superintendent registrars, who, in turn, are under An tArd-Chlaraitheoir (the Registrar General).

Registration of births: the local registrar has the duty of registering all births in his district. He keeps the register in local premises and the informant attends there to give the information necessary for registration and sign the register. The duty of doing this rests primarily on the parents and, in their default, on the occupier of the house where the child was born, on each person present at the birth and on the person in charge of the child. [Section 1 of the Births and Deaths Registration Act (Ireland) 1880]. The information recorded is the date and place of birth, the name and sex of the child, the name, surname and dwelling-place of the father, the name, surname of the mother and the rank or profession of the father.

Each quarter, the registrar sends to the superintendent registrar a copy of the entries made by him in his register. The superintendent checks and certifies these and sends them to An tArd-Chlaraitheoir. The local registrar keeps the register-book until it is filled, when he sends it to the superintendent registrar for retention. The copies of the entries in the local registers which are received in Oifig an Ard-Chlaraitheora (the General Register Office) are there bound into volumes and indexed.

The clerk of the Local Poor Law Union was named by section 22 of the Registration of Births and Deaths (Ireland) Act 1863, as superintendent registrar. His successor in the public assistance administration was later designated to act as superintendent. Under section 10 of the Vital Statistics and Births, Deaths and Marriages Registration Act 1952, the public assistance authority itself took over the functions of the superintendent registrar whenever a vacancy occurred. The health boards have now replaced the public assistance authorities as superintendent registrars (section 6 of the Health Act 1970) and discharge this function through nominated officers.

Birth certificates: birth certificates are issued by Oifig an Ard-Charaitheora, the superintendent registrars and the local registrars (the last named can, of course, only issue certificates of comparatively recent registrations as their completed register books will have been sent to the superintendent registrar). Any member of the public is entitled, on paying a fee, to a certificate relating to any entry in a register.

Registration of deaths and issue of death certificates: the duty of registering all deaths in his district also falls on the local registrar. In the case of a death taking place in a house, the obligation to register a death rests, in the order of priority shown, on:

1. the nearest relatives of the deceased who were present at his death or in attendance during his last illness;
2. every other relative living or being in the same district;
3. each person present at the death;
4. the occupier of the house where the death took place;
5. each other inmate of the house;

6. the person causing the body to be buried.

Rather similar priorities of obligation to register apply where a death occurs elsewhere than in a house. Sections 10 and 11 of Births and Deaths Registration Act (Ireland) 1880. The cause of death is usually certified by the medical practitioner who attended the deceased. Where an inquest has been held, a coroner's certificate as to the cause is received by the registrar. The death registers are checked, copied and indexed in the same way as the registers of births and the procedure and charges for the issue of certificates from the registrars are similar.

Statistics of births and deaths. The Vital Statistics Regulations 1954: From 1 January 1955, an improved system was introduced for collecting statistics of births and deaths. Before then only the information required to be given for registering a birth or death was available to the statistical service. This was not sufficient to allow for the production of some desirable statistical tables and indices.

Fetal deaths. The collection of information on foetal deaths is a feature of the vital statistics in most modern states. Comprehensive, systematic collection of these statistics commenced in Ireland from 1 January 1957. [Vital Statistics (Fetal Deaths) Regulations 1956]. When a fetal death (or stillbirth—although it is with the death and not the birth that the statistician is concerned) occurs after the 28th week of pregnancy, the medical practitioner or midwife (or medical student or pupil mid-wife) is required to send information about it to the local medical officer.

INFANT DEATH

Natural death. Sudden infant death syndrome (**SIDS**)

Introduction

Since the beginnings of scientifically orientated medical research, in most parts of the world, man has attempted to explain the sudden unexpected death of infants.

The sudden and unexpected death of a seemingly healthy baby is one of the most distressing experiences that can happen to young parents and the most puzzling to doctors. It is not a new problem but has been thrown into greater prominence as formerly fatal diseases in young infants have been successfully eradicated or brought under control.

Every year about 2000 babies in Britain die suddenly and unexpectedly of the sudden infant death syndrome, which makes it the most common cause of death in this age group, representing as it does approximately 15% of total infant mortality. The label 'cot death' appears more than twice as often on death certificates today as it did 10 years ago. Where pneumonia once appeared on the certificate to spare all concerned the embarrassment and trauma of an inquest for an unexplained death, sudden infant death syndrome has taken its place.

Indeed the pendulum has swung in the other direction, with cot death being over-reported where post-mortem facilities are not sufficient to establish the true cause of death.

The higher incidence of cot deaths is not surprising. After all, there is even disagreement over the terminology itself. Some believe that the phrase 'sudden infant death' includes children who die after a minor illness insufficient to kill in itself; others say the term refers only to those babies whose deaths are inexplicable and where no abnormality can be found.

The whole area of sudden infant deaths is controversial, with leading authorities taking entrenched positions. Some believe that all the theories of the past few years should go back into the melting pot.

In the Anglo-American literature several terms are used synonymously: cot death, crib death, sudden unexpected or unexplained death syndrome, as well as sudden infant death syndrome (SIDS). The last term mentioned has achieved world-wide use in the medical field, probably because of its compact form, although, like other terms, it fails to convey anything about the aetiology or pathology of the functional disturbances which may have caused death: it remains purely a description of the sudden appearance of death or its unexpected discovery. In all cases a natural death from internal causes is assumed. However, it is the view of many that, until proved otherwise, all sudden unexpected deaths should be regarded with suspicion.

It is estimated that the incidence of death from the sudden infant death syndrome is about 1.8 per 1000 live births in the United Kingdom, 90% of all infants who die being less than eight months.[1] The syndrome is also a recognised problem in other countries, although results of national comparisons cannot be too strictly interpreted because of differences in definition. Rates in the range 1.5–3 per 1000 live births are quoted for countries with an infant mortality rate of 15 to 20 live births (for example New Zealand, USA, Ireland and Canada); rates as low as 0.5 for countries with infant mortality rates less than 15 (for example, Finland, Sweden, The Netherlands). There are exceptions to this general pattern. Israel and Czechoslovakia with comparatively high infant mortality rates have a reported cot death rate of less than 1 per 1000 live births.[2]

Sudden unexpected death has been recognised since Biblical times, the most famous case being recorded as presented to Solomon: 'this woman's child died in the night because she overlaid it' (1 Kings, 3:19). Until comparatively recently overlaying or suffocation were widely considered to be the causes of sudden infant death. Only in the last 20 years has rational research been able to discredit these and other erroneous theories and led to more acceptable reasons for the deaths of these infants. Increased knowledge has been followed by a greater sensitivity to the needs of the bereaved parents and efforts to alleviate their suffering.[2,3]

It goes beyond the boundaries of this chapter to even begin to list the authors who have dedicated all their scientific endeavours to this problem. However, extensive listings of the literature have been compiled, among others by Barbey,[4] Kendell & Ferris,[5] Mahnke,[6] Maresch,[7–10] Valdes-Dapena[11] Shannon & Kelly.[3]

Unexpected death is defined as death when the cause cannot be satisfactorily explained by the previous state or condition of the child.[12] The difficulties establishing a common definition are made worse when the physicians who certify death are unable to rely on their own negative findings or experience and are forced to rely on the barely objective symptoms reported by relatives to the reporting officer or coroner's officer.

Nowadays, the definition most commonly accepted by researchers into the problem was proposed by Beckwith[13]—'the sudden death of any infant which is unexpected by history and in which a thorough post-mortem fails to demonstrate an adequate cause of death'. Since 1971 this syndrome had been a registerable cause of death in Britain. Although this definition is useful to focus research it leaves unanswered the questions of what is an adequate history and what is considered a sufficient cause for death by an individual pathologist.

Characteristics identified include a higher winter incidence; death occurring particularly during the regional occurrence of respiratory disease; a male preponderance; a higher incidence in cities than in rural areas; a characteristic age distribution with three-quarters of the cases between four and six months and a few outside these limits; an increased incidence in twins; in babies of low birthweight; among offspring of young mothers who have had several children; in poor living conditions and in bottle fed babies.[2]

Most fatalities seem to have occurred during the night, the babies being found dead in the morning.[14, 15] Many of these features are common to other causes of infant death, but the age distribution with a pronounced peak between two or four months is peculiar to this syndrome.

It had often been reported that most infants who die in this manner seem to have been healthy or only mildly unwell shortly prior to death, death occurring suddenly, and usually unobserved, and more often than not during sleep. The child is found lifeless without any evidence of a struggle or violence being applied. The increased awareness of the syndrome is now a great cause of anxiety to both mothers and doctors.

The paucity of symptoms in these infants before death has been repeatedly emphasised. However, this does not necessarily prove that they had been healthy.[16–19]

Causes

There is a multiplicity of theories about what causes sudden infant death. There is evidence to support many of these theories but each one provides the possible cause in only a proportion of the infants. Recent research has discredited many myths surrounding these deaths—often attributed to overlaying, suffocation or inhalation of vomit which account for a small proportion of unexpected infant deaths. In 1972,[20] experiments showed that exhaled air in carry cots does *not* accumulate and

cause danger to babies. It is generally agreed by researchers working in the field that sudden infant death probably results not from a single cause but from a variety of different factors which combine fatally while a child is passing through a vulnerable period of development.

Current research is approaching the problem from several directions. The physiological development of normal infants, focusing on breathing patterns and upper airway function in different depths of sleep, is being studied.

Prolonged sleep apnoea (cessation of breathing)[3] associated with age, low birthweight and infection[21] may be the mechanism of death in some cases. Apnoea produced in young lambs by introducing water or the milk of a different animal into the larynx is thought to have significance for some infant deaths as it has been observed that human infants given cow's milk or water at the first feed tend to choke more frequently than those given human milk, but this effect is absent in older infants. The studies suggest that the control of breathing of human infants depends on multiple factors which change with age.[22]

Again, airway obstruction from a blocked nose has been shown to be a possible cause of some deaths.[23] Other investigators currently believe that viruses have a significant role in the pathogenesis of sudden infant deaths. Respiratory viruses found in about 25% of cot deaths[24] may cause a rapidly fatal infection or, it is suggested, trigger sudden apnoea.

In addition to these physio-pathological investigations into the mechanism of sudden infant death, several local social and pathological studies have been undertaken which are throwing increasing light on its aetiology. A detailed investigation into all sudden infant deaths reported to the Inner North London Coroner (London, England) revealed the presence of pathological lesions sufficient to account for death in a proportion of cases notified as sudden infant deaths. In addition, a high rate of symptoms was recorded at the interview and by means of a rigorous interviewing schedule an inadequate response to these symptoms was demonstrated.[17] This method of investigation was later adopted by a number of other Area Health Authorities wishing to undertake detailed studies of their sudden infant deaths.[25]

In Sheffield, England, a multi-stage scoring system was devised to measure selected factors at birth and again at one month of age. In trials in which extra health care attention was given by a paediatrician by means of two examinations, 'special' health visiting and speedy access to hospital if the baby was unwell, some unexpected deaths are alleged to have been prevented.[26]

The London and Sheffield studies have both shown that some mothers may be unaware of illness in their infants, and that some cases previously considered 'unexpected' might have been 'expected' if more skilled observers had been present. Some cases of sudden infant death appear to be due to social pathology rather than specific disease.[27]

When these cases are autopsied they deserve a much more thorough investigation than that usually afforded adults.[16] This is not only true for the technique of the autopsy itself, but also holds true for further investigation into radiology, histology, microbiology, virology, serology and even toxicology.

In agreement with Müller[28] and Althoff,[16] the results of an autopsy should not and cannot be used as the final criterion for the definition because they can be strongly subjectively influenced. On the other hand, cases with an objectively negative history have resulted in extensively positive pathological changes being found, and the converse likewise with virtual negative autopsy findings.

In 1963,[29] it was suggested differentiality between:
1. death during syncope;
2. found dead in bed, no previous symptoms of illness or behavioural disturbances;
3. history of banal symptoms not going further back than 48 h before death,
4. peracute, dramatic illnesses leading to death within a few hours, accompanied by febrile convulsions, loss of consciousness, etc.

The findings of most studies,[17, 30, 31] support the view that sudden infant death is essentially a mode of death in children suffering from occult illness. There is no evidence however, to suggest that different standards of pre-death health care would have affected that outcome and the vast majority of babies from such backgrounds survive similar illnesses. This fact alone stresses that importance of continuing the search for abnormalities, e.g., in respiratory reflexes or in the immune response which might predispose to a fatal outcome and for more information about infection in the age group concerned.[17]

Most forensic pathologists and paediatric pathologists would agree with Althoff[16] when he states that there is no single causal or pathogenetic principle behind the sudden infant death syndrome and that it is of multifactoral occurrence with a high incidence of certain types of findings specific to one region or another. In the experience of most, the majority of the sudden infant death syndrome cases investigated reveal a predominance of interference with respiration.

There is, however, small evidence that children from abusing families may be at greater risk of death in infancy, not necessarily as a result of abuse.[32-34] In addition, previous research on the sudden infant death syndrome has highlighted associated factors such as a young maternal age, premature delivery and neonatal mortality,[26, 31, 35] all of which are also associated with child abuse and neglect.[36, 37]

Effect of a cot death bereavement on the family

Whilst research programmes are apparently throwing increasing light on the aetiology of sudden infant death, the greatest significance of these deaths lies in their impact on the bereaved parents. Any death of a young child is a tragedy, but the death has a particular poignancy when it is that of a young baby who has survived birth, appears perfectly normal, and is then found 'inexplicably' dead. The unexpectedness of the tragedy and the absence of any convincing explanation leaves the parents much more shocked than if the child had been known to be ill or to have had a congenital malfunction. Their anxieties and concerns, although well documented,[38] have received too little attention from health care professionals[3].

Parkes,[39] who has contributed extensively to the study of bereavement, puts forward the view that changes in family size have resulted in closer attachment to those few children one now has, which makes the loss of a child a much greater tragedy. Emery,[40] was one of the first investigators into sudden infant death to identify the unnecessary psychological trauma to which they are often subjected as part of the process of the exclusion of unnatural death. He described the role that paediatricians could adopt in helping parents come to terms with their grief and unnecessary guilt feelings.

Reassurance and comfort for many families bereaved in this way has been increasingly supplied in Britain by the Foundation for the Study of Infant Deaths, a registered charity founded in 1971. Support has been given by letter or telephone and to many more by its leaflets 'Information for the Parents of a Child who had Died Suddenly and Unexpectedly in Infancy' and 'Your Next Child'. The Foundation offers to put parents in touch with other suitable parents in their area or with one of the 25 parent groups associated with the Foundation, who offer a befriending service. Nevertheless, as Limerick & Downham point out,[41] supporting bereaved families by means of leaflets and self-help groups cannot entirely replace the help that can easily be given by a specially interested paediatrician who works closely with the primary care team.[3]

Reaction to the loss

Similar reactions to the loss are observed in all social classes and in widely differing areas from the most socially deprived to the most affluent. Over 70% of parents mention anger, bewilderment, self-blame and anxiety about a possible recurrence; guilt feelings are particularly apparent where abortion had been considered or the pregnancy unplanned.[25] Neighbours' comments can be very upsetting in some cases. More than one family has been accused of murdering their baby after a report of the death has appeared in the newspaper. Several families blame medical care, particularly when it is their second cot death.

Families with a strong religious faith, the Sikh, Bangladeshi and Hassidic Jewish families accept the death more readily and seem to have felt protected by their religion.[2]

Cause of death on the death certificate

The cause of death given on the death certificate when a baby dies suddenly and unexpectedly varies widely, depending on the personal interpretation of the individual pathologist. Because of the vagaries of certification, it is not possible to distinguish between the explained, partially explained or unexplained from death certificates. Some pathologists use the term 'sudden infant death' for any sudden, unexpected death of a baby between one week and two years, while others prefer to reserve the term for those unexpected deaths which on post-mortem examination reveal no microscopic pathology sufficient to account for death and generally prefer to give a definitive cause such as tracheo-bronchitis or bronchopneumonia.

To the parents in this tragic situation, fearful about what they did or did not do, which may have contributed to the death, the cause of death is vitally important. Over 60% of parents admit to not understanding the cause of death given on the death certificate.[2] Where the term 'sudden infant death syndrome' has been given even more anxieties in the parents was recorded by Watson.[2] This supports Emery's contention[40] that to register sudden infant deaths as 'cot death syndrome' except as a supplementary registration, may increase parental anxieties.

Problems with other children

According to Watson,[2] over 50% of families reported that they had behaviour problems with other siblings after the death of the baby. Problems included insomnia, sleep walking, nightmares, bedwetting, regression in toilet training to more babyish habits, refusal to leave parents to go to play groups or allow the mother out of sight.

Summary

In spite of the network of medical observation and treatment being improved in the last few years in many countries, the number of cases of sudden infant death syndrome have not been substantially reduced. Regular check-ups, such as described by Emery & Carpenter,[42] have the positive side-effect of better informed parents who more conscientiously observe their children, care for them and feed them adequately.

One of the most difficult questions is with what symptoms should parents and physicians exercise particular care over, or even institute prophylactic procedures? One can only make suggestions here, e.g., diarrhoea, vomiting, respiratory infections or obstructions and viraemia to mention but a few.

Finally, the parents of such cases are themselves in need of medical attention and comfort.[2]

Unnatural death. Child abuse

Introduction

One of our cherished folk beliefs is that human nature compels parents to rear their young with solicitousness and concern, good intentions and tender and loving care.[43] Evidence to the contrary—the rather alarming frequency with which parents harm or fail to adequately care for their offspring—has forced the recognition that child abuse and neglect are well within the repertoire of human behaviour.

The maltreatment of children is an issue that has always been with us and civilised societies provide a range of services, both social and medical, to care for the children and families afflicted. Violence and agression are aspects of human behaviour which have always interested psychologists and psychiatrists.[44] Today, however, with the increase in violent crime and the wide coverage given to such problems by all the media, we are perhaps more aware of violence and more concerned about it than ever before. However, one aspect of our social development, the protection of children from abuse, has shown a marked lack of progress until the very recent past.[45] Child abuse is only now becoming a major issue of concern. Though child abuse in industry no longer occurs in Britain, the pattern of injuries in the home is little different now from 1881—when a meeting organised by the Society for the Prevention of Cruelty to Animals for an appeal for a dogs' home extended its appeal for the protection of children.[46] In May 1889 the National Society for the Prevention of Cruelty to Children (NSPCC) was formed.

While it is true that child abuse has existed for centuries with varying degrees of acceptance by society, one of the greatest stumbling blocks has been the difficulties in reaching an agreed definition of child abuse—a fact clearly illustrated in the writings of those working in the field. Some consider the problem in terms of a spectrum of abuse,[47] while others take a much narrower medical view.[48]

Non-accidental injury is a socially defined phenomenon and therefore its boundaries cannot be stated as if they were fixed and permanent. This is the very reason for the difficulty in producing accurate statistical estimates of the extent of abuse and of the problem in general.

The condition is a major problem for accident and emergency departments, children's hospitals, general practitioners, social workers, the police and many others concerned with the welfare of children.[49] The injuries seen may include, for example, fractures, soft tissue injuries, bruises, lacerations, burns and scalds, to mention but a few. Most victims of child abuse are under four years old (i.e., usually pre-school), and many under two years. The majority of 'battering parents' are more or less normal parents who are worn out by their small children—parents who are lonely, poorly, immature or under emotional or financial stress, with no-one to turn to for help. The batterer is usually the mother or father, but sometimes the grandparent, co-habitee, baby-minder or older child. If one parent batters the child, the other one almost certainly knows about it and aids and abets.[50] Every parent is a potential baby-basher (Kempe, unpublished data 1970).

The diagnosis can be difficult to reach and almost impossible to prove. Cases which come to light are merely the 'tip of the iceberg'.[51]

Since 1946,[52] attention has been drawn to the increasing number of children who have received bodily injuries for which the clinical picture bore no relation to the medical history given by the parent or guardian. Other reports after this time referred to the pattern of injuries as 'unrecognised trauma',[53, 54] and it was not until 1962 that Kempe and his associates,[55] first called the clinical condition of the injuries of maltreatment the 'battered child syndrome'.

It is not easy to give a simple definition of the battered child syndrome. It is a term used to define a clinical condition in young children, usually under three years of age, who have been the victims of non-accidental, wholly inexcusable violence or injury on one or more occasions. The injury may be minimal, severe or fatal trauma for what is often the most trivial provocation, and administered by the hand of an adult in a position of trust, generally a parent, guardian or foster parent. In addition to physical injury, there may be deprivation of nutrition, care and affection in circumstances indicating that such deprivation is non-accidental.[56–58]

The battered baby produces such an emotional reaction of revulsion that it may well be rejected as improbable by both the legal profession, who tend to require a high standard of proof in many cases, and the medical profession. The term 'battered baby' is so emotive[59] that perhaps it should be dropped, yet it describes the actual situation very clearly and is useful diagnostically. Other terms that have been suggested include the physically abused child, the maltreated child or the ill-treated child syndrome.

Taking care of 'crying children' under five years of age evokes distress for the parents as well as for the infant. Nearly every week there are press reports of cruelty to children by their parents or guardians resulting in either irreparable brain or eye damage, skeletal trauma or death.

As soon as non-accidental injury is suspected by the family doctor, casualty officer, health visitor or social worker, the child should always be referred to hospital for study and for safety. If not already involved, the family doctor and health visitor should be notified, so that they may discuss any information in their possession. The paediatrician, radiologist and medico-legist should call in other colleagues, such as a neurosurgeon, when appropriate. He should also discuss the findings with the parents who occasionally admit part of the true story, especially if they see the paediatrician as someone who helps rather than accuses or condemns.

The thought that an adult in a position of trust could be responsible for the injury is so repugnant to natural feeling that it does not come to mind. Despite published efforts in the lay and medical press to clarify and define the legal, medical and social issues associated with the syndrome, some doctors still find it hard to accept the reality of wilful abuse of children. This may be due to lack of confidence in their own judgement, fear that such suspicion would necessitate violating the ethics of their oath of secrecy, or because it may jeopardise their doctor-patient relationship. They may feel that a threat of criminal investigation in any case would increase the danger of other parents not bringing their children to a hospital when battered.

Obviously no one wants to split up families if it can be avoided. One solution, after careful assessment, may be to return the child to his home and parents, making certain that they have adequate support and treatment[60] from the medical and nursing profession, the children's department, the National Society for Prevention of Cruelty to Children and other social services. Numerous battered babies are at present simply accepted as accident cases, treated and promptly returned to the possibly fatal hazards of their homes.

In serious cases criminal proceedings against the parent(s) are taken for the appropriate offence. Provided that a conviction is secured, disposal is a matter for the court acting upon the available evidence. There should, however, be concern for the discrepancy in sentence from one case to another, one Court to another and one part of the country to another.

The 'battered child syndrome' is a problem of increasing importance, calling for full co-operation of the medical, social and legal authorities in the country. There is a definite lack in medical education concerning ill-treatment in children. According to some authorities, less than a third of such cases seen by doctors are reported to the authorities.

There seems little doubt that the present situation shows an explosive increase of a certain type of traumatic clinical picture. The extent of the explosion is underlined by the fact that until recently it was not included in the punch diagnostic records of one of the most important children's hospitals in the country. There can be little doubt that in the early stages of the escalation it was missed by clinicians and unacceptable both to magistrates and judges because of the emotional rejection of such violence being inflicted upon babies. Although the findings are quite variable, the syndrome should be considered in any child exhibiting evidence of possible trauma or neglect (fractures in various stages of resolution, subdural haematoma, multiple soft tissue injuries including laceration of the mouth, poor skin hygiene or unexplained malnutrition) or where there is a marked discrepancy between the clinical findings and the past history as supplied by the parents. In all such cases the doctor should have a low threshold of suspicion and order a radiographic study of the whole skeleton. In this way the presence or absence of the characteristic multiple bony lesions in various stages of healing can be ascertained. A negative X-ray does not exclude the diagnosis, the basis of which depends upon the nature and recurrence of injuries, the time taken to seek medical advice and a discrepant history.

No one wants to believe or even think that the ordinary young man or woman one passes in the street could, driven by some terrible impulse, swing their baby by the ankles and bash his head against the wall and furniture; shake or jump on his chest until his ribs are crushed, his diaphragm torn, or his liver and intestines ruptured; or burn or knock him into unconsciousness, coma and death. There can be few who at one time or another have not been exasperated beyond endurance by the behaviour of their children.[61] Fortunately for most, the expression of their exasperation stops short of real violence. However, there must be a spectrum of violence ranging from corrective trauma from a zealous parent to deliberate cruelty. Parental discipline has consistently alternated between complete abandonment of physical punishment and its excessive use to a point of savagery.

Psychiatric knowledge pertaining to the problem is relatively meagre,[62] and the type and degree of physical attack varies greatly. Parents who inflict such abuse on their offspring do not necessarily have psychopathic or socio-pathic personalities, or come from one particular social class more than another. In a number of cases there is some defect in the parental character structure present, while not infrequently the infant is the product of an unwanted pregnancy—a pregnancy that began before marriage, or at some other time when it was felt to be extremely inconvenient.

Regardless of the doctor's personal reluctance to become involved in such cases, he should remember that his moral obligation is to the child and he should be aware that at least 60% of these children are liable to further injuries or death if not fully investigated. Complete investigation, including a full radiographic study and ophthalmological examination therefore are necessary for the child's protection, together with steps to prevent repetition of the ill treatment through normal medical channels, social services, and in extreme cases by legal sanctions. Clearly the general practitioner, casualty officer and paediatrician have a clear responsibility both to the child and his family as a total unit. In dealing with the abused, maltreated or battered child, the general practitioner has one of his most difficult roles to play, for he may find himself emotionally involved. In such an event, he should immediately refer the case to someone less involved, possibly at a distance, particularly if it is a small town or community.

In 1946 Caffey[63] drew attention to the apparently increasing frequency of subdural haematoma in infants accompanied by fractures of long bones, and he later[52] offered the possible explanation of parental neglect and abuse as a cause of this association of symptoms. Although other reports have referred to this disease of maltreatment as 'unrecognised trauma' it was Kempe and his associates[55] who first called it the battered child syndrome.

When a doctor is called to see an injured child, particularly under the age of three, he must always consider the diagnosis of a 'battered baby'. Nevertheless he should not on the slightest provocation start a 'witch-hunt'.

Although the safety of the child must be the primary consideration one must remember that battering parents need help and, above all, a good relationship with a helping person, with a priority in many cases for re-housing, day nursery placement, and even temporary reception of the children into care during periods of stress and crisis. Legislation can provide an effective instrument for preventing or mitigating child neglect, while abuse calls for attention to psychological stresses rather than to material needs. It has been suggested[64] that child guidance treatment may be necessary to help parents understand a child's behaviour. Close co-operation between doctors and social agencies is essential at all stages. Mutual respect for the duties, responsibilities and professional practices of the several disciplines involved in the management of the battered child and his family is an important aspect of the problem that is solved only by understanding its underlying causation. If this succeeds, there will be less cause for the almost hysterical demand for legislation to introduce obligatory reporting of cases when a child is found to be injured—accidents can happen. The most exciting and encouraging aspect of this problem must lie in the area of prevention, particularly looking for a reliable means of identifying parents who demonstrate a potential for child abuse. Such parents could then be given help and support in order to prevent another battered child.

Examination

No other entity better illustrates the need for a comprehensive approach to the investigation of non-accidental injuries or unnatural death and no other calls for better teamwork. No matter how straightforward the findings may appear initially, or how elaborate and complete a confession is, one must assume that the 'confession' may well be discounted or that some subsequent findings in the investigation may well reverse the hypothesis it had evolved at the initial investigation. The absence of overt trauma on the exterior of the body should in no instance be considered a contraindication for a full clinical examination, or in a dead child an autopsy, since it often bears no relationship to the trauma to the interior of the body. One should initially inspect the body carefully to note the nature of the clothing, the degree of its cleanliness, and the state of repair or disrepair. This, together with the general external characteristics (including height, weight and state of nutrition) and any discrepancy, no matter how subtle, in the clinical and pathological findings with the alleged statement by the parent(s) or guardian should be carefully followed up. Photographs with careful drawings or even tracings (especially of bite marks) may afford an opportunity to reach a conclusion concerning the nature of the weapon used to inflict such wounds and to the subsequent investigation. In cases of autopsy, routine histological examination should be carried out on every organ in all cases, particularly the eyes.

Recent contributions to the literature point out the importance, in addition, of a general toxicological examination to rule out the introduction of exogenous poisons or overdoses of therapeutic agents as contributory factors to the injury or death of these children. The toxicological assay should be qualitative as well as quantitative and as comprehensive as possible.

Clinicians have a duty and a responsibility to the child to evaluate the problem fully and to guarantee that no repetition of the trauma, either in this child or to any other child, will be permitted to occur. Unfortunately the condition is frequently not recognised or, if diagnosed, is inadequately handled by the clinician because of either hesitation to bring the case to the attention of the proper authorities, or the doctor's reluctance to report such a case since it may involve entanglement in legal matters. A major diagnostic feature of this syndrome is the marked discrepancy between the clinical findings and the historical data as supplied by the parents. Because of this there is a reluctance on the part of many clinicians to accept the radiological signs as indicative of repetitive trauma and possible abuse. To the informed clinician the bones tell a story the child is too young or too frightened to tell.[65] There can be little difficulty in differentiation between disease and trauma if proper laboratory investigations are available, although it must be stressed that trauma may occur to a child which is not healthy. In fact, it may be the ill child whose crying precipitates violence.

Variations of the 'syndrome'

In a condition such as child abuse there must be, and there are, a number of different variants, most of which overlap and many of which show an element of more than two types. For the sake of discussion let us consider seven principle groups (Table 15.3).

Table 15.3 Variations of non-accidental injury/death

Infanticide
Sadistic variant
Deprivation variant
Classical 'battered baby syndrome'
'Battered child syndrome'
Psychological maltreatment
Sexually abused child

Infanticide. One includes infanticide in this table because a number of cases of infanticide may exhibit a degree of maltreatment by the mother leading to its death. Infanticide itself is discussed on page 336.

Sadistic variant. Such cases are subjected to episodes of almost uncontrolled violence by a parent, who is usually under the influence of alcohol at the time and who may well be a 'wife-batterer' or 'husband-basher' as well.

Deprivation variant. Acts of omission can be equally as deleterious to a child's health as acts of violent commission. There is the problem of the ambiguous case where 'deliberate intent' cannot be confidently inferred or where unconscious motives may be in operation. The broadening of the initial definition to include acts of 'omission' or neglect in such cases was suggested by Gil.[66, 67]

Giovannoni[68] argues that one must distinguish between neglect and abuse for the purpose of explanation, but in agreement with Allan,[44] such a distinction has no practical value at the level of intervention. A clear distinction is misleading since it often occurs that severe abuse cases also include elements of neglect. In such family groups it is frequently noted that the family pets are beautifully cared for, whilst the child is allowed to develop into a totally emaciated state, occasionally being given scraps of unsuitable food, in some cases, pet food. Figure 15.1 illustrates such a case.

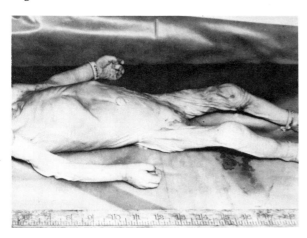

Fig. 15.1 An emaciated child.

Classical 'battered baby syndrome'. One child taken out of the family, unwanted for one reason or another, and who receives physical abuse. All the classical features, which will be discussed later, are present. If the mother is the perpetrator it is not uncommon to find that the assaults are associated with pre-menstrual tension and can be aged roughly every four weeks. Although physical injuries are the first signs of abuse to be recognised,

only later is it recognised that the injuries are but a signpost to a family with severe internal stress needing urgent diagnosis and treatment.[69] Roberts & Hawton[70] draw attention to the fact that attempted suicide in parents of young children considerably increases the risk of child abuse. Which comes first, the chicken or the egg? Whichever, help should be directed at these problems at the time of the suicide attempt which may possibly prevent child abuse.

'Battered child syndrome'. Such cases occur in children in the school-child age group—say three to 10 years of age. Here the injuries are primarily soft tissue and are normally covered when the child wears outdoor clothing. Teachers and the like should be extremely cautious of young children who frequently present themselves with a letter from a parent to excuse them from partaking in physical exercise and gymnasium activities because if they were to undress, bruises, etc., may be seen. Frequently the perpetrator is a common-law father or co-habitee, who abuses his alleged spouse's children, whilst his own are properly cared for.

Psychological maltreatment. Not all women or men were intended to be parents, and, as in the animal world, there must be good and bad parents. This may lead to a lack of 'mothering', with lack or deprivation of love, care and attention, possibly without intent, to their offspring.

The effect of emotional (or psycho-social) abuse on a child includes failure to thrive and various learning problems.[45] Diagnosis is difficult because there are no dramatic bruises or marks of violence to be detected.

Sexually abused child. Little is known about the prevalence of sexual mistreatment of children or how it is being dealt with. Kempe,[71] in a survey of child abuse, postulated five stages of recognition, of which the 5th was adequate understanding and recognition of the problem of sexual abuse. He suggested that the 5th stage had been reached in the United States of America but not yet in the United Kingdom.

Reports of sexually abused children in the United States have increased dramatically in the last few years as a result of child abuse legislation and public awareness campaigns. The National

Centre on Child Abuse and Neglect in Washington D C estimates that the current annual incidence is between 60 000 and 100 000 cases per year in the United States.[72]

A recent study[73] estimates that 1 in 5 girls and 1 in 11 boys in the United States have had sexual experience with a much older person and that 5% of children have been victimised by a much older person within the nuclear family.

Comparable statistics are not available in Britain. Recorded figures from the Home Office for 1980 report 312 cases of incest and 254 cases of unlawful sexual intercourse with children under 13 years in England and Wales. A current survey in Britain of professionals who work with children may more accurately reflect the extent of recognised child sexual abuse in this country.[74]

In a series of 80 abused children referred in 1979, Cameron found that 10 (12%) of these children were also sexually abused, four of these by the age of six months (unpublished data).

Mrajek reports that physicians identify a relatively small percentage of reported child sexual abuse cases. In part this is because of the infrequency of positive findings. Bennett & Pettybridge[75] in a study of 83 abused and neglected children consecutively admitted to the childrens' wards of the Royal Naval Hospital, Haslar, reported only one case of sexual abuse which could indicate that others had been missed. Orr[76] has stressed the necessity of gathering pertinent psycho-social data during the medical evaluation to make the correct diagnosis.

There is no evidence that any particular unit of treatment is specifically indicated in the treatment of child sexual abuse. Few treatment programmes for child sexual abuse have reported their results. Because of this paucity of information health care professionals face a dilemma of what to do when they encounter a sexually abused child and its family. Suffice it to say that any case of non-accidental injury must now be examined to exclude any sexual connotation.

Characteristic injuries

The serious injuries are subdural haemorrhage with or without a fractured skull and injuries in the abdomen such as a rupture of the liver or bruising of the intestine. The diagnosis is confused by denial of any accident or explanations by the parent such as the following:

1. he bumped his head against the cot;
2. he bruises easily;
3. he fell downstair;
4. he fell off the bed;
5. a swing hit him in the tummy.

On some occasions the injuries will speak for themselves, either by their nature or pattern. In others, the mechanism of a fracture may be capable of interpretation. Injury to the mucosa of the upper lip seen in some cases is almost diagnostic (Figs 15.2 and 15.3).

Although bruises are a prominent feature and give rise to the statement 'he bruises easily', care must be given in interpreting their cause. Gripping a child will cause four or five bruises, and these, as well as photographs of them, can give a false impression. The serious ones are those that matter, and their age. Clearly the basis of approach to each case must be first to save the life of the child by treating the immediate injury, while at the same time being awake to the fact of possible aggravation of an older lesion such as secondary bleeding from a subdural haemorrhage.

In the case of post-mortem examination, upon completion and ideally after a period of 12 to 24 h

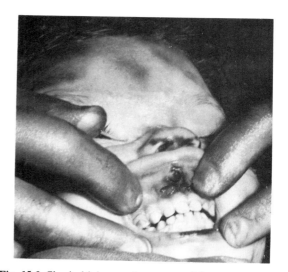

Fig. 15.2 Classical injury to the mucosa of the upper lip as a result of an upward blow to the face.

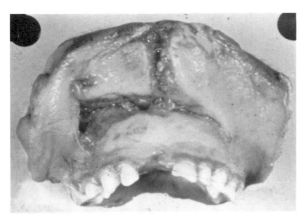

Fig. 15.3 A severe example of the tearing of the upper lip extending along the alveolar margin which occurred 3 days prior to death. There is also evidence of an older injury to the mouth in the form of a tooth having been knocked out and scarring of the gum as a result, approximately 3–4 months earlier.

of refrigeration, it is of value to re-examine the exterior of the child's body, for frequently with the progressive blanching of the skin the surface bruises beneath the skin surface are better delineated; even pattern injuries not noted on earlier examination are seen then.

The clinical pathology typical of the battered child can be summarised as follows:

Surface marks. These consist of bruises (Fig. 15.4), abrasions and burns, of different colours and clearly of different ages, indicative of repeated incidents (Fig. 15.5). They may, however, give an exaggerated idea of the degree of violence due to the fact that children do bruise easily. The important factor is their distribution. Bruises of the scalp are not always clearly visible but may be discovered by palpation and by reaction to tenderness. At autopsy, however, on reflection of the scalp deep bruising is often detected (Fig. 15.6). The presence, in almost 50% of cases, of laceration of the mucosa of the inner aspect of the upper lip, near the frenulum sometimes with tearing of the lip from the alveolar margin of the gum (Figs 15.2 and 15.3), is now considered almost pathognomonic.[65] This injury is thought to be the result of a blow on the mouth or of other efforts to silence a screaming or crying child.

The limbs frequently show 'finger-tip' bruises, commonly grouped around the elbows and knees, due to gripping of the child so as to shake or pull

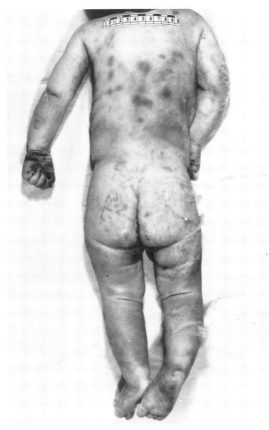

Fig. 15.4 The back of a child showing the classical areas of bruising of varying age over the body together with a moderate nappy rash.

him, or hurl him into his cot or against furniture, while more diffuse bruises may be due to blows or impact against a surface. Bruising of the chest and trunk may be due to blows, while bruising of the abdominal wall is often minimal, in spite of severe intra-abdominal injury. It is often difficult, due to shock and peripheral vascular failure, to age the bruises with accuracy. Recent cases showed an increasing incidence of bite marks.[77, 78]

Since 1969 one has been increasingly aware that bite marks figure significantly as a feature of this syndrome. The entire surface of the child's body is available to the assailant and bite marks may be found on the cheeks, shoulders, chest, abdomen, arms, legs and buttocks. These appear to be the most common sites for biting and there may be single or multiple bites on one particular area or generalised biting over all areas. The investigation

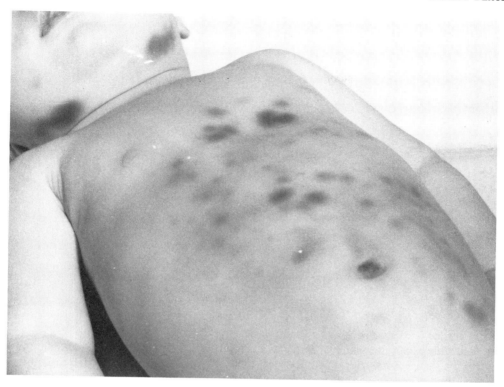

Fig. 15.5 Shows an area of bruising of varying age (similar to that shown in Fig. 15.4) over the front of the upper chest and lower face.

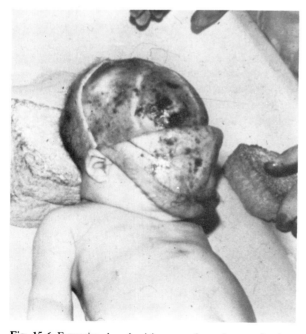

Fig. 15.6 Extensive deep bruising over the scalp on reflection.

and evaluation of such marks follows the normal methods one would employ for investigations of marks on adults. However, the bite marks on children do appear to present some common features, namely that they tend to be poor in definition and detail and have diffuse areas of bruising. Routinely one examines the entire body with an ultraviolet lamp in order to elicit previous areas of bruising,[79, 80] and the body is viewed at intervals of 24 h in order to ascertain if the marks will develop further in detail. The distortion of tissues does not appear to be so evident in children as it sometimes is in adults when the marks are examined in situ, but there is shrinkage when a portion of tissue containing the bite mark is removed from the body. Even so, the marks do provide valuable information concerning the possible perpetrator because the number of suspects is limited to those persons with close access to the child. In the living children that have been examined it has been found on many occasions that other children have been responsible for biting in play or jealousy and

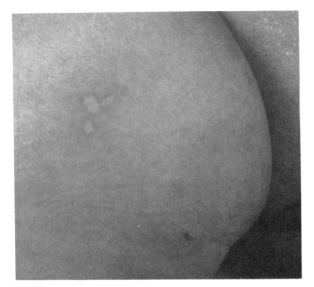

Fig. 15.7 Cigarette burns.

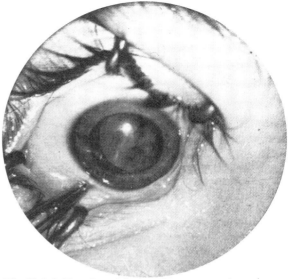

Fig. 15.9 Subluxation of the lens due to trauma (note the pigment dispersal on the detached retina behind the lens).

are limited to brothers or sisters or playmates in a nursery where the supervisor, or the foster-parent, or the guardian is not present the whole time.

Such methods of refracted ultra-violet photography can be of considerable value in interpreting the presence of older scars—such as cigarette burns (Fig. 15.7)—which are not visible to the naked eye.

Having mentioned the eyes, recently it has been found that in addition to the facial injuries described in the literature, there are marked subcutaneous and subconjunctival haemorrhages (Fig. 15.8), detached retinae, and in very severe cases, displaced lenses (Fig. 15.9) of the eyes.[81–83]

Clinically, one should remember that bilateral 'black eyes' (Fig. 15.10), even in adults, are, until proved otherwise, non-accidental. Permanent impairment of vision affecting one or both eyes is now a well-recognised complication of battered children.[84, 85] Trauma should be especially considered in pseudoglioma, Coat's disease, lens dislocation and all forms of old or recent intra-ocular haemorrhage.

Mention has already been made of cigarette or cigar burns, and they are frequently associated with scalds. Placing a child in hot water—i.e., 'hot' to an adult skin, but 'boiling' to a child's skin—is a frequent finding. One must differentiate from plac-

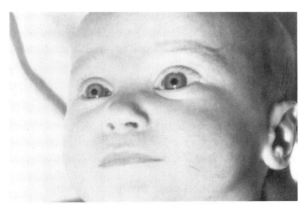

Fig. 15.8 Subconjunctival haemorrhage.

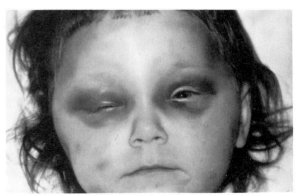

Fig. 15.10 Example of bilateral 'black eyes'.

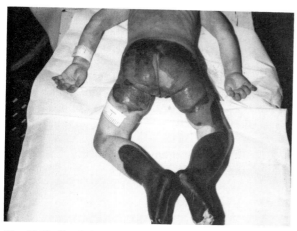

Fig. 15.11 Classical scald burns as a result of immersion in boiling water. Note the absence of burning on reflection of the legs but nevertheless the extensive bruising associated with the outer aspect of the left knee.

ing in a bath of hot water, when the soles of the feet are scalded (Fig. 15.11), from being put in a bath and hot water 'turned on', when a natural reflex is for the child to try and avoid being scalded and if he is held forcibly in the bath there will be bruising of the shoulder where forced to sit, and lack of scalding on the soles of feet and cheeks of the buttocks. Scalding is also frequently used as a technique to cover up a cigarette burn—say in the palm of the hand where the hand has been immersed in very hot water or corrosive solution.

Frequently the back, buttocks and lower extremities show a severe weeping, infected napkin erythema (Fig. 15.12), that in some cases even extends over the soles of the feet, which are secondarily infected with 'pox-like' scars of healed ulceration, often associated with weeping denudation of the skin of the genitalia and perineum.

Skeletal injuries. In view of the usual intermittent nature of the trauma, radiological examination of fractures may reveal various stages of reparative change. On the other hand, if no fractures or dislocations are apparent on examination, it must always be remembered that bone injury may be difficult to detect during the first few days after inflicted trauma. In life, as documented in the historical observations of the classical description of the battered baby, the radiologist may be the first to call attention to the existence of pre-existing trauma in a child suffering from acute violence.[49]

It should be clearly understood, however, by all working in the field that the assistance of the radiologist is invaluable; not only may he date and serialise bone injuries on the trunk more accurately than the pathologist, but in those portions of the body which the pathologist is often reluctant for aesthetic reasons to examine, he may document injuries hitherto unsuspected.

The forces applied in grasping and seizing the child usually involve traction and torsion; such strains and stresses produce epiphyseal separations and periosteal shearing, while fractures of the shafts of the long bones may result from direct trauma, bending, compressing or twisting.

Metaphyseal fragmentation may also be produced mechanically. As the periosteum of infants is not securely attached to the underlying bone, periosteal haemorrhages may well be responsible for a number of irregular changes seen, particularly with secondary periosteal calcification.

The mechanism by which some of the fractures occur is not always easy to determine. The type of fracture should be noted. Oblique and greenstick fractures are caused by indirect violence, whereas transverse fractures are caused by violence directed at the site of fracture.

Radiology plays an essential part in the investigation and diagnosis of non-accidental injury in children.

There is no standard appearance of the progress and consolidation of new bone, so that one can only

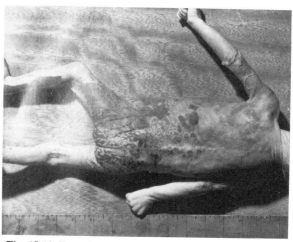

Fig. 15.12 Extensive napkin erythema with pock-like scars from old healed ulceration extending over the genitalia, perineum and the soles of the feet.

give a rough estimate as to the age of the injuries according to one's experience.[49]

It is the custom nowadays to radiograph the whole body when non-accidental injury is suspected, prior to autopsy, and then to dissect out and re-radiograph any bone that appears to be damaged. This makes it possible for the smallest of injuries to be detected in detail, even by taking macroradiographs. The radiographic study of the 'dead battered child' has helped to piece together a comprehensive picture of the type of skeletal injuries that one should look for in the live suspect battered child where the small injuries may not be so clearly demonstrated radiographically. There are two principle reasons why one wishes to understand the mechanism by which these injuries were caused: firstly to establish where possible and confirm the diagnosis in cases in which there is a discrepancy between the history as given and the radiographic findings; secondly, one should in most cases be able to give an opinion as to how such injuries were caused. Any unusual skeletal injury or an injury, the severity of which is not consistent with the history given, demands a complete radiographic skeletal survey.[58] This establishes the full extent of the injuries with special reference to the metaphyses and ribs; and ascertains whether there

are any old injuries, indicative or previous trauma.

The presence of multiple fractures of the long bones in various stages of healing (Fig. 15.13), implying more than one traumatic incident, may suggest to the experienced eye a case of child abuse but this need not necessarily be definite proof alone of non-accidental injury. One must exclude natural bone disease which can resemble non-accidental injury.

When the periosteum has been lifted from the underlying bone by a haematoma, periosteal new bone formation occurs normally and can be seen in over 40% of such cases within seven days.[58] In a case of injury, a distinction must be made between the normal bone layer and the pathological new bone resulting from the trauma. In the case of trauma, the normal layer may be interrupted by a fracture or by haemorrhage. When the pathological new bone forms later it will be as a continuous, unbroken layer superimposed upon the normal one. This distinction is of importance when estimating the age of the injury. Deformities resulting from metaphyseal injuries may persist for some time and it is important that they should be recognised. In a case of non-accidental injury to children, any deformity, however slight, should not be disregarded.[58] The older the injury the less notice-

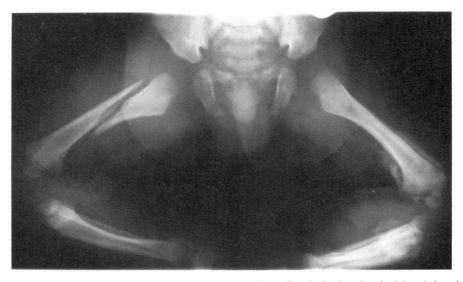

Fig. 15.13 Oblique fractures of the shaft of the right femur with no visible callus, indicating that the injury is less than a week old. This is the torsion-type fracture which could be caused by an accidental fall. The presence of metaphyseal injuries with callus formation in the distal end of the left femur and in the proximal end of the tibia indicate that the fractures of the right femur could be the result of a non-accidental injury. Judging by the amount of callus present, these metaphyseal injuries are about 2–3 weeks old.

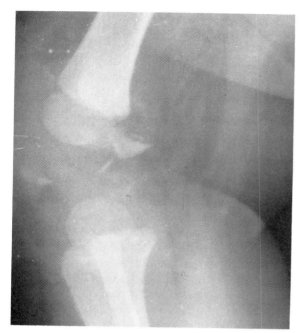

Fig. 15.14. Loose piece of bone lying by the distal end of the femur. It will be noticed that there is a dislocation of the tibiofibular joint.

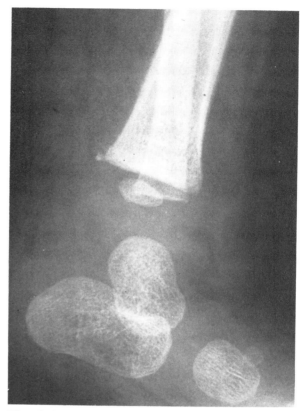

Fig. 15.15 Loose piece of bone at posterior aspect of distal end of tibia.

able will the deformity become. Any metaphyseal injury may be so small as to be considered of no importance, but it cannot be emphasised too strongly that any injury in the region of the metaphysis—be it a crack or a small piece of detached bone in a suspected case of child abuse—should in the first instance be regarded as a result of non-accidental injury.[49, 58]

It is unusual for a baby to sustain multiple fractures of the ribs merely by falling from a cot or a pram, or by being dropped and it is very rare to sustain multiple fractures. Multiple fractures can occur in automobile accidents and in cases where there is a pathological lesion, such as osteogenesis imperfecta ('brittle bone disease'). In cases of child abuse (Figs 15.14 and 15.15), a common site of these fractures is in the posterior aspect of the rib, often close to the spine and frequently bilateral. These are caused by direct violence against the ribs.[49] Fractures of the costochondral junctions may be associated, though less commonly, and are caused frequently by violent squeezing of the chest from side to side. The reason for this action is that it tends to make the ribs spring and fracture at their fixed points. Antero-posterior compression is more likely to cause fractures underneath the armpits (i.e., in the midaxillary line), but one must remember that fractures can also occur as a result of cardiac resuscitation. Direct violence, as distinct from compression, can also cause fractures of the ribs, such as striking the chest with the fists, with a boot or by swinging the child by the foot and causing the chest to come into contact with some hard object. The site of a fracture caused in this way will usually be at the point where the violence is applied and is usually associated externally by a bruise. Many cases when first radiographed show multiple fractures of the ribs in varying stages of healing indicative of more than one traumatic incident.

As further healing takes place, the nodules (callus formation) become contracted and less dense (Figs 15.16 and 15.17). They may even become almost indistinguishable from normal. It is well known that cases return to normal some six months after an injury, although in some cases they may

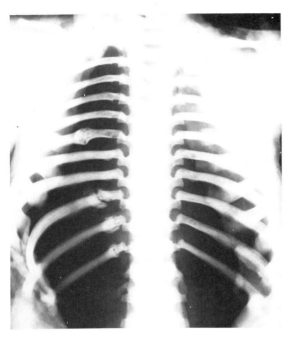

Fig. 15.16 As healing progresses, the nodules become contracted and less dense.

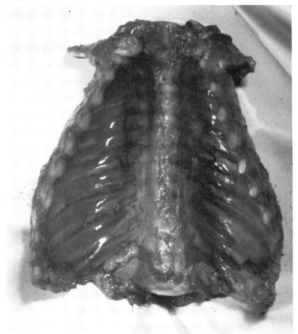

Fig. 15.17 Post-mortem specimen which shows the extent of the osteomyelitis of the right middle and left lower ribs. The previous well—formed callus in the posterior aspects of the left lower ribs has been eroded. The upper fractured left ribs and the fractured costochondral junctions on both sides show no evidence of osteomyelitis.

well retain the fracture deformities. In some cases it must be noted that recent fractures are not demonstrated unless a number of views are taken from varying angles, hence the reason for removing the rib cage in death following alleged non-accidental injury and violence so that the rib cage itself can be radiographed in three dimensions. In every case of suspected battered child syndrome where there are no obvious fractured ribs, the whole length of the rib should be carefully examined for evidence of old fractures. The presence of multiple rib fractures must be considered as having resulted from non-accidental trauma after the exclusion of such causes as a vehicular accident or manual compression in an attempt to revive the child either by a doctor or a parent. Proven bone disease must also be excluded, but it should be remembered that even a baby with a bone disease can be battered or subjected to non-accidental violence.

A fracture of a long bone occurring as the only skeletal injury in suspected battering usually cannot be distinguished from one resulting from an accident, such as falling from a cot, but when it occurs in conjuction with a metaphyseal injury or with multiple rib fractures, it should be considered as non-accidental injury, unless there is definite proof to the contrary. The age of the injury and the mechanism by which it was caused are important in establishing the diagnosis, particularly in cases where legal proceedings have been instituted.

Any fracture occurring in a child under 18 months that is of the spiral variety in the long bone should be regarded as being suspicious until proven otherwise,[58] for such a fracture can be caused by a torsion force applied to a limb as when a baby is forcibly jerked upwards and rotated whilst held by the wrist or ankle. Similarly, when a spiral fracture of the humerus occurs, this may result when the wrist is held or a fracture of the femur when the child is held by the ankle. In the absence of any corroborative evidence, one cannot, however, say how this type of fracture was caused, but the presence of an associated metaphyseal avulsion injury, as in the wrist, is conclusive evidence of non-accidental trauma. A transverse fracture usually is the result of a direct blow. Avulsion of a muscle from its attachment to a long bone can result in the so-called traumatic myositis ossificans, which is ossification of a periosteal haematoma (Fig. 15.18).

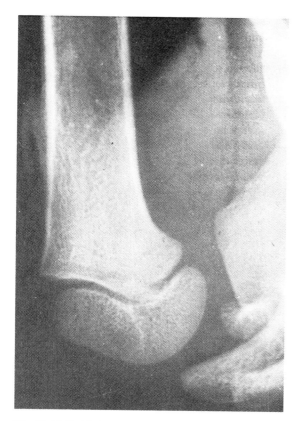

Fig. 15.18 Ossified subperiosteal haematoma on the shaft of the humerus resulting from an avulsion injury in a known case of an abused 3-year-old girl. Eight months previously there was extensive swelling of the whole arm.

As regards the estimation of age of the fracture of a long bone, the same criteria apply as in the case of a metaphyseal injury and in multiple rib fractures; that is, callus not visible on the radiograph for seven to ten days following the injury and the subsequent estimation of age becomes a matter of natural experience. In a case of a fracture of the skull, it is unusual for any notable healing change to take place for four to six weeks following the injury. The fracture may become more definite in the days following the injury, especially if increased cranial pressure in the form of a subdural haematoma develops. A fracture of the spine may also occur more often that one would give it credit for and, if it is an isolated injury, it may not be diagnostic, as it will not differ from that sustained by accidental injury. If, however, it is associated with other skeletal injuries, the diagnosis of abuse will probably be made in the presence of these injuries and particularly if associated with a heel mark in the back of the child.

Differential radiological diagnosis

There are several diseases where bone injuries can simulate those seen in non-accidental cases in children but, in most of these, the clinical examination should establish the diagnosis. It is important, however, that the medical practitioner should be conversant with these radiological appearances when examining a suspected case of non-accidental injury and when giving evidence in a Court of law on such a case.

Osteogenesis imperfecta

In the majority of cases, the diagnosis is not in doubt and in the neonatal type (Figs 15.19 and 15.20), there are multiple fractures of the tubular-shaped long bones or multiple fractures where the bones are thin and bowed. In severe cases the bones may be thin and not fractured (Fig. 15.21). Cases which simulate the battered child syndrome are those when the bones appear normal and fractures occur several months later and although a special test has been described in which the collagenous tissue of the body is examined, this is of negative value because it provides only negative proof. It is, however, frequently found where a suggestion is made to the Court that the case could be one of 'brittle bone disease' in spite of the fact that the children concerned improve on hospital therapy, and sustain fractures only when at home. It should be noted, however, that the fractures of the long bones involve the diaphyses and not the metaphyses, as occurs in the avulsion-type injury. These are not avulsion fractures, but fractures occurring in porotic bones, either spontaneously or as a result of slight trauma. A similar type of fracture is seen in the porotic bones of a case of spina bifida, although exuberant callus (Fig. 15.22) is seen to be a feature of 'brittle bone disease' (osteogenesis imperfecta). Nevertheless, one must state categorically that excessive new bone formation is not an uncommon feature following injury to the distal end of the femur in a case of spina bifida

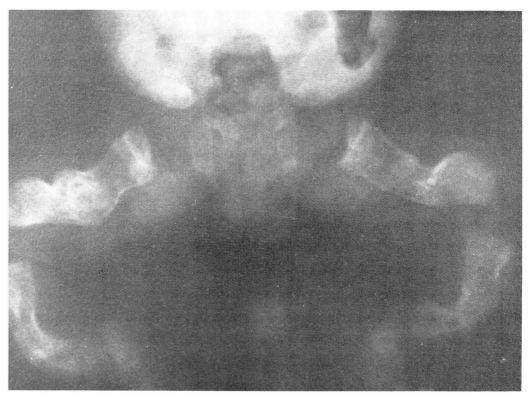

Fig. 15.19 Osteogenesis imperfecta—neonatal type with multiple fractures in tubular-shaped long bones.

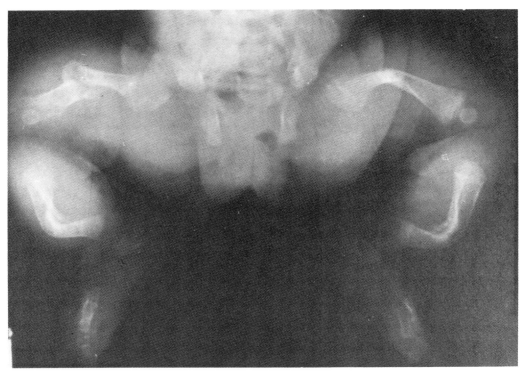

Fig. 15.20 Osteogenesis imperfecta—neonatal type with multiple fractures in thin and bowed bones.

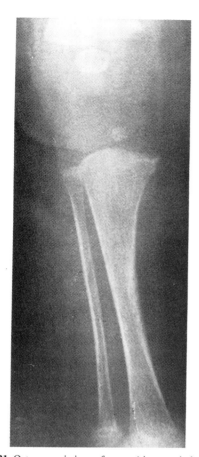

Fig. 15.21 Osteogenesis imperfecta—thin porotic bones with no fractures.

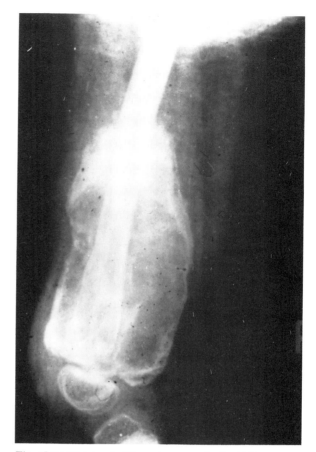

Fig. 15.23 Distal end of femur in a case of spina bifida.

(Fig. 15.23). It can occur in cases of osteomyelitis involving the metaphysis (Fig. 15.24) and also in cases of non-accidental injury to children in which there has been no immobilisation. There are, however, other features which are diagnostic of osteogenesis imperfecta such as blue sclerotics and a mosaic pattern in the posterior aspect of the skull (Fig. 15.25). The possibility that skeletal injuries in the case of osteogenesis imperfecta may have resulted from non-accidental trauma should, however, not be overlooked because even children suffering from abnormal bone disease can be battered.

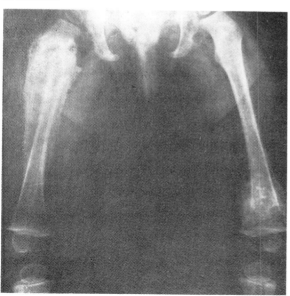

Fig. 15.22 Osteogenesis imperfecta—exuberant callus formation around the proximal aspect of the right femure, 6 weeks after the injury. Note that the callus at the distal end of the left femur (Fig. 15.21) has resolved in 3 weeks.

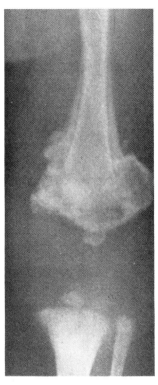

Scurvy

The changes occurring in scurvy with the fractured metaphysis and calcification in the subperiosteal haematoma (Fig. 15.26) closely resemble the appearances of metaphyseal injuries in non-accidental injury. In theory, however, there is a generalised osteoporosis and the metaphyses of most of the long bones will be involved.[49]

Congenital syphilis

In congenital syphilis there may be a fractured and separated metaphysis of a long bone with periosteal new bone along the shaft. Extensive periosteal new bone is a common feature of the shafts of the limb bones and this tends to be symmetrical (Fig. 15.27).

Fig. 15.24 Osteomyelitis of distal end of a femur with extensive calcification in the surrounding soft tissues and with periosteal new bone formation on the shaft. These appearances simulate those caused by a severe metaphyseal injury.

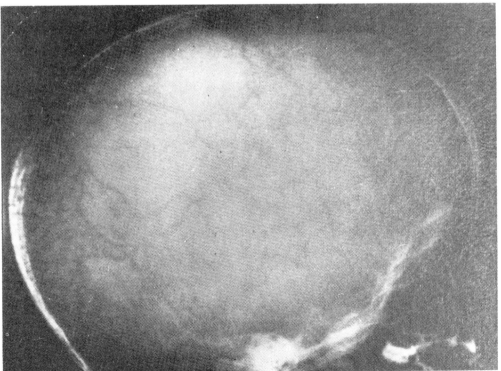

Fig. 15.25 Osteogenesis imperfecta—mosaic pattern in the posterior aspect of the skull.

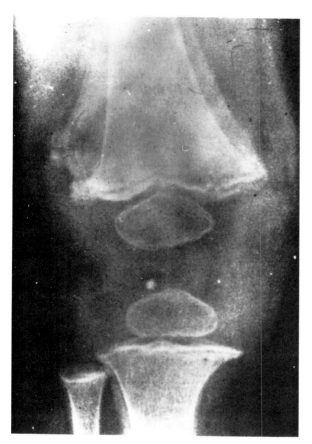

Fig. 15.26 Scurvy—the distal end of the femur showing a fractured and separated metaphysis with calcification in the subperiosteal haematoma. Similar, but less extensive, changes are present in the tibia.

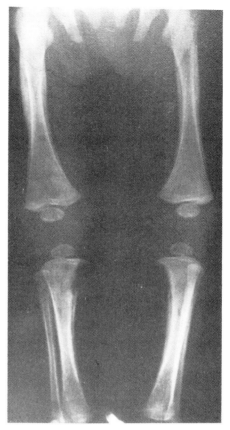

Fig. 15.27 Congenital syphilis—erosion of the proximal end of the medial border of each tibia, Wimberger's sign. This appearance is diagnostic of congenital syphilis and bears no resemblance to an avulsion injury. Periosteal new bone on the shafts of the femora and tibiae does not extend to the metaphyses. In the main the lesions in congenital syphilis tend to be symmetrical.

It tends to extend the metaphysis, though the bone adjacent to the metaphysis is often porotic. There are no changes in the metaphysis as would be seen in cases of an avulsion injury. Occasionally, however, the metaphyseal border may be eroded by the syphilitic inflammation and in such a case it may be difficult to exclude superimposed trauma.[49]

Infantile cortical hyperostosis of Caffey (Caffey's disease)

In this condition periosteal new bone forms along the shafts of several long bones (Figs 15.28 and 15.29). Where this new bone extends to the metaphyses, it may occasionally resemble the periosteal

new bone resulting from an avulsion injury, especially when the injury involves the proximal and distal metaphyses of the long bone. In Caffey's disease, the metaphyses will show no evidence of injury. One will see, however, a fracture of either a short oblique or transverse type and the callus is more localised. In a large proportion of Caffey's disease the mandible will show cortical thickening.[49]

Osteomyelitis

When the metaphyses of a long bone is affected by osteomyelitis, the appearances resemble those of metaphyseal avulsion injury (Fig. 15.30). The

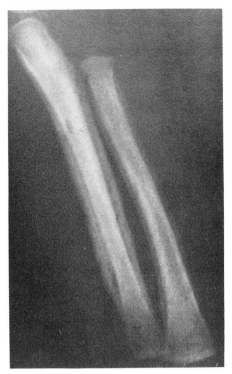

Fig. 15.28 Caffey's disease—periosteal new bone formation along the shafts of the radius and ulna; this does not extend to the metaphyses, which are normal.

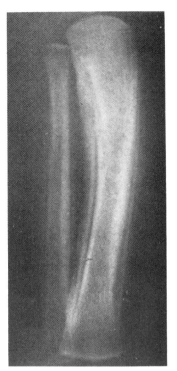

Fig. 15.29 Caffey's disease—the tibia and fibula of the same case as in Fig. 15.28.

metaphyses may become irregular and periosteal new bone may form along the shaft. In some cases there may be excessive calcification of the surrounding soft tissues resembling a severe avulsion injury. Such deformity resulting from the osteomyelitis in the region of the metaphysis, with thickening of the cortex, could in some cases simulate the thickened cortex of an old subperiosteal haematoma. There is, however, no metaphyseal damage (Fig. 15.31) and the soft tissue swelling would probably be more extensive than that resulting from a haematoma.[49]

Spina bifida

In cases of spina bifida where the legs are paralysed

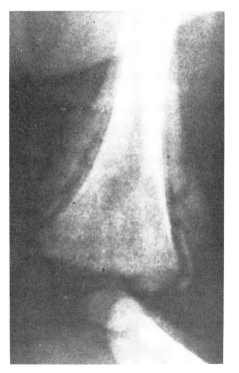

Fig. 15.30 Metaphyseal injury of the distal end of the femur with extensive calcification in the surrounding soft tissues in a male infant aged 4 months. These appearances resemble those occurring in a case of scurvy (see Fig. 15.26), but it should be remembered that scurvy is uncommon under the age of 5 months. A similar appearance can occur following an avulsion injury caused during labour where the leg presents.

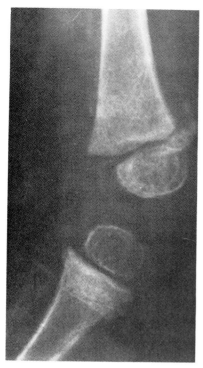

Fig. 15.31. Spina bifida—dislocation of the distal epiphysis of the femur following slight trauma. There is also a fracture of the proximal end of the tibia.

and the bones are porotic, very slight trauma can cause a fracture, but it is usually transverse at the distal end of the shaft of the femur or causes a dislocation of the epiphysis with associated damage to the metaphysis. These injuries are frequently accompanied by excessive haemorrhage and subsequent new bone formation in the adjacent soft tissues. This creates an appearance not unlike that seen in a case of child abuse, except that this degree of dislocation of the epiphysis is uncommon as a result of non-accidental injury. As in 'brittle bone disease' (osteogenesis imperfecta), the fact that the slight trauma can be non-accidental should not be overlooked. It should also be remembered that fractures in both these cases can occur spontaneously.[49]

Visceral injuries. Analysis of the fatal injuries show that they are associated predominantly with the head and secondarily with a ruptured liver. If proper objective consideration is given to this pattern, the terminal injuries are nearly always a subdural haemorrhage with or without a fractured

skull and, at the same time, in many cases compression of the chest with fractured ribs and ruptured viscera. The commonest cause of infantile subdural haemorrhage[86] is rupture of one or more of the delicate bridging veins which run from the cerebral cortex to the venous sinuses, the mode of injury being either a single acceleration or deceleration due to a heavy moving object striking the head or the rapidly moving head being brought into contact by or against a stationary mass; multiple applications might result in an increased incidence of rupture. Subdural haematoma is one of the commonest features of the battered child syndrome, yet by no means do all the patients so affected have external injury marks on the head. This suggests that in some cases repeated acceleration/deceleration rather than direct violence is the cause of the haemorrhage, the infant having been shaken rather than struck by its parent. Such a hypothesis might also explain the remarkable frequency of the finding of subdural haemorrhage in battered children as compared with its incidence in head injuries of other origin and the fact that it is so often bilateral.[58, 87] Rupture of the liver and abdominal viscera with tearing of the mesentery (Fig. 15.32) is seen, but external bruising of the abdominal wall is not necessarily present, a reminder that a diffuse blow to the relaxed abdomen may cause severe internal injury and yet leave no external mark.[57, 88]

An explanation for the high incidence of visceral injuries near a relatively fixed point in the mid-

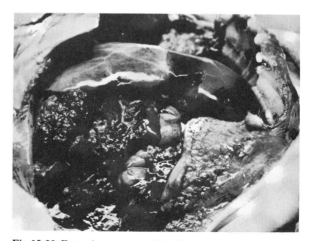

Fig 15.32 Extensive rupture of the liver and bruising of the mesentery as a result of violence having been applied to the upper abdomen.

abdomen is offered by Haller[89] who distinguishes the causes of blunt abdominal trauma by the mechanism of injury. Crushing or compression forces produce bursting injuries of the liver or spleen, or they may cause perforation of a distended hollow viscus, such as the stomach, intestine or bladder. Intestinal injuries are usually on the antimesenteric surface. A decelerating force such as a punch or blow tears the mesentery and may disrupt the small intestine at the site of ligamental support. The galaxy of visceral injuries in battered children best fits the latter category.[90]

The possibility of visceral injury from blunt trauma should be eliminated in any child with abdominal complaints who has characteristic bruising regardless of whether skeletal fractures or a head injury are present. A specific history of abdominal trauma may be remote or non-existent. Even if it is elicited, there may be a variable period of well-being preceding the onset of abdominal complaints.

Social aspects

If anyone has a right to be loved, a baby does. It is well known how vital it is for a human being to have a good start in life and for this it is essential that one should be wanted and loved when one first enters the world, frail and helpless. People sometimes think that they have a right to be loved and that it is the duty of their husbands, wives, children, parents and friends to love them. Frequently they expect this to happen without any effort on their part to make themselves lovable. Asked about this, many of those who complain of being unloved would be horrified and even resentful.[58]

Sadly, we are all somewhat afraid of being criticised and this is what sometimes makes us behave in a disagreeable or aggressive manner. On the other hand, it has some advantages because it makes us more willing to compromise in order to be accepted and wanted. As far as a child is concerned, the mother is the baby's life-line, both from the physical and psychological point of view. A baby or a small child cannot realise the effect it is having on others and it has very little control over its behaviour or emotions.

It sometimes happens that children with the most lovable natures do not get their due, whilst those less deserving receive far more than enough love, and this is by no means always fair. No one can love to order, simply because someone deserves love or needs it. On the whole, we have to work hard to make ourselves lovable if we want to be loved! Over the age of seven, this is relatively easy, but under that age a child, or baby, has no control. In a family there are, of course, natural bonds of affection between husband and wife, parents and children, and between the children themselves. At the same time, one is apt to show one's worst side to one's family, e.g., children usually behave worse at home than outside; the husband and wife may exhibit less charm and grace in their home lives, particularly to their children, than they show to outsiders, for frequently those who are the life and soul of the party may be irritable and morose in the family circle. The love parents feel for their baby may not be less, but it is certainly different from the love they feel towards an adolescent or married son or daughter. In the same way, children's love for their parents undergoes many changes as they develop from complete acceptance of them to the critical and independent attitude of youth.

It is in this climate that children are battered. There are still many people—doctors, lawyers and social workers among them—who even today deny that battering exists at all.[58] They cannot bring themselves to accept that 'ordinary' people could ever attack their own children.

Ill treatment of children by parental abuse or neglect may occur at any age; when under three years of age, however, the child cannot relate how the trauma was inflicted and older children in the family are reluctant or afraid to tell the story. Hence the age is significant, especially when the history given by the parents is at variance with the clinical picture and the physical signs noted on objective examination of the child, together with the knowledge that no new lesions occur during the child's hospitalisation. Close questioning frequently reveals that the child has been taken to various hospitals and doctors in an attempt to negate any suspicion of parental abuse. Often the parents completely deny any knowledge of inflicted trauma. This difficulty in obtaining any type of history leaves the diagnosis dependent upon physical examination, radiological findings, and a low threshold of suspicion on the part of the clinician, pathologist or police.

Often the victim is an unwanted child, e.g., the result of pregnancy before marriage, where there is doubt of the father's paternity, where the child is 'in the way' or where there is infidelity or suspicion of it.

There is frequently a history of family discord, long-standing emotional problems, or financial stress, although the character and personality of the guilty parent, commonly aged between 20 and 30, need not give outward signs of neurosis or psychosis; on the contrary, he or she may present the rather disarming attitude of co-operativeness, over-protectiveness and neatness. Many of the fathers have, or are alleged to have, criminal records and are unemployed at the time of the incident,[91] and the mother is frequently pregnant or in the pre-menstrual period at the time of battering.

Court[92] reports that many support the view that the 'innocent' partner in a battering situation is always consciously or unconsciously aware of what is happening. In many cases the partner was present when the actual episode took place.

Parents who mistreat their children in the manner characteristic of battering are rarely schizophrenic or psychopathic. They are generally young and are found in all levels of social class, intelligence and education. Characteristically their standards of appearance, speech and social manner are high. The underlying personality defect appears to be a temporary or permanent deficiency of the feelings of affection, acceptance and approval which normal parents have toward children, combined with a positive tendency to give violent expression to tension.[58]

Battering can and occasionally does occur in well-to-do families who do not have any adverse social problems. However, most of those involved come from the lower income groups where social deprivation adds greatly to the danger of child battering in families in which the parents are psychologically at risk. Financial hardship and intolerable housing conditions add to the strains and tensions in any marriage and place impossible demands on the vulnerable parents' already limited reserves. The difficulties of tolerating a crying baby at night

and the consequent loss of sleep may increase the possibility of aggressive outbursts to such an extent as to produce the 'crying child syndrome'.

The syndrome is not confined to children of parents with a psychopathic or a borderline socio-economic status, but in most cases there is some defect in the character structure. According to Fairburn & Hunt,[93] the rejection of the child is probably a constant feature starting either with the first realisation of pregnancy, during an anxious or painful puerperium, or when the infant is fractious for long periods; or it is sometimes rejected by the father who for some reason doubts the child's paternity. Guilt amnesia is a well recognised condition in most abusive parents.[56,57,65]

Dawson[94] added another view when she pointed out that the state of motherhood had undergone a change during the previous two decades. On the one hand the mother's and her baby's health have received more attention through the National Health Service, but on the other a mother has never before been left so alone. Modern life has placed intolerable burdens on the mother of a young family—burdens she frequently has to carry alone. There appear to be certain periods when the risk is greater, such as during pregnancy or in the pre-menstrual phase of her cycle. The child is also at risk during early infancy, particularly if persistently crying, wet or dirty. His very inability to co-operate can easily evoke rage rather than under-standing and love. Help is what is required.

Pathologist's role

The absence of overt trauma on the exterior of the body should in no instance be considered a contraindication for a full autopsy on a dead child, since it often bears no relationship to the trauma on the interior of the body. One should initially inspect the body carefully to note the nature of the clothing, the degree of its cleanliness and its state of repair or disrepair. This should be noted, together with the general external characteristics, including height, weight, state of nutrition (including any suggestion of apparent selective nutritional deficiency). Any discrepancy, no matter how subtle—such as a discrepancy between the distribution of the hypostasis and the alleged terminal position of the body; taking the body temperature; and the alleged final care by the parents; or between the obvious state of nutrition and/or the well being of the infant or child; and the alleged concern of the parents—should be carefully followed up. Photographs, with careful drawings or sketches and, in some cases, even tracing (such as in teeth marks) may afford an opportunity to reach a conclusion concerning the nature of the weapon used to inflict the wounds that are found. Each wound should be specifically topographically located on the body with reference to known anatomical landmarks. One must remember, however, that the umbilicus and the nipples vary regarding the position of the body. Measurements should be taken from a fixed point, namely the heel and from the midline of the body in cases of autopsy, routine histological examination should be carried out on every organ in all cases and particularly, the eyes.[58]

Recent contributions to the literature point out the importance, in addition, of a general toxicological examination to rule out the introduction of noxious poisons or overdoses of therapeutic agents. The toxicological assay should be qualitative as well as quantitative and should be as comprehensive as the scope of the toxicological laboratory will allow. Naturally, this part will depend on the degree or level of suspicion of the pathologist.

On many occasions the injuries all speak for themselves, either by their nature or pattern. In other words, the mechanism of a fracture may be capable of interpretation. Injury of the mucosa of the upper lip, seen in numerous cases, is almost diagnostic or pathognomonic of the condition. Care must always be taken in interpreting the presence of bruising, but 'finger-tip' type bruises are always highly suggestive and one cannot take too many photographs during an autopsy because frequently one cannot go back and re-photograph.

Following an autopsy on an alleged 'battered child' one must remember, on completion of the examination, particularly after a period of say, some 12 to 24 h refrigeration, that it is of value to re-examine the exterior of the child's body, for, frequently, with progressing blanching of the skin, clearer demarcation of surface bruises of the skin surface can be revealed and even patterned injuries not noted on earlier examination may have become more apparent. One may fail to see bruising exter-nally on the scalp, yet at autopsy, on reflection of the scalp, deep bruising is often detected. The limbs frequently show 'finger-tip' type bruising; commonly grouped around the elbows and knees, due to gripping of the child in order to shake or pull him or her, or to hurl him or her into his or her cot or against furniture, while more diffuse bruising may be due to blows or impacts by or against a flat surface. Bruising of the chest and trunk may be due to blows, whilst severe bruising of the abdomen is often minimal, in spite of a severe intra-abdominal injury, due to the laxity of the abdominal muscles. It is often difficult, due to shock and peripheral vascular failure, to age bruises with accuracy, and this is one advantage of using colour photography, where one can leave it for the Court to decide the age of bruising. Recently it has been shown that there has been an increasing incidence of bite marks. Radiological examination should exclude conditions of a differential diagnosis, including rickets, congenital syphilis, osteogenesis imperfecta and various other bony abnormalities which have been described elsewhere.

Analysis of the fatal injuries show predominantly that they are associated with the head or, as an alternative, with a ruptured liver. If proper objective consideration is given to this pattern, the terminal injuries are nearly always seen to be a subdural haemorrhage, with or without a fractured skull, and at the same time, in many cases, compression of the chest with fractured ribs and ruptured viscera. The commonest cause of infantile subdural haemorrhage[86] is rupture of one or more of the delicate bridging veins which run from the cerebral cortex to the venous sinuses, the mode of injury being either a single acceleration or deceleration due to a heavy moving object striking the head, or the rapidly moving head being brought up against a stationary mass; multiple applications of force would increase the total strain on the bridging veins and might result in an increase of rupture. Subdural haematoma is one of the commonest features of the 'battered child syndrome'—seen in approximately 40% of cases—yet by no means all the patients so affected have external marks of injury to the head, suggesting that the child might well have been shaken rather than struck. In such cases ophthalmic damage is far more common.

Rupture of the liver and abdominal viscera with tearing of the mesentery is seen, but external bruising of the abdominal wall is not necessarily present—a reminder that a diffuse blow to the relaxed abdomen may cause severe internal injury and yet leave no mark. Explanation for the high incidence of visceral injuries near a relatively fixed point in the abdomen has been offered by Haller[89], who distinguished the cause of blunt abdominal injury by the mechanism of the injury. He noted that crushing or compressing forces produced bursting injuries of the liver or spleen or they might cause perforation of distended hollow viscus, such as the stomach, intestine or bladder. Intestinal injuries are usually on the antimesenteric surface.[49] A deceleration force, such as a punch or blow, tears the mesentery and may rupture the small intestine at sites of the ligamental support. The galaxy of visceral injuries in fatally battered children fits the latter category.[90] The possibility of visceral injuries from apparent blunt trauma should be eliminated in any child with abdominal complaints who has characteristic bruising, whether or not skeletal fractures or head injury are present. Increasing observation of permanent impairment of vision affecting one or both eyes in cases of subsequently proven battered children reminds one that at autopsy one should remove the eyes for ophthalmic pathological opinion.[58]

The autopsy

As in all medico-legal cases, photography is essential and photographs should be taken at all stages in the investigation of a suspected battered child, at the request and under the direction of the pathologist. Obviously, the first object is to have a photograph of both the front and the back of the child and of the facial views in case one had to damage any of the facial features subsequently. The body, having been identified by the relatives, can then be subjected to the necessary examinations as are required in all child deaths. A full antero-posterior skeletal radiological survey and a lateral view of the skull must be taken, realising the fact that a negative radiograph of the chest need not necessarily mean that there are no fractures, either old or recent, of the rib cage. Using a diagram to assist as an *aide-mémoire*, the bruises and injuries, as seen

externally, are noted and recorded, taking the heel and the midline as the fixed points of the body. Marks that resemble bite marks should be treated as an actual bite mark, namely a swab should be taken to test for secretor status in case the assailant is not related to the deceased.[78] Petechial haemorrhages may be indicative of an asphyxial element in the cause of death. After all the injuries and bruises have been noted externally, and the body has been skeletally surveyed radiologically, the internal examination can commence, provided that any marks resembling those caused by human dentition have been examined by a forensic odontologist before dissection. It is of minimal value for a forensic odontologist to examine any mark resembling human dentition after any incision has been made, because such an incision might reduce the elasticity of the skin and alter the shape of the 'bite mark'. Any unusual mark should be photographed with a scale, particularly those resembling bite marks, which can be blown up to a 1 to 1 scale, in order that a forensic odontologist might compare it with casts of the teeth of the potential assailants.[78]

Swabs should be taken of every orifice, as if it were a case of sexual assault, to exclude the possibility of necrophilia or a sexual element in the cause of death. In the United Kingdom the usual Y-shaped incision from both ears to the top of the sternum should be used, extending down the midline to the pubis. Next, the ear to ear incision must be used for the removal of the vault of the cranium. When one reflects the skin of the scalp, one can note whether there are any subaponeurotic haemorrhages to exclude the element of asphyxia or deep bruises. Thereafter, even though the child might be under three months, a saw-cut should be made around the head to remove the vault of the skull, contrary to the usual practise of incising down the suture lines. This excludes the possibility of any fractures that might have extended into the suture lines. On removal of the skull vault, if necessity arises, namely by the presence of a subdural haemorrhage or subarachnoid haemorrhage, further photographs should be taken. The brain should be removed and retained for fixation and subsequent examination. It is the writer's belief that it is far wiser to examine a 'dry' brain than a 'wet' brain.[58]

The incisions, i.e., head and body post-mortem incisions, having met, it is relatively easy to reflect the skin of the face over to the point of the nose, thus exposing not only the angle of the jaw, the upper and lower jaw, the sublingual region, the supraclavicular region, but also around the orbit and the bridge of the nose. This makes it considerably easier to enucleate the eyes. The eyes should then be sent, after fixation, for ophthalmological pathological opinion. By this manoeuvre of the reflection of the skin of the face, one incorporates reflection of the 'V' in the neck, over the chin cutting through the mucosal membranes of the lips at the edges and thus exposing the inner aspect of the lips, to see whether there is any bruising of the lips following a blow or blows to the face impinging the gums against the teeth and also to see whether there are underlying bruises of the chin. It also makes removal of the tongue more easy and exposure of the neck more readily available and, in addition, samples of blood can be taken from the vessels in the neck. It is the writer's preference to take all his samples from the right side of the body, working from that side. Samples of blood should be taken as they might later prove to be of value in cases of alleged disputed paternity. Disputed paternity might well prove the exclusion of an individual from being a potential assailant.[58]

Such a manoeuvre can be done without defacing the face because most mortuary superintendents can correct such defects by their training and technique. The rib cage is opened by using a scalpel and by dissecting through the sternoclavicular joint, where it can be disarticulated, thus freeing the clavicles from the rib cage, and retaining them within the skeleton.

Using the classical Rokitansky post-mortem techniques, the organs are removed in toto and observation can be made as to whether there is free blood or fluid, pus or stomach contents present in the thoracic cavities or in the abdominal cavity and as to whether the diaphragm is ruptured or not. Should there be any fractures of the ribs, this should be noted. After total evisceration of the body, any evidence of fractures of the ribs is detected macroscopically although not radiologically. The rib cage should be dissected by cutting through the intervertebral disc between the 12th thoracic and 1st lumbar vertebra and, by cutting round the body next to the skin, one can remove the rib cage intact, leaving the skin whole. The rib cage can then be X-rayed in at least three dimensions in order to visualise and confirm any fractures.[49] Such fractures should be subjected to histological examination as well as to this radiological examination, in order to age them. Histological sections must naturally be taken of all the thoracic organs.

As far as the abdominal cavity is concerned, it is very difficult to offer advice as to what should be done when there is a ruptured mesentery or ruptured intra-abdominal viscera. According to Cameron,[58] it is wiser to fix the abdominal cavity in toto for subsequent examination should there be any possibility or question as to any ruptured viscera or mesentery. Otherwise, the organs are dissected in a normal manner, as described in any normal pathology textbook. Naturally, samples of liver blood, bile and stomach contents and the usual samples for any medico-legal autopsy are taken at the appropriate time. Should, however, there be a fracture of a limb, of which one feels, as a result of one's examination, it would be advantageous to know its age, one should remove that limb, i.e., the skeletal and muscular attachments thereof, leaving the skin to be reconstructed by the mortuary superintendent/technician, for radiological and histological examination. Whilst one realises that such a technique is radical, one can never be challenged with being negligent in one's approach nor can the fairness of specimens (as retained in England and Wales under the Coroner's Rules 1963) be questioned. Naturally, this technique must be modified for every country in which autopsies are requested by law to be carried out in cases of alleged child abuse. By and large the technique which one does carry out in such cases can prove a guilty case. If there is any doubt, it is the duty of the forensic pathologist, or medico-legist, to give the benefit of the doubt to the accused, remembering that the autopsy room is the Temple of Truth.

REFERENCES

1. Gardner, A. & Carpenter, R. G. (1974) Proc. Francis E. Camps Int. Symp. on Sudden and Unexpected Death in Infancy, Toronto, Canada.
2. Watson, E. (1980) Personal Communication.
3. Shannon, D. C. & Kelly, D. H. (1982) New J. Med., **306**, 1022.
4. Barbey, I. (1978) Bundesgesundheitsbl., **21**, 5.
5. Kendall, S. R. M. & Ferris, J. A. J. (1977) J. For. Sci. Soc., **17**, 223.
6. Mahnke, P. F. (1966) Dtsch. Gesundh. Wochenschr., **21**, 2188.
7. Maresch, W. (1960) Z. Kindesheilk., **84**, 565.
8. Maresch, W. (1961) Schweiz. Rdsch. Med., **32**, 804.
9. Maresch, W. (1962) Wein. Klin. Wochenschr., **74**, 21.
10. Maresch, W. (1968) Dtsch. Ges. Gerichtl. Soziale Medizin, Innsbruck.
11. Valdes-Dapena, M. A. (1977) In: Pathology Annual, part 1. New York: Appleton-Century Crofts.
12. Masshoff, W. (1957) Plötzlicher natürlicher Tod bei Säugling und Kind- in A. Ponsold: Lehrbuch Der gerichtlichen Medizin. Stuttgart: Thieme.
13. Beckwith, J. B. (1969, 1970) Proc. 2nd Int. Conf. on Causes of Sudden Deaths in Infants, Seattle.
14. Froggatt, P. (1969) Proc. 2nd Int. Conf. on Causes of Sudden Death in Infants, Seattle, p. 32.
15. Froggatt, P., Lynas, M. A. & MacKenzie, G. (1971) Br. Med. J., **1**, 612.
16. Althoff, H. (1980) Sudden Infant Death Syndrome (SIDS) Forensic Medical Experience, Research and Conclusions Regarding a General Medical Problem, 2nd edn. Stuttgart: Gustov Fisher Verlag.
17. Cameron, J. M. & Watson, D. (1975) J. Pathol., **117**, 55.
18. Sinclair-Smith, C., Dinsdale, F. & Emery, J. L. (1976) Arch. Dis. Child., **51**, 424.
19. Maeye, R. L., Ladus, B. & Drage, J. S. (1976) Am. J. Dis. Child., **130**, 1207.
20. Bolton, D. P. G., Cross, K. W. & McKettrick, A. C. (1972) Br. Med. J., **4**, 80.
21. Steinschneider, A. (1972) Pediatrics, **50**, 646.
22. Johnson, P. (1974) Proc. Francis E. Camps Int. Symp. on Sudden and Unexpected Death in Infancy, Toronto, Canada, p. 143.
23. Cross, K. W. (1974) Proc. Francis E. Camps Int. Symp. on Sudden and Unexpected Deaths in Infancy, Toronto, Canada, p. 269.
24. Scott, D. J. (1972) Br. Med. J., **2**, 12.
25. Watson, E. (1978) Med. Sci. Law, **18**, 271.
26. Carpenter, R. G., Gardner, A., McWeeny, P. M. & Emery, J. L. (1977) Arch. Dis. Child., **52**, 606.
27. Valman, H. B. (1977) Update, **14**, 11.
28. Müller, G. (1971) Dtsch. Ges. Path., **55**, 537.
29. Müller, G. (1963) Der plötzliche kindstod. Stuttgart: Thieme.
30. McWeeny, P. M. & Emery, J. L. (1975) Arch. Dis. Child., **48**, 835.
31. Protestos, C. D., Carpenter, R. G., McWeeny, P. M. & Emery, J. L. (1975) Arch. Dis. Child., **48**, 835.
32. Baldwin, J. A. & Oliver, J. E. (1975) Br. J. Prev. Soc. Med., **29**, 205.
33. McRae, K. N. & Ferguson, C. A. (1973) Can. Med. Assoc. J., **108**, 859.
34. Roberts, J., Lynch, M. A. & Golding, J. (1980) Br. Med. J., **2**, 102.
35. Frederick, J. (1974) Br. J. Prev. Soc. Med., **28**, 164.
36. Lynch, M. A. (1975) Lancet, **2**, 317.
37. Lynch, M. A. & Roberts, J. (1977) Br. Med. J., **1**, 624.
38. Limerick, S. R. (1977) Midwives Chronicle and Nursing Notes, October.
39. Parkes, C. M. (1972) Bereavement—Studies of Grief in Adult Life. London: Tavistock.
40. Emery, J. L. (1972) Br. Med. J., **1**, 612.
41. Limerick, S. R. & Downham, M. A. P. S. (1978) Br. Med. J., **1**, 1527.
42. Emery, J. L. & Carpenter, R. G. (1974) Proc. Francis E. Camps Int. Symp. on Sudden and Unexpected Death in Infancy, Toronto, Canada.
43. Korbin, J. E. (1980) Child Abuse and Neglect, **4**, 3.
44. Allan, L. J. (1978) In: Martin, J. P. Violence and the Family, ch. 3. Chichester: John Wiley & Sons.
45. McNeese, M. C. & Hebeler, J. R. (1977) Clinical Symp., **29**, 5. NJ: Ciba Pharmaceutical Co.
46. Pinchbeck, I. & Hewitt, M. (1973) Children in English Society, Vol. 2. London: Routledge and Kegan Paul, p. 621.
47. Steele, B. F. (1968) Child's Guardian, September, p. 16.
48. Oppe, T. E. (1968) Address given at Annual Council Meeting, NSPCC.
49. Cameron, J. M. & Rae, L. J. (1975) Atlas of the Battered Child Syndrome. Edinburgh: Churchill Livingstone.
50. Kempe, C. H. (1971) Arch. Dis. Child., **46**, 28.
51. Simpson, C. K. (1965) The Battered Child Syndrome. London: NSPCC.
52. Caffey, J. (1957) Br. J. Radiol., **30**, 225.
53. Altman, D. H. & Smith, R. L. (1960) J. Bone Joint Surg., **42A**, 407.
54. Gwinn, J. L., Lewin, J. W. & Patterson, H. G. Jr. (1961) J. Am. Med. Assoc., **176**, 926.
55. Kempe, C. H., Silverman, F. N., Steele, B. F., Droegmueller, W. & Silver, H. K. (1962) J. Am. Med. Assoc., **181**, 17.
56. Cameron, J. M. (1970) Br. J. Hosp. Med., **4**, 769.
57. Cameron, J. M. (1972) Practitioner, **209**, 302.
58. Cameron, J. M. (1978) In: Smith, S. M., ed. The Maltreatment of Children. Lancaster: MTP Press.
59. Cooper, C. E. (1970) J. Med. Wom. Fed., **52**, 93.
60. Antice, E. (1968) World Med., **4**, 50.
61. Fleming, G. M. (1967) Br. Med. J., **2**, 421.
62. Helfer, R. E. & Kempe, C. H. (1968) The Battered Child. Chicago: University Press.
63. Caffey, J. (1946) Am. J. Roentg., **56**, 163.
64. Gibbens, T. C. N. & Walker, A. (1956) Cruel Parents. London: Institute for Study and Treatment of Delinquency.
65. Cameron, J. M., Johnson, H. R. M. & Camps, F. E. (1966) Med. Sci. Law. **6**, 2.
66. Gill, D. G. (1970) Violence against Children. Harvard: University Press.
67. Gill, D. G. (1971) Violence to Children. J. Marriage Fam., **33**, 639.
68. Giovannoni, J. M. (1971) J. Marriage Fam., **33**, 649.
69. Smith, S. M. (1978) The Maltreatment of Children. Lancaster: MTP Press Ltd.

70. Roberts, J. C. & Hawton, K. (1980) Lancet, 1, 882.
71. Kempe, C. H. (1979) Child Abuse and Neglect, 3, 9.
72. Special Report (1978) United States DHEW Publ. No. (OHDS) 79–30166.
73. Finkelhor, D. (1979) Sexually Victimised (1980) Children. London: Macmillan.
74. Beyley Mrajek, P. M., Lynch, M. A. & Bentovin, A. (1980) In: Beyley Mrajek, P. M. & Kempe, C. H., eds. Sexually Abused Children and their Families. New York: Garland.
75. Bennett, A. N. & Pettybridge, R. (1979) J. R. Soc. Med., 72, 743.
76. Orr, D. P. (1978) Am. J. Dis. Child., 132, 873.
77. Sims, B. G., Grant, J. H. & Cameron, J. M. (1973) Med. Sci. Law, 13, 207.
78. Cameron, J. M. & Sims, B. G. (1973) Forensic Dentistry. Edinburgh: Churchill Livingstone.
79. Cameron, J. M., Grant, J. H. & Ruddick, R. (1973) J. For. Photogr., 2, 9.
80. Ruddick, R. (1974) Med. Biol. Illus., 25, 128.
81. Mushin, A. S. (1971) Br., Med. J., 3, 402.
82. Mushin, A. S. (1975) In: Cameron, J. M. & Rae, L. J., eds. Atlas of the Battered Child Syndrome, ch. 6. Edinburgh: Churchill Livingstone.
83. Mushin, A. S. & Morgan, G. (1971) Ocular injury in the battered baby syndrome. Brit. J. Opthalmol. 55, 353.
84. Kiffney, G. J. Jr. (1964) Arch. Ophthal., 72, 231.
85. Gilkes, M. J. & Mann, T. P. (1967) Lancet, 2, 468.
86. Guthkelch, A. N. (1971) Br. Med. J., 1, 430.
87. Adams, J. H., Graham, D. I. & Genarelli, T. A. (1981) Acta Neuropathol. supp. (Bal) 7, 26.
88. Cameron, J. M. (1972/73) Practitioner, 1, 59.
89. Haller, J. A. Jr. (1966) Clin. Pediatr., 5, 476.
90. Touloukian J. (1968) Paediatrics 42, 642.
91. Skinner, A. E. & Castle, R. L. (1969) 78 Battered Children: A Retrospective Study. London: NSPCC.
92. Court, J. (1970) J. Med. Wom. Fed., 52, 99.
93. Fairburn, A. C. & Hunt, A. C. (1964) Med. Sci. Law, 4, 123.
94. Dawson, D. (1970) Leader. The Scotsman, 19 January.

FURTHER READING

Fontana, V. J., Donovan, D. & Wong, R. J. (1963) N. Engl. J. Med., 269, 1389.
Mrajek, P. M. (1980) J. Child Psychol. Psychiat., 21, 91.

16

Psychiatry and the law

Psychiatry concerns the law in a number of ways, in relation to the compulsory detention of the mentally abnormal in mental hospitals, the psychiatric aspects of crime, criminal responsibility of the mentally abnormal and the imprisonment or medical detention of abnormal offenders. Mental abnormality may affect the validity of contracts, wills and the contract of marriage. Many psychiatrists have little to do with civil contracts apart from quite rare litigation and those dealing with offenders and the Courts are relatively few. Nearly all, however, are concerned with the compulsory detention of the mentally ill or handicapped.

The Mental Health Act of 1959 was a far-sighted measure which looked forward to the time when mental illness would be regarded as similar to physical illness as far as arrangements for treatment are concerned. To a large extent this has come about. The overwhelming majority of psychiatric patients who enter hospital do so voluntarily. Moreover, great progress with drug treatment has had the result that the severely ill have recovered sufficiently in a few weeks to become voluntary patients with the understanding that they are ill and need treatment, so that short-term compulsion and admission for assessment for 28 days is sufficient to restore voluntary status. Compulsory patients have tended to be discharged for out-patient treatment and if necessary voluntarily re-admitted without appeal to the Mental Health Review Tribunal. For some years most referrals to the Mental Health Review Tribunal have been in relation to dangerous mentally abnormal offenders in special hospitals or severely mentally handicapped patients where there is a difference of opinion about their capacity to manage their lives outside these insti-

tutions or be cared for adequately. Meanwhile the number of individuals who have lost their fear of mental disorder and seek at least out-patient treatment for their sufferings has greatly increased until the psychiatric services have become the most expensive section of the National Health Service.

In the course of 30 years the various defects in the Act have naturally emerged, but the most powerful motives for change probably come from two sources. First, the growing realisation that prolonged institutionalisation was psychologically destructive to the personality as well as being very expensive. Shortage of staff as well as the occasionally excessive use of powers given to doctors led to the deterioration below acceptable standards of some institutions for chronic patients. The second motive for change was the 'human rights' movement, a change in social attitudes extending far beyond the problems of psychiatry. The Mental Health (Amendment) Act of 1982 made changes, incorporated in what follows, which increased the rights of detained patients to give or withhold consent for the treatment advised.

The Mental Health Act and the Amendment Act are long and detailed. It is necessary to provide only a summary of their main provisions, sometimes in the words of the Act but often in paraphrase, emphasising the main changes introduced by the Amendment Act.

Since there is still some confusion about the nature and variety of serious mental disorder, a short description may be helpful.

The concept of mental illness can gain from clarification: excluding all those varieties which do not impair the individual's contact with reality, and which are therefore outside the essentially legal

terms of reference of this chapter, there remain:
1. functional psychoses, and
2. structural or organic psychoses.

FUNCTIONAL PSYCHOSES

These include such illnesses as schizophrenia and severe depression whose basis is to be understood in disturbance of function of the brain and central nervous system rather than in structural damage or disease. They represent essentially severe impairments of the patient's contact with and appreciation of reality which are not attributable either to mental defect or to structural degeneration of brain and nervous tissue. All forms of mental illness which exhibit such symptoms of mental disturbance in the absence of such structural immaturity or decay may come under this heading. Their separate description and diagnosis would be out of place in this chapter, and the reader is referred to textbooks of psychiatry for their elucidation.

It remains, however, helpful to have a few concepts of the principal types of symptoms which may be seen in any of the forms of mental illness and these will be given here.

Depression of mood

This is obviously not necessarily a sign of madness, for it may be justified by the patient's life situation. However, it may appear without such apparent external justification, or it may be continued after some external catastrophe such as bereavement, or personal loss, or disaster, to a point where the patient is clearly no longer reacting in a normal way. If such depression cannot be recognised by the patient as without justification and cannot be modified or mitigated by any form of comfort or reasonable reassurance, it strongly suggests mental illness. The importance of this lies in the fact that a depression which involves a divorce of the patient's judgement from reality is more than likely to induce a state of sufficient suffering and hopelessness to lead to suicide.

Exaltation or pathological elation

To be distinguished from sheer excitement, this represents the opposite kind of disorder of mood. Once again, when justified and normally short-lived, it may be clearly separable from any form of mental imbalance. But if not related to the reality of the patient's personal situation, it will again frequently be seen to overthrow judgment and lead to conduct which is manifestly abnormal and due to illness.

Excitement and stupor

These are both essentially disturbances of conduct. We may presume in both cases that there is a corresponding underlying disturbance of mind, but often the patient is inaccessible to discussion or even emotional contact with others, and we can only proceed upon the basis of treating the condition as the patient's behaviour demands, bearing in mind the provisions mentioned above, that any action which is taken must be justified by being required for the safety and well-being of the patient himself, or for the safety and well-being of others. After recovery from excitement or stupor, the patient who was previously inaccessible may say that despite his inability at that time to communicate with others, or to modify his conduct, he was aware of what was going on, and may have been helped by the calmness and confident acceptance of his needs by those who dealt with him during his critical illness.

Delusions, hallucinations and illusions

These may all occur as symptoms of dementia or other psychotic illness. A delusion may be defined as a mistaken belief which has for the patient the force of conviction, and is firmly held despite all evidence to the contrary. A hallucination is a sensory perception which does not correspond to any stimulus from the outside world; whereas an illusion is a sensory perception, which although produced by external stimulus, is misinterpreted by the patient in purely subjective terms.

Examples will make these three descriptive terms clear. If a man believes that he has lost all his money, and is suffering from a fatal illness, despite the production of concrete evidence that he is still solvent, and has no demonstrable physical disease, then he is suffering from delusions. If he hears voices or sees visions which no one else can hear or see, and which are in fact projections of his own fantasy, then he is hallucinated; while if he mistakes his physician or nurse for his father or mother, or for the devil come to take him away, then he is suffering from illusions, which are grafted on to the normal experience of seeing the people whose identity he miscontrues.

All these symptoms will be seen to have in common that severance of the patient's subjective experience from external reality which is characteristic of mental illness. Under the influence of such severance from reality the patient's conduct is naturally disordered, and in this way his mental illness may be made manifest. It remains important to realise that some forms of abnormal behaviour may be the outcome of purely temporary, acute and short-lived confusion or delirium; for example in delirium tremens from the toxic confusional state produced after long addiction to alcohol, or from any of the other acute illnesses which may be accompanied by toxic confusional episodes. These can be regarded as varieties of acute dementia. Dementia is more commonly recognised as the chronic deteriorative outcome of progressive degeneration of brain structure or function. But when seen in its acute and reversible form, it retains the same clinical characteristics, although these are of course telescoped together, so that their individual recognition tends to be obscured. The general clinical characteristics of such states include:
1. clouding of consciousness;
2. failure of recent memory;
3. failure of attention, concentration and judgement.

All these three features tend to produce:
4. disorientation of space and time; to which are added,
5. emotional lability, and finally
6. hallucinations, and misinterpretations of external reality.

From these six spring all the rest: delusions, excitement, panic, disturbance of behaviour, and the entire phenomenon of the frightened and frightening patient who is temporarily out of touch and beyond control. The importance to patient and doctor of an understanding of these matters is of course that adequate and humanely efficient man-agement depends upon professional recognition *that this is part of every doctor's and nurse's job*, not a disgraceful or embarrassing catastrophe for which responsibility can be shelved, or shoved elsewhere. Given such recognition, the outlook for such conditions is usually excellent: the same unfortunately cannot be said for chronic dementia, in the majority of cases.

STRUCTURAL PSYCHOSES

These are exemplified by varieties of chronic dementia. These are forms of mental illness associated with structural damage, disease, or degeneration of brain and nervous tissue. They are usually characterised by the progressive development of the following symptoms:
1. diminution of intellectual performance and capacity, with particular reference to the capacity for attention, concentration and balanced judgement.
2. confusion in the patient's relationship with external reality, particularly in his orientation in time and space.
3. the loss or failure of recent memory, with comparative retention of memory for earlier events in life.
4. blunting or excessive lability of emotional response.
5. comparable blunting or deterioration of behaviour, usually in the direction of apparently grosser, cruder or more primitive habits.

Insight for all these aspects of deterioration may or may not be present in any particular case, but in either event the patient's capacity to convey awareness of such deterioration may itself be impaired by the degenerative process.

PSYCHOPATHIC PERSONALITY

The Mental Health Act was highly original in England (but not in Scotland) in defining this further type of abnormality. The psychiatric section of the International Classification of Diseases (ICD) does not recognise the term, which acquired medical and indeed popular currency in the Second World War when used by the medical services of the forces as a basis for excluding individuals from useful military service. The ICD lists eight varieties of 'pathological personality', referring to marked anomalies or deviations of personality which are not the result of psychosis or any other 'illness', though they consult or are brought to doctors because of a suspicion that they are psychotic or neurotic. They include such varieties as manic depressive, schizoid, obsessional, hysterial, paranoid personalities, etc., relating to forms of psychosis or neurosis. Those with the manic depressive (cyclothymic) variety show wide and sometimes prolonged swings of mood from elation to depression though not to a degree preventing perception of reality or requiring hospitalisation or protection. Many creative geniuses have shown such an extreme of personality, bursts of elated creativeness being followed by perhaps years of depressed lack of 'inspiration', as seen for example in the life of the song writer Hugo Wolf.

The 'psychopathic' personality referred to in the Act is described in the ICD as 'anti social personality'. They offend against society, show a lack of sympathetic feeling, and their behaviour is apparently unmodified by experience or punishment. Emotionally cold and callous, they are so egocentric that they appear incapable of understanding the feelings and motivation of others. They are described in the Act as either 'abnormally aggressive' or 'seriously irresponsible'. Henderson[1] divided them descriptively into three groups—the aggressive, the inadequate and the creative. They may have any level of intelligence. The first is characterised by excessively aggressive behaviour, impulsiveness and callousness. The inadequates include many who, without being overtly aggressive, often respond with a similar degree of hostility but react to life situations by abandoning a job or a wife in an excessive response to mild criticism; others overlap with the 'asthenic' (weak) group of personality disorders, characterised by excessive lack of energy or capacity to cope with normal demands of life but in the anti-social group because of a tendency to exist by petty stealing. Others in the inadequate group overlap with hysterical personality disorder, continually defrauding and lying, but acting the part of a millionaire with such conviction and success that it is doubtful if they are temporarily self-deluded.

Three aspects should be especially noted.

1. Immaturity, shown in many instances in the electroencephalogram which has characteristics in much younger people. Emotionally they behave like young children with impulsiveness and temper trantrums though they frequently 'mature' in later life.

2. The doctor's conviction that they show a pathological state is frequently supported by a definitive previous mental illness. For example, a highly skilled journalist many times in prison for passing bad cheques over which he apparently had no control, had suffered in early life from panic attacks of such severity that he required hospital treatment; but on recovery developed his fraudulent personality. Other inadequate psychopaths sometimes finally drift into overt schizophrenia.

3. All types of personality disorder exist in mild, moderate or severe grades, and psychiatrists are concerned only with the severest who are not in a special category of their own with clear definition.

THE MENTAL HEALTH ACT 1959 AND THE MENTAL HEALTH (AMENDMENT) ACT 1982

Definitions of varieties of mental disorder

The definitions of the variety of mental disorder, and especially the degree of severity which would justify interference with liberty, presents great difficulties. Technical terms are unsuitable for the law since their meaning can change suddenly and produce effects quite contrary to the intentions of Parliament.

The Acts describe four varieties of mental disorder; mental illness, psychopathic disorder, mental handicap and severe mental handicap—and a residual category of 'any other disorder or disability of mind'. The importance of this distinction is that no one can be compulsorily detained in hospital for more than quite short periods without medical evidence that the patient belongs to one of these categories, to which different conditions apply.

Mental illness

This is not itself defined but compulsion is usually

only contemplated when the patient is so ill that he cannot make rational decisions in his own interests.

Psychopathic disorder

This means a persistent disorder or disability of mind (whether or not including significant impairment of intelligence) which results in abnormally aggressive or seriously irresponsible conduct on the part of the patient.

No one can be described as mentally disordered or suffering from any form of mental disorder by reason only of *promiscuity or other immoral conduct, sexual deviancy or dependence on alcohol or drugs.*

Severe mental handicap

This means a state of arrested or incomplete development of mind which includes severe impairment of intelligence and *social functioning.*

Mental handicap

This means a state of arrested or incomplete development of mind (not amounting to severe mental handicap) which includes *significant impairment of intelligence* and *social functioning.*

This inclusion of a criterion of social functioning by the Amendment Act will have the effect of freeing some patients previously regarded as severely subnormal on grounds of intelligence alone from compulsory control, considered previously to be in their interests. It is likely for example that criminal law, which prohibits the severely subnormal from ever having sexual intercourse (surely an unacceptable interference of human rights by modern standards) and anyone having intercourse with them guilty of a serious offence, may come to be modified to allow them to have persistent relationships in hostels, etc., and even at times to marry. The balance between protection and deprivation is delicate and variable.

The Act provides for 3 forms of compulsory admission to hospital.

Procedure for admission

Admission for assessment (Section 25)

Application for admission for assessment may be made in respect of a patient on the grounds that

1. he is suffering from a mental disorder of a nature and degree which warrants the detention of the patient in a hospital for assessment for at least a limited period, and

2. that he ought to be so detained in the interests of his own health or safety or with a view to the protection of other persons.

Application for admission shall be founded upon the written recommendation on the prescribed form of two medical practitioners, including in each case a statement that the conditions set out in (1) and (2) above apply.

The patient admitted for assessment may be detained for a period not exceeding 28 days unless, before the expiration of that period, he has become liable to be detained by virtue of a subsequent application order or direction in any of the following provisions.

The application for admission may be made either by the nearest relative of the patient or by the mental welfare officer, and shall be addressed to the managers of the hospital to which admission is sought and shall specify the qualification of the applicant to make the application. Before or within a reasonable time after an application is made by the mental welfare officer the officer shall take such steps as are practicable to inform the person (if any) appearing to be the nearest relative of the patient that the application is to be or has been made and of the power of the nearest relative under Section 47 of the Act to discharge the patient. (The Amendment Act uses the title of mental welfare officer but provides that within two years of it being enacted the term approved social worker shall be used.)

A patient admitted for assessment may apply to the Mental Health Review Tribunal within 14 days of the day of admission.

Admission for treatment (Section 26)

A patient may be admitted and detained for the period allowed by the following provisions. He may be admitted on the grounds

1. that he is suffering from mental illness, severe mental handicap, psychopathic disorder or mental handicap;

2. a mental disorder of a nature or degree which

makes it appropriate for him to receive medical treatment in hospital;

3. in the case of psychopathic disorder of mental handicap such treatment is likely to alleviate or prevent a deterioration in his condition, and

4. that it is necessary for the health or safety of the patient or for the protection of other persons that he should receive such treatment, and that the treatment cannot be provided unless he is detained under this Section.

The application for admission shall be founded upon the written recommendation on the prescribed form of two medical practitioners, including in each case a statement that in the opinion of the practitioner the conditions set out in paragraphs (1), (2) and (3) above apply and each such recommendation shall include

a. such particulars as may be presented of the grounds for that opinion so far as it relates to the conditions set out in paragraph (1), and

b. specifying whether other methods of dealing with the patient are available and if so why they are not appropriate.

Any recommendation for the purposes of such an application may describe the patient as suffering from more than one of the forms of mental disorder referred to above; but the application shall be of no effect unless the patient is described in each of the recommendations as suffering from the same one of these forms of mental disorder, whether or not he is also described in either of the recommendations as suffering from another of these forms.

If recommendations describe the patient as suffering from only psychopathic disorder or mental handicap, they must state the age of the patient, or if not exactly known must state (if it is the fact) that the patient is under 21. The Mental Health (Amendment) Act 1982 makes changes in the status of the medical practitioners who can sign an application. Of the two medical recommendations one must be made by a practitioner approved for the purpose of the order by the local authority as having special experience in the diagnosis and treatment of mental disorder; the second application may be made by a medical practitioner who, if possible, has had previous acquaintance with the patient. They may both be on the staff of the hospital (but not if the intention is to admit the patient to a bed for private patients) provided one has worked at the hospital for less than half the time which he is bound by contract to devote to work in the Health Service, and, where one is a consultant, the other does not work in the hospital in a grade in which he is under the consultant's direction. A general practitioner employed part-time in the hospital shall not, however, for the purposes of this Section be regarded as a practitioner on its staff. The two practitioners making the recommendation may have examined the patient together or separately; but if separately within five days of one another. No recommendation for admission can be made unless both practitioners have examined the patient in the previous 14 days.

Application for admission for treatment shall not be made by a mental welfare officer if the nearest relative has notified the officer (or the local authority who employs him) that he objects to the application being made and the officer will not make the application except after consultation with the person (if any) appearing to be the nearest relative, unless in the circumstances it appears to the officer that such a consultation is not reasonably practicable or would involve unreasonable delay.

Emergency admission for assessment (Section 29)

In any case of urgent necessity, application for admission for assessment may be made as follows. The mental welfare officer or the nearest relative to the patient can make an application for emergency admission for assessment, including a statement (to be verified by the medical recommendation) that it is urgently necessary for the patient to be admitted and detained under Section 25 and that compliance with the usual procedure for Section 25 would involve unnecessary delay.

For the application to be effective it is sufficient if one medical practitioner, preferably one who has had previous acquaintance with the patient, but conforming to the conditions required for making a recommendation, certifies that it is urgent and necessary for admission and detention for assessment to take place. The order ceases to have effect 72 h after the patient is admitted unless a second recommendation for an assessment order is received by the managers of the hospital.

Practitioners making the application must have examined the patient not more than 24 h previously.

Patients already in hospital

An application of admission and detention of a patient may be made notwithstanding that he is already a patient in hospital not subject to be detained, or in the case of a treatment order, that he is subject to an order for assessment.

If, in such a case, it appears to the medical practitioner in charge of the treatment of the patient (or any medical practitioner on the staff of that hospital nominated by him to act under this subsection) that an application under this part of the act should be made, he may furnish the managers with a report in writing to that effect. The patient then may be detained for a period of 72 h from the receipt of the report.

If the application for the recommendation for an assessment or treatment is found, within 14 days, to be incorrect or defective, it may, with the consent of the managers, be amended by the person who signed it, and it will then be deemed to have the effect originally intended.

If, in the case of a patient who is receiving treatment for mental disorder as an in-patient and is not liable to be detained, it appears to a nurse of the prescribed class that
1. the patient is suffering from mental disorder to such a degree that it is necessary for his health and safety or for the protection of others for him to be immediately restrained from leaving the hospital, and
2. that it is not practicable to secure the immediate attendance of a practitioner for the purpose of making a report (described above), the nurse may record the fact in writing and in that event the patient may be detained in the hospital for a period of 6 h from time of the record.

Reception into guardianship

Application for reception into guardianship may be made in a similar way to recommendations for treatment, but referring to guardianship. Any person or the local authority may be the guardian but an individual must be accepted as suitable by the local health authority. The local authority may refuse to accept the recommendation to become a guardian.

The mentally disordered person received into guardianship is subject to regulations made by the Minister, but in all cases the following powers are conferred:
1. power to require the patient to reside at a place specified by the authority or person named as guardian;
2. power to require the patient to attend at places and times so specified for the purpose of medical treatment, occupation or training;
3. power to require access to the patient to be given, at any place where the patient is residing, to any registered medical practitioner, mental welfare officer or other persons so specified.

Aspects of hospital care

The Amendment Act makes important changes.

Correspondence (Section 37)

1. A postal packet addressed to any person by a patient detained in a hospital under the principal Act or Amendment Act and delivered by the patient for dispatch may be withheld from the Post Office if that person has requested that communications addressed to him by the patient should be withheld; and any such request shall be made by a notice in writing given to the managers, the medical practitioner in charge of the patient's treatment, or the Secretary of State.
2. The postal packet addressed to the patient in a *special hospital* may be withheld from the patient if, in the opinion of a person on the staff appointed for the purpose by the managers, it is necessary to do so in the interests of the safety of the patient or the protection of other persons.

The person appointed for the purpose of (2) may inspect and open any post to see if it should be withheld; this includes power to withhold anything that it contains.
3. The above paragraph does not apply to postal packets sent to the patient by any Minister or member of either House of Parliament, the master or

deputy master or other officer of the Court of Protection, the Parliamentary Commissioner for Administration, the Health Services Commissioners for England and Wales, the Mental Health Tribunal, a health authority or local social services authority, the managers, any legally qualified person who is instructed by the patient, the European Commission of Human Rights or the European Court of Human Rights.

Section 36 of the principal Act and Section 134 of that Act shall cease to have effect.

Where a packet or its contents are withheld the patient shall be informed of his rights under the following sections in 24 h. Such a patient may make oral or written representations to the managers within 14 days of being so informed or, if he is entitled to apply to the Mental Health Review Tribunal, to that tribunal.

The Secretary of State may make regulations with respect to the exercise of the powers conferred by this section.

Visits

A medical officer or other person duly authorised to visit the patient to report upon his condition may visit the patient at any reasonable time, and examine the patient in private. If a medical practitioner he may examine the treatment notes at the hospital, or records relating to the treatment of the patient in *any* hospital.

Reclassification

The responsible medical officer may report to the managers that he has reclassified the patient. When a change from mental illness or severe mental handicap is to psychopathic disorder or mental handicap, the patient must be discharged unless he certifies that further medical treatment in hospital is likely to alleviate or prevent deterioration in the patient's condition. The Mental Health Review Tribunal may reclassify the patient.

Absence without leave

A patient under compulsory treatment may be given leave of absence for a definite period. If absent without leave he may be brought back by a constable or a member of the staff of the hospital in the next 28 days.

When a condition of leave is that he resides in another hospital he may be detained in that hospital. If absent without leave the reference to recovery by the staff of the hospital refers to this hospital and includes the staff of the hospital which allows the condition of leave.

Duration of authority or detection or guardianship

Within two months within the period of six months following the patient's detention for treatment it shall be the duty of a responsible medical officer to examine the patient; and if it appears to him that it is necessary in the interest of the patient's health or safety or for the protection of other persons that the patient should continue to be liable to be detained, he shall furnish the managers of the hospital with a report to that effect on a prescribed form. This will be authority for the patient's detention for one year, when a further examination and report shall be made. If not discharged, subsequent examinations and reports shall be made in successive periods of one year.

The report shall also state the classification of the patient, that it is of a nature and degree which makes it appropriate for him to receive treatment in a hospital; that such treatment is likely to alleviate or prevent the deterioration of his condition; and that such treatment cannot be provided unless he continues to be detained. In the case of mental illness or severe subnormality an alternative to the condition above is that if discharged he is unlikely to be able to care for himself, to obtain the care he needs or to guard himself against serious exploitation. If such report is made the patient shall be informed and he may, within a period for which detention has been renewed, apply to the Mental Health Tribunal.

A patient detained as suffering from psychopathic disorder must be discharged when he reaches the age of 25 unless it is reported that he would be liable to act in a manner dangerous to other persons or to himself. If such a report is made the patient and the nearest relative of the patient shall be informed and the patient and relative may apply to the Mental Health Review Tribunal in the 28 days following the day the patient is 25.

Discharge

An order to discharge may be made, where the patient is liable to be detained in a hospital in pursuance of an application of an admission for assessment or for treatment, by the responsible medical officer, the managers, or by the nearest relative.

An order for discharge shall not be made by the nearest relative except after giving not less than 72 h in writing to the managers of the hospital. If within 72 h of such notice the responsible medical officer furnishes the managers with a report certifying that in his opinion the patient, if discharged, would be likely to act in a manner injurious to other persons or to himself, the order of discharge of the relative will have no effect and no further order for discharge by the relative shall be made for a period of six months following the report. In any case where such a report is made the managers shall cause the nearest relative to be informed and within a period of 28 days the relative so informed may apply to the Mental Health Review Tribunal.

Mentally abnormal offenders

Hospital orders

Where a person is convicted before a Court of Assize or Quarter Sessions of an offence punishable by imprisonment (other than an offence the sentence for which is fixed by law) or is convicted by a Magistrates' Court of an offence punishable on summary conviction with imprisonment and the following conditions are satisfied. The Court is satisfied on the written or oral evidence of two medical practitioners (one of whom is recognised as experienced in the treatment of mental disorder by the local authority):
1. that the offender is suffering from mental illness, psychopathic disorder, mental handicap or severe mental handicap, and
2. that the mental disorder from which the offender is suffering is of a nature and degree which makes it appropriate for him to be detained in a hospital for medical treatment and, in the case of psychopathic disorder or mental handicap that such treatment is likely to alleviate or prevent a deterioration of his condition, the Court may make a hospital order.

Where a person is charged before the Magistrates' Court with an act or omission as an offence and the Court would have power, on convicting him of such offence, to make an order under the above section as a person suffering from mental illness or severe mental handicap, then if the Court is satisfied that the accused did the act, or made the omission charged, the Court may, if it thinks fit, make such an order without convicting him. (This provision, often neglected by counsel or solicitors, is important if after complete recovery the patient subsequently wishes to obtain a visa or emigrate to countries which prohibit those with criminal convictions.)

The Court shall not make a hospital order unless it is satisfied on written or oral evidence that arrangements have been made for the admission of the offender to hospital within a period of 28 days beginning from the date of the order. The evidence required shall be given by the medical practitioner who would be in charge of the offender's treatment or some other person representing the managers of the hospital in question.

Both the medical practitioners must agree that the same one of the disorders is present, whether or not one or both mention the presence of a second disorder as well.

When the order is made the Court may not at the same time also impose a sentence of imprisonment, impose a fine or make a probation order or any other order which the Court has the power to make. A sentence of imprisonment includes any form of detention or committal to an approved school.

In the case of a child or young person brought before the Juvenile Court as in need of care or protection or beyond the control of parents or guardian the Court may make a hospital order under the same provisions above as would apply to such a person who had committed an offence punishable in an adult by imprisonment. The provisions for making an order apply with the necessary modifications. The Court, however, would not make the order unless it is satisfied that the offender's parents or guardian understands what will follow from the order and consents to it being made.

When the Court makes a hospital order in respect of a child or young person it may at the same time commit him to the care of the local authority as a fit person under the Children and Young Persons Act of 1933. When a hospital order is made for an adult, the Court may direct how the offender is to be detained in the subsequent 28 days or less before admission. If, in an emergency, the hospital named cannot receive the offender, the Minister may arrange for him to be admitted to another hospital.

The Court may receive a medical report in writing without proof of the signature or qualifications of the practitioner but may in any case require the practitioner to give oral evidence.

When, in pursuance of the directions of the Court, any such report is tendered in evidence, otherwise than by or on behalf of the accused, then
1. a copy of the report shall be supplied to defending counsel or solicitor, if any;
2. if the offender is not represented, the substance of the report shall be disclosed to the offender or in the case of a child or young person to his parents or guardian.

The accused, or his legal representative, may require the practitioner signing the report to give oral evidence; and evidence to rebut the evidence contained in the report may be called by or on behalf of the accused. The hospital order shall be sufficient authority (Section 63) for a constable or mental welfare officer or a person directed to do so, to take the patient to the hospital within the period of 28 days and for the hospital to receive and detain him.

A patient admitted under a hospital order will be dealt with as if he were admitted under a Part 4 order for compulsory treatment (Section 26) except that
1. the nearest relative cannot exercise his power of discharge, and
2. the special provisions relating to the expiry of the order for psychopathic or mentally handicapped patients at the age of 25 do not apply.

When a hospital order is made an application may be made to the Mental Health Review Tribunal:
1. by the patient within six months of the order or the day he reaches the age of 16, whichever is later;
2. by the nearest relative of the patient within one year of the date of the order, or in any subsequent period of 12 months.

Restriction orders (Section 65)

Where a hospital order is made in respect of an offender by a Court of Assize or Quarter Sessions, and it appears to the Court, having regard to the nature of the offence, the antecedence of the offender, and the risk of his committing a further offence if set at large, that it is necessary for the protection of the public from serious harm so to do, the Court may, subject to the provisions of this section, further order that the offender shall be subject to the special restrictions set out below, either without limit of time or during such period as may be specified in the order.

(The Lord Chief Justice in the Court of Criminal Appeal made a practice direction in 1967 that since it was impossible to decide when a patient would become no longer dangerous, orders of unlimited duration were to be preferred, and this has subsequently followed in most cases. The Amendment Act, however, continues to provide for orders of limited duration. For a practitioner to state that a patient is too dangerous to be discharged after a fixed period is a different decision from a statement that he has become fit for discharge after an indefinite period.) An order may not be made unless at least one of the medical practitioners whose evidence is taken into account has given evidence orally.

The special restrictions are that the provisions of Part 4 for duration, renewal and expiration of authority to detain the patient for treatment do not apply, nor entitlement to apply to the Mental Health Review Tribunal. The power to grant leave of absence, with or without conditions, or transfer the patient, is vested in the Secretary of State and the power of recall from leave may be exercised by him and by the responsible medical officer.

If the restrictions cease or the Secretary of State decides to remove them the patient remains under an ordinary hospital order with appropriate conditions. At any time the Secretary of State may discharge the patient absolutely or conditionally in which case the hospital order is discharged. A patient discharged conditionally may be recalled by warrant to any hospital named in the warrant and for that purpose be taken into custody. A patient conditionally discharged who is subject to restrictions of a limited duration will not be discharged from them unless he returns to hospital.

The Secretary of State may require the attendance of a restricted patient at any place in the interests of justice or for the purposes of any public enquiry. If directed to attend the patient remains in custody.

The Secretary of State may at any time refer the case of a patient to the Mental Health Review Tribunal for their advice. After he has been under restriction for a year the patient may make a request for such a referral. Action on such a request will follow in under two months of it being made. He may make one such request in each subsequent year.

Where a person over the age of 14 is convicted of an offence, punishable by imprisonment by a Magistrates' Court, fulfils all the conditions for making a restriction order, the Court may commit him in custody to the Crown Court. The Crown Court will enquire into the circumstances, and may make a hospital order or a restriction order or deal with the offender in any way which is within the power of the Magistrates' Court.

The magistrates also have power to commit to a Crown Court an offender whose offence appears to them to call for a more severe sentence than they can impose, unless a hospital order is made with restrictions of discharge.

Where an offender is committed under the previous section and the Magistrates' Court is satisfied on written or oral evidence that arrangements have been made for the admission of the offender to hospital in the event of an order being made under this section, the Court may, instead of committing him in custody, by order direct him to be admitted to that hospital, specifying it, to be detained there until the case is disposed of by the Crown Court, and may give directions as it thinks fit for his production at the Crown Court. The evidence required for this section shall be given by the medical practitioner who would be in charge of the offender's treatment or by some other person representing the managers of the hospital in question.

Transfer directions (Section 72)

If in the case of a person serving a sentence of imprisonment the Secretary of State is satisfied by the report of two medical practitioners (complying with the provisions of this section) that:

1. the person is suffering from mental illness, psychopathic disorder, mental handicap or severe mental handicap, and
2. that the mental disorder is of the nature or degree which makes it appropriate for him to be detained in a hospital for medical treatment and (in the case of psychopathic disorder or mental handicap, that such treatment is likely to alleviate or prevent a deterioration of his condition),

the Secretary of State may, having regard to the public's interest and all the circumstances that it is expedient so to do, by warrant direct that that person be remanded to and detained in such hospital (not being a mental nursing home) as may be specified in the direction. The direction under this section shall cease to have effect at the expiration of 14 days from the day it is given.

Section 73. If the court is satisfied that an offender is suffering from mental illness or severe mental handicap of a nature or degree which makes it appropriate for him to be detained in a hospital for medical treatment and that the patient is *in urgent need of such treatment*, transfer orders may be made for persons detained in a prison or remand centre who have not been sentenced to imprisonment, or some other categories (e.g., civil prisoners committed to prison for a limited term by a Court under a writ of attachment, persons detained under the Immigration Act 1971).

Section 74. Where a transfer direction is made in respect of any person the Secretary of State by warrant may impose restrictions on discharge.

Section 75. If before the expiration of the prisoner's sentence, the Secretary of State is notified by the responsible medical officer, any other medical practitioner, or the Mental Health Review Tribunal that the person no longer requires treatment in hospital for mental disorder, the Secretary of State can direct by warrant that he be removed to any other institution to which he could originally have been sent and authorise the Prison Commissioners or managers of an approved school to exercise any power of release on licence or discharge under supervision which they would have possessed. The restrictions will then cease.

Restriction orders in such a transferred case cease at the end of the sentence, and the period will be calculated to end when he would have been discharged if he had lost no remission.

Section 76. When a person transferred during remand has his case disposed of by the Court, the transfer order ceases but the Court may make a hospital order with or without restriction.

If the Secretary of State is notified at any time before the offender is disposed of by the Court that he no longer requires treatment in hospital for mental disorder or that no effective treatment can be given at the hospital to which he has been removed, he may be remitted to the place where he was originally detained and dealt with as if never transferred.

If such a direction is not given and it appears impractical or inappropriate to bring the offender to Court, a hospital order with or without restriction may be made in his absence, provided two medical practitioners have certified that he suffers from mental illness or a severe mental handicap and it is appropriate that he be treated in hospital.

Apart from amendments to the principal Act of which the main ones have been incorporated in the above, the Mental Health (Amendment) Act 1982 makes some valuable new provisions which will relate to a much larger section of the mentally abnormal population than previous provisions.

Remands to hospital

Section 27 of the Amendment Act provides that the Crown Court or Magistrates' Court may remand an accused person to a hospital specified by the Court for a report on his mental condition. An accused person means that:
1. in relation to the Crown Court, the accused is any person arraigned for an offence punishable by imprisonment (other than an offence for which the sentence is fixed by law) and has not yet been sentenced or otherwise dealt with for his offence;
2. in relation to the Magistrates' Court, any person who has been convicted for an offence punishable on summary conviction with imprisonment and any person with such an offence if the Court is satisfied that he did the act or made the omission charge or he has consented to the exercise by the

Court of the powers conferred by this section.

This power can be exercised if:
1. the Court is satisfied on the written or oral evidence of a medical practitioner approved as experienced under Section 26 of the principal Act, that there is reason to suspect that the accused is suffering from mental illness, psychopathic disorder, mental handicap or severe mental handicap; and
2. the Court is of the opinion that it would be impracticable for a report on his mental condition to be made if he were remanded on bail.

The Court shall not remand the accused to a hospital unless satisfied on the written or oral evidence of the medical practitioner who would be responsible for making the report or some other person representing the managers of the hospital that arrangements have been made to admit him to the hospital within seven days of the remand being made; if so satisfied the Court can give direction for his conveyance to, and his detention in, a place of safety. The offender may be further remanded if it appears to the Court on written or oral evidence of the practitioner making the report, that a further remand is necessary for completing the assessment. The Court may make the further remand without requiring the accused to attend Court if he is represented by counsel or solicitor who is given the opportunity to be heard.

The remand or further remand shall not be for more than 28 days at a time or 12 weeks in all; and the Court may end the remand at any time if informed that the practitioner has completed his assessment.

A constable or other person directed by the Court shall convey the accused to the hospital within seven days and the hospital will thereafter detain him in accordance with the provisions.

If the accused absconds from hospital or from conveyance he may be arrested without warrant and taken as soon as practicable before the Court which remanded him, and the Court may terminate the remand and deal with him as if he had not been remanded.

Section 28. A Crown Court may remand an accused person to a hospital specified if satisfied on the written or oral evidence of two medical practitioners (of which one must be approved as experienced) that he is suffering from mental illness of severe mental handicap of a nature or degree which makes it appropriate for him to be detained in hospital for treatment.

The accused person may be in custody awaiting trial or a person who before sentence is in custody in the course of a trial. The Court shall not remand him unless it has written or oral evidence from the medical practitioner who would be in charge of his treatment or some other person representing the managers that arrangements have been made for a hospital to admit him within seven days; pending his admission it may direct that he be taken to a place of safety.

Where a Court has remanded an accused person under this section it may further remand him on the written or oral evidence of the responsible medical officer that a further remand is warranted. The accused shall not be remanded under this section for longer than 28 days at a time or for more than 12 weeks in all, and it may terminate the remand at any time if satisfied on the written or oral evidence of the responsible medical officer:
1. that the accused person no longer requires treatment in hospital for mental disorder, or
2. that no effective treatment for his disorder can be given in the hospital to which he has been remanded.

Interim hospital orders [Section 29 Mental Health (Amendment) Act]

Where an offender has been convicted before the Crown Court or convicted by a Magistrates' Court as in the previous section and the Court is satisfied on the written or oral evidence of two medical practitioners (one approved as experienced) that
1. the offender is suffering from mental illness, psychopathic disorder, mental handicap or severe mental handicap; and
2. that there is reason to suppose that the mental disorder from which the offender is suffering is such that it may be appropriate for a hospital order to be made in his case,
the Court may before making a hospital order or dealing with him in some other way make an *interim hospital order* authorising his admission to a hospital specified and his detention there in accordance with this section.

The order shall not be made unless written or oral evidence is given by the practitioner who

would be in charge of his treatment, or a representative of the managers, that arrangements have been made to admit him within 28 days.

During the interim order a hospital order may be made without the accused being brought to Court, provided he is represented by counsel or solicitors who are given the opportunity of being heard.

The interim order shall be enforced *for such period not exceeding 12 weeks* as the Court may specify but may be renewed for further periods of not more than 28 days at a time, on receipt of written or oral evidence from the responsible medical officer that it is warranted, but shall not *continue in force for more than six months in all.*

Provisions for conveying the accused to hospital and dealing with absconding are similar to those for remands to hospital; as well as acceptance of the practitioner's report and provision for distribution.

Special hospitals

The Minister shall provide such institution as appear to him to be necessary for persons subject to detention under this Act, being persons who, in the opinion of the Minister, require treatment under conditions of special security on account of their dangerous, violent or criminal propensities.

The special hospitals shall be under the control and management of the Minister, who is entitled to acquire land for the purpose of the Act. Any patient who is for the time being liable to be detained under this Act in the special hospital may, on the direction of the Minister, at any time be removed to any other special hospital.

Management of property and affairs of patients

The Lord Chancellor shall from time to time nominate one or more judges of the Supreme Court to act for the purposes of this Act. There shall continue to be an Office of the Supreme Court called the Court of Protection for the protection and management of the property of persons under disability. The functions shall be exercisable by the Lord Chancellor or any nominated judge and also by the Master or Deputy Master of the Court of Protection. The judge may, with respect to the property and affairs of the patient do or secure the doing of all such things as appear to be necessary or expedient for the maintenance and other benefit of the patient and members of the patient's family; for making provision for other persons or purposes for whom or which the patient might be expected to provide if he were not mentally disordered, or otherwise for administering the patient's affairs.

Mental Health Review Tribunals

Where a person is entitled to make an application to the Mental Health Review Tribunal within a certain period, he shall only make one application during this period but may do so again if he withdraws the first application. Where an application is made to the Tribunal it may in any case direct the patient be discharged but shall do so if:

1. he is not then suffering from mental illness, psychopathic disorder, mental handicap or severe mental handicap or any of those forms of disorder of a nature and/or degree which makes it appropriate for him to be detained in hospital for medical treatment, or

2. that it is not necessary for the health or safety of the patient or for the protection of other persons that he should receive such treatment or, in relation to other sections would not be liable to act in a manner dangerous to other persons or himself.

In determining whether to direct the discharge of a patient of a case not falling within paragraphs (1), (2) and (3) above the Tribunal shall have regard

a. to the likelihood of medical treatment alleviating or preventing a deterioration of the patient's condition, and

b. in the case of a patient suffering from mental illness or severe mental handicap, to the likelihood of the patient, if discharged, being able to care for himself, to obtain the care he needs or to guard himself against serious exploitation.

A number of rules governing the Tribunals have been laid down.

Consent to treatment

The Mental Health Amendment Act 1982 makes new provisions which are so complex that the section must be quoted in full.

Section 38

1. Subject to the provisions of this section the consent of a detained patient shall not be required for any medical treatment given to him for his mental disorder if the treatment is given by or under the direction of the responsible medical officer.

2. Subject to subsection (7) below, a patient detained as aforesaid shall not be given any form of treatment to which this subsection applies unless:

a. either the responsible medical officer or a medical practitioner appointed for the purpose of this section by the Secretary of State has certified in writing that the patient is capable of consenting to that form of treatment and has consented to it, or

b. the medical practitioner appointed as aforesaid (not being the responsible medical officer) has certified in writing that the patient is not capable of consenting and has not consented as aforesaid but that the treatment should nevertheless be given.

3. Subject to subsection (4) below, subsection (2) above applies to:

a. a single treatment including any diagnostic procedure involving physical interference;

b. the administration of medicine by any means, and

c. electroconvulsive therapy.

4. Subsection (2) above does not apply to any form of treatment specified for the purposes of this subsection by the Secretary of State; and subject to subsection (7) below no such treatment shall be given to any patient detained under the Act until a medical practitioner appointed for the purpose of the section by the Secretary of State (not being the responsible medical officer) has certified in writing

a. that the patient is capable of consenting to the treatment in question and has consented, and

b. that the treatment should be given.

5. Any certificate given for the purposes of section (2) or (4) shall be in such a form as may be prescribed by the Secretary of State.

6. Where the consent of a patient to any treatment has been given for the purposes of subsection (2) or (4) the patient at any time before the completion of the treatment may withdraw his consent and subject to subsection (7) below those subsections

shall then apply as if the remainder of the treatment were a separate form of treatment.

7. Subsections (2) and (4) shall not apply to any treatment

a. which is immediately necessary to save the patient's life, or

b. which (not being irreversible) is immediately necessary to prevent a serious deterioration of his condition, or

c. which (not being irreversible or hazardous) represents the minimum interference necessary to prevent the patient behaving violently or being a danger to himself or others;

and subsection (6) above shall not preclude the continuation of any treatment pending compliance with subsection (2) or (4) above if the responsible medical officer considers that its discontinuance would cause serious suffering to the patient.

8. For the purposes of subsection (7) above treatment is irreversible if it has unfavourable, irreversible, physical or psychological consequences and hazardous if it entails immediate significant hazard.

The responsible medical officer means the practitioner in charge of the treatment of the patient.

Section 39

1. The Secretary of State shall prepare and from time to time revise a code of practice for the guidance of medical practitioners and members of the other professions concerned in the medical treatment of detained patients.

2. The code shall specify forms of medical treatment in addition to any specified by regulations made for the purposes of Section 38 (4) which in the opinion of the Secretary of State give rise to special concern and should accordingly not be given by any medical practitioner, unless a medical practitioner appointed for the purposes by the Secretary of State has given such a certificate as mentioned in that section.

Before preparing the code the Secretary of State will consult relevant professions and lay a copy before both Houses of Parliament.

Section 40

The medical practitioner appointed by the Secretary of State under this section may visit, interview privately, and examine the treatment notes of any patient detained in a mental nursing home.

Section 41

The Secretary of State shall keep under review the exercise of powers concerned by these Acts and shall make arrangements for the persons authorised by him to interview privately patients detained in hospitals and mental nursing homes and investigate any complaint which such a patient considers has not been satisfactorily dealt with by the managers of the hospital or mental nursing home in which he is detained.

Section 42

The Secretary of State shall establish a special authority to be known as the *Mental Health Act Commission*. He will direct them to appoint medical practitioners for the purposes of Section 38 and 39 above and perform the functions of the Secretary of State unless under Section 41 above. The medical practitioners appointed for the purpose of Section 41 may include members of the Commission.

Section 135

If it appears to a Justice of the Peace, on information on oath laid by a mental welfare officer, that there is reasonable cause to suspect that a person believed to be suffering from mental disorder:

1. has been, or is being, ill-treated, neglected or kept otherwise than under proper control, in any place within the jurisdiction of the justice, or

2. being unable to care for himself, is living alone in any such place,

the justices may issue a warrant authorising any named constable to enter, if need be by force, and remove him to a place of safety.

The patient subsequently may be detained for 72 h. For the execution of the warrant the constable shall be accompanied by a mental welfare officer or a medical practitioner.

Similarly a warrant may be issued if an absconded patient is thought to be in certain premises and admission has been refused or refusal is expected.

Section 136

If a constable finds in a place to which the public have access a person who appears to him to be suffering from mental disorder and to be in immediate need of care or control, the constable may, if he thinks it necessary to do so in the interests of that person or the protection of other persons, remove that person to a place of safety. He may be detained there for not more than 72 h to enable him to be examined by a medical practitioner and interviewed by a mental welfare officer and to make any necessary arrangements for his treatment or care. The use of this section is largely confined to the Metropolitan Police Area and the Durham area. Big cities and London especially attract the vagrant chronic psychotic and in London there is a special responsibility to keep chronic psychotics clear of Parliament, the Palace and Whitehall. David McNaughton was himself an example of the delusional protester. Many hospitals, however, refuse to accept an admission under this section; the police must than take the patient to a police station, make out all the documents, and call a police surgeon to sign an emergency admission for assessment.

MENTAL DISORDER AND RESPONSIBILITY

This may be divided into civil and criminal responsibility. The law presumes that every man is mentally sound until he is proved mentally disordered, but the degree and nature of any disorder which should free a man from a contract, render him incompetent to bear witness or be held responsible for his offences is somewhat variable. Since psychiatric knowledge constantly advances, issues of this sort are likely to be constantly reviewed.

Competency as a witness

The effect of even the most serious mental illnesses, the psychoses, upon different mental functions is extremely variable. The paranoid psychotic may be only deluded about one or two matters, such as his wife's infidelity, while remaining quite competent to carry out complex and skilled pro-fessional tasks; while the first sign of an organic psychosis may be in a failure of memory, attention and habits of personal hygiene, which are not affected in the first case. A psychotic individual is capable of giving valid evidence if in the opinion of the judge, upon the evidence of a medical practitioner, he is considered capable of giving an account of a transaction which happened before his eyes and of understanding the obligation of an oath. Before he is sworn, however, the person of unsound mind may be cross-examined, and witnesses called to prove circumstances which tend to show that he is competent to give evidence; but in the absence of such evidence he may be allowed to give evidence, and it must be left to a Court to measure the value of his testimony. Under any other view quite serious crimes might be openly perpetrated in mental hospitals without the possibility of conviction of an offender.

Marriage and mental disorder

Problems of mental health occur in a number of circumstances in the law relating to marriage. The Matrimonial Causes Act of 1973 consolidated previous acts and laid down an important new principle: 'A petition for divorce may be presented to the Court by either party to a marriage on the ground that the marriage has *broken down irretrievably*'; the former principle of the matrimonial offence, with a guilty and injured party was thereby greatly modified. It also deals with nullity and judicial separation.

Nullity

Any marriage celebrated after 31 July 1971 could be declared void under several circumstances: that the parties were within the prohibited degrees of relationship, that either was under 16, or already married, or was not respectively male and female, had not followed the regulations with regard to a legal marriage, etc. A marriage celebrated after that date is voidable if either party is incapable of consummating it, wilfully refuses to consummate it, or was pregnant or suffering from venereal disease at the time (provided the petitioner did not know this at the time). It is also voidable if either party did not validly consent to it, whether in consequence of duress, mistake, unsoundness of mind or otherwise, or, though capable of giving valid consent, was suffering (whether continuously or intermittently) from mental disorder within the meaning of the Mental Health Act 1959 of such a kind or to such an extent as to be unfitted for marriage. A degree of nullity, however, may not be granted if the respondent satisfies the Court that the petitioner, with knowledge that it was open to him to have the marriage avoided, so conducts himself as to lead the respondent reasonably to believe that he would not seek to do so, or it would be unjust to grant the decree.

In petitioning for divorce, which cannot take place within three years of marriage except in special circumstances of hardship, 'irretrievable breakdown' will only be found provided one or more of five circumstances obtains:
1. that the petitioner finds it intolerable to live with the respondent;
2. that the respondent has behaved in such a way that the petitioner cannot reasonably be expected to live with the respondent; or
3. has deserted the petitioner for a continuous period of at least two years immediately preceding the petition;
4. that the parties have lived apart continuously for two years immediately preceding the petition ('two years separation') and the respondent consents to the divorce; or
5. have lived apart for a continuous period of five years immediately preceding the application.
If granted, a decree nisi will be made and not declared absolute until six months have passed, unless there are special circumstances. The Court must be satisfied that the marriage has broken down irretrievably and may require evidence that attempts at reconcilation have been made.

There are many provisions to take account of misunderstanding, deceptions, or changes of attitude, as well as detailed arrangements for the disposition of property and of the custody of any children. But the many roads that may be taken to obtain a divorce have somewhat reduced the importance of psychiatric evidence. The doctor should note, however, that the Court has ultimate power to order the production of any case notes of treatment which has taken place. With regard to psychiatric evidence about custody and the best interests of the child or step-children of the marriage, living in the home, the Courts have quite rightly been at times severely critical of psychiatric evidence derived from interviewing only one parent with the child, rather than both. A recent decision that psychiatric evidence in this matter is only acceptable with regard to what the doctor directly observes or hears from the child in assessing the child's attitude is understandable in view of the severely biased account which one or other parent may give as the child's history; but this imposes a severe burden upon thorough assessment which traditionally in psychiatry is based upon the history combined with the observed mental state.

The Matrimonial Causes Rules (April 1977) published under the Act provides that in proceedings for nullity on the grounds of incapacity to consummate the marriage the petitioner may apply to the registrar to appoint medical inspectors to examine the parties, with certain limitations in undefended cases. In proceedings for wilful refusal to consummate, either party may apply for medical inspectors to examine both parties and report the result to the Court confidentially. Each party must be supplied with a copy of the report. The Rules also provide that a patient under disability who by reason of mental disorder within the meaning of the Mental Health Act 1959 is incapable of managing and administering his property and affairs may prosecute any matrimonial proceedings by his next friend and defend any such proceedings by a guardian *ad litem*, to be appointed. Children, if necessary, may be separately represented.

Responsibility in ordinary contracts

The validity of ordinary contracts entered into by persons of unsound mind will depend mainly on the circumstances which accompany the act. If there is nothing unreasonable in the conduct of the person of unsound mind and the party with whom he contracts has no knowledge or suspicion of his mental disorder, then the contract will be binding on the person of unsound mind and his representatives.

In *Molton* v. *Camroux* (1849, 4 Exch., 17), the administrator of a deceased person sued the secretary of an insurance office for a sum paid by the deceased as the consideration for two annuities, it being alleged that at the time when the agreement was made the deceased was not of sound mind. It appeared that the negotiation had been conducted by the deceased 'with apparent prudence, sanity, and judgement', although, in fact, the deceased (who died very soon after the business had been arranged) 'was insane both before and after the transaction'.

In the above case it was laid down as a general rule, that when a person of apparently sound intellect enters into an ordinary contract, and the parties cannot be restored to their former condition, the mere fact that one of them was at the time *non compos mentis* is no ground for setting aside the contract.

Every person dealing with a person of unsound mind with knowledge of his incapacity is deemed to perpetrate upon him a fraud which avoids the contract.

Molton v. *Camroux* was followed in *The Imperial Loan Co.* v. *Stone* (1892, IQ.B.D. 599), where a promissory note had been signed by a person of unsound mind as surety. The defence was that the person sued was 'so insane when he signed the note as to be incapable of understanding what he was doing, and that such insanity was known to the plaintiffs'. The case was taken to the Court of Appeal, where it was held that the contracts of a person who is *non compos mentis* may be avoided when there is proof that his condition was known to the other party.

In *York Glass Co.* v. *Jubb* (1925, 25 T.L.R.I), the Court of Appeal held that there is no right to avoid a contract made with a person of unsound mind unless it be proved that the other party either knew that he was of unsound mind or knew such facts about him that the other party must be taken to have been aware that he was of unsound mind.

It is significant that the Judicial Committee of the Privy Council upon at least two occasions since the decision in *The Imperial Loan Co.* v. *Stone* have refused to follow that decision. The two cases referred to are *Daily Telegraph Newspaper Co. Ltd.* v. *McLaughlin* (1904, A.C. 776) and *Molyneux* v. *Natal Land and Colonisation Co. Ltd* (1905, A.C. 555).

Supervening mental disorder does not release a person from his obligations under a contract unless the nature of the mental disorder renders the performance of the contract impossible (*Hall* v. *Warren*, 1804, 9 Vas. 605).

The general law of agency is not invalidated by the mental disorder of one of the parties; and in *Yonge* v. *Toynbee* (1910, I K.B. 215) the Court of Appeal decided that an agency created during mental health will be determined *ipso facto* by the mental disorder of the principal or of the agent. So that where an authority given to an agent has, without his knowledge, been determined by the mental disorder of the principal, and, subsequently to such mental disorder the agent has, in the belief that he was acting on behalf of the principal, made contract with a third person, the agent will be liable in respect of any damage which may be sustained by the third party by reason of the non-existence of the principal's authority.

The mental disorder of a partner does not *of itself* dissolve the partnership, unless the articles of partnership contain a provision to that effect; hence, unless steps be taken for dissolution, the mentally disordered partner continues to be entitled to share the profits and to be liable for the losses of the firm.

Where necessaries are supplied to a person of unsound mind, the law raises an implied obligation to pay a reasonable price therefor, 'provided that the necessaries supplied are suitable to the position in life of the person of unsound mind' (*In re Rhodes*, 44 Ch. D. 94, and Sale of Goods Act 1893).

A husband is liable for necessaries supplied to his wife during his mental disorder inasmuch as the wife's authority to pledge her husband's credit for necessaries is not a mere agency, but springs from the relation of husband and wife, and is not revoked by the fact of the husband's mental disorder (*Drew* v. *Nunn*, 4 Q.B.D. 661).

Torts and mental disorder

To define a tort is difficult and unsatisfactory; a good description is: 'A tort is an infringement of a general right, or right *in rem*'. An alternative definition which may be easier for the layman to comprehend, although less legally formal and precise, is that a tort is a failure to respect the general rights of others, independently of contract.

An examination of the leading English textbooks on the law of torts shows that there has been little authority on the question whether a person of unsound mind is liable for his torts. Lord Esher in *Hanbury* v. *Hanbury* (1892, 8 T.L.R. 559), said that he was 'prepared to lay down as the law of England that whenever a person does an act which is either a criminal or a culpable act, which act, if done by a person with a perfect mind, would make him civilly or criminally responsible to the law, that was an act for which he could be civilly or criminally responsible to the law, *provided the disease of the mind of the person doing the act be not so great as to make him unable to understand the nature and consequence of the act which he is doing'*. In the latest decision on the subject (*Morris* v. *Marsden*, 1952, 1 ALL E.R. 925), when a person suffering from mental disease attacked and injured the plaintiff, the latter recovered damages from him for assault and battery, since he knew the nature and quality of his tortious act even though he did not know that what he was doing was wrong. The McNaghten Rules were held not to apply to this tort in the circumstances. Asking himself the question, 'whether granted that the defendant knew the nature and quality of his act, it is a defence in this action that, owing to mental infirmity, he was incapable of knowing that his act was wrong', Mr Justice Stable said: 'If the basis of liability be that it depends not in the injury to the victim, but on the culpability of the wrongdoer, there is considerable force in the argument that it is; but I have come to the conclusion that knowledge of wrongdoing is an immaterial averment, and that, where there is the capacity to know the nature and quality of the act, that is sufficient although the mind directing the hand that did the wrong was diseased'.

Testamentary capacity

This is discussed under the following headings:
1. A disposing mind.
2. Aphasia and will-making.
3. Delusions and will-making.
4. Eccentricity and will-making.
5. Undue influence and will-making.
6. Suicide and will-making.
7. Wills *in extremis*.

A disposing mind

Questions involving the testamentary capacity of persons arise frequently, and medical evidence is usually required. When the testator disposes of his estate in an abnormal manner, it may be alleged by the relatives that he was wholly incompetent to understand the nature of his act—either from mental disorder, dementia as a result of disease or on the approach of death. The law requires a *disposing mind* in order to render a will valid. The practical test is: did the testator, at the time of executing the will, know the nature and amount of his property and was he able to recognise the just and reasonable claims of others upon him? It has been said truly that the evidence on this matter of the will is of greater value than the opinions of experts or of witnesses who may have seen the testator at other times and in other circumstances. The capacity for making a will does not depend solely upon the testator's mental health or mental disorder, but rather upon the proof of competency or incompetency on the part of the testator at the time when he made the will.

The general test is: was the testator, *at the time of making the will*, labouring under a delusion material to his judgement and decision with regard to the disposal of his property? 'It is essential to the exercise of the power of making a will that the testator shall not be suffering from any disorder of the mind, which would poison the affections, pervert his sense of right, or prevent the exercise of his natural faculties; that no insane delusion shall influence his mind in disposing of his property in such a way as would not have been done if the mind had been sound' (*Banks* v. *Goodfellow*, 1870, L.R.5 Q.B. 549).

A medical man is often asked to witness a will. He should remember that when he signs his name as a witness, he is regarded as testifying to the testator's competency to make a will.

Bodily disease or incapacity does not affect the validity of a will, unless the mind be directly or indirectly disturbed thereby.

In all cases of this kind the law looks exclusively to the actual *effect* of the bodily disease upon *conduct*; and this is a question for the determination of the Court from the evidence of those who attended the deceased, as well as from the evidence of medical experts; but, so far as a disposing mind is concerned, judges look very much more to the actual distribution of the property than to anything else; and, so long as the terms of the will do not seem to inflict any substantial injustice upon any near relatives, it is probable that the will will be upheld.

An attempt to deal with the situation created by the moral incapacity of a testator is made by the Inheritance (Family Provision) Act, 1938, whereby a surviving spouse or other dependent of a testator or testatrix who dies domiciled in England or Wales, may apply to the Court for an order for reasonable provision to be made for his or her maintenance in cases where the deceased by his will has failed to make reasonable provision for the maintenance of the applicant. Many successful ·applications have been made under this statute.

Where the validity of a will is contested on the ground of incapacity, the issue is not whether the testator could have made a will, but whether he had capacity to make the particular will in dispute; and in order to form a proper judgement on this matter, a medical expert intended to be called as a witness should read the instrument before he gives an opinion.

Aphasia and will-making

The fact that certain structural lesions of the brain may affect a patient's powers of communication and comprehension without otherwise impairing his soundness of mind, may be of particular importance in regard to the making of a will.

Aphasia is one of a series of terms used to describe specific failure of communication or comprehension of this nature; aphasia may be subdivided into motor aphasia, which means inability to communicate accurately by speech; and sensory or auditory aphasia, standing for a corresponding inability to comprehend the spoken word. Similarly, agraphia signifies a comparable failure to communicate by writing, and alexia is failure to comprehend by reading. It is important to realise that each of these types of failure of communication or comprehension may occur separately or in combination with others; but that they all have in common a failure of the powers to recognise or reproduce the normal symbols of communication of human thought, without necessarily implying any impairment of the underlying thought processes themselves. A patient suffering from any

form of aphasia, agraphia, alexia or similar disability, may therefore possess a perfectly sound disposing mind, but be incapable of communicating his wishes through the normal channels of speech or writing. Equally, although capable of understanding his obligations to others, he may not be able to comprehend written instructions or spoken advice as to how he should carry them out.

In general these specific disturbances of a patient's powers of communication or comprehension can be correlated with some accuracy with lesions in various parts of his brain. These are of no importance in the present context, except in so far as recognition of the essentially localised basis of this particular form of mental disturbance will prevent the avoidable error of confusing such disability with incapacitating mental disorder.

When a will has been written by a testator in his own handwriting (holograph wills), the only points which need be considered are:

1. Is the document written in such a manner as to be legible and capable of clear construction?
2. Does it express the wishes of the testator without doubt or ambiguity?
3. Was the testator suffering from any ·material delusion of the kind considered in the preceding section?

The fact that the will has been written legibly and clearly, and appears to be sensible and free from delusion, excludes the possibility of agraphia and renders irrelevant the possibility of aphasia. But where the will is more or less formally written by others and then submitted to the testator to read and to sign, or is read over to him aloud before signature, difficulties in connection with the possibility of aphasia or agraphia are clearly material. In such cases it is necessary to explore carefully ways of getting into communication with the patient which are reliable; and where such ways can be found, the patient's capacity to make use of them in a reasonable manner can be accepted as evidence of a disposing mind.

An example is provided by the case of a man suffering from disease affecting the brain which rendered him unable to write and only able with difficulty to understand what was said. This man was able by gestures to make it clear that he wished to make a will. ·He would read and could understand what was written. The doctor in attendance had the name of possible legatees written each on a separate card, and the main items of the testator's estate also written, each on a separate card; the patient was then able to put a name and piece of property together by means of these cards. Probate in the sense of these terms was in fact granted.

Delusions and will-making

A dispute may arise about the validity of a will executed by a person suffering from delusions. The mere existence of a delusion in the mind of a person does not of itself necessarily vitiate a will, unless conclusive evidence be given that, at the time of executing the will, the testator's mind was influenced by the delusion in making the will (*Banks* v. *Goodfellow*, 1870, L.R. 5 Q.B. 549).

Although a will may be manifestly unjust to the surviving relatives of a testator, and it may indicate that the testator held extraordinary views, it will not necessarily be void unless the testamentary dispositions clearly indicate that the testator's mind was affected by his *delusions*.

Delusions may co-exist with testamentary capacity: so that, if the testator comprehends the extent of the property to be disposed of, and the nature of the claims of those whom he excludes, mental illness not affecting the general faculties, nor operating in regard to testamentary disposition, is insufficient to render him incapable of making a will (*Pilkington* v. *Gray*, 1899, A.C. 401).

Eccentricity and will-making

Whereas the will of an eccentric man would probably be such a will as might have been expected from him, the will of a person who is suffering from delusions is different from that which could have been expected had he not been deluded. While it is admittedly sometimes difficult to define precisely the distinction between eccentricity and mental disorder, or to draw the exact line between mental health and mental disorder, it is normally possible to determine in a particular instance whether a man is mentally healthy or mentally disordered or merely eccentric.

Sane childless women who live solitary or secluded lives are often very fond of animals. One old lady used to keep her sitting-room full of mon-

keys, to the great annoyance of her visitors. She was a woman of shrewd and strong mind, well able to look after her affairs and to dispose of her property. She was considered to be eccentric, but there was no indication of insanity. Other women are only happy when surrounded by parrots, or when their sitting-rooms are converted into aviaries for all kinds of birds. In one case, a woman whose mental health was disputed, was very fond of cats, for which she provided meals at regular hours, complete with plates and napkins. In that case mental disorder was established, not so much on the ground of the special attention which she had given to the cats, as from her acts in regard to her property, and from the history of her association with certain persons who took advantage of her mental weakness. It remains true that eccentricity is in no way necessarily incompatible with testamentary capacity.

From the judgement delivered in *Smith* v. *Tebbitt* (1870, L.R.1 P. & D. 398) it appears that to the legal mind, the question of 'insanity' is a mixed one, partly within the range of common observation and partly within the range of special experience; and it is the duty of the Court to inform itself of the general results of medical observation. A medical expert may give an opinion as to whether the acts of an eccentric testator are evidence of delusions. He may also be able to say, from a consideration of the previous habits and manner of life of the testator, whether at or before the making of the will there has been any change of habits or character which would indicate mental disorder such as the existence of an unaccountable hatred of members of the family who are not mentioned in the will, and a suspicion and distrust of all around him. Cruelty to children, unnatural conduct towards a wife, and the keeping and feeding of animals as pets, are matters which are finally considered in relation to testamentary capacity by a learned judge who is bound to assess them in the light of his own views and opinions, as well as the medical evidence.

Undue influence in will-making

'Undue influence' is frequently alleged as a ground for having a will set aside. The exercise of undue influence by one person over a testator, in order to procure a will in favour of himself or of some third person, renders the will invalid. What amounts to undue influence depends upon the circumstances of each particular case.

In order to set aside a will on this ground, it must be shown that the circumstances in which the will was executed are inconsistent with any hypothesis other than of undue influence. The exercise of undue influence must be proved to have been exercised in relation to the will itself, and not merely to other transactions (*Boyse* v. *Rossborough*, 1857, 6 H.L.C 2).

'Undue influence' is possible as a rule only when the testator is below the average mentally; for example, when he is suffering from incipient dementia, such as often accompanies old age. In such cases, however, it frequently happens that someone (daughter, second wife, niece or stranger) takes special care in looking after the testator, and when the devoted nurse benefits under the will, disappointed relatives sometimes raise the question of undue influence. In these cases, if a medical man is present when a will is executed, he may easily satisfy himself as to the state of mind of a testator, by requiring him to state from memory the manner in which he has disposed of the bulk of his property.

A person may resort to honest intercession and persuasion quite properly in order to procure a will in favour of himself; but persuasion brought to bear upon a testator who is on his deathbed, or in a weak state of health, may be equivalent to force inspiring fear, e.g., if such persuasion amounts to importunity which the testator is too weak to resist, and which renders the making of the will no longer the offspring of his own volition (*Wingrove* v. *Wingrove*, 1885, 11 P.D. 81).

If a medical man be disinterested, he may be of great service in the case of a disputed will; but when a medical man takes a direct benefit under the will, the Court will inquire very closely into all the circumstances connected with the drawing up and execution of the will. The Court may set aside such a will on the ground of undue influence, in as much as the position of a medical attendant is very similar to that of a trusted friend, nurse or adviser.

If a medical man expects to benefit under the will

of a patient with whom he is on familiar terms, he should take the greatest care to secure the intervention of a professional lawyer, with a view to placing his own position above suspicion.

If a beneficiary under a will, or his or her spouse, signs his or her name as a witness to the will, the gift to such beneficiary will be void (Wills Act 1837, s. 15).

Suicide and will-making

The act of suicide is not accepted as conclusive proof of mental disorder even where the testator took his life shortly after the execution of his will. A testator committed suicide three days after having given instructions for his will; but, in the absence of other evidence of mental disorder, the will was pronounced valid. In *Edwards* v. *Edwards*, the testator committed suicide three days after the execution of his will, and there was some evidence of eccentric habits; the will was pronounced to be valid.

Wills in extremis

Where a person whose mental capacity during life has never been doubted makes a will while lying at the point of death (*in extremis*), such will may be regarded with suspicion; and may be set aside if there is medical evidence that the testator had not a disposing mind at the time of the execution of the will. Many diseases, particularly those which affect the brain or nervous system directly or indirectly, produce a dullness or confusion of intellect which may deprive the patient of his testamentary capacity.

A will was set aside because it was executed by the testatrix while she was suffering from an attack of cholera, and proper means had not been taken to test her capacity. At the time of the execution of the will the testatrix was reduced to such an extreme state of weakness that her mental powers were impaired. The validity of another will was contested on the ground that the testator was at the time of execution suffering from gastritis. The will was witnessed by the medical attendant and by the solicitor, both of whom deposed to the competency of the testator, i.e., that the disease had not reached that point where the brain was affected or the mind disturbed. In all cases of this nature *integritas mentis non corporis sanitas exigenda est.*

A will executed by a dying person during delirium would be pronounced invalid. On the other hand, on some occasions, when the mind has been weakened by disease or infirmity from age, it has suddenly become clear before death; and the person has unexpectedly shown a disposing capacity.

Where a testator made his will when on his deathbed, his medical attendant took his instructions, and shortly afterwards a solicitor drew the will in accordance therewith. The medical attendant and the solicitor attested the will, but it was alleged that, although he was conscious when instructions were given, the testator was unconscious when the will was executed. The solicitor thought that he was quite unconscious at the time of execution. The physician and the nurse thought that he was conscious.

The law requires not only that a man should be conscious at the time of execution of the will, but that he should have a sound and disposing mind. The party propounding the will is bound to establish this; and, where he fails to do so, the will must be declared invalid. It would appear from the evidence in the above case that the will was signed *within 10 min* of the time at which the testator was known to have lost consciousness. His property was bequeathed to a stranger. At the time of executing the will the deceased said nothing, did nothing, and made no movement to indicate that he was aware of what he was doing.

A relative of the husband of a dying woman (who was aged 76) took instructions from her for her will which was drawn in his favour. The medical man gave evidence that the deceased had died from apoplexy, and that at the time of executing the will she was so exhausted by illness and by the near approach of death as to be incompetent. On the day of the execution of the will, the deceased retained in some measure her consciousness; it was very doubtful whether she had sufficient capacity to make a will. No other person was present when the instructions were given, and the husband's relative did not even take the precaution of reading the will over in the presence of the witnesses. Even if the deceased had full possession of her faculties at the time, there was some doubt whether she was fully aware of the contents of the will when she signed it. The relative of the husband failed to satisfy the Court that the deceased knew and approved the contents of the will, and the Court therefore pronounced against it.

Whenever possible, care should be taken to make certain that the testator is able to state the provisions of the will, and to repeat them substantially from memory.

If the testator, at the time of giving instructions to a solicitor to prepare his will, is competent to make a will, it will be valid although *at the time of execution* he may be too ill to understand the contents thereof, provided that he is conscious of having given the instructions and believes that the will has been prepared in accordance with them (*Thomas* v. *Jones*, 1928, 139 L.T. 214).

CRIMINAL RESPONSIBILITY IN MENTAL DISORDER

There are several ways in which a mentally disordered offender may be found to be irresponsible (i.e., not liable to punishment) or only partially responsible for his offence.

1. The oldest procedure, under the Criminal Lunatics Act of 1800, is that the offender should be found 'unfit to plead' or 'insane on arraignment', nowadays referred to as 'under disability'. In the words of Sir Norwood East a prisoner 'is unfit to plead to an indictment when he suffers from such disease of the mind as prevents him from challenging a juror, from understanding the nature of the proceedings in Court, from distinguishing between a plea of guilty and not guilty, from examining witnesses or instructing counsel on his behalf or otherwise making a proper defence or from following the evidence intelligently'. This is still subsumed in the legal description that the offender is 'under disability' in conducting his defence. If found unfit to plead or under disability the offender is detained indefinitely during Her Majesty's pleasure. The issue can be raised by the offender, his defence, prosecution or the judge. In practice, the prison doctor and a second psychiatrist for the prosecution and a psychiatrist appointed by the

defence interview the prisoner and all agree that he is too ill to be tried according to East's criteria and often that it would be scandalous to bring him to Court.

The plea is unsatisfactory since no proof that the offender committed the crime is necessary, though this has been partially remedied by allowing the plea to be raised at the completion of evidence for the prosecution. The importance of the proof of guilt was demonstrated in a recent case in which a chronic psychotic patient in a mental hospital was accused of murdering another patient. Preparations were made to regard him as under disability, until it emerged that he could not have been involved in the offence. Even more dramatically, a Zulu woman, a qualified barrister, had suffered from paranoid schizophrenia for many years but had eked out a simple existence in a rooming house. When a neighbour insisted on having noisy late night parties, she broke a panel in his door and threatened him with a knife. She insisted on going for trial, dismissed two groups of counsel for the defence and insisted on conducting her own defence, rebuking the judge when he tried to help her. She examined the chief witness with such vigour that he nearly fainted in the dock and virtually withdrew his evidence. The jury acquitted her.

The most awkward cases concern calm, intelligent, apparently rational psychotics who dismiss defence counsel repeatedly because they will not defend them on the basis that their delusions are true. They insist on conducting their own defence and a doctor giving evidence that they are unfit to plead may be examined by them in Court as to why he thinks the delusions are not true.

In the case of Podola, he shot two policeman during a robbery and was later knocked out when police burst into his room. He claimed to have a total amnesia of all that had happened before and so claimed that he was unfit to plead and to defend himself. He was nevertheless convicted. On appeal it was decided that since it had always been legal to convict a man who is unable to trace an important witness for his defence, it was legal to convict a man who had lost the witness of his own memory.

Deaf mutes or mutes or those with severe mental handicap may sometimes be found to be unfit to plead. Mute defendants are traditionally divided

into those 'mute by malice' (i.e., unco-operative) and those mute by the grace of God (i.e. genuine cases). The latter may be found unfit to plead.

2. *The MacNaghten rules.* For many years the most frequent (and most satisfactory because it provided a full trial) method of dealing with abnormal offences entailed the use of the MacNaghten Rules. These rest upon the answers of the judges consulted by the House of Lords in 1843 after the murder of Mr Edward Drummond, private secretary to Sir Robert Peel. Drummond was shot dead by McNaghten, who was suffering from delusions of persecution and who killed Drummond in mistake for Sir Robert Peel himself. McNaghten was tried and after evidence about his delusions had been heard was acquitted on grounds of insanity on the judges' direction. The public reaction to this acquittal was most unfavourable probably because it had political overtones—McNaghten's delusion was that 'the Tories in his native city of Glasgow made him do it'—and eventually led to a debate in the House of Lords when a number of questions were put to its judicial members with regard to what was (not what should be) the law. They were not unanimous and some of the answers have been allowed to lapse in force, notably their views on 'partial delusions', which meant a delusion apparently unrelated to the crime which they felt should not excuse it. It has been generally accepted that psychosis affects the whole mind and not merely areas of the mind, though this may seem contrary to the rule about the ability of the psychotic to be a valid witness of a crime.

Essentially the rules provide that in order to establish a *defence* on the grounds of insanity, it must be clearly proved 'that at the time of committing the act (or making the omission) the accused was labouring under such a defect of reason from disease of the mind as not to know the nature and quality of the act he was doing, or if he knew what he was doing, that he did not know it was wrong'. It was soon established that 'nature and quality' referred to the physical nature of the act; in an example often quoted, that a man knew he was cutting somebody's throat and was not under the impression that he was slicing a loaf (a confusion only possible in a state of delirium). But whether 'wrong' meant morally wrong or merely that it was illegal was carefully left undecided until as late as 1956 when Lord Goddard CJ ruled on appeal that it meant only illegal; and everyone may be presumed to know that, even though like many insane murderers they believed they were carrying out the instructions of God, which supplant those of the law of man.

The Rules have always been very unpopular with doctors, and indeed many judges, mainly on the grounds, in the words of Lord Bramwell, 'no one is hardly ever mad enough to satisfy them' if looked at logically. Their practical effect was to enable the judge to decide the question of irresponsibility because, if he did not accept the defence's view, he could nearly always ask questions to show that it was untenable. The main criticism is that it makes no allowance for the fact that the essential disorder in psychosis is usually one of emotion and impulse rather than of reason or knowledge.

Nowadays they are only invoked in about half a dozen cases a year, while many hundreds of psychotic offenders are dealt with justly and compassionately by other methods. Following the abolition of the death penalty they are no longer a vital defence in murder trials, and since it is a defence which must be raised with the offender's consent and makes him eligible for indefinite detention instead of a (probably) quite short sentence if convicted of the crime, few can be persuaded to make such a choice.

The existence of the Rules, however, exercises a powerful and in many respects necessary, influence on the criminal law. The Rules do not seek to define sanity but rather the degree and practical effects of any mental disorder on the behaviour of the accused. The decision is for the jury of laymen, with (or if necessary without) medical evidence, as in other criminal trials.

It can be argued that anyone, whatever his mental state, who breaks the law in any serious degree should be answerable to a Court of law for his actions even though the Court should take just and appropriate action as a result. If there were no test or criterion of irresponsibility in law, it would be open to any offender who felt, with or without any real justification, that he had not been responsible for his actions, to argue his case before a jury of laymen. The number of cases contested in the higher Courts might reach quite unmanageable proportions and justice come to depend mainly on the eloquence of defending counsel or doctors.

Even if it accepted that there must be some test or criterion of criminal responsibility, its form is still a controversial matter. The doctor is competent to describe the nature and degree of mental disorder, but not to answer the questions implied in the McNaghten Rules. In practice, the majority of insane offenders are dealt with quite simply, and by the lower Courts, without overt reference to criminal responsibility. On the evidence of two doctors, as we have seen, a mentally ill offender who is in need of hospital treatment can be committed to hospital by the Magistrates under Section 60 of the Mental Health Act of 1959. When they have refused to do so in strongly supported cases, the Appeal Court has tended to uphold the views of the doctors. If magistrates are reluctant to agree for fear that hospital admission will not protect the public sufficiently because the patient may abscond or be released too early, they may remit the case to a higher Court, which has power to add an order under Section 65 restricting discharge for a definite or indefinite period until the Home Secretary is satisfied that there is no further risk. The existence of a lack of criminal responsibility is implied, however, in the provision that those offenders (only) who are mentally ill or severely subnormal may be committed to hospital under Section 60 *without recording a conviction* if the magistrates so decide. Application for such a decision is often omitted by those defending, although it may have important consequences for the accused if, for example, he wishes to emigrate when recovered. The wide use of this convenient procedure of making a hospital order might not have occurred if the legal barriers presented by the McNaghten Rules had not continued to exist in some form.

The Homicide Act of 1957, introduced while the death penalty was still in existence, provided a welcome relief from the rigours of the McNaghten rules. It provides (Section 2) that where a person kills or is a party to the killing of another, he shall not be convicted of murder if he was suffering from such abnormality of mind (whether arising from a condition of arrested or retarded development or any inherent causes, or induced by disease or injury) as substantially to impair his mental responsibility for his acts and omissions in doing or being party to the killing. In practice the decision whether impairment was 'substantial' has usually been left to the jury without explanation or persuasion by the judge. If the offender is found to have diminished responsibility in this way, he is convicted of manslaughter rather than murder, is then not eligible for the death penalty, but eligible as now for any form of sentence from probation to life imprisonment or committal to hospital under the Mental Health Act. Since the abolition of the death penalty it has less importance but it still can be conveniently used in murder trials as a defence in preference to the complexities of the McNaghten rules even when they could apply.

It is convenient to mention here that in relation to the last paragraph the Committee on Mentally Abnormal Offenders (Butler Committee) recommended that murder should no longer carry a statutory life sentence, but that all the sentences should be available at the judge's discretion except absolute discharge. If accepted, this might render the Homicide Act redundant.

CRIMINAL RESPONSIBILITY IN AUTOMATISM

To be convicted of any of the great bulk of criminal offences within the common law two conditions have to be proved: that the offender committed the act (*actus reus*) and also that he had a 'guilty mind', having criminal intent or awareness of acting illegally. The McNaghten Rules refer to defective reason due to disease of the mind but there are a number of disorders in which a criminal act may be carried out while in a state of absent or clouded consciousness in which the offender is not aware or fully aware of what he is doing, and is entitled to be acquitted. They include such conditions such as epileptic automatism, in which after an epileptic fit a man may carry out a series of acts while still quite unconscious. The variety called temporal lobe epilepsy is particularly likely to cause disturbed sensations and sounds, and to give rise to automatic behaviour. Other conditions such as unconsciousness due to head injury or arteriosclerosis of the brain (hardening of the arteries), hypoglycemia (low blood sugar) in diabetes due to overdosage with insulin or a normal dose of insulin

not followed by an expected meal, or sleep walking may lead to non-insane automatism. The Butler Committee gave as an example a motorist who owing to an uncontrollable fit of sneezing fatally injured a pedestrian.

An offender found not guilty by reason of insanity under the McNaghten Rules is liable to indefinite detention in a mental hospital, but this is manifestly absurd in the case of a sane and law-abiding citizen such as the motorist mentioned above. Nevertheless the object of the criminal law is to protect the public and where, as in cerebral arteriosclerosis the offender is not mentally ill before and after the offence but suffers from a progressive condition or one liable to recur, absolute acquittal is clearly inappropriate. The problem of legal differentiation of such circumstances is not altogether resolved.

The case of Bratty (*R. v. Bratty*, 1961, 3 ALL E.R. 523) established the general principle for a decade. Bratty murdered a girl in a state of what the defence claimed was automatism due to psychomotor epilepsy. The evidence was unconvincing, the judge withdrew the plea of automatism from the jury, and Bratty was convicted of murder. The Appeal Court upheld the conviction, but on appeal to the House of Lords, which also upheld the conviction, Lord Denning extensively reviewed the law. He observed, 'It seems to me that any mental disorder which has manifested itself in violence and is prone to recur is a disease of the mind. At any rate it is the sort of disease for which a person should be detained in hospital rather than given an unqualified acquittal'. Nevertheless he drew a distinction between 'non-insane' and insane automatism. The procedure in several cases since this appeal is that if a plea of non-insane automatism is raised, and the medical evidence is consistent, thorough and impressive, the judge will decide to give the jury the discretion to acquit absolutely or to convict. If he does not so rule, the McNaghten Rules will be invoked by the defence's claim. The judgement also made it clear that when the plea of automatism is raised the prosecution has the onus of disproving it. In the case of Sell, who offered the unsuccessful and somewhat forlorn defence that he obtained money by false pretences on several occasions in a state of epileptic automatism, the Appeal

Court quashed the conviction on five counts on the basis of misdirection by the judge as to the burden of proof, though they upheld the conviction on one count (*R*. v. *Sell*, 1962, Cr. L.R. 463).

The problem still remains that nearly all the undoubted causes of non-insane automatism must be regarded as being 'prone to recur', though it is extremely unlikely that a similar set of circumstances will recur with a similar result. In the case of Quick (*R*. v. *Quick*, 1973, 1 Q.B. 910), involving a nurse who assaulted a patient in a hypoglycaemic state of automatism, it was established that non-insane automatism could lead to an acquittal, not withstanding that it is 'prone to recur'. The defence of automatism is perhaps most often raised in relation to motoring offences when a driver falls asleep through fatigue, or the effects of antihistamines for hayfever, or under the influence of carbon monoxide poisoning from a leaky exhaust; but the circumstances are different, for motoring offences are not common law offences, but statutory offences of absolute prohibition, requiring no *mens rea*. As long as one is driving, one is responsible for all that happens in general and the usual judgement is that a motorist who feels fatigue or dizziness coming on should immediately stop. If unconsciousness is sudden and has never occurred before, as in some cases of epilepsy, the accused might claim to be 'not driving', but otherwise he will be convicted, apart from some exceptions such as the sneezing motorist or the motorcyclist who swerves and strikes a pedestrian when stung by a bee which got under his helmet.

RESPONSIBILITY WHEN INTOXICATED BY DRINK OR DRUGS

Acute intoxication with alcohol is not to be equated with insanity. Chronic alcoholism may lead ultimately to transitory acute psychoses such as delirium tremens, or alcoholic hallucinosis; in such cases the McNaghten Rules apply. But in the case of Beard (*DPP* v. *Beard*, 1920, A.C. 479), who murdered a girl in the course of rape when severely intoxicated, the prosecution was first quashed on the basis that the McNaghten Rules should not have been applied, but was re-instated by the House of Lords, who stated the principle that the charge could only be reduced to manslaughter if the accused has been so drunk as to have been incapable of forming the necessary criminal intent, which clearly had not been the case in this instance. In all other cases a man is held at least partly responsible for what he does when drunk.

People accused of rape are unlikely nowadays to succeed by claiming incapacity to form the necessary intent, for they would then probably be physically incapable of rape. But they may claim to have believed, in their intoxicated state, that the woman was consenting. The Sexual Offences (Amendment) Act of 1975 which followed the recommendations of the Heilbron Committee on the Law of Rape, defined rape for the first time as sexual intercourse with a woman who does not consent, knowing that she was not consenting or being reckless as to whether she consented or not. The latter circumstances would apply usually to those who are intoxicated.

In the case of intoxication with other drugs, the same principles apply; murder may be reduced to manslaughter if, for example, a hallucinatory drug such as LSD so affects the individual that he is incapable of forming the intent. There is a difficulty, however, that whereas most people know the effects of drink, people increasingly take unknown tablets or especially mixture of tablets, given to them with an explanation that it will make them feel good. Occasionally they induce a state of mind, especially the illusion that they are being threatened, which leads to murder or other serious violence. Presumably the principle applies that they are not entitled to acquittal because they did not apply reasonable precautions as to the possible consequences, although they could not have known them. Lipman, for example, an American citizen visiting London, was familiar with the use of LSD (a hallucinatory drug) (*R*. v. *Lipman*). One day someone gave him in addition a large and different tablet saying it was particularly effective. It was possibly one of the new hallucinogens STP or some allied drug. After taking half and giving half to his girlfriend he became hallucinated, went up into the stratosphere, saw the world miles below, then descended to the bowels of the earth where he felt terrified at being attacked by writhing snakes which he fought off. After some hours sleep he awoke to find the girl dead beside him, asphyxiated by sheets stuffed in her mouth, and her skull fractured probably by a broken tumbler which was nearby. He was not regarded as totally reasonable ble but guilty of manslaughter and sentenced to three years imprisonment and ordered to be subsequently deported—a sentence which one may think entirely just. Offences of a similar kind are increasing. Moreover, chronic alcoholism may produce permanent disturbances in the blood sugar metabolism so that even in an unintoxicated state the alcoholic may have a level of blood sugar so low that in most people it would lead to a feeling of faintness. The effects of subsequent drinking are very difficult to calculate. The Courts have many times shown themselves remarkably adaptable to these new situations since the range of sentences available on conviction of manslaughter is so wide. But the issue becomes very difficult if a person quite properly is prescribed a drug by his doctor without forewarning that it should not be taken with alcohol or some other drugs. The Butler Committee paid special attention to this dilemma which is occurring with greater frequency nowadays.

FUTURE TRENDS

The Butler Committee on Abnormal Offenders made several recommendations with regard to murder and other crimes of violence. They suggested a new test to replace the MacNaghten Rules, that those found 'not guilty on evidence of mental disorder' should be triable in the Magistrates' Courts when mentally ill or with severe mental handicap and awarded a Section 60 hospital order in appropriate cases. Like many others they suggested that the fixed term of life imprisonment for murder should be abolished, allowing the judge to pass any sentence, or that the differentiation between murder and manslaughter should be abolished, making one crime of homicide, with the same effect. The crime of infanticide, they suggested, should be abolished since the law of diminished responsibility for murder covered the situation.

The recent report of the Criminal Law Revision Committee on offences against the person does not adopt any of these suggestions and in particular recommends that infanticide should continue as a special offence, since it is more flexible than murder with diminished responsibility. The Committee makes one recommendation of great interest to doctors—that it should be possible to combine the defences of provocation *and* diminished responsibility on the grounds of mental disorder. Provocation at present applies only to a normal or reasonable man who is so provoked by word or deed that he is unable to control his violent impulses, and any mental abnormality reducing responsibility must be 'substantial' and sufficient defence on its own. But there are fairly frequent cases which cannot be successfully or justly defended on either ground—e.g., a homosexual excessively taunted by his lover in a way which would reduce the responsibility if the pair were heterosexual. Homosexuality in itself is not a mental abnormality in law.

None of these changes has so far been enacted.

MEDICAL EVIDENCE TO COURTS

The doctor who assists a Court, whether in written reports or in oral evidence, has to remember that a trial, especially a criminal trial, is a highly technical process, though this is not apparent from the non-technical language used. When examining a patient in his consulting room a doctor expects him to answer the strangest questions with confidence that they are relevant; the doctor must similarly recognise that counsel has his reasons for asking questions in Court which may also seem irrelevant to the doctor and he must answer them honestly without elaboration. Lengthy elaboration of what the doctor thinks are relevant matters provides opposing counsel with opportunity to suggest that he is wrong or unreliable in certain particulars. When a doctor feels that not enough attention has been paid to his evidence, it is usually because there has been inadequate preparation and preliminary consultation, and in difficult cases he should make sure that his views are thoroughly understood before trial. In civil cases the rules of evidence are much less rigid.

In adult Courts the accused or his counsel is entitled to read any medical report, and the doctor preparing them should ask himself 'whether it is clearly understandable, accurate, logical, modest and appearing to be made by a physician and therefore by one who is impartial and genuinely concerned for the welfare of the offender'.[2] The test is whether the doctor is confident that the accused, if he read it, would agree that this is the case. Circumlocutions, e.g., 'if the court takes a certain course', should be avoided and the doctor state clearly what he means, showing that he recognises that the Court also has the public interest to take into account.[3] If the report is on behalf of the prosecution, the doctor must recognise that the prosecution in the Crown Court is based upon the depositions, and counsel's role is strictly to lay the evidence before the court, test any defence evidence, and is not to secure a conviction. If the report contains a great deal of additional information about the crime counsel may forget where the information has come from and unwittingly exceed his duty. There are cases in which it is essential to discuss the details of the crime in order to establish the diagnosis but the reasons for this must be quite clear. Medical reports immediately before the crime was committed, and which are therefore not liable to prejudice, may be especially valuable and should clearly be quoted at some length. Otherwise doctors should in general confine their report to well-chosen words not exceeding $1\frac{1}{2}$ to 2 pages.

FORENSIC PSYCHOLOGY

A psychologist is a person without medical qualifications who has a degree in psychology, which concerns the study of normal and abnormal mental functioning usually by means of tests of intelligence, personality, etc.; a psychiatrist is a person with a medical degree. In the best practice there is mutual appreciation by the psychiatrist and the psychologist of the scope of the other's skills. Psychologists have contributed notably to such matters as the reliability of evidence by experimental study, e.g., reproducing the exact circumstances of an alleged crime in the presence of a dozen or so members of the public and showing that the majority have made the wrong interpretation of events. Evidence of identification is notoriously unreliable and contributions have also been made in this field. In some civil litigation, e.g., claims that head injury has produced permanent brain damage, it has occurred that neurologists have found no evidence of damage while psychologists have sought successfully to show that psychological tests reveal permanent damage. In such cases it is important that opposing counsel should obtain the evidence of another psychologist to consider the reliability of the tests employed, and the extent to which they can measure changes in mental activity.

REFERENCES

1. Henderson p. 6.
2. Scott, P.D. (1953) Br. J. Delinquency, **4**, 82.
3. Gibbens, T.C.N. (1974) Br. J. Hosp. Med., 278.

17

Forensic blood, breath and urine alcohol determinations

ROAD TRAFFIC ACT (1967)

There are two essential parts to the scientific determination of the alcohol concentration in the blood or urine of a person suspected of driving under the influence of drink. The first is the preliminary roadside breathalyser test, along with the second breathalyser test at the police station (should the first one prove positive), and the subsequent quantitative determination of the blood or urine alcohol content. The first breath test is the screening device for the whole determination and is the new element in the procedure. Blood and urine alcohol measurements have always been made for many years, though their statistical evaluation has not been challenged, until the mandatory 80 mg/100 ml limit for blood or 107 in urine arrived in 1967.

The breathalyser test is not usually afforded a wealth of scientific examination because it is simply a means of screening in order that a particular defendant can be apprehended under Section 1. The breathalyser test cannot be made the subject of an earnest scientific debate, however, as it uses a relatively crude semi-quantitative technique for the determination of breath alcohol content. Under very carefully controlled laboratory conditions with the Cavett Flask method, the assay can, with care, be very precise, in the hands of an experienced worker. However, more modern breath analysers mean that it may technically be possible to dispense with the subsequent blood or urine tests and rely on a breath test performed in the local police station. This will leave the statistical discussion of any borderline results in the hands of the policeman carrying out the test.

The gas chromatographic determination of alcohol ensures that very precise measurements can be made of this substance, particularly employed with n-propanol as an internal standard as outlined in the method of Curry[1].

A gas chromatographic determination of alcohol in mixtures of pure alcohol and water solutions, as well as alcohol in blood, was made in the writer's laboratory, with the following results (Table 17.1). It can be seen that in the case of fresh blood samples taken in the laboratory from subjects who had been given alcoholic drinks or where fresh alcohol solutions had been added to freshly collected blood taken from laboratory staff (not from patients) there is no difference in the assay results. Then the two gas chromatographic results were in excellent agreement with the Cavett Flask method and the enzymatic alcohol determination.

Table 17.1

| Aqueous alcoholic solution | | | | Blood samples (mg/100 ml) | | | |
A	B	C	D	A	B	C	D
62	59	64	67	150	148	149	161
103	107	97	109	168	160	165	168
108	112	102	110	60	61	55	65
54	52	49	60	34	31	36	40
91	90	93	95	82	85	78	80

A = gas chromatographic column PEG 400; B = gas chromatographic column 20% SP 2100 0.1% Carbowax 1500; C = Cavett Flask method; D = enzymatic alcohol determination.

However, when these particular methods of analysis were applied to the blood of patients with:
1. known diabetes mellitus and a corresponding high blood sugar, and
2. patients with chronic renal failure and a plasma creatinine in excess of 450 mmol,
then it can be seen that the Cavett Flask method and the enzymatic alcohol assay may, with some patients, produce results (Table 17.2) that are not exactly the same as those produced by the gas chromatographic methods. This means that the biological fluid is having some influence on the assay, particularly the Cavett Flask method and the enzymatic determination of alcohol.

Table 17.2 Blood alcohol determination, made by additions of aqueous ethanol solutions

	A	B	C	D
Diabetic patients	150	169	184	202
Renal patients	150	155	194	132

Values are mg/100 ml.

A comparison of the determinations made by the two gas chromatographic methods reveal that there is still excellent agreement between these assays. In some samples the gas chromatographic methods are influenced differently with respect to one another; however, this only happened in samples of blood collected from patients who were critically ill, and most unlikely to be the subject of driving under the influence.

ACCURACY OF THE BREATHALYSER

In the examination of a range of blood alcohol determinations in non-patients, made by gas chromatography and correlated to the breath alcohol determinations calculated from the breathalyser 'Alcotest Kit', it can be seen that (Table 17.3) some

Table 17.3

Breathalyser test	Blood alcohol (mg/100 ml)
1. Negative	83
2. Positive	55
3. Negative	105
4. Positive	62

Note the samples were taken simultaneously.

blood alcohol concentrations that would result in a positive breath test are sometimes well below the blood alcohol minimum of 80 mg/100 ml of blood. Furthermore, it should be noted that some test cases (students given fixed amounts of dilute alcohol) had a negative breath test even though their blood alcohol determinations—measured at the same time—were in excess of the blood alcohol limit. In other words some people 'get away with it' at the screening stage, either because of the inadequacy of the 'kit' or the possibility of an incorrect 'blowing procedure'.

These problems are essentially those of any chemical screening device not being applied in ideally standard controlled conditions. With policemen all over the country giving such tests to a wide range of subjects—in a variety of alcohol states—it is hardly surprising that there is a fail rate of the breathalyser technique, either through operation or fault of the device itself. In our estimation in an entirely artificial laboratory situation the fail rate is approximately 8%, though the total numbers in the survey were very small indeed. During this small survey it should be noted that the technique of breath test and blood alcohol determination cannot be reproduced at the side of the road as this is an entirely artificial laboratory operation. There must always be a delay in taking a suspect to the station, informing him of his rights and then calling a doctor to take the blood sample. However, any delay between the breath test and the blood alcohol quantitative sampling—which can be several hours—in my opinion always operates in the favour of the defendant. In all the work that we have carried out with normal laboratory volunteers all the discrepancies have always operated in the defendant's favour.

In the case of urine samples when examined by the four techniques, i.e., two different gas chromatographic columns, the enzymic method and the Cavett Flask method, all showed excellent agreement in normal urine samples. Normal is defined in this case again, as urine taken from a hospital laboratory worker to which alcohol has been added, or the urine has been collected from laboratory personnel who have been consuming alcoholic drinks. In the case of urine samples collected from patients, again particularly with diabetes mellitus or urinary tract infections, there were wild fluctuations in some of the results. In such patients a duplicate determination using the two gas chromatographic columns would resolve any question of the validity of urine alcohol determinations.

COLLECTION AND PRESERVATION OF THE BLOOD SAMPLE AND URINE SAMPLES

In practice at the present time, when a person is apprehended because he or she has failed a roadside breathalyser test, then a blood or urine sample is collected at the police station, following a further breathalyser test. Blood or urine selection is a matter for the person apprehended. In the case of a urine sample, the first urine voided is rejected and the next urine collected is the sample that is sent to the appropriate Home Office Forensic Science Laboratory. The collection of the second urine sample is a perfectly reasonable procedure in that it is the sample of urine that was most recently in equilibrium with the current blood concentration. Without the diuretic effect of a large amount of water plus alcohol—as in normal beer consumption—then it is possible that the urine sample currently contained within the bladder may have been diluted with the urine from a period prior to that when the last alcohol consumption had started, and the second urine sample is the more significant one from the point of view of the most recently consumed alcohol. The second urine sample cannot contain any alcohol from a previous bout of high alcoholic consumption, involved in the story 'I had a lot to drink last night'. Again the taking of two urine samples ideally removes any possibility of there being any factors operating against the accused person.

The blood sample, which must always be taken by a registered medical practitioner, cannot in any way, because of sampling time differences, be unfair to a defendant. Residual alcohol in the blood from a previous bout of high consumption is still in equilibrium with the brain and the clinical behaviour of any person correlates with that concentration that is affecting the brain.

The taking of the blood sample itself has been subject to some disasters, for example, in those cases where a person's arm, prior to the collection of the blood from the antecubital fossa has been swabbed with alcohol. In hospital cases this occurs where a junior hospital casualty officer, under pressure to obtain a quick blood sample, has swabbed a patient's arm with ethyl alcohol prior to taking the sample. These cases are particularly easy to spot in hospital as the alcohol concentration thereby reported invariably exceeds the fatal limit. Although such cases have been noted in the writer's laboratory in the past, more recently the use of swabs containing isopropylalcohol or more commonly dry swabbing (or none at all) has now ensured that such problems have passed into toxicological folk lore.

Where contamination with a large quantity of isopropylalcohol occurs then a gas chromatographic trace of such a sample is easy to detect. Cases of isopropanol consumption itself have been reported; however, these are rare and are either suicide attempts or occur amongst a group of consumers who are not likely to be found in the car driving population.

Collected blood samples are divided equally between two glass containers containing sodium fluoride as preservative. These containers are sterile and must be filled via a septum cap that is rigidly retained by a metal ring. It is important that any independant laboratory making a blood alcohol analysis should remove the blood from the container using the method whereby it was filled, i.e., with a hypodermic needle and syringe for collection. This means that the metal retaining ring is unmarked in any way. Any attempt to withdraw the blood sample by removing the ring ensures that the latter is destroyed and any marks of interference with the ring are likewise obliterated. Any analyst who is without such needles and syringes would be advised to keep a large store handy. In the case of an urgent request for analysis the analyst should make a particularly thorough examination of the security of the container before damaging it, on opening. The vials are now retained in a plastic 'Securitainer' which cannot be opened unless the retaining seal is broken. Again before any analysis is performed by an independent analyst it is advisable to pay particular attention to the containers. Several containers arrived in the authors's laboratory where independent analysis has been refused because of strange marks that have appeared on both the plastic and the metal retaining ring. The first container to be examined by the independent analyst is the brown envelope holding the plastic container for any signs of 'deterioration' in the envelope seal. Opening the envelope is best performed by a simple straight scissor cut about one-third along the length of the envelope. In this way the seal of the envelope either at the side or the top are not interfered with in any way and that, if necessary, such seals are still available for examination in Court. In the early days of such tests two samples were received in the author's laboratory, in which it was subsequently demonstrated beyond doubt that containers had been opened and samples had been interfered with; however, no such cases have been found since the combined septum-vial and plastic 'Securitainer' have been in operation.

PRESERVATION OF SAMPLES

The two preservatives, sodium fluoride and phenyl mercuric nitrate, have been used in blood and urine, respectively, as alcohol stabilisers. The sodium fluoride performs the function of enzyme inhibition and prevention of clotting of the sample. Phenyl mercuric nitrate has the properties of bacterial inhibition. Although it is reported[2] that both these compounds together do not inhibit activity, no problems of this nature have been recognised by this author. Though in comparison to the normal forensic science laboratory, the writer is largely concerned with an alcohol sample workload not exceeding 100 samples per week, which is very much smaller than the lowest workload of a Home Office laboratory.

The clotting of blood samples has been reported[3-5] as producing inaccurate alcohol results in that the then uneven red cell:plasma distribution means that the resulting remaining liquid sample could somehow manage to yield an alcohol determination in excess of the original whole blood. A little credence is possibly lent to this idea by the fact that instructions for dissolving or disposing of the clots are contained on each official blood sample envelope, i.e., the restoration of a total liquid sample without clotting ensures the attainment of the 'correct' blood alcohol level. Even though there are grounds for assuming that the alcohol determination in plasma water is not the same as that in whole blood, because the two components of blood, plasma and red cells contain different amounts of protein, these assumptions ignore the practicalitites of the situation, in fact there is no significant difference between the two. In the writer's laboratory we have shown that in a range of differently preserved blood samples (taken fresh in the laboratory from normal healthy volunteers), producing either plasma, serum or whole blood give what is practically the same answer. This means that there is no *practical* difference to the separate alcohol determinations whether the sample is completely clotted (i.e., thus producing serum), or as plasma from whole blood produced via fluoride, lithium heparin or EDTA-treated blood. The small clots that seldom occur in a perfectly well preserved sample of blood can sometimes prove to be a problem if automatic sampling and dispensing are employed, because of the possibility of clogging the apparatus. However, duplicate determinations on the same sample quickly reveal this source of error. For the highest precision it should be stated that automatic sampling and dispensing are essential.

If the fluoride has not prevented clotting it cannot also be acting as a preservative. The question of production of alcohol in blood samples taken from live and apparently well persons, is in the writer's opinion an entirely different phenomena to the production of alcohol in non-preserved post-mortem samples of blood and also the question of the production of alcohol in the body (post-mortem) is another field of study. There is no authenticated example of a properly preserved sample of blood taken from a living person and stored in a refrigerator at 4°C that has been demonstrated to produce alcohol to such a level as to nullify the findings of a blood alcohol determination to any significant extent.

Two questions of production of alcohol in blood samples that have received a great deal of attention are:
1. the production of alcohol in the body of a deceased person that remains several days at normal or elevated temperatures prior to post-mortem examination (the Moorgate Tube disaster), and
2. the production of alcohol in samples left exposed at ambient temperatures.

Table 17.4

Samples	3 days later A	30 days later A	B	C
1	21	47	35	17
2	5	22	29	39
3	7	16	31	4
4	Nil	112	137	145
5	Nil	32	37	14
6	262	230	212	192

A = GLC (1) 20% SP–2100 0.1% Carbowax 1500; B = GLC (2) PEG 400; C = enzymatic alcohol.

Although it is certain that unpreserved samples of blood allowed to remain for several days in a normal laboratory not refrigerated will produce a peak in a gas chromatographic trace that will sometimes appear in the position of ethyl alcohol, Table 17.4 gives some small idea of the complexities of the problem. The blood alcohol concentrations listed in the table are all genuine figures taken from a train crash of a few years ago. The evidence presented left no doubt that only one of the persons involved had been drinking and this is demonstrated in the first column. The other levels are those which would normally be seen in unpreserved samples, i.e., post-mortem production of alcohol in the body. The second series of columns represent the subsequent production of 'alcohol' in the samples allowed to remain at ambient temperature over a month and their subsequent analyses using three different methods of 'specific' ethyl alcohol determination. Two separate gas chromatographic columns were employed along with the enzymatic determination of alcohol using a perchloric acid deproteinised sample. The production of alcohol in the samples (and it is certainly not established that it is all alcohol) certainly accorded with the bacterial contamination in each blood sample. What can be deduced to some extent from this small sample is that:

1. the problem of alcohol production in such a heterogeneous mixture as normal human blood is very complex, and
2. other substances apart from ethyl alcohol are recorded in the gas chromatograph as ethyl alcohol (or the two separate gas chromatographic columns would be much closer in agreement).

In cases where the enzymatic alcohol determination gives a lower figure than the gas chromatograph, it may mean that substances are produced in the samples that inhibit the enzyme alcohol dehydrogenase. This thesis was tested by adding further quantities of pure ethyl alcohol solutions in order to test the recovery rate. The recovery rate exceeds 92% in the case of samples added to whole blood and those added to the perchloric acid deproteinised material exceeded 90%. Again it must be stated that this study represents a very small statistical sample and any conclusions drawn can only be noted as pointers for future work.

The question of ethyl alcohol production within the body after death is a phenomenon that is recognised by forensic toxicologists the world over. This is a problem that in fact most toxicologists will have recognised and accepted that in 'old post-mortem samples', cases that have remained for many days do in fact produce peaks in a gas chromatographic trace that appear in the position of ethanol. Most workers in the field have now recognised that these peaks and many others can occur in samples where the person under investigation has been a teetotal for many years. Levels of 'reported alcohol' generally are in the range of 20–30 mg/100 ml of blood. These levels have been suggested as arising from the actual sugar, or glucose, content in the body, although there is no evidence for this, and Blackmore[6] has shown that alcohol can be produced from a wide range of endogenous molecules in the body and that an immediate supply of glucose is unnecessary. Whatever the merits may be of a particular case, to decide if a deceased person has been drinking or not when the blood level is found to be low, less than 40 mg/100 ml of blood, cannot be decided on the blood level alone.[7] If a urine sample is available and the level correlates with the corresponding blood level, then a case for consumption becomes stronger. Urine is a far more reliable biological fluid for deciding[8] in cases of whether a small amount of alcohol has been consumed or not. Urine samples obtained from patients having a positive glucose reaction that are allowed to remain at ambient temperature in a normal laboratory, have not shown any evidence of alcohol production. Furthermore, the urine of patients with evidence of urinary tract infections to which glucose has been added in "diabetic mellitus' amounts have in the writer's laboratory failed to produce a significant level of ethyl alcohol when measured using two separate gas chromatography columns. The specific determination of alcohol in the blood can have a considerable bearing on determining the cause of death in the case of a 'query suicide', in those cases where the level of drug determined is in the overdose but not in the fatal range. For example, a low overdose level of an intermediate or fast-acting barbiturate drug can so very easily become a fatal level, if the blood alcohol level that is determined can be shown to have been the result of alcohol consumption before death and not merely the post-mortem production of alcohol. Again high overdose levels of the benzodiazepine drugs are very rarely established as being the cause of death in the case where it is clearly established that those particular compounds can be shown to be the only ones that have been taken. However, in the presence of even a relatively small amount of alcohol (corresponding perhaps to that maximum level of alcohol that can be produced endogenously), then benzodiazepine drugs in some overdose quantity can prove fatal. The use of the expression 'can prove fatal' is meant to cover those cases where an overdose of such drugs are consumed without any real intention of taking one's life, a 'cry for help' case. However, sometimes alcohol consumption, the 'courage catalyst' to the attempt, can transform such a dose into a fatal combination.

Another fluid that deserves a great deal more attention than it has had in the recent past is vitreous humour. In a few cases examined thus far from such cases of 'drinking or not', the vitreous humour appears to be an excellent source of information. Recommendations for its correct preservation are as yet still required. The author favours simply the use of small fluoride containers. This is not to imply that ordinary fluoride-preserved material has been proved to be the best, but that most toxicologists throughout the world will have examined so many samples contained in fluoride bottles that we are aware of the pitfalls and problems associated with these samples.

BLOOD ALCOHOL LEVEL AND ALCOHOL CONSUMPTION

So much has been written about this subject that it would not be profitable to repeat again the problems of relating amount consumed to a particular blood or urine alcohol level. However, I will confine my remarks to those subjects that have been discussed, sometimes at great length, with members of the legal profession. Curry[2] points out that the main problems in any calculation relating consumption to blood alcohol figure, is that one is always dealing with an accurate chemical assay and trying to correlate that with an estimate sometimes from a person whose memory may be slightly impaired by alcohol, and who reports to consuming, for example, two pints of brown ale, one vodka and martini, two 'Manhattans' and two glasses of wine. How can any assessment be made of this consumption in terms of the classical pint of beer or single whisky for an 11 stone or 70 kg average male? In the laboratory we have carried out a few simple experiments in alcoholic consumption with a wide variety of drinks and a variety of glasses. The material point about glasses is that it affects greatly the quantity of a 'single' drink actually delivered. For example, a recent holiday in France enabled the writer at first hand to compare a 'Manhattan' made in the U S A and France. Although both were prepared with the same ingredients, the American variety had nearly $2\frac{1}{2}$ times the volume of the French one.

A glass of wine, poured at random in a series of wine glasses in the laboratory, showed that the volume varied from 76 to 134 ml. The different wines could, even on a conservative selection, vary from nearly 7–14% of alcohol, in other words, one person's glass of wine could contain almost as much as four times the alcohol of another 'glass'. Measures of whisky poured at home are usually double the quantity that are given as single whiskies in a public house, for example.

In one very interesting biochemical laboratory experiment we invited a group of people to partake of drinks available whilst using at least two non-drinkers to note the consumption of the others and warning the participants to remember what they had consumed. In the main, poor memory correlated very closely with subsequent blood alcohol level, i.e., the higher the alcohol level the worse was their estimate of the amount of drink that they had consumed. Oddly people below the level of 80 mg/100 ml gave the best estimates of the consumption that they had had previously.

In the calculation of time of consumption and blood alcohol level, we have found that during a large number of alcohol tolerance tests, performed with 100 ml of a 70% proof spirit, and with a series of experiments conducted with randomly consumed alcoholic drinks, that most subjects, following fasting for at least 8 h, reached their alcohol peak between 30 and 72 min. The timing of the peak greatly increased with the quantity and type of food in the stomach. For example, a heavy meal containing a lot of fat often delayed their alcohol peak for several hours and that the level of alcohol was very much lower than if no food whatsoever had been taken. Whatever the timing and height of the peak of alcohol in the blood, all the people tested oxidised the alcohol in their livers at a mean rate of 17 mg/100 ml/h. The range was 13–19 mg with by far the majority between 16–17 mg. This figure was constant whether dealing with near-teetotallers or hardened rugby players. There was no correlation between the mean oxidation rate and the gamma-glutamyl transpeptidase enzyme activity (GT). The latter enzyme has been used as a guide to the level of social drinking[9] and an excellent guide to the prognosis of the allegedly cured 'alcoholic'.

We cannot find any biochemical basis for the expression 'ability to hold one's liquor', in that the oxidation rate is any faster. Six people, who were obviously alcoholics, arrived for testing with small amounts of alcohol in their blood (usually equivalent to one to two singles) and they had enzyme levels of gamma-GT greater than 150 (normal less than 36). They had no other biochemical signs of disordered liver function. These small amounts of alcohol were present in spite of the fact that very specific instructions had been given, not to consume any alcohol during the previous 12 h. One feature noticed in this group was that they tended to have slightly lower peak alcohol levels than the non-teetotaller group. It is possible that this is due to impaired absorption of alcohol in the group of alcoholics. Alcoholics as a group tend to be less fit than normal social drinkers, though whether this is due to the actual consumption of alcohol or their concomitant poor dietary habits is outside the scope of this dissertation. It is not surprising, however, that some alcoholics exhibit signs of malabsorption.

DRUGS AND DRIVING

In a few cases, very low alcohol levels have been found in blood samples taken from persons whose driving has not satisfied a particular police officer. It may well be worthy of consideration in fact as to how some of these people managed to produce a significant reading on the roadside 'Alcotest'. Firstly there may have been several hours between the roadside breathalyser and the taking of the blood sample. An actual blood alcohol reading of 15 mg/100 ml plus 2 h of oxidation (assuming the peak was reached) could mean a blood alcohol at the time of driving of 52 mg/100 ml. This is just within the limit at which some 'Alcotest' kits have given positive results in the author's laboratory. However, some blood samples have contained as little as 5 mg/100 ml; this level would have required an oxidation of 17 mg/100 ml of blood for an interval of 3 h plus the unfortunate combination of a very low threshold 'Alcotest' kit.

Aside from these anomalies of subsequent blood alcohol finding and breathalyser screening, some of these 'odd' blood samples have been further examined for the level of particular drugs, especially if the suspected person has exhibited signs of clinical intoxication, or has been in possession of that particular drug. These drugs have covered a wide range of therapeutic agents, sedatives, anticonvulsant and psychotropic drugs, as well as, in the extreme case, narcotic drugs. Further, prosecutions have been brought against several persons for driving under the influence of drugs, with attempts being made to correlate a particular drug level to a certain clinical state.

Because of the variation in metabolism, conjugation and excretion of different drugs, it would be a very difficult exercise to attempt to correlate the urine level of a particular drug (or its metabolites) with that of any level of driving skill.

ACCURACY AND PRECISION OF ALCOHOL DETERMINATIONS

In any laboratory performing quantitative analytical determinations, it is essential to check the reliability of the results. Reliability is expressed in terms of the two parameters 'accuracy' and 'precision'. Unfortunately in Courts of law, in the author's experience, the two terms are interchanged and are often assumed to be the same thing.

The laboratory term precision is the function of the scatter of individual values about a mean. The smaller the scatter, the better is the precision and the reliability. The precision, however, does not give any information about the accuracy of a determination. In spite of good precision, the value found could be a long way from the 'true' value. The greater the deviation of the 'found' value from the 'true' value then the lower is the accuracy. Precision is simply the ability to get a constant answer in a particular set of determinations in the same analytical technique, accuracy is the ability to get the right answer. A measure of the individual values about the mean is in the 'standard deviation' of that method which can be determined mathematically. The standard deviation of a particular method shows how large the unavoidable error is in that method. With the best scientific apparatus and the highest quality personnel, for example, determining a true blood alcohol of 81 mg/100 ml, will get answers ranging from 75–87 mg/100 ml. These are the unavoidable errors of a particular set of determinations, or the systematic error, the error one can do nothing about. The errors are influenced by the number of steps in the procedure, the method itself, the quality of the reagents and the analytical technique. Thus precision may differ widely from laboratory to laboratory.

As stated earlier the standard deviation is the unavoidable error of individual scatter. The standard deviation can be derived for a particular assay technique, by a particular person and at a particular concentration level of the sample. It can vary as well with the time of the day that the test is performed. Tests carried out at the end of the day rarely exceed the quality of results performed earlier that day. The standard deviation has a particular value with each technique and can be determined normally for that method by carrying out the same assay at least 10 times. About 68% of all these scattered values fall within ±1 standard deviation (1 SD), and 95% will fall within 2 SD. According to the laws of statistics one value in every 20 will still fall outside ±2 SD thus ±3 SD

are normally selected, because they will include 99.7% of all unavoidable results.

This is the reason why results of a particular blood (or urine) estimation are expressed as not less than × mg/100 ml. This will normally mean that the average of that particular determination is × + 6 mg and that 6 mg is deducted in order to cover 3 SD. This is normally allowed by the forensic science laboratories around the level of 100 mg/100 ml.

BREATH ALCOHOL OF THE TRANSPORT ACT OF 1981

The Transport Act of 1981 changed the whole procedure for the investigation of drinking and driving. Breath analyses were introduced for the first time into legislation not simply as screening devices, as the previously mentioned dichromate tube (i.e. turning the crystals green) but as a means for measuring accurately the breath alcohol level. The amount of alcohol eliminated in the breath is directly proportional to the blood alcohol concentration. Alcohol is eliminated in the breath with various volatile substances contained in the ingested alcohol, especially in the case of disease. The practical importance of these substances is that they are not normally present in the blood, with the exception of acetone in the breath of diabetics.

Following the important work of Dubowski[10] and the study of the breath testing meters at the Karolinska Institute in Stockholm[11], quantitative breath analysers are in current use. There are several systems available for the measurement of breath alcohol, involving:
1. fuel-cell sensing,
2. electrochemical oxidation and
3. infra-red photometry

The fuel-cell device lends itself readily to adaption as a pocket alcohol-meter, it can be carried by the patrolling policeman and it can produce a more reliable indication of the breath alcohol level than previously. It is important to note that this fuel-cell device, carrying out frequent tests with short intervals between, can become 'exhausted' and will need a recovery time for accurate work.

Thus, such a device is ideal for a policeman who is not liable to encounter a large number of cases on a particular spell of duty. However, in a busy police station, the 'exhaustible' nature of the fuel-cell device could prove a problem. Hence, the machines in current use at particular stations, are based on the infra-red photometry principle.

Proper breath sampling is essential to the correct analysis of breath alcohol. For correct sampling the operating procedure is performed so as to obtain what is described as alveolar air or deep-lung breath. This requires the collection of the end-portion of a prolonged forced expiration, or that breath sample that is nearest to equilibrium with the corresponding blood alcohol level. This sampling of the alveolar air is considered necessary to avoid too much mixing with dead-space air, i.e. air that is not totally in equilibrium with the blood alcohol concentration.

However, not all investigators are in agreement that such sampling of the deep-lung air is the only reliable portion. From the many experiments conducted, it is evident that under carefully controlled sampling conditions, there is an excellent correlation between the breath and blood level. This ratio is generally calculated in the range of 2100 : 1 to 2500 : 1. Thus, in order to avoid any assumed gross variation in this ratio, an actual breath alcohol limit is set at 35 μg/100 mm of breath. Again, in order to avoid the confusion of each police operator being therefore required to calibrate and describe his particular standard deviation, a breath alcohol can be supported by a concomitant blood sample. The latter is transferred to the appropriate Forensic Science Laboratory and is analyzed by gas chromatography. This determination is subject to rigorous statistical analysis and in this case, the defendant can receive his own sample for separate analysis. However, it is difficult to see how a defendant can be given a separate breath sample. Defendants in the defined range 35–45 μg are allowed the option of a further blood or urine test. Above this range, a defendant must call his own physician, at his own expense, in order to provide his own separate blood sample. Accordingly, the later arrival of his physician (i.e. at a finite time after the breath test) means that oxidation of alcohol in the body results in an almost certainly lower reading.

The greatest advantage of the new breath test ensures that a defendant knows his fate, immediately, and does not wait for several weeks.

REFERENCES

1. Curry, A. S., Walker, G. W. & Simpson G. S. (1966) Analyst, 91, 742.
2. Curry, A. S. (1972) In: Advances in Forensic and Clinical Toxicology. Cleveland: CRC Press, p. 28.
3. Barnett, C. W. H. (1970) New Law J., October 15.
4. Robinson, A. E. & Camps F. (1970) Med. Sci. Law, 10, 69.
5. Rudram, D. A. (1974) J. For. Sci. Soc., 14, 19.
6. Blackmore, D. J. (1974) J. For. Sci. Soc., 8, 73.
7. Plueckhahn, V. D. & Ballard B. (1968) Med. J. Aust., 1, 940.
8. Mueller, B. (1975) In: Gerichtliche Medizin. Berlin: Springer-Verlag, p. 1005.
9. Whitfield, J. B., Hensley W. J., Bryden D. & Gallagher H. (1978) Ann. Clin. Biochem., 15, 297.
10. Dubowski, K. M. (1975) Z. Rechtsmed., 76, 93.
11. Jones, A. W. & Goldberg, L. (1978) For. Sci. Int., 12, 1.

Index